Recent Developments in Insulin Resistance

Recent Developments in Insulin Resistance

Edited by Jessica Morris

hayle medical
New York

Hayle Medical,
750 Third Avenue, 9th Floor,
New York, NY 10017, USA

Visit us on the World Wide Web at:
www.haylemedical.com

ISBN: 978-1-63241-908-8

Cataloging-in-Publication Data

Recent developments in insulin resistance / edited by Jessica Morris.
p. cm.
Includes bibliographical references and index.
ISBN 978-1-63241-908-8
1. Insulin resistance. 2. Insulin antibodies. 3. Diabetes--Complications. 4. Hormone resistance. I. Morris, Jessica.
RC662.4 .R43 2020
616.46--dc23

Table of Contents

Preface

In my initial years as a student, I used to run to the library at every possible instance to grab a book and learn something new. Books were my primary source of knowledge and I would not have come such a long way without all that I learnt from them. Thus, when I was approached to edit this book; I became understandably nostalgic. It was an absolute honor to be considered worthy of guiding the current generation as well as those to come. I put all my knowledge and hard work into making this book most beneficial for its readers.

Insulin resistance (IR) is a pathological condition characterized by the failure of the cells of the human body to respond normally to the hormone insulin. When the carbohydrate in food is digested, glucose gets released into the bloodstream, thus triggering the release of insulin. Normally, this activity initiates glucose absorption by the body cells which is used for energy, thus causing blood glucose levels to decrease and stay within an acceptable range even with a high carbohydrate intake. In the case of insulin resistance, cells are resistant to insulin and therefore cannot use it efficiently. This leads to high blood sugar. The body thus increases insulin production, which can contribute to obesity, type 2 diabetes or latent autoimmune diabetes in adults. Insulin resistance may arise due to pathologies such as liver diseases, hemochromatosis, obesity, metabolic syndrome, etc. It can also have genetic influences and be triggered by environmental factors, lifestyle choices or lack of a proper diet. This book discusses the fundamentals as well as modern approaches in the management of insulin resistance. It unravels the recent studies in the pathophysiology of insulin resistance. This book is a vital tool for all researching or studying this medical condition.

I wish to thank my publisher for supporting me at every step. I would also like to thank all the authors who have contributed their researches in this book. I hope this book will be a valuable contribution to the progress of the field.

Editor

HCC Development is Associated to Peripheral Insulin Resistance in a Mouse Model of NASH

Samuele De Minicis[1]*, Laura Agostinelli[1], Chiara Rychlicki[1], Gian Pio Sorice[2,3], Stefania Saccomanno[1], Cinzia Candelaresi[1], Andrea Giaccari[2,4], Luciano Trozzi[1], Irene Pierantonelli[1], Eleonora Mingarelli[1], Marco Marzioni[1], Giovanna Muscogiuri[2], Melania Gaggini[5], Antonio Benedetti[1], Amalia Gastaldelli[5], Maria Guido[6], Gianluca Svegliati-Baroni[1,7]*

1 Università Politecnica delle Marche, Department of Gastroenterology, Ancona, Italy, **2** Università Cattolica del Sacro Cuore, Policlinico Gemelli, Division of Endocrinology and Metabolic Disease, Rome, Italy, **3** Diabetic Care Clinics, ACISMOM, Rome, Italy, **4** Don Gnocchi Foundation Onlus, Milan, Italy, **5** Institute of Clinical Physiology, Head of Cardiometabolic Risk Unit, Pisa, Italy, **6** Università di Padova, Department of Medicine Anatomic Pathology Unit, Padova, Italy, **7** Università Politecnica delle Marche, Obesity Center, Ancona, Italy

Abstract

NAFLD is the most common liver disease worldwide but it is the potential evolution to NASH and eventually to hepatocellular carcinoma (HCC), even in the absence of cirrhosis, that makes NAFLD of such clinical importance. Aim: we aimed to create a mouse model reproducing the pathological spectrum of NAFLD and to investigate the role of possible co-factors in promoting HCC. Methods: mice were treated with a choline-deficient L-amino-acid-defined-diet (CDAA) or its control (CSAA diet) and subjected to a low-dose i.p. injection of CCl_4 or vehicle. Insulin resistance was measured by the euglycemic-hyperinsulinemic clamp method. Steatosis, fibrosis and HCC were evaluated by histological and molecular analysis. Results: CDAA-treated mice showed peripheral insulin resistance at 1 month. At 1–3 months, extensive steatosis and fibrosis were observed in CDAA and CDAA+CCl_4 groups. At 6 months, equal increase in steatosis and fibrosis was observed between the two groups, together with the appearance of tumor. At 9 months of treatment, the 100% of CDAA+ CCl_4 treated mice revealed tumor versus 40% of CDAA mice. Insulin-like Growth Factor-2 (IGF-2) and Osteopontin (SPP-1) were increased in CDAA mice versus CSAA. Furthermore, Immunostaining for p-AKT, p-c-Myc and Glypican-3 revealed increased positivity in the tumors. Conclusions: the CDAA model promotes the development of HCC from NAFLD-NASH in the presence of insulin resistance but in the absence of cirrhosis. Since this condition is increasingly recognized in humans, our study provides a model that may help understanding mechanisms of carcinogenesis in NAFLD.

Editor: Birke Bartosch, Inserm, U1052, UMR 5286, France

Funding: The research leading to these results has received funding from the European Community's Seventh Framework Programme (FP7/2007–2013) under grant agreement n° HEALTH-F2-2009-241762 for the project FLIP, from MIUR grant PRIN 2009 - prot. 2009X84L84_003 and Ministero della Salute grant GR-2010-2306996 to MM, from MIUR grant PRIN 2009 - prot. 2009YNERCE_002, FIRB 2010 - prot RBAP10MY35_001 to GS-B. The funders had no role in study design, data collection and analysis, decision to publish, or preparation of the manuscript.

Competing Interests: The authors have declared that no competing interests exist.

* E-mail: g.svegliati@univpm.it (GS-B); s.deminicis@yahoo.it (SDM)

Background

Hepatocellular carcinoma (HCC) is the third most common cause of cancer-related death worldwide. [1,2]. Moreover, several studies have shown that 5% to 30% of patients with HCC lack a readily identifiable risk factor for their cancer [1]. Most of these "cryptogenic" HCC might be attributed to Non-Alcoholic Fatty Liver Disease (NAFLD) and the concomitant metabolic syndrome [2,3], nevertheless it is not yet clear what predisposes to the progression of the disease [4].

On this regard, NAFLD is a major health problem that integrates several liver conditions ranging from simple fatty liver to Non-Alcoholic Steatohepatitis (NASH), which is associated with fibrosis that may evolve into cirrhosis and results into HCC [5]. How HCC develops from NASH livers is still obscure. Some hypotheses suggest that obesity, insulin resistance, release of inflammatory cytokines and autophagy can contribute to the carcinogenic potential in NASH liver, where HCC can occur in 65% of patients without an over cirrhosis in the background liver [6]. However, no direct link has been provided yet. Studies that aim to link HCC and NAFLD are blunted by the lack of reliable animal models. The use of a choline-deficient L-aminoacid-defined diet (CDAA) in rats provided the most interesting results inducing steatohepatitis [7]. Concerning this issue, a still unresolved question is however related to the potential of CDAA diet in inducing insulin resistance [8,9]. The purpose of this study is to develop a mouse model of liver injury which mimics NASH features that lead to HCC.

Materials and Methods

Animals and Treatment

Male 6 to 8 weeks old C57BL/6 mice were purchased from Charles River Laboratories International, Inc. (Wilmington, MA). Animals were fed a CDAA diet or its control diet, CSAA diet (Laboratorio Dottori Piccioni, Milano, Italy). In parallel experiments, starting simultaneously to the diet administration, liver fibrosis was enhanced by weekly intraperitoneal injections of Carbon Tetrachloride (CCl_4) at the dose of 0.2 µl/g of body weight. Mice (8 mice/group) were sacrificed at 1, 3, 6 and 9 months of treatment and samples processed for histopathology, serological and molecular analysis.

All animal work has been conducted according to the local committee for care and use of laboratory animals. The study protocol was approved by the Ethical Committee for animal experimentations of the "Università Politecnica delle Marche" under the protocol named FIRB07/2011GE.

Evaluation of Peripheral Insulin Resistance

After 1 month of treatment, we evaluated peripheral insulin resistance by the euglycemic-hyperinsulinemic clamp method [10]. Surgery for the positioning of catheters was performed 3 to 5 days prior to the insulin clamp procedure as previously described [11]. The euglycemic-hyperinsulinemic clamp was performed in the awake unrestrained state after 6 hour-fast. At time 0, a primed continuous (4.0 mU/kg/min, Actrapid 100U, Novo Nordisk, Copenhagen, Denmark) infusion of human insulin was started simultaneously with a variable infusion of 10% dextrose in order to maintain the plasma glucose concentration constant at its basal level (80–100 mg/dl). Fasting Plasma Glucose (FPG) was measured at time 0. Subsequently, blood samples were taken from the tail vein at 10 min intervals for at least 2 hours to measure glucose concentration and adjust dextrose infusion rates. Insulin sensitivity was calculated as M value (rate of peripheral glucose uptake) from average glucose concentrations and dextrose infusion rates during the last 30 min of the steady-state clamp period. Fasting insulin concentrations were measured using an ELISA kit (Merck Millipore, Darmstadt, Germany).

Triglyceride Measurement

Hepatic triglyceride content was measured as previously reported [12].

Liver Histology and Immunohistochemistry

Mice liver tissues were fixed in 10% buffered formalin and embedded in paraffin. Liver sections were routinely stained Hematoxylin and Eosin and Sirius Red. Frozen sections from the different groups of mice were stained for Oil Red O. Diagnosis of NASH was based on the presence of steatosis, inflammation and hepatocyte ballooning. The severity was assessed by using the NAS scoring system [13].

For Immunohistochemistry, liver sections were incubated with primary monoclonal antibodies against Alpha-Smooth Muscle Actin (αSMA) (DakoCytomation, Carpinteria, CA), p-AKT Ser473, β-Catenin (Cell Signaling, Boston, MA), p-c-Myc Ser373 (Biorbyt, Cambridge, UK) and Glypican-3 (Cell Marque, Rocklin, CA). Antibodies against Ki67 and F4/80 were from ABCAM, Cambridge, UK. In Situ Cell Death (TUNEL) kit was from Roche, Manneheim, Germany. Detection of positive staining was performed by using DAB reagent (Sigma-Aldrich, St. Louis, MO).

Quantitative morphometry was performed as previously described [14,15].

Quantitative Real-time Reverse Transcription-Polymerase Chain Reaction (qRT-PCR)

Total RNA was extracted from mice liver using TRIzol Reagent (Life Technologies Corporation, Woburn, MA). Total RNA was reverse-transcribed to complementary DNA [14]. qRT-PCR was performed using Rotor-Gene 6000 instrument (Corbett Life Science Pty. Ltd., Mortlake, NSW, Australia). The relative abundance of the target genes was normalized to 18S rRNA as internal control.

Statistical Methods

Results are expressed as mean ± SEM. The results were analyzed using ANOVA test. A p value of less than 0.05 was considered statistically significant.

Results

Treatment with CDAA Induces Insulin Resistance

We evaluated the effects of CSAA and CDAA diets with the association of CCl_4 on peripheral insulin resistance by the euglycemic-hyperinsulinemic clamp method. After 1 month of treatment, mice treated with CDAA diet develop peripheral insulin resistance as shown higher fasting plasma insulin concentrations (Fig. 1C) and the lower glucose uptake in comparison to CSAA-treated mice (M value, Fig. 1B), despite a similar level of FPG between the two diets evaluated at time 0 (Fig. 1A). Conversely, CCl_4 treatment induces a significant increase in FPG levels and potentiates the lowering of peripheral glucose uptake both in CSAA and CDAA diets (Fig. 1A–B). The above mentioned experiments were performed by infusing insulin at a very high rate, which is associated to a complete suppression of hepatic glucose production. Insulin levels increased in animals treated with CDAA (Fig. 1C).

Moreover, both CSAA and CDAA diets lead to a progressive and time-dependent increase in body weight (Fig. 1D). This was associated to a constant amount of caloric intake that did not differ between CSAA- and CDAA-treated animals at all time points, not significantly affected by CCl_4 administration (data not shown). Furthermore, mice treated with a concomitant chronic low-dose injection of CCl_4 show a significant reduction in body weight in comparison to not injected-mice (Fig. 1D).

The epididymal fat/body weight ratio strongly confirms the previous results (Fig. 1E), showing a significant increase from 3 to 9 months with both diets, with similar reduction in the presence of CCl_4.

Treatment with CDAA Determines a Progressive Increase of Hepatic Steatosis

CDAA diet-treated mice show an increase in liver/body weight ratio (Fig. 2A), compared to CSAA diet, starting already at 1 month. No significant differences are observed in association to CCl_4.

Oil Red O staining in mice treated with CDAA shows significantly higher lipid deposition in comparison to mice treated with CSAA as can be observed in the representative pictures at 3 months treatment and quantified by the morphometric analysis for each time point (Fig. 2B). Furthermore, hepatic triglyceride content is increased in CDAA- and CDAA+CCl_4-treated animals but not in its control diet alone or together with CCl_4 (Fig. 2C).

Gene Expression Modifications of Enzymes of Carbohydrate and Lipid Metabolism

Hepatic steatosis was associated to specific modifications in gene expression of elements involved in carbohydrate and lipid metabolism (Figure 3). The expression of enzymes associated with gluconeogenesis, as Phosphoenolpyruvate Carboxykinase (PEPCK) and glucose production, as Glucose 6-phosphatase (G6PC) was reduced in the liver of CDAA-treated animals starting

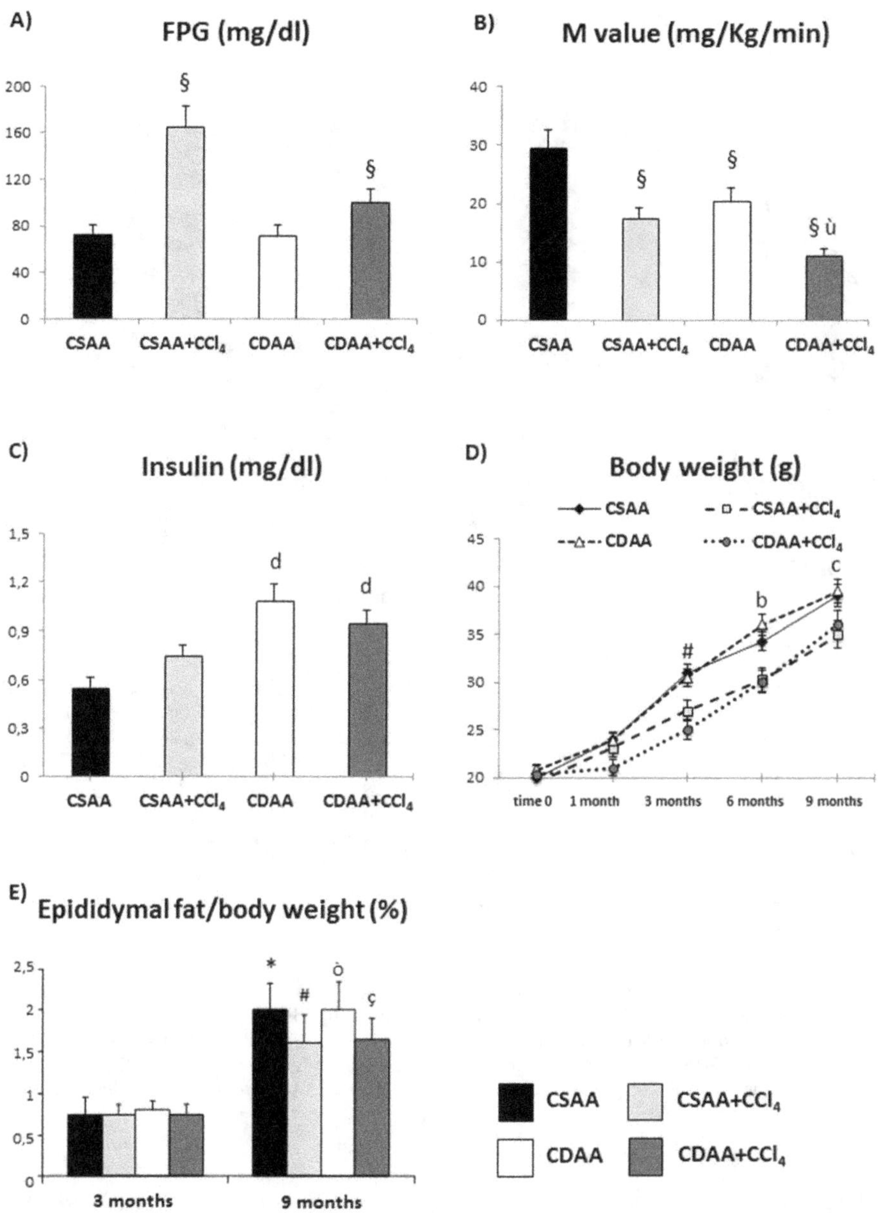

Figure 1. Effect of diet treatment on metabolic parameters and body weight. A–B) Mice treated with CDAA diet for 1 month develop peripheral insulin resistance as shown by the lower glucose uptake vs CSAA-treated mice (M value) with similar levels of FPG. CCl_4 treatment induces an increase in fasting plasma glucose and enhances the condition of insulin resistance, reducing M value. C) Insulin levels measured at 1 month of treatment. D) The graphic shows a gradual increase in body weight in both CDAA and CSAA diet. CCl_4 injection similarly reduces body weight in both diets. E) Epididymal fat/body weight ratio appears to be similar between the two different diets both at 3 and 9 months of treatment, with similar reduction in the presence of CCl_4. Data represent mean ± SD; §$p<0.05$ vs CSAA; ù $p<0.05$ vs CDAA; *$p<0.05$ vs CSAA 3 months; #$p<0.05$ vs CSAA+ CCl_4 3 months; ò $p<0.05$ vs CDAA 3 months; ç $p<0.05$ vs CDAA+CCl_4 3 months; b $p<0.05$ vs CSAA+CCl_4 6 months; c $p<0.05$ vs CSAA+CCl_4 9 months; d $p<0.05$ vs CSAA.

at 1 months, and further decreased at 9 months, independently from CCl_4 administration indicating that hepatic insulin resistance was not increased by CDAA (Fig. 3A–B).

On the other hand, the hepatic expression of the Sterol Regulatory Element Binding Protein-1c (SREBP-1c), that is the transcription factor activating all genes required for lipogenesis [16], was slightly reduced by CDAA treatment without major modifications induced by CCl_4 administration in our experimental model (Fig. 3C). Furthermore, the Carbohydrate-Responsive Element-Binding Protein (ChREBP), a key element of glucose-mediated stimulation of lipogenesis [16] progressively decreased in CDAA-treated animals, independently from CCl_4 administration, starting at 1 month (Fig. 3D). These data indicate that the development of steatosis in CDAA model was not associated with an increased lipogenesis.

Thus, we analyzed the pathways related to FA oxidation, finding a decreased expression of both ACOX-1 (a rate-limiting enzyme in peroxisomal fatty acids β-oxidation) and CPT1A (a key enzyme in mitochondrial fatty acids β-oxidation) [12] observed in CDAA+CCl_4-treated animals at 1 months and in CDAA mice thereafter, indicates that reduced fatty acid oxidation could be one of the mechanisms of hepatic steatosis (Fig. 3E–F).

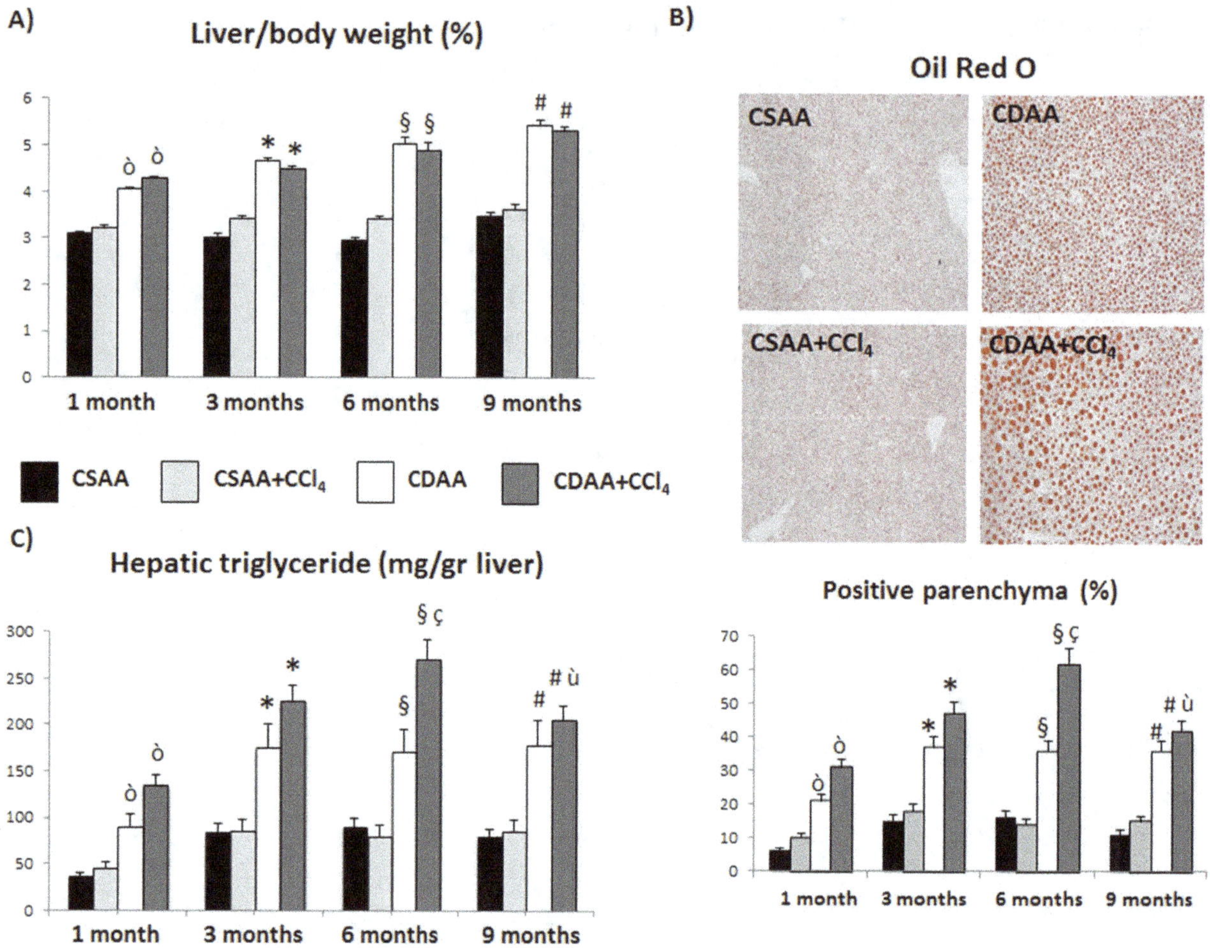

Figure 2. Treatment with CDAA determines a progressive increase of hepatic steatosis. A) Increased levels of liver/body weight fraction are observed in the group of mice treated with CDAA diet, either with or without CCl_4 administration, in comparison to mice treated with control diet, starting at 1 month. B) Histochemical staining and relative morphometric evaluation for Oil Red O and C) hepatic triglyceride measurement show increased deposition of lipids in the liver parenchyma of CDAA and CDAA+CCl_4 treated animals in comparison to CSAA treated mice. Data represent mean ± SD; ò $p<0.05$ vs CSAA 1 month; *$p<0.05$ vs CSAA 3 months; §$p<0.05$ vs CSAA 6 months; #$p<0.05$ vs CSAA 9 months; ç $p<0.05$ vs CDAA 6 months; ù $p<0.05$ vs CDAA 9 months.

Treatment with CDAA or CDAA+CCL$_4$ Induces Liver Damage and Hepatic Fibrosis in Mice

The effect of CDAA diet in terms of liver injury and fibrosis was analyzed at the level of both gene expression and histological analysis for different aspects of liver injury, inflammation, and fibrosis (Fig. 4–6).

Concerning inflammation, at the histological level, by Immunohistochemistry, the pan-macrophage marker F4/80 increased at all time points tested, reaching the highest level in CDAA+CCl_4-treated animals at 3 months (Fig. 4A). In addition, CDAA feeding increases at early stage the expression of genes related to liver injury and inflammation, such as the Tumor Necrosis Factor Alpha (TNFα) (Fig. 4B), the Monocyte Chemotactic Protein-1 (MCP-1) (Fig. 4C) and the Inflammasome components as the Apoptosis-associated Speck-like protein containing a CARD (ASC), Caspase-1 and Interleukin-1 beta (IL-1β) (Fig. 4D–F).

After blind evaluation by an expert liver pathologist (M.G.), treatment with CSAA+CCl_4 induces different degrees of hepatocyte necrosis and lobular inflammation. A more severe degree of steatosis and necrosis is observed at histology in mice treated with CDAA+CCl_4. The CDAA+CCl_4 treatment, already at 3 months, is able to create a condition that resembles the human NASH with a NAS score >5 (Fig. 5A). This was associated to a light but significant increase in the number of apoptotic cells as measured by TUNEL staining (Fig. 5B). We further investigated the expression of fibrogenic markers at each time point. CDAA+CCl_4 treatment induced a stable and significant increase of the Metallopeptidase Inhibitor-1 (TIMP-1) (Fig. 5C) and cytokines involved in collagen synthesis stimulation such as the Connective Tissue Growth Factor (CTGF) and the Transforming Growth Factor β (TGFβ) starting at 3 months (Fig. 5D–E). Notably, CDAA+CCl_4 treatment shows the higher increase in mRNA expression of Collagen α1(I) in a time-dependent manner (Fig. 6A). Additionally, qRT-PCR analysis shows in the CDAA+CCl_4 group a time-dependent increase of mRNA levels of αSMA, a marker of Hepatic Stellate Cell (HSC) activation and fibrogenesis, reaching the highest levels at 9 months of treatment (Fig. 6B). The CDAA diet alone is also able to induce fibrogenesis, but the increase is significantly lower than in the CDAA+CCl_4 group. Conversely, the CSAA diet determined a modest increase in fibrogenesis only in the presence of CCl_4 (Fig. 6A–B).

Similar results were obtained from the morphometric analysis of the Sirius Red-positive parenchyma that reveals at 6 months the

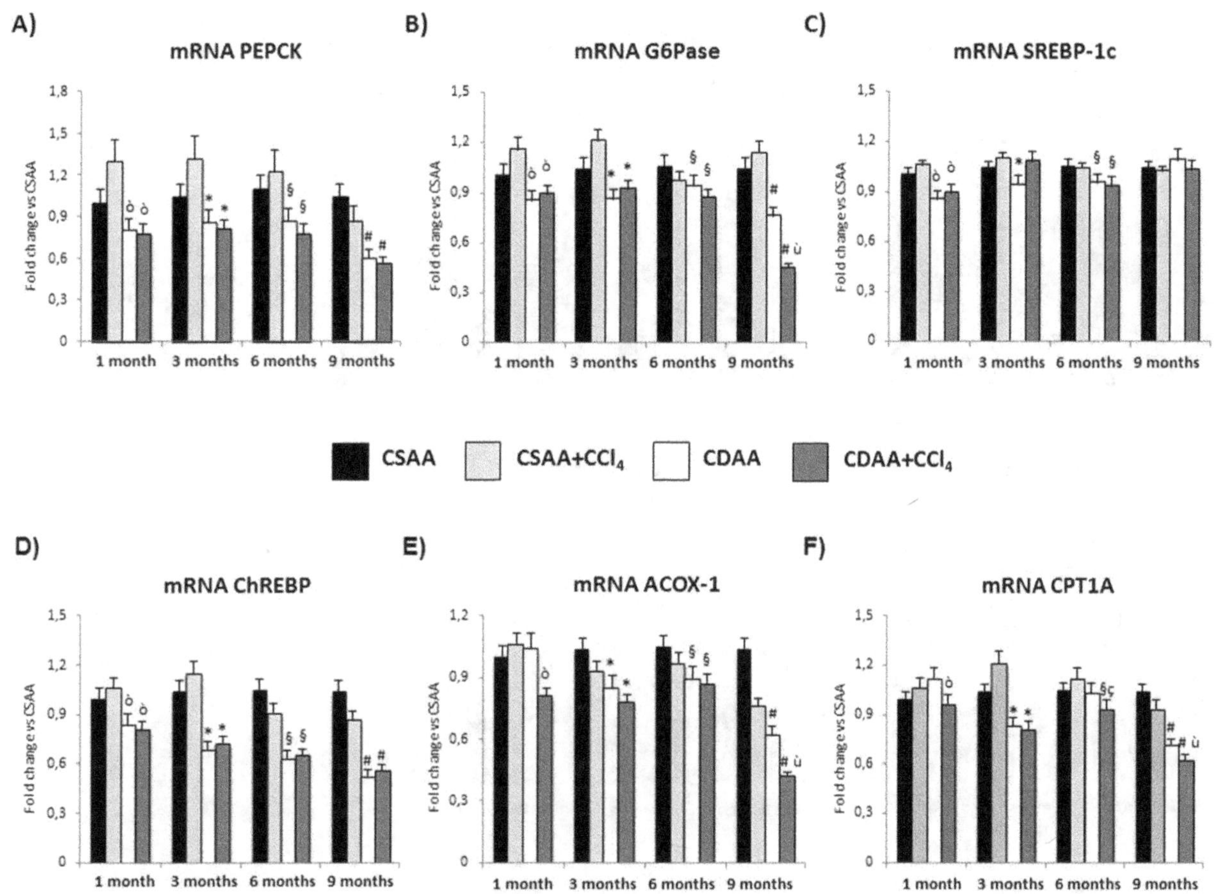

Figure 3. Gene expression of elements involved in carbohydrate and lipid metabolism. qRT-PCR expression shows a progressive decrease of the amount of PEPCK (A), G6Pase (B), ChREBP (D), ACOX-1 (E) and CPT1A (F) mRNA expression in the groups of CDAA or CDAA+ CCl_4, while only a slight decrease is observed for mRNA expression of SREBP-1c (C). Data represent mean ± SD; ò $p<0.05$ vs CSAA 1 month; *$p<0.05$ vs CSAA 3 months; §$p<0.05$ vs CSAA 6 months; #$p<0.05$ vs CSAA 9 months; ç $p<0.05$ vs CDAA 6 months; ù $p<0.05$ vs CDAA 9 months.

higher collagen deposition in the liver of mice treated with CDAA+CCl_4 (Fig. 6C). The CDAA diet alone is able to induce collagen deposition, even if at lower levels compared to the CDAA+CCl_4 group. More importantly, only low collagen deposition is observed in mice subjected to CCl_4 and treated with CSAA diet. Similar data were obtained by αSMA Immunohistochemistry, which shows the highest level of myofibroblast activation in the group of mice treated with CDAA+CCl_4 at 6 and 9 months (Fig. 6D).

Treatment with CDAA+CCL_4 Induces HCC Development after 9 Months

No tumor development was observed in mice treated with CSAA diet up to 9 months, not even when associated to CCl_4 injection.

At 6 months of treatment, almost 30% of mice treated with CDAA and CDAA+CCl_4 diets develop at least one nodule of tumor in the liver, with no statistically significant differences between the two groups (Fig. 7A–C). Although there are no differences at 6 months of treatment in the percentage of mice developing tumors, significant differences are observed in the size of the tumors (Fig. 7D).

Notably, after 9 months of treatment, all mice from CDAA+ CCl_4 group show the presence of at least one tumor nodule, with a median dimension of 9 mm. On the other hand, CDAA-fed mice with no CCl_4 support show HCC in only 35% of cases with a significantly lower average diameter (Fig. 7C–D).

Microscopically, cancer areas appear completely free from collagen deposition (Fig. 7B). Furthermore, Immunohistochemical evaluation of p-AKT, p-c-Myc and Glypican-3, that are associated to diagnosis and classification of human HCC, reveals a positive staining also in our mouse model [17–19]. Specifically, after 9 months of treatment a positive staining for p-AKT and p-c-Myc in the areas of liver parenchyma that were recognized as HCC, was evident in the CDAA+CCl_4 group, differently from all the other groups (Fig. 8A). Glypican-3 Immunohistochemistry reveals positive staining in the tumor nodules, similarly to what happens in humans, and in the zone 3 of the parenchyma of damaged liver in the CDAA+CCl_4 group [20] (Fig. 8B). In addition to these data, we did not observe any nuclear staining for β-Catenin (data not shown).

Changes in Pro-carcinogenic Gene Expression Anticipate Tumor Formation

In CDAA and CDAA+CCl_4 groups we observed a significant increase in the mRNA expression starting at 3 months of the pro-carcinogenic genes such as the Insulin-like Growth Factor-2 (IGF-2) and Osteopontin (SPP-1), respectively involved in angiogenesis and migration/metastasis (Fig. 8C–D). In the same groups, the expression of the tumor suppressor gene Phosphatase and Tensin

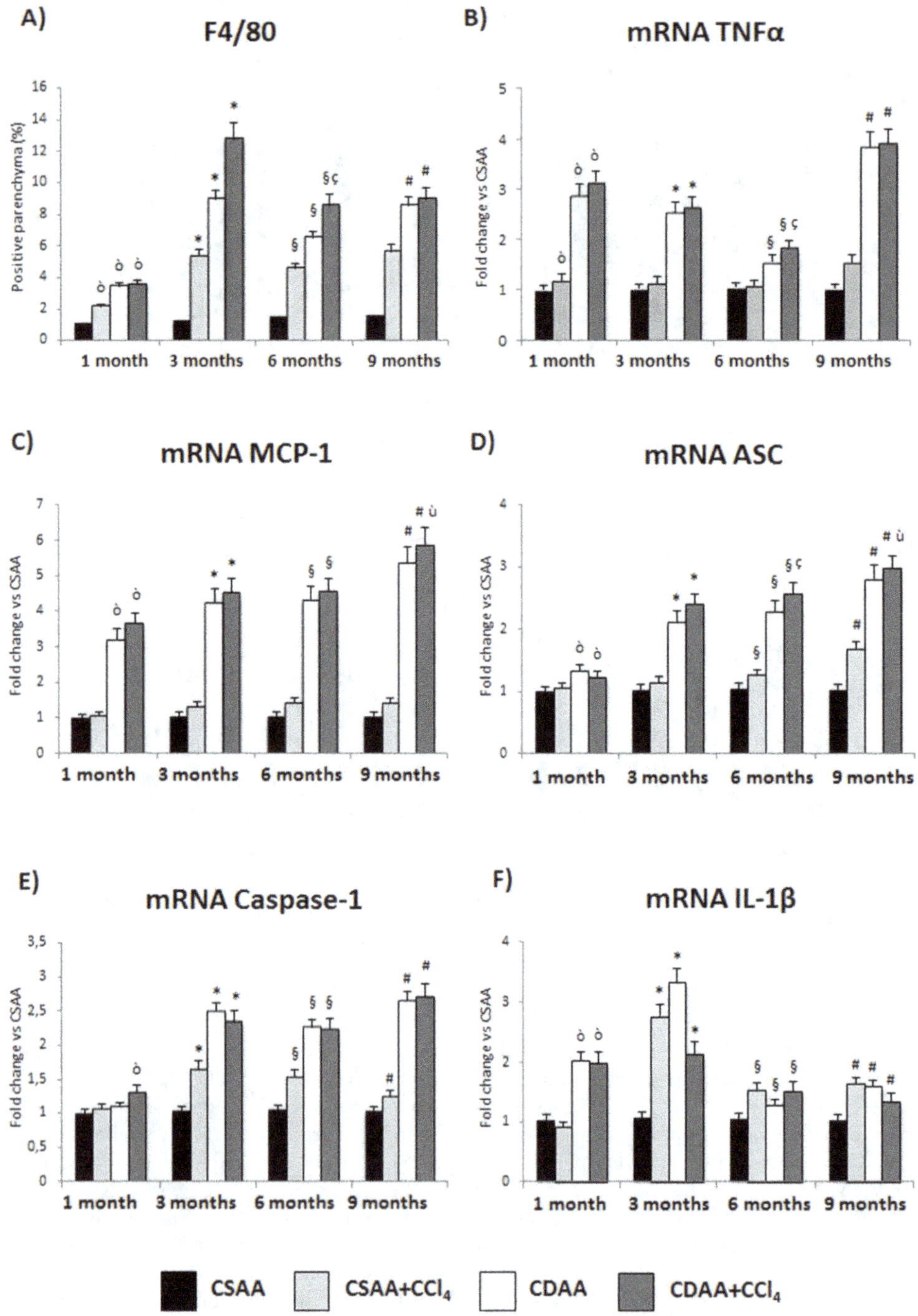

Figure 4. Treatment with CDAA or CDAA+CCl$_4$ induces hepatic inflammation in mice. A) Immunohistochemistry for pan-macrophage marker F4/80. B) TNFα and (C) MCP-1 mRNA levels are increased in CDAA or CDAA+ CCl$_4$ already after 1 month of treament. D–F) Markers of Inflammasome activation ASC, Caspase-1 and IL-1β show increased expression in CDAA or CDAA+ CCl$_4$ groups. Data represent mean ± SD; ò $p<0.05$ vs CSAA 1 month; *$p<0.05$ vs CSAA 3 months; §$p<0.05$ vs CSAA 6 months; #$p<0.05$ vs CSAA 9 months; ç $p<0.05$ vs CDAA 6 months; ù $p<0.05$ vs CDAA 9 months.

Homolog (PTEN) is significantly reduced again starting at 3 months (Fig. 8E). The expression of pro-carcinogenic genes was associated to a progressive increase in hepatocyte proliferation in CDAA+CCl$_4$ group as measured by Ki67 labeling that significantly increased at 6 months and reached the highest levels at 9 months (3.8±0.5 labeled parenchymal cell/field vs 2.2±0.5 in CDAA-treated animals, $p<0.05$ and data not shown).

Discussion

In this study, we have provided evidences that CDAA diet induces peripheral insulin resistance already in the first month after treatment, and this was associated to the pathological spectrum of NAFLD, including NASH and HCC. Peripheral insulin resistance is a primary feature of NAFLD/NASH, and is probably one of the main co-factors involved in the worsening of

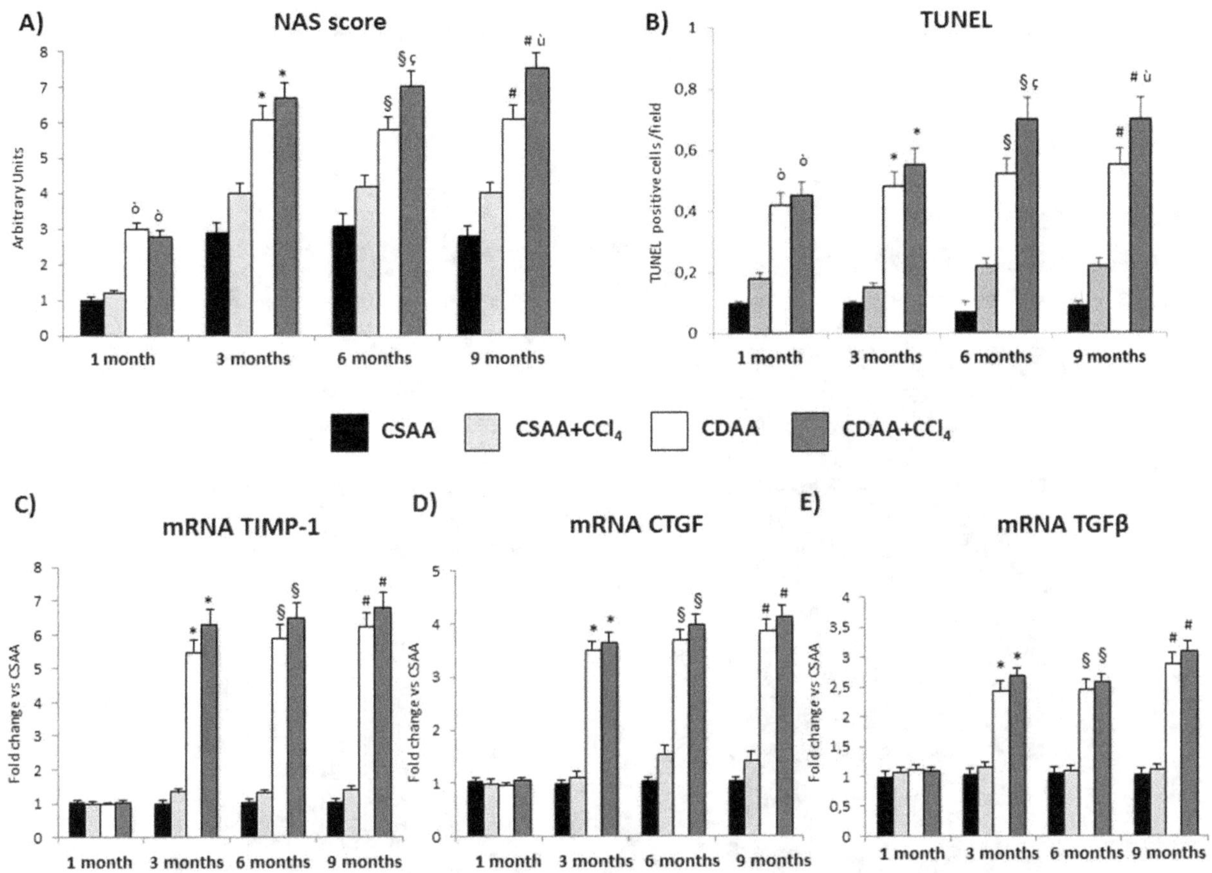

Figure 5. Treatment with CDAA or CDAA+CCl_4 induces liver injury and expression of markers of hepatic fibrogenesis in mice. A) The total degree of liver injury (hepatic steatosis and necroinflammation) was determined according to the NAS score. B) The number of apoptotic cells was measured with TUNEL and expressed as apoptotic cell/field. C–E) qRT-PCR shows a progressive increase, in a time dependent manner, of the amount of TIMP-1 (C), CTGF (D) and TGFβ (E) mRNA expression in the group of CDAA, with the evidence of a promoting effect exerted by CCl_4 starting from month 3. Data represent mean ± SD; ò $p<0.05$ vs CSAA 1 month; *$p<0.05$ vs CSAA 3 months; §$p<0.05$ vs CSAA 6 months; #$p<0.05$ vs CSAA 9 months; ç $p<0.05$ vs CDAA 6 months; ù $p<0.05$ vs CDAA 9 months.

the disease [8,21]. Thus the novelty of our results is the demonstration that the CDAA+CCl_4 model determines peripheral insulin resistance, NAFLD and its progression to HCC. Using this novel experimental approach we observed: a) development of peripheral insulin resistance already after 1 month; b) entire spectrum of lesions ranging from simple steatosis to NASH and HCC; c) development of HCC after 9 months of treatment in all mice; d) association of HCC development to increased extracellular matrix deposition; e) significant modification of oncogenic genes expression already after 3 months of treatment. Thus, this experimental model is able to guarantee in 9 months the development of HCC in almost 100% of animals and to early resemble the main features of the progression from NAFLD to NASH and HCC.

In the majority of human cases, HCC arises in patients with advanced chronic liver injury and/or cirrhosis [1]. NAFLD, which is present in up to 90% of all obese persons and in up to 70% of persons with type 2 diabetes, is a recognized risk factor for HCC, that may develop in NASH in the absence of cirrhosis [1]. However, the study of the molecular mechanisms linking steatosis development to chronic liver injury and HCC is hampered by the lack of adequate experimental models that often do not resemble the human situation [22], either are not associated to a significant development of chronic liver injury or lead to a cachectic phenotype that does not allow a long period of observation, as needed for carcinogenesis. In the CDAA model, mice develop steatosis in the absence of a high fat diet, mice continue to eat, do not reduce the appetite and the amount of calories introduced and weight changes are similar to control diet. Furthermore, in comparison to other existing rodent models, CDAA is able to drive the progression of steatosis (NAFLD) toward a condition of inflammation and fibrosis (NASH).

We have investigated the potential mechanisms that could explain the hepatic steatosis. First of all we demonstrated that CDAA-treated mice were more insulin resistant (in the periphery) already at one month as compared to the control CSAA diet-treated mice. Data in the literature show controversial results concerning the potential condition of insulin resistance in the course of CDAA treatment in rodents [23,24], mainly based on methods that provide only a partial and indirect measurement of insulin resistance, and related to the fasting glycemic and insulinemic state [24,25]. Here insulin resistance was measured by the euglycemic-hyperinsulinemic clamp, which represents the gold standard for the evaluation of insulin sensitivity [26], and the results were confirmed by finding increased fasting insulin concentrations (Figure 1). This condition was even enhanced by the addition of CCl_4 to the diet. The mechanisms by which CDAA diet induces insulin resistance are unknown but could be related to

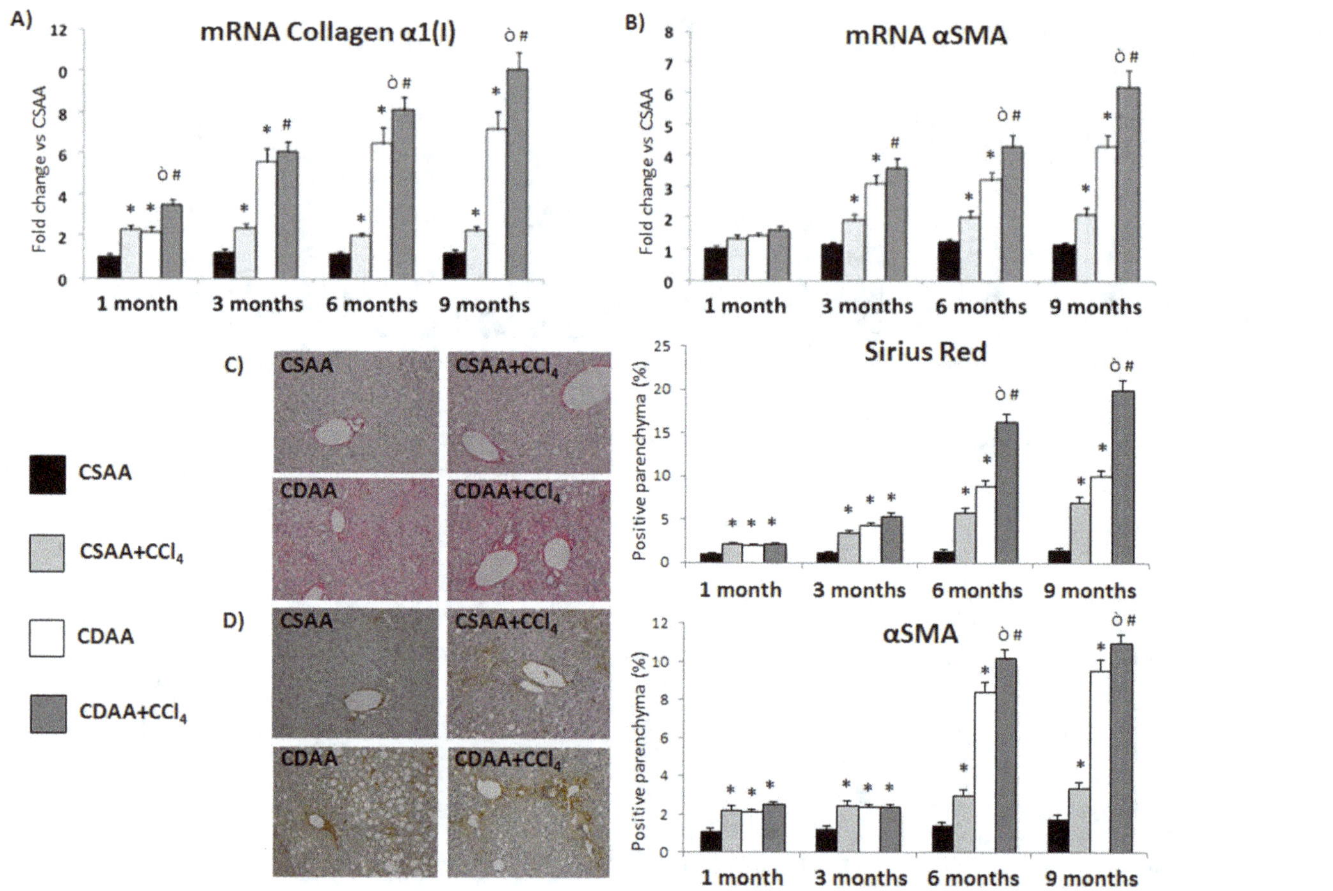

Figure 6. Treatment with CDAA or CDAA+CCl$_4$ induces hepatic fibrosis in mice. A–B) qRT-PCR expression shows a progressive increase, in a time dependent manner, of the amount of Collagen α1(I) (A) and αSMA (B) mRNA in the group of CDAA, with the evidence of a promoting effect exerted by CCl$_4$ starting from month 6. Conversely, mice treated with control diet (CSAA) do not show any time-dependent increase neither in the level of Collagen α1(I) nor of αSMA, not even after chronic CCl$_4$ injection. C–D) Morphometric analysis shows increased collagen deposition by Sirius Red staining (C) and increased HSC activation by αSMA Immunohistochemistry (D) in the liver of CDAA treated mice in comparison to CSAA treated mice. This condition is even enhanced in the liver of mice treated with CDAA+CCl$_4$. Data represent mean ± SD; *$p<0.05$ vs CSAA; #$p<0.05$ vs CSAA+CCl$_4$; ò $p<0.05$ vs CDAA.

the gut microbiota metabolism of choline as shown in humans [27]. Metabolomics data have indicated that reduced concentrations of lysophosphocholine, in particular reduced lyso-PC C18:2, and lyso-PC C16:0, are associated with peripheral insulin resistance [28] and hepatic steatosis [29,30] [31]. Moreover, we found that CDAA diet increases Inflammasome components in the liver, which supports our hypothesis of a possible link between gut microbiota modifications, insulin resistance and progression of liver injury [32,33]. The discovery that CDAA diet induces peripheral insulin resistance is important for the translation of this animal model to the human studies. To our knowledge, this is the first experimental model where a clear link between peripheral insulin resistance, NASH development and HCC formation has been established. In human patients with NAFLD/NASH, peripheral insulin resistance is a primary feature of the disease, even in lean subjects that do not present the characteristics of metabolic syndrome [34]. Moreover, a worse peripheral insulin resistance state has been associated with the presence of fibrosis [8]. To investigate if CDAA was worsening also hepatic insulin resistance, we have measured the expression of liver enzymes associated with glucose production (G6Pase), gluconeogenesis (PEPCK) and de-novo lipogenesis as SREBP-1c and ChREBP [16,35]. The results show that G6Pase and PEPCK mRNA expression was decreased, indicating a parallel decrease in glucose production. This is in agreement with the observed reduction in FPG and possibly due to the increase in fasting plasma insulin that is known to suppress both glucose production and gluconeogenesis [36]. ChREBP and SREBP-1c expressions were also reduced indicating that de-novo lipogenesis was not directly implicated in the development of liver steatosis. On the other hand, the reduction in ACOX-1 and CPT1A indicates that CDAA diet reduced hepatic fatty acid oxidation and this could be one of the mechanisms for hepatic triglyceride deposition and for the higher lipid deposition in CDAA+CCl$_4$ treated animals, presumably mediated by TGFβ signaling in hepatocytes [12] [37]. Thus, we can conclude that CDAA induces steatosis mainly by reducing FFA oxidation, while neither de novo lipogenesis nor glucose production seem to play an important role.

Despite the intrinsic differences among etiological factors for HCC, a common denominator at the origin of this neoplasia is the perpetuation of a wound-healing response triggered by parenchymal cell death, the ensuing inflammatory reaction and the concomitant fibrosis progression [38]. Indeed, HCC almost always develops on a background of chronic liver injury including chronic hepatitis and cirrhosis, conditions referred as preneoplastic stages [39]. Accumulating evidences indicate that the inflammatory

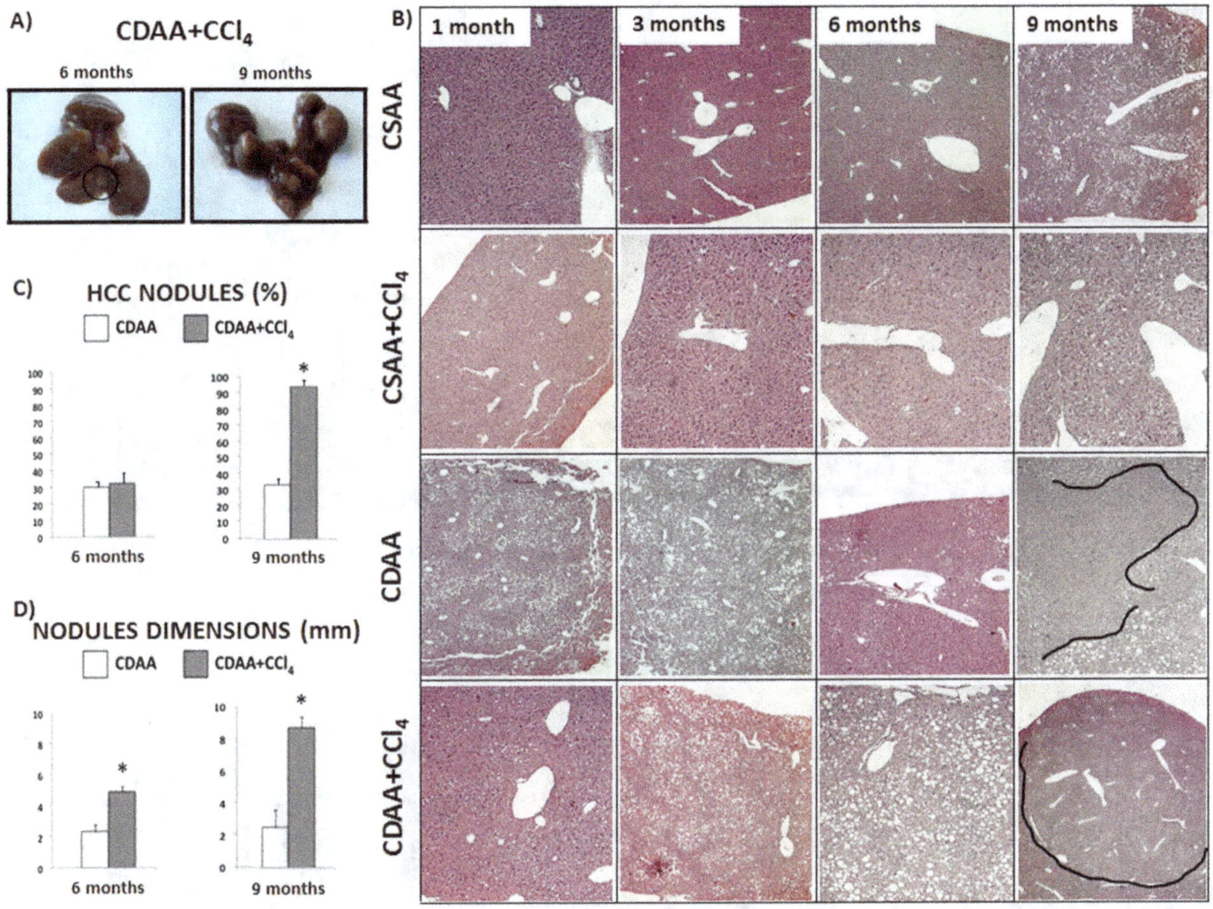

Figure 7. Treatment with $CDAA+CCl_4$ induces development of HCC after 9 months. A) Mice sacrificed after 1 and 3 months from the beginning of the treatment do not show any nodular lesions in the parenchyma. Conversely, mice sacrificed after 6 months of treatment show few nodular lesions compatible with HCC. After 9 months of treatment mice show a liver parenchyma completely damaged. B) Histochemical staining for H&E and Sirius Red show respectively no fat deposition and absence of collagen content into the nodules. C) After 6 months of treatment, about 30% of mice show HCC development both with CDAA and $CDAA+CCl_4$. After 9 months of treatment, 100% of mice from the $CDAA+CCl_4$ group show at least one nodule into the liver parenchyma. D) After 6 months, the average of nodules dimension in the group of CDAA mice is significantly lower in comparison to that of the group of $CDAA+CCl_4$ mice. After 9 months, the average of nodules dimension in the group of $CDAA+CCl_4$ mice results of 9 mm, in comparison to 3 mm of the group of mice treated with CDAA alone. Data represent mean ± SD; $^*p<0.05$ vs CDAA.

reaction characteristic of chronic liver injury actively participates in the development of hepatic fibrosis, as well as in the activation of the potent regenerative response of liver parenchyma, ultimately leading to HCC development [40,41]. For instance, the production of cytokines such as TNFα and IL-6 is essential to trigger hepatocyte proliferation, liver regeneration and animal survival after partial hepatectomy [41]. On this regard, in our model we observed an higher number of infiltrating macrophages (significantly increased in $CDAA+CCl_4$-treated mice compared to all other groups) and this was accompanied by a complete repertoire of the inflammatory response such as apoptotic cells, TNFα, MCP-1 and components of the Inflammasome pathway (ASC, Caspase-1, IL-1β) gene expression. Inflammasomes are intracellular multiprotein complexes expressed in both parenchymal and non-parenchymal cells of the liver that in response to cellular danger signals activate Caspase-1 and release the pro-inflammatory cytokine IL-1β, and their role in NASH development is controversial [42]. In a majority of Inflammasomes, activation of Caspase-1 requires interaction with the adaptor protein ASC and this leads to increased IL-1β synthesis and secretion, that finally synergizes with TNFα to induce cytotoxicity, HSC activation and maintenance of macrophages in inflammatory state [43]. Thus, it is possible that the inflammatory milieu occurring in the damaged liver in our model favors survival of preneoplastic hepatocytes, promotes the generation of a fibrotic substrate and eventually contributes to carcinogenesis [44].

As known from the literature, both hepatic steatosis and fibrosis represent independent risk factors for HCC development [45,46]. In our hands, HCC development was associated to steatosis and fibrosis in 35% of mice in the CDAA alone-treated group. Recent studies used CDAA diet in mice: Denda et al. reported a 100% incidence in preneoplastic foci after 65 weeks of treatment, with no further information on the presence of lesions at earlier time points [47]. In the study from Kodama et al. mice fed CDAA diet up to 20 weeks showed steatosis and fibrosis, with no mention on the development of carcinogetic foci [23]. In our study the addition of a low-chronic dose of CCl_4 to the CDAA administration promoted HCC development in 100% of mice after 9 months of treatment. This was associated to increased extracellular matrix deposition. Thus, CCl_4 should be considered as a promoting factor in CDAA diet-induced liver damage. It could be hypothesized that, even at low doses, CCl_4 synergizes with hepatic steatosis in the develop-

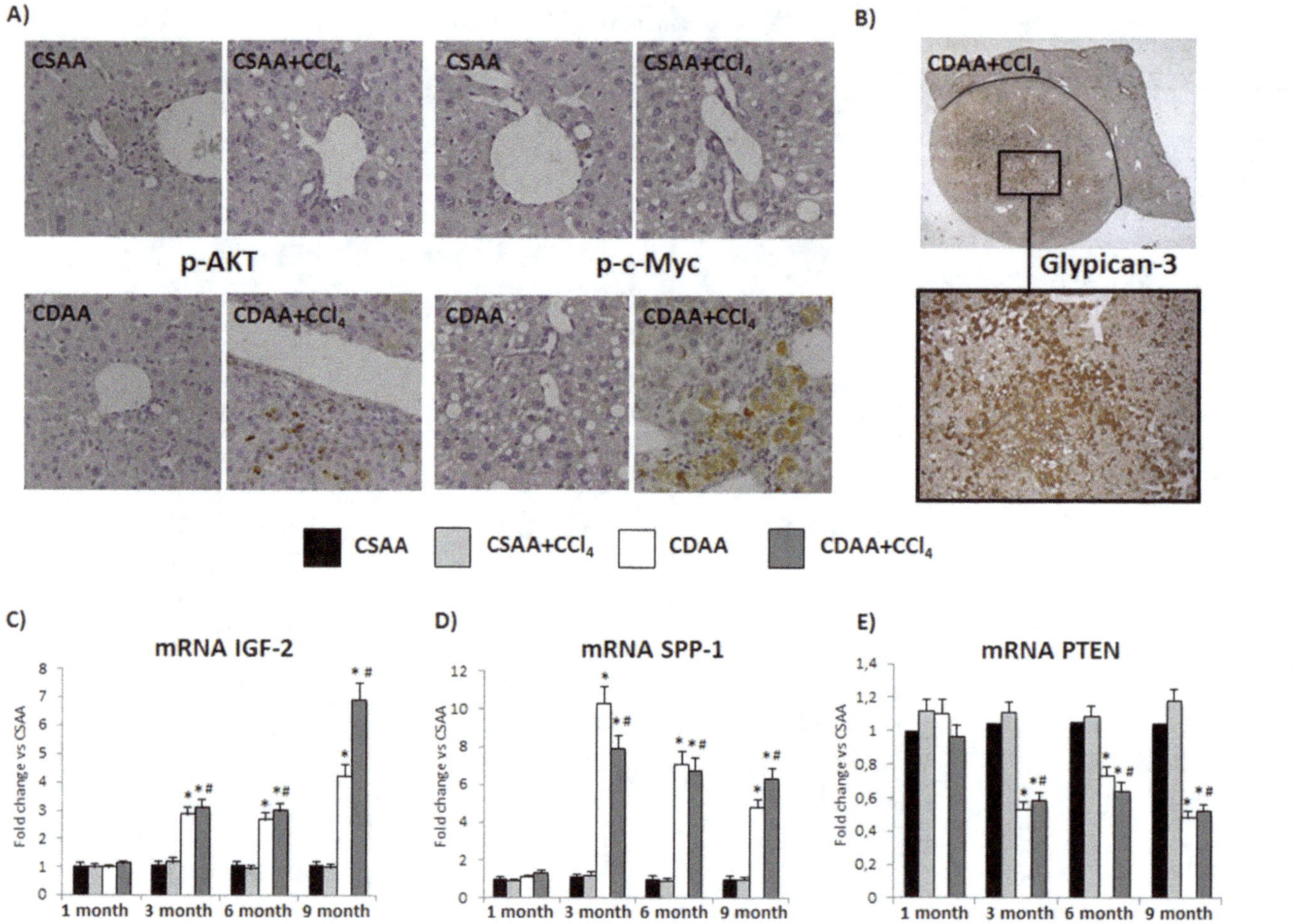

Figure 8. The expression of pro-carcinogenic genes is modified already after 3 months of treatment. A) Immunohistochemistry for p-AKT and p-c-Myc shows positive staining in the liver parenchyma of CDAA+CCl_4 mice, in correspondence of HCC foci (20X magnification) B) Glypican-3 Immunohistochemistry shows positive staining in the tumor area (5X and 20X magnification). C) Mice treated with CDAA or CDAA+CCl_4 show, starting at 3 months, increased levels of mRNA for IGF-2 and (D) SPP-1 and (E) decreased mRNA levels of PTEN. Data represent mean ± SD; *$p<0.05$ vs CSAA; #$p<0.05$ vs CSAA+CCl_4.

ment of liver injury and HCC, as shown by increased fibrosis deposition at 6 months and increased nodules formation at 9 months in CDAA+CCl_4-treated mice. On this regard, in our model we observed higher macrophages infiltration at 3 months in CDAA+CCl_4-treated animals, followed by increased liver injury (as determined by the NAS score), markers of fibrogenesis (type I collagen gene expression and HSC activation) and extracellular matrix deposition starting from 6 months in CDAA+CCl_4-treated mice.

Thus our model shows all the main features of the typical condition of HCC development, including the early modification in the expression of pro-carcinogenetic genes, increased hepatocyte proliferation and the expression of markers in the tumor parenchyma, similarly to the human condition. Specifically, both in the CDAA and CDAA+CCl_4 groups increased mRNA levels of IGF-2 and SPP-1 genes, respectively involved in angiogenesis and migration/metastasis [48], and decreased mRNA levels of the oncosoppressor gene PTEN were observed at 3 and 9 months [49,50], additionally confirming the neoplastic potential of our model even at early stages. In addition to the current data, several similarities with the human pattern of HCC have been shown in our model, by the positive staining for p-AKT, p-c-Myc and Glypican-3 distribution observed in the tumor parenchyma of mice treated for 9 months with CDAA and CCl_4. Furthermore, the absence of any nuclear stain for β-Catenin, which is usually observed in poorly differentiated HCC is consistent with the histopathological diagnosis of well differentiated HCC in our mouse model.

In conclusion, our study provides a reproducible model that recapitulate the pathological spectrum of human NALFD evolving towards HCC, highlighting the potential role of peripheral vs hepatic insulin resistance and may therefore represent an ideal tool to investigate the interaction mechanisms and new potential genes hypothetically involved in HCC development.

Author Contributions

Conceived and designed the experiments: SDM GS-B. Performed the experiments: LA CR EM IP GPS LT. Analyzed the data: SDM CR LA CC. Contributed reagents/materials/analysis tools: SDM LT SS GM. Wrote the paper: SDM CR LA GS-B MG AG AG AB MM.

References

1. El-Serag HB (2011) Hepatocellular carcinoma. N Engl J Med 365: 1118–1127.
2. Page JM, Harrison SA (2009) NASH and HCC. Clin Liver Dis 13: 631–647.
3. Marchesini G, Brizi M, Bianchi G, Tomassetti S, Bugianesi E, et al. (2001) Nonalcoholic fatty liver disease: a feature of the metabolic syndrome. Diabetes 50: 1844–1850.
4. Day CP (2005) Natural history of NAFLD: remarkably benign in the absence of cirrhosis. Gastroenterology 129: 375–378.
5. Nobili V, Svegliati-Baroni G, Alisi A, Miele L, Valenti L, et al. (2013) A 360-degree overview of paediatric NAFLD: recent insights. J Hepatol 58: 1218–1229.
6. De Minicis S, Day C, Svegliati-Baroni G (2013) From NAFLD to NASH and HCC: pathogenetic mechanisms and therapeutic insights. Curr Pharm Des 19: 5239–5249.
7. Koteish A, Diehl AM (2001) Animal models of steatosis. Semin Liver Dis 21: 89–104.
8. Svegliati-Baroni G, Bugianesi E, Bouserhal T, Marini F, Ridolfi F, et al. (2007) Post-load insulin resistance is an independent predictor of hepatic fibrosis in virus C chronic hepatitis and in non-alcoholic fatty liver disease. Gut 56: 1296–1301.
9. Vanni E, Bugianesi E, Kotronen A, De Minicis S, Yki-Jarvinen H, et al. (2010) From the metabolic syndrome to NAFLD or vice versa? Dig Liver Dis 42: 320–330.
10. Giaccari A, Rossetti L (1992) Predominant role of gluconeogenesis in the hepatic glycogen repletion of diabetic rats. J Clin Invest 89: 36–45.
11. Giaccari A, Morviducci L, Zorretta D, Sbraccia P, Leonetti F, et al. (1995) In vivo effects of glucosamine on insulin secretion and insulin sensitivity in the rat: possible relevance to the maladaptive responses to chronic hyperglycaemia. Diabetologia 38: 518–524.
12. Svegliati-Baroni G, Saccomanno S, Rychlicki C, Agostinelli L, De Minicis S, et al. (2011) Glucagon-like peptide-1 receptor activation stimulates hepatic lipid oxidation and restores hepatic signalling alteration induced by a high-fat diet in nonalcoholic steatohepatitis. Liver Int 31: 1285–1297.
13. Kleiner DE, Brunt EM, Van Natta M, Behling C, Contos MJ, et al. (2005) Design and validation of a histological scoring system for nonalcoholic fatty liver disease. Hepatology 41: 1313–1321.
14. De Minicis S, Candelaresi C, Agostinelli L, Taffetani S, Saccomanno S, et al. (2012) Endoplasmic Reticulum stress induces hepatic stellate cell apoptosis and contributes to fibrosis resolution. Liver Int.
15. Svegliati-Baroni G, Ghiselli R, Marzioni M, Alvaro D, Mocchegiani F, et al. (2006) Estrogens maintain bile duct mass and reduce apoptosis after biliodigestive anastomosis in bile duct ligated rats. J Hepatol 44: 1158–1166.
16. Browning JD, Horton JD (2004) Molecular mediators of hepatic steatosis and liver injury. J Clin Invest 114: 147–152.
17. Calvisi DF, Wang C, Ho C, Ladu S, Lee SA, et al. (2011) Increased lipogenesis, induced by AKT-mTORC1-RPS6 signaling, promotes development of human hepatocellular carcinoma. Gastroenterology 140: 1071–1083.
18. Boyault S, Rickman DS, de Reynies A, Balabaud C, Rebouissou S, et al. (2007) Transcriptome classification of HCC is related to gene alterations and to new therapeutic targets. Hepatology 45: 42–52.
19. Bruix J, Sherman M, American Association for the Study of Liver D (2011) Management of hepatocellular carcinoma: an update. Hepatology 53: 1020–1022.
20. Suzuki M, Sugimoto K, Tanaka J, Tameda M, Inagaki Y, et al. (2010) Up-regulation of glypican-3 in human hepatocellular carcinoma. Anticancer Res 30: 5055–5061.
21. Svegliati-Baroni G, Faraci G, Fabris L, Saccomanno S, Cadamuro M, et al. (2011) Insulin resistance and necroinflammation drives ductular reaction and epithelial-mesenchymal transition in chronic hepatitis C. Gut 60: 108–115.
22. Marra F, Gastaldelli A, Svegliati Baroni G, Tell G, Tiribelli C (2008) Molecular basis and mechanisms of progression of non-alcoholic steatohepatitis. Trends Mol Med 14: 72–81.
23. Kodama Y, Kisseleva T, Iwaisako K, Miura K, Taura K, et al. (2009) c-Jun N-terminal kinase-1 from hematopoietic cells mediates progression from hepatic steatosis to steatohepatitis and fibrosis in mice. Gastroenterology 137: 1467–1477 e1465.
24. Miura K, Kodama Y, Inokuchi S, Schnabl B, Aoyama T, et al. (2010) Toll-like receptor 9 promotes steatohepatitis by induction of interleukin-1beta in mice. Gastroenterology 139: 323–334 e327.
25. Nakano T, Cheng YF, Lai CY, Hsu LW, Chang YC, et al. (2011) Impact of artificial sunlight therapy on the progress of non-alcoholic fatty liver disease in rats. J Hepatol 55: 415–425.
26. Wang L, Balas B, Christ-Roberts CY, Kim RY, Ramos FJ, et al. (2007) Peripheral disruption of the Grb10 gene enhances insulin signaling and sensitivity in vivo. Mol Cell Biol 27: 6497–6505.
27. Spencer MD, Hamp TJ, Reid RW, Fischer LM, Zeisel SH, et al. (2011) Association between composition of the human gastrointestinal microbiome and development of fatty liver with choline deficiency. Gastroenterology 140: 976–986.
28. Gall WE, Beebe K, Lawton KA, Adam KP, Mitchell MW, et al. (2010) alpha-hydroxybutyrate is an early biomarker of insulin resistance and glucose intolerance in a nondiabetic population. PLoS One 5: e10883.
29. Ferrannini E, Natali A, Camastra S, Nannipieri M, Mari A, et al. (2012) Early Metabolic Markers of the Development of Dysglycemia and Type 2 Diabetes and Their Physiological Significance. Diabetes.
30. Gastaldelli A (2011) Role of beta-cell dysfunction, ectopic fat accumulation and insulin resistance in the pathogenesis of type 2 diabetes mellitus. Diabetes Res Clin Pract 93 Suppl 1: S60–65.
31. Lehmann R, Franken H, Dammeier S, Rosenbaum L, Kantartzis K, et al. (2013) Circulating lysophosphatidylcholines are markers of a metabolically benign nonalcoholic fatty liver. Diabetes Care 36: 2331–2338.
32. De Minicis S, Rychlicki C, Agostinelli L, Saccomanno S, Candelaresi C, et al. (2013) Dysbiosis contributes to fibrogenesis in the course of chronic liver injury in mice. Hepatology.
33. Henao-Mejia J, Elinav E, Jin C, Hao L, Mehal WZ, et al. (2012) Inflammasome-mediated dysbiosis regulates progression of NAFLD and obesity. Nature 482: 179–185.
34. Bugianesi E, Gastaldelli A, Vanni E, Gambino R, Cassader M, et al. (2005) Insulin resistance in non-diabetic patients with non-alcoholic fatty liver disease: sites and mechanisms. Diabetologia 48: 634–642.
35. Burgess A, Vanella L, Bellner L, Schwartzman ML, Abraham NG (2012) Epoxyeicosatrienoic acids and heme oxygenase-1 interaction attenuates diabetes and metabolic syndrome complications. Prostaglandins Other Lipid Mediat 97: 1–16.
36. Gastaldelli A, Toschi E, Pettiti M, Frascerra S, Quinones-Galvan A, et al. (2001) Effect of physiological hyperinsulinemia on gluconeogenesis in nondiabetic subjects and in type 2 diabetic patients. Diabetes 50: 1807–1812.
37. Yang L, Roh YS, Song J, Zhang B, Liu C, et al. (2014) Transforming growth factor beta signaling in hepatocytes participates in steatohepatitis through regulation of cell death and lipid metabolism in mice. Hepatology 59: 483–495.
38. Berasain C, Castillo J, Perugorria MJ, Latasa MU, Prieto J, et al. (2009) Inflammation and liver cancer: new molecular links. Ann N Y Acad Sci 1155: 206–221.
39. Farazi PA, DePinho RA (2006) Hepatocellular carcinoma pathogenesis: from genes to environment. Nat Rev Cancer 6: 674–687.
40. Friedman SL (2008) Mechanisms of hepatic fibrogenesis. Gastroenterology 134: 1655–1669.
41. Fausto N, Campbell JS, Riehle KJ (2006) Liver regeneration. Hepatology 43: S45–53.
42. Szabo G, Csak T (2012) Inflammasomes in liver diseases. J Hepatol 57: 642–654.
43. Kubes P, Mehal WZ (2012) Sterile inflammation in the liver. Gastroenterology 143: 1158–1172.
44. Sun B, Karin M (2012) Obesity, inflammation, and liver cancer. J Hepatol 56: 704–713.
45. Pekow JR, Bhan AK, Zheng H, Chung RT (2007) Hepatic steatosis is associated with increased frequency of hepatocellular carcinoma in patients with hepatitis C-related cirrhosis. Cancer 109: 2490–2496.
46. Baud V, Karin M (2009) Is NF-kappaB a good target for cancer therapy? Hopes and pitfalls. Nat Rev Drug Discov 8: 33–40.
47. Denda A, Kitayama W, Kishida H, Murata N, Tsutsumi M, et al. (2002) Development of hepatocellular adenomas and carcinomas associated with fibrosis in C57BL/6J male mice given a choline-deficient, L-amino acid-defined diet. Jpn J Cancer Res 93: 125–132.
48. Chao W, D'Amore PA (2008) IGF2: epigenetic regulation and role in development and disease. Cytokine Growth Factor Rev 19: 111–120.
49. Peyrou M, Bourgoin L, Foti M (2010) PTEN in liver diseases and cancer. World J Gastroenterol 16: 4627–4633.
50. Vinciguerra M, Foti M (2008) PTEN at the crossroad of metabolic diseases and cancer in the liver. Ann Hepatol 7: 192–199.

2

Silymarin Induces Insulin Resistance through an Increase of Phosphatase and Tensin Homolog in Wistar Rats

Kai-Chun Cheng[1], Akihiro Asakawa[1], Ying-Xiao Li[1], Hsien-Hui Chung[2], Haruka Amitani[1], Takatoshi Ueki[3], Juei-Tang Cheng[4], Akio Inui[1]*

1 Department of Psychosomatic Internal Medicine, Kagoshima University Graduate School of Medical and Dental Sciences, Kagoshima, Japan, **2** Institute of Basic Medical Sciences, College of Medicine, National Cheng Kung University, Tainan City, Taiwan, **3** Department of Neuroanatomy, Hamamatsu University School of Medicine. Hamamatsu, Japan, **4** Department of Medical Research, Chi-Mei Medical Center, Yong Kang, Tainan City, Taiwan

Abstract

Background and aims: Phosphatase and tensin homolog (PTEN) is a phosphoinositide phosphatase that regulates crucial cellular functions, including insulin signaling, lipid and glucose metabolism, as well as survival and apoptosis. Silymarin is the active ingredient in milk thistle and exerts numerous effects through the activation of PTEN. However, the effect of silymarin on the development of insulin resistance remains unknown.

Methods: Wistar rats fed fructose-rich chow or normal chow were administered oral silymarin to identify the development of insulin resistance using the homeostasis model assessment of insulin resistance and hyperinsulinemic- euglycemic clamping. Changes in PTEN expression in skeletal muscle and liver were compared using western blotting analysis. Further investigation was performed in L6 cells to check the expression of PTEN and insulin-related signals. PTEN deletion in L6 cells was achieved by small interfering ribonucleic acid transfection.

Results: Oral administration of silymarin at a dose of 200 mg/kg once daily induced insulin resistance in normal rats and enhanced insulin resistance in fructose-rich chow-fed rats. An increase of PTEN expression was observed in the skeletal muscle and liver of rats with insulin resistance. A decrease in the phosphorylation of Akt in L6 myotube cells, which was maintained in a high-glucose condition, was also observed. Treatment with silymarin aggravated high-glucose-induced insulin resistance. Deletion of PTEN in L6 cells reversed silymarin-induced impaired insulin signaling and glucose uptake.

Conclusions: Silymarin has the ability to disrupt insulin signaling through increased PTEN expression. Therefore, silymarin should be used carefully in type-2 diabetic patients.

Editor: Marcia B. Aguila, State University of Rio de Janeiro, Biomedical Center, Institute of Biology, Brazil

Funding: This work was supported by the Young Researcher Overseas Visits Program for Vitalizing Brain Circulation by the Japan society for the promotion of science. The funders had no role in study design, data collection and analysis, decision to publish, or preparation of the manuscript.

Competing Interests: The authors have declared that no competing interests exist.

* E-mail: inui@m.kufm.kagoshima-u.ac.jp

Introduction

Hepatic pathologies, ranging from hepatic steatosis to steatohepatitis, fibrosis, and cirrhosis are commonly associated with metabolic disorders such as insulin resistance and dyslipidemia [1]. Obesity and metabolic syndrome are major etiological factors that contribute to the development of severe liver diseases [2,3]. Although the development of metabolic and hepatic diseases is highly correlated, the effects of the medications prescribed for hepatic protection on glucose homeostasis remain unknown.

Milk thistle (*Silybum marianum*) is a dietary supplement that provides hepatic protection against drug- or alcohol-related injury [4]. Silymarin is an active mixture of flavonolignane diastereomers found in milk thistle extract, and reportedly acts as a strong antioxidant and free radical scavenger [5,6], as well as exerts a liver-protective action without notable adverse effects. In addition, silymarin has demonstrated an inhibitory effect on multiple cancer cell lines, including prostate, lung, colon, skin, and bladder cancers [7–12], as well as hepatocellular carcinoma [13,14]. The mechanism for the silymarin-mediated anti-tumorigenic effect is associated with increased activity of phosphatase and tensin homolog (PTEN) and the decreased phosphorylation of Akt [13].

The PTEN protein is a phosphoinositide phosphatase that dephosphorylates the phosphatidylinositol 3,4-bisphosphate and phosphatidylinositol 3,4,5-trisphosphate second messengers on the 3′-position of the inositol ring [15]. PTEN is frequently mutated in hepatocellular carcinoma [16]. PTEN antagonizes phosphoinositide 3-kinase (PI3K) activation and acts as a potent regulator of growth factor signaling in the insulin signal pathway [17]. PTEN-specific deletion in muscle improves skeletal muscle insulin sensitivity and to protect mice from insulin resistance [18]. Treatment with PTEN antisense oligonucleotides in db/db mice normalized plasma glucose levels [19]. Thus, a crucial role for PTEN in insulin sensitivity has been established.

Although silymarin is known to upregulate PTEN, causing its anti-tumor action, the effect of silymarin on insulin sensitivity remains unknown. In the present study, we used Wistar rats to

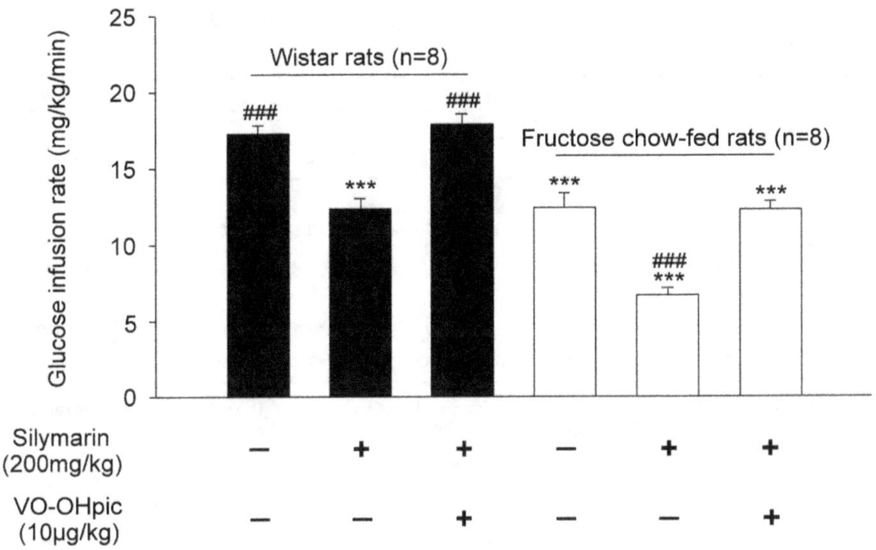

Figure 1. Mean values for the direct measure of insulin sensitivity, as assessed by the glucose infusion rate during the last 20 min of a 2-h hyperinsulinemic-euglycemic clamp. Silymarin (200 mg/kg body weight) was orally administered once daily to Wistar rats for 2 weeks. A glucose clamp was performed 30 min after the oral intake of silymarin (200 mg/kg) in Wistar rats fed normal or fructose-rich chow. VO-OHpic (PTEN inhibitor, 10 μg/kg) was i.p. injected 30 min before administration of silymarin. The vehicle used to dissolve the testing drugs was given at the same volume. Values (mean ± SE) were obtained from each group of 8 animals. ***$P<0.001$ compared with vehicle-treated normal chow-fed group. ###$P<0.001$ compared with the vehicle-treated fructose-rich chow-fed group.

evaluate the effect of silymarin on insulin sensitivity and clarify the role of PTEN in silymarin-induced insulin resistance.

Materials and Methods

Animals

Male Wistar rats weighing 200–250 g were purchased from the Animal Center of National Cheng Kung University Medical College. The rats were housed in a temperature-controlled room (25°C) and kept on a 12:12 light/dark cycle (lights on at 6:00 a.m.). Fructose-rich chow (Teklad Laboratory Diets, Madison, WI, USA) containing 60% fructose was fed for 4 weeks to induce insulin resistance according to our previously described method [20]. Development of insulin resistance in rats was characterized by loss of the tolbutamide-induced glucose-lowering lowering action. In brief, tolbutamide (10 mg/kg, i.p.) was injected into rats receiving fructose-rich chow to determine the change in blood glucose levels. Rats were treated independently through intragastric administration of silymarin (Sigma-Aldrich, St. Louis, MO, USA) dissolved in saline at 200 mg/kg once daily. Each rat was fasted overnight prior to all experiments. All animal procedures were performed according to the Guide for the Care and Use of Laboratory Animals of the National Institutes of Health and the guidelines of the Animal Welfare Act. The animal experiments were approved by the Regional Ethics Committee for Animal Research in Chi-Mei Medical Center (Tainan, Taiwan).

Measuring the Body Weight and Biochemical Analysis

Body weights of the rats were measured first. Blood samples were collected from the femoral veins of rats under sodium pentobarbital anesthesia (30 mg/kg, i.p.), and serum was analyzed to determine levels of triglycerides, total cholesterol, low-density lipoprotein-cholesterol and high-density lipoprotein cholesterol using an automatic analyzer.

Identification of Insulin Resistance

Insulin resistance was assessed using the homeostasis model assessment of insulin resistance (HOMA-IR) index according to previous reports [21,22]. In brief, the HOMA-IR was calculated as fasting glucose (mmol/L)×fasting insulin (mU/L)/22.5. Plasma glucose concentrations were obtained using a commercial kit (Biosystems, Costa Brava, Barcelona, Spain) in an automatic analyzer (Quik-Lab; Ames, Miles Inc., Elkhart, IN, USA). Plasma insulin levels (pmol/L) were determined by an insulin enzyme-linked immunoassay (ELISA) kit (Mercodia AB, Uppsala, Sweden).

Hyperinsulinemic-euglycemic Clamping

The hyperinsulinemic-euglycemic clamping was performed as described previously [23] with some modifications. Before the hyperinsulinemic-euglycemic clamping was perfomed, food was withdrawn for 12 h. Rats were then anesthetized with sodium pentobarbital (30 mg/kg, i.p.) and cannulated in the femoral vein for infusion of glucose and insulin and in the femoral artery for sampling. Animals were weighed and placed in a restrainer to which they were accustomed before the clamp procedure. At 0 min, rats were randomly assigned to be infused with regular human insulin (Novo Industries, Bagsvaerd, Denmark) at 40 mU/(kg·min). The infusate of insulin was diluted with saline containing 0.5% human serum albumin (Baxter, Glendale, CA, USA). Blood samples (10 μL) were withdrawn at 10-min intervals for the immediate determination of plasma glucose. On the basis of these values, 20% dextrose (Abbott, Chicago, IL, USA) was variably infused to maintain the plasma glucose concentration at approximately 5.5 mmol/L. The steady state was generally achieved within 70–90 min, whereupon a blood sample was collected to determine the glucose concentration. After terminal blood sampling at 120 min, the animals were killed with a lethal dose of sodium pentobarbital (100 mg/kg, i.p.). The glucose infusion rate at steady state was calculated using Steele's equation [24].

Table 1. Effects of silymarin on body weight, biochemical indicators and HOMA-IR) in Wistar rats receiving fed fructose-rich chow or normal chow.

	HOMA-IR index	Cholesterol (mg/dL)	TG (mg/dL)	LDL (mg/dL)	HDL (mg/dL)	LDL/HDL	Body weight
Normal chow-fed rats (n = 8)							
+Vehicle	6.47±0.27	97.13±7.22	93.13±15.17	63.37±6.44	16.88±2.11	4.12±0.79	288.20±6.27
+Silymarin (200 mg/kg)	13.00±0.51	100.38±10.52	116.38±32.62	61.10±11.62	16.00±2.01	4.27±1.05	288.42±8.45
Fructose-rich chow-fed rats (n = 8)							
+Vehicle	18.68±0.49***	111.45±8.78	176.25±22.79**	63.83±5.95	12.38±2.46	6.35±1.06	304.62±10.96
+Silymarin (200 mg/kg)	21.82±0.62***###	116.43±11.35	175.38±23.66**	62.55±9.83	12.50±2.76	6.36±1.49	305.91±12.12

Silymarin (200 mg/kg body weight) was orally administerated once daily to Wistar rats fed fructose-rich or normal chow for 2 weeks. The HOMA-IR index was calculated as fasting glucose (mmol/L)×fasting insulin (mU/L)/22.5. Data represent mean ± standard error of mean of 8 animals.
***P<0.001 compared with normal chow-fed rats receiving vehicle;
###P<0.001 compared with fructose-rich chow-fed rats receiving vehicle.

Cell Cultures

The L6 cell line was purchased from the American Type Culture Collection (Manassas, VA, USA). The cells were maintained at 37°C and 5% CO2 in Dulbecco's modified Eagle's medium (DMEM; HyClone, South Logan, UT, USA) supplemented with 10% fetal bovine serum (FBS). Cells (1×106) were plated on 60-mm culture dishes, and at 80% confluence, they were differentiated by culturing for 6–7 days in DMEM containing 2% fetal bovine serum. Medium was changed every other day.

Glucose Uptake

A glucose uptake assay using 2-[*N*-(7-nitrobenz-2-oxa-1,3-diazol-4-yl)amino]-2-deoxy-D-glucose (2-NBDG; Invitrogen, Carlsbad, CA, USA) was performed according to a previously described method [25] with some modifications. Briefly, differentiated L6 cells were treated with or without a given concentration of silymarin and 1 μM insulin in the absence or presence of 200 μM 2-NBDG for 1 h. After the cells were washed, fluorescence intensity of 2-NBDG at 520–560-nm wavelength (480-nm excitation wavelength) was measured by the SPECTRA max 340PC ELISA reader (Molecular Devices Corporation, Union City, CA, USA). All cell culture results represent at least 2 independent experiments.

Western Blotting Analysis

Total protein lysates from tissues or cells were extracted in lysis buffer (1% Triton X-100, 150 mM NaCl, 10 mM Tris [pH 7.5], and 5 mM ethylenediaminetetraacetic acid) containing a protease and phosphatase inhibitor cocktail (Sigma-Aldrich). Protein concentration was determined by the BCA assay kit (Pierce Biotechnology, Rockford, IL, USA). Protein lysates (50 μg) were separated using 10% sodium dodecyl-polyacrylamide gel electrophoresis and transferred to a polyvinylidene difluoride membrane (Millipore, Billerica, MA, USA). The membrane was blocked at 25°C for 1 h in Tris buffered saline with Tween (TBS-T; 10 mM Tris [pH 7.6], 150 mM NaCl, and 0.05% Tween 20), containing 3% bovine serum albumin, and probed with primary antibodies (1:1000), such as those against PTEN, phospho-Akt, and Akt (Cell Signaling Technology, Beverly, MA, USA) at 4°C overnight. After the membrane had been washed with TBS-T, the blots were incubated with a 1/5000 dilution of horseradish peroxidase-conjugated secondary antibodies at 25°C for 1 h. Protein bands were visualized using the enhanced chemiluminescence kit (PerkinElmer, Boston, MA, USA). Actin (Millipore) was used as an internal control. The optical densities of the bands were determined using software (Gel-Pro Analyzer version 4.0 software (; Media Cybernetics Inc., Silver Spring, MD, USA).

Small Interfering Ribonucleic Acid Transfection

L6 cells were grown in 6-well culture plates at a density of 2×105 cells/well and transfected with duplexed RNA oligonucleotides (Stealth RNAi^{TM}; Invitrogen) of PTEN or scrambled small interfering RNA (siRNA) (as negative control) using Lipofectamine 2000TM (Invitrogen) according to the manufacturer's instructions. The cells were used at 48-h after-transfection.

Statistical Analysis

Data are expressed as means ± standard error of means. An analysis of variance and Dunnett's post hoc range comparisons were used to determine the source of significant differences where appropriate. Significance is defined as a P-value <0.05.

Results

Silymarin Induces Insulin Resistance in Wistar Rats

Oral administration of silymarin at 200 mg/kg body weight once daily for 14 days as described previously [25] produced insulin resistance in the Wistar rats, which was identified using the HOMA-IR or hyperinsulinemic-euglycemic clamping. In preliminary experiments, various doses of silymarin were administered to Wistar rats, and we found that 200 mg/kg body weight as most reliable dose to induce insulin resistance in rats. Therefore, we used this dose in all following studies. No intolerance, side effects, or allergic reactions were observed.

In rats receiving fructose-rich chow for the induction of insulin resistance, similar treatment with silymarin significantly enhanced insulin resistance (Tab. 1). In addition to HOMA-IR, the exacerbation of insulin resistance by silymarin in rats receiving fructose-rich chow was also evident by the hyperinsulinemic-euglycemic clamping method (Fig. 1).

Interestingly, this action of silymarin was impeded by a PTEN inhibitor (VO-OHpic) at the effective dose as described in a previous report [26]. Moreover, this action of silymarin disap-

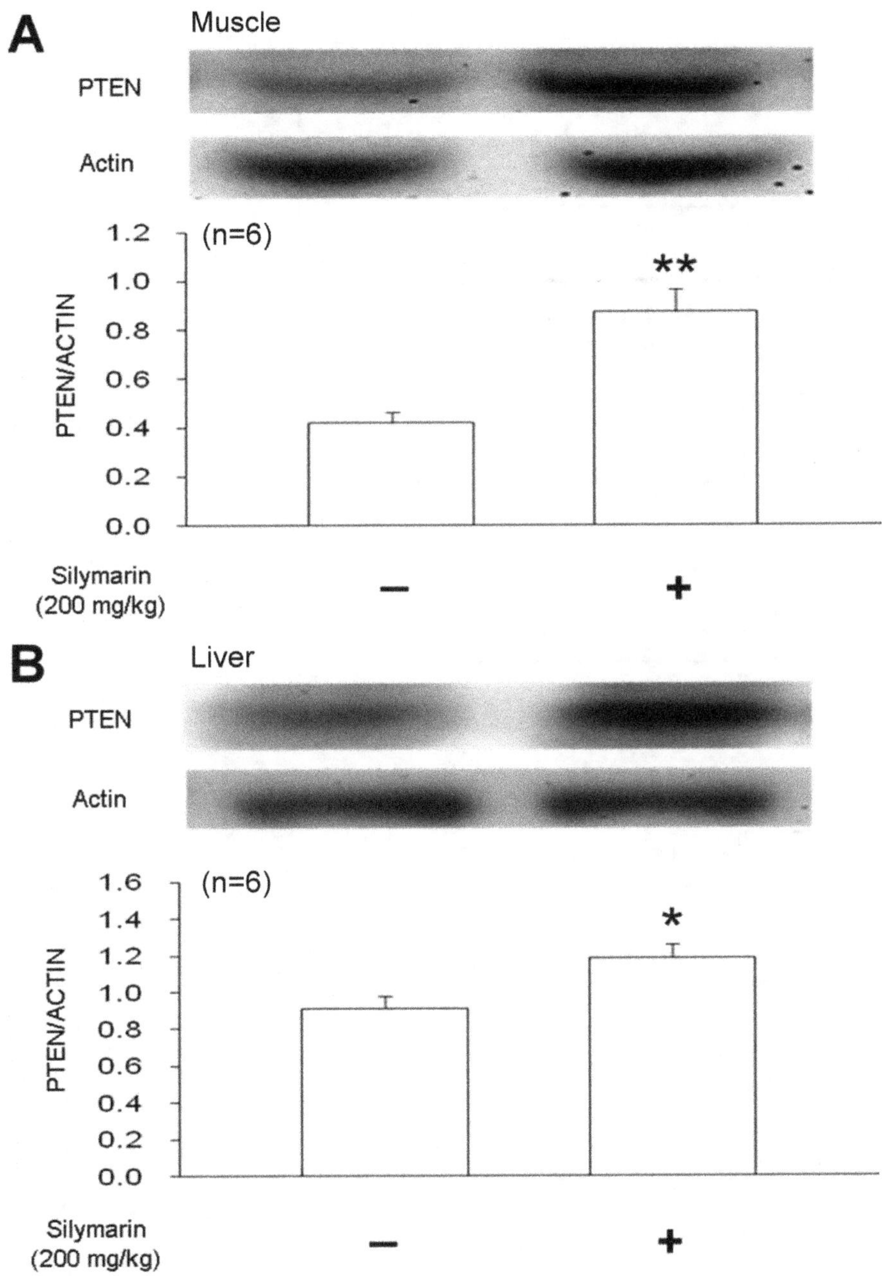

Figure 2. The effect of silymarin on the expression of PTEN. Silymarin (200 mg/kg body weight) was orally administered once daily to Wistar rats for 2 weeks. Skeletal muscle (A) and liver (B) were isolated for identification of PTEN expression using western blotting analysis. Data are obtained from 6 individual experiments and expressed as mean $\pm$ standard error of mean. **P*<0.05; ***P*<0.01 compared with the vehicle-treated group (first column).

peared within 2 or 3 days following the termination of dosing in rats. Thus, an irreversible action of silymarin was negligible.

Increased PTEN Expression by Silymarin in Wistar Rats

Skeletal muscle and the liver are widely used to identify insulin resistance. Therefore, both tissues were used to investigate the changes in PTEN expression using western blotting analysis. Silymarin significantly increased PTEN expression in skeletal muscle and the liver as shown in Fig. 2; PTEN expression was increased 2.03-fold by silymarin in skeletal muscle and 1.27-fold the in the liver.

Silymarin Disrupts Insulin Signaling to Decrease Glucose Uptake in Cultured L6 Myotube Cells

Insulin significantly increased the phosphorylation of Akt in cultured L6 cells, maintained in low-glucose condition (5 mM), whereas the elevated phosphor-Akt levels were decreased in high-glucose (25 mM) condition, implying the development of insulin resistance in cells. Pretreatment with silymarin aggravated high glucose-induced insulin resistance (Fig. 3A). To further confirm the development of insulin resistance, glucose uptake ability was assessed. Decreased glucose uptake was observed in cells

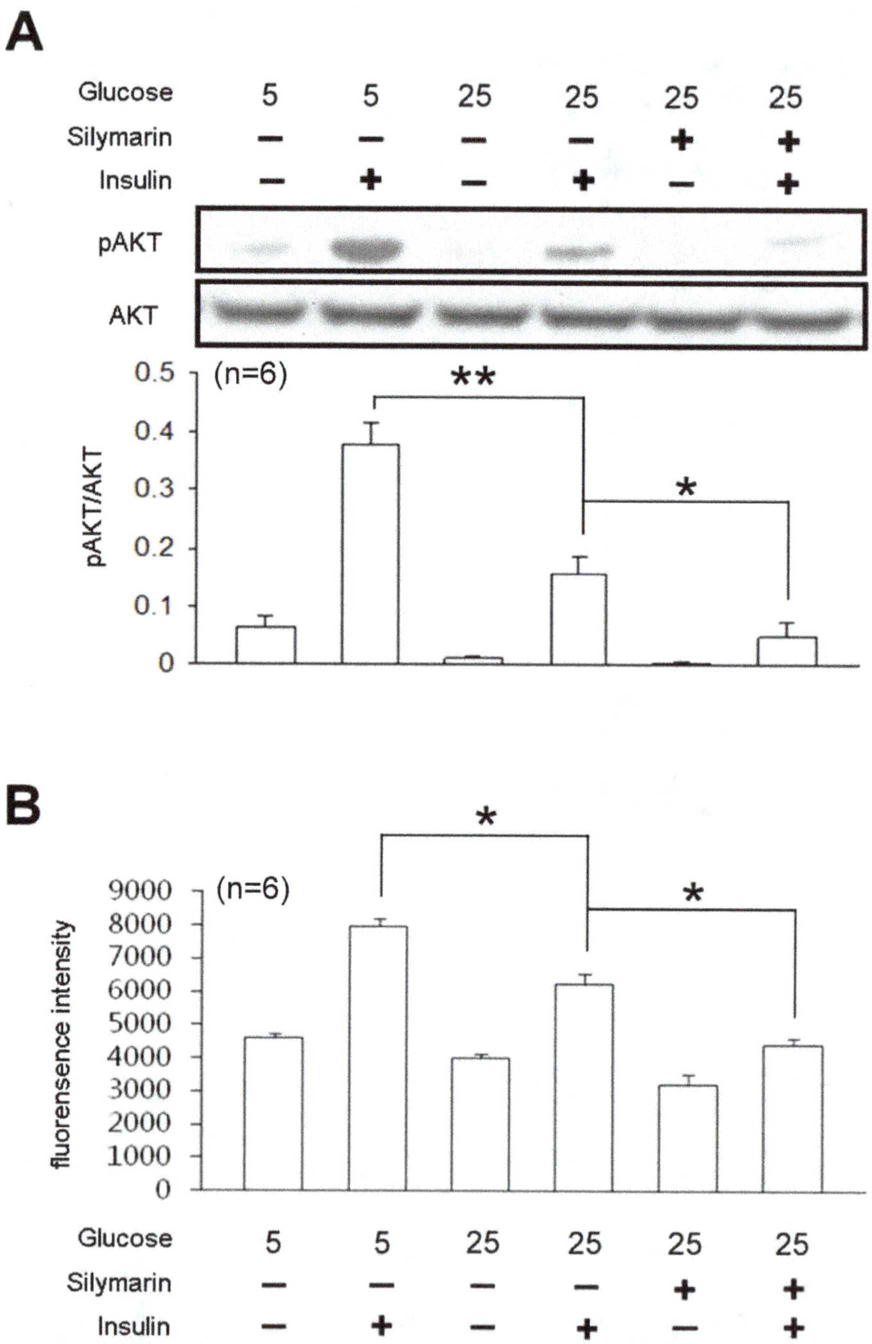

Figure 3. Silymarin disrupted insulin signaling to decrease glucose uptake in L6 myotube cells. L6 cells were maintained in normal-glucose (5 mM) or high-glucose (25 mM) medium. Cells were treated with 1 μM silymarin, and each group was exposed or not to 0.1 μM insulin for 30 min. Equal amounts of the total lysates of each group were immunoblotted with anti-phospho-Akt (pAkt) or Akt (A). The L6 cells were then treated with 200 μM 2-NBDG for 10 min to evaluate the glucose uptake ability of each group (B). Values represent means ± standard error of mean of 3 independent experiments. *$P<0.05$; **$P<0.01$ compared with the control group.

maintained in high-glucose conditions and silymarin exacerbated this effect of high glucose on glucose uptake (Fig. 3B).

Deletion of PTEN in Cultured L6 Myotube Cells Reversed Silymarin-induced Insulin Resistance

To confirm the role of PTEN in silymarin-induced insulin resistance, siRNA specific to PTEN was used. Transfection with this specific siRNA for PTEN significantly decreased the expression of PTEN in L6 cells, whereas scrambled siRNA had no effect (Fig. 4A). Disruption of insulin signaling by silymarin was reversed in L6 cells with specific PTEN deletion, whereas scrambled siRNA failed to affect the silymarin-induced effects (Fig. 4B).

Moreover, glucose uptake showed similar changes. In the presence of PTEN-specific siRNA, the effect of silymarin on

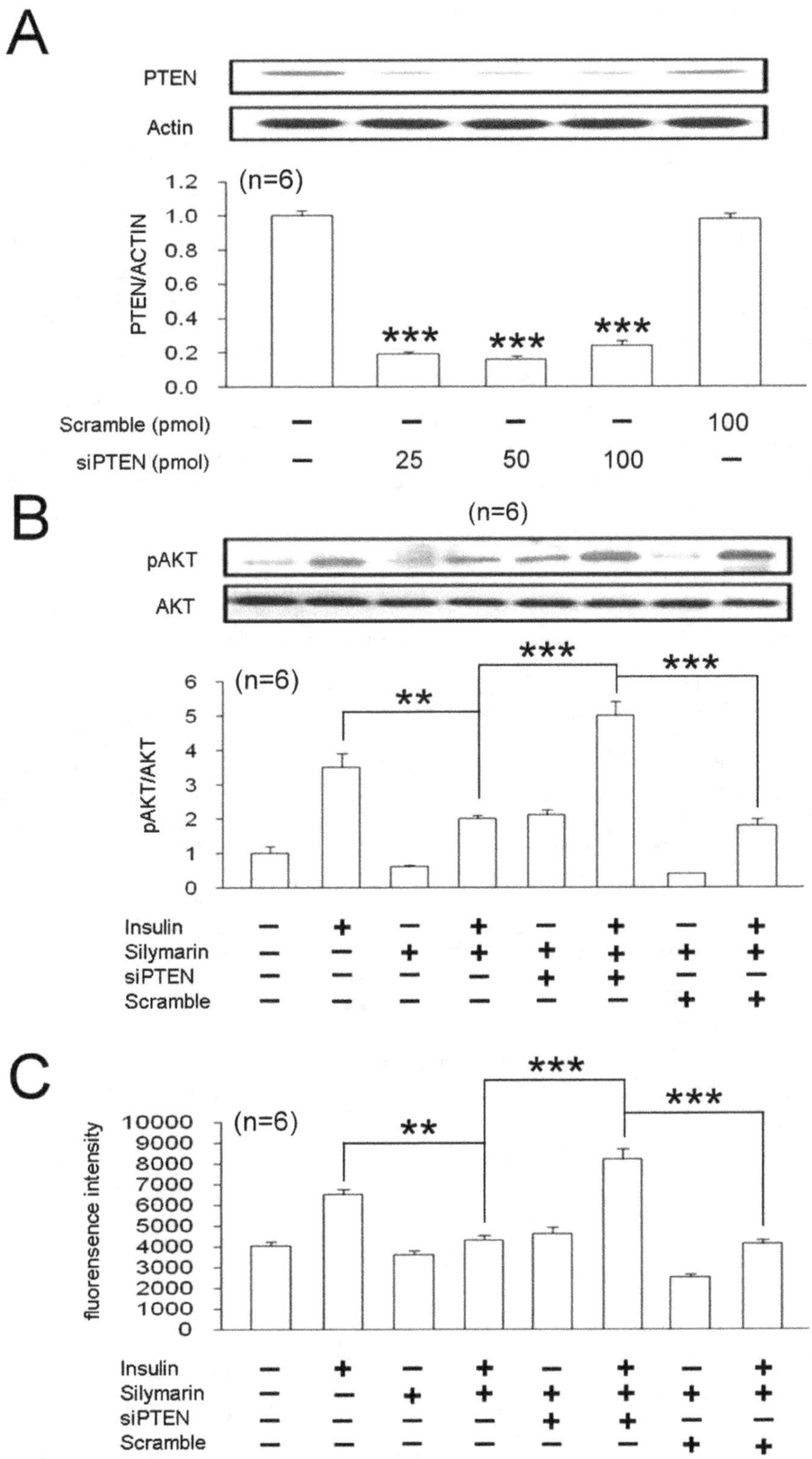

Figure 4. PTEN deletion in L6 cells reversed the effect of silymarin on insulin sensitivity and glucose uptake. Cells were transfected for 48 h with the indicated doses of PTEN siRNA or scramble siRNA. The total protein was extracted and blotted with PTEN or actin antibodies (A). Cells treated with 1 μM silymarin for 6 h with or without specific PTEN siRNA were exposed or not to 0.1 μM insulin. Equal amounts of the total lysates of each group were immunoblotted with anti-phospho-Akt (pAkt) or Akt (B). Cells were transfected for 48 h with 50 pmol PTEN siRNA or scramble siRNA were treated with 1 μM silymarin 6 h with or without specific PTEN siRNA and exposed or not to 0.1 μM insulin for 30 min. The L6 cells were then treated with 200 μM 2-NBDG for 1 h to evaluate the glucose uptake ability of each group (C). Values represent means ± standard error of mean for 3 independent.

glucose uptake was significantly reversed in L6 cells, wheras scrambled siRNA was not effective (Fig. 4C).

Discussion

In the present study, we found that silymarin induced insulin resistance in normal rats and enhanced insulin resistance in rats receiving fructose-rich chow. Insulin resistance was characterized using the HOMA-IR and hyperinsulinemic-euglycemic clamping. HOMA-IR is widely used clinically to identify the presence of insulin resistance [27–29], and hyperinsulinemic-euglycemic clamping is reported as a reliable tool in research for the estimation of insulin resistance in animals [30,31]. To the best of our knowledge, this is the first study to show that silymarin may induce insulin resistance. In this report, we demonstrated the presence of insulin resistance using HOMA-IR as described previously [32] while the values were different with that in clinics [28,29]. In addition, the effective dose in rats was not the same as that used in clinics; oral dose of silymarin in human subjects was 420–1680 mg/day [33,34] whereas the dose for cancer-resistance was 13000 mg/day [35].

It has been established that silymarin is a safe and well-tolerated dietary food supplement [4] and is widely used to protect against liver damage induced by chemicals [36,37]. In addition, the ability of silymarin to lower blood glucose and cholesterol has been documented in type-1 like diabetic rats [38]. However, another study indicated that silymarin had no significant effect on blood glucose [39]. Therefore, the effect on silymarin on blood glucose in diabetic animals remains obscure. The difference seems related to the dose used in the animals as the anti-diabetic action of silymarin was observed in lower doses through antioxidant-like actions [38]. Indeed, silymarin shows multiple actions related to the treatment dose [40,41]. Thus, silymarin-induced insulin resistance seems different from that described in previous reports [42,43] owing to the variation in dosing.

The anti-cancer action of silymarin is associate with an increase of PTEN [13]. Moreover, PTEN specific deletion in muscle improves skeletal muscle insulin sensitivity and protects mice from insulin resistance [18]. A crucial role for PTEN in insulin sensitivity has been documented [44,45]. Interesting, the effect of silymarin was reduced by a PTEN inhibitor, VO-OHpic, which has been used in previous studies [26,46]. Furthermore, PTEN expression identified by western blot was markedly increased by silymarin (Fig. 2), Thus revealing mediation of PTEN in the action of silymarin.

Glucose uptake in skeletal muscle plays an important role in glucose homeostasis [47], and we used L6 cells to investigate the potential underlying mechanism(s). Because isolated skeletal muscle preparations are short-lived during experimental manipulation [48] and nedds to be obtained from freshly killed animals, we used L6 cells as an alternative to investigate glucose uptake. Radioactive tracers are also widely employed glucose uptake assays [49]. To avoid radioactive damage, a fluorescence indicator, 2-NBDG, has been developed [50], and is generally measured by a fluorescence spectrofluorometer [51] or by an ELISA reader [52]. Similar to previous studies [25,53], we determined the changes in 2-NBDG uptake using an ELISA reader.

High glucose significantly impaired insulin signaling in L6 cells, whereas silymarin augmented high glucose-induced insulin resistance (Fig. 3A). To confirm the development of insulin resistance, glucose uptake in L6 cells was investigated. In parallel with the impaired insulin signaling as shown in Fig. 3A, glucose uptake was also impaired in silymarin-treated L6 cells under the high glucose condition, similar to that observed in rats receiving fructose-rich chow. It has been reported that silymarin induces the expression/activity of PTEN, [13] and that PTEN is responsible for the disruption of insulin signaling [15]. This view is consistent with our data that deletion of PTEN using siRNA reverses both silymarin-induced insulin resistance and impaired glucose uptake in L6 cells (Fig. 4). There is no doubt that the action of silymarin is produced though a PTEN-dependent pathway. However, the present study is mainly focused on the insulin sensitivity in muscle. Effect of silymarin on the insulin signals in liver shall be characterized in the future.

Taken together, PTEN loss is considered as a biomarker for activated PI3K/AKT, a pathway frequently mutated in cancer [16]. A previous study has demonstrated that silymarin could inhibit the Akt signaling pathway through increased PTEN expression, indicating its potential for suppressing migration and invasion of cancer cells [54]. Therefore, we should be aware of the possibility of insulin resistance when using silymarin for cancer therapy in patients with diabetes or with family history of diabetes.

In conclusion, we suggest that silymarin induces insulin resistance in Wistar rats and enhances insulin resistance in rats fed fructose-rich chow through an increase of PTEN. Administration of silymarin to cancer patients may affect insulin sensitivity, which should not be ignored clinically.

Acknowledgments

We thank Dr. H.T. Wu to help in this research.

Author Contributions

Conceived and designed the experiments: AA JC AI. Performed the experiments: AA HC KC YL. Analyzed the data: AA HC KC YL. Contributed reagents/materials/analysis tools: HC HA TU. Wrote the paper: AA HC KC YL.

References

1. Contos MJ, Choudhury J, Mills AS, Sanyal AJ (2004) The histologic spectrum of nonalcoholic fatty liver disease. Clin Liver Dis 8: 481–500.
2. Marchesini G, Babini M (2006) Nonalcoholic fatty liver disease and the metabolic syndrome. Minerva Cardioangiol 54: 229–239.
3. Williams R (2006) Global challenges in liver disease. Hepatology 44: 521–526.
4. Flora K, Hahn M, Rosen H, Benner K (1998) Milk thistle (Silybum marianum) for the therapy of liver disease. Am J Gastroenterol 93: 139–143.
5. Jacobs BP, Dennehy C, Ramirez G, Sapp J, Lawrence VA (2002) Milk thistle for the treatment of liver disease: a systematic review and meta-analysis. Am J Med 113: 506–515.
6. Lieber CS, Leo MA, Cao Q, Ren C, DeCarli LM (2003) Silymarin retards the progression of alcohol-induced hepatic fibrosis in baboons. J Clin Gastroenterol 37: 336–339.
7. Singh RP, Dhanalakshmi S, Tyagi AK, Chan DC, Agarwal C, et al. (2002) Dietary feeding of silibinin inhibits advance human prostate carcinoma growth in athymic nude mice and increases plasma insulin-like growth factor-binding protein-3 levels. Cancer Res 62: 3063–3069.
8. Singh RP, Gu M, Agarwal R (2008) Silibinin inhibits colorectal cancer growth by inhibiting tumor cell proliferation and angiogenesis. Cancer Res 68: 2043–2050.
9. Singh RP, Sharma G, Dhanalakshmi S, Agarwal C, Agarwal R (2003) Suppression of advanced human prostate tumor growth in athymic mice by silibinin feeding is associated with reduced cell proliferation, increased apoptosis, and inhibition of angiogenesis. Cancer Epidemiol Biomarkers Prev 12: 933–939.
10. Singh RP, Tyagi A, Sharma G, Mohan S, Agarwal R (2008) Oral silibinin inhibits in vivo human bladder tumor xenograft growth involving down-regulation of survivin. Clin Cancer Res 14: 300–308.
11. Tyagi A, Agarwal C, Agarwal R (2002) Inhibition of retinoblastoma protein (Rb) phosphorylation at serine sites and an increase in Rb-E2F complex formation by silibinin in androgen-dependent human prostate carcinoma LNCaP cells: role in prostate cancer prevention. Mol Cancer Ther 1: 525–532.
12. Tyagi A, Bhatia N, Condon MS, Bosland MC, Agarwal C, et al. (2002) Antiproliferative and apoptotic effects of silibinin in rat prostate cancer cells. Prostate 53: 211–217.

13. Lah JJ, Cui W, Hu KQ (2007) Effects and mechanisms of silibinin on human hepatoma cell lines. World J Gastroenterol 13: 5299–5305.
14. Varghese L, Agarwal C, Tyagi A, Singh RP, Agarwal R (2005) Silibinin efficacy against human hepatocellular carcinoma. Clin Cancer Res 11: 8441–8448.
15. Peyrou M, Bourgoin L, Foti M (2010) PTEN in liver diseases and cancer. World J Gastroenterol 16: 4627–4633.
16. Wang L, Wang WL, Zhang Y, Guo SP, Zhang J, et al. (2007) Epigenetic and genetic alterations of PTEN in hepatocellular carcinoma. Hepatol Res 37: 389–396.
17. Vinciguerra M, Foti M (2006) PTEN and SHIP2 phosphoinositide phosphatases as negative regulators of insulin signalling. Arch Physiol Biochem 112: 89–104.
18. Wijesekara N, Konrad D, Eweida M, Jefferies C, Liadis N, et al. (2005) Muscle-specific Pten deletion protects against insulin resistance and diabetes. Mol Cell Biol 25: 1135–1145.
19. Butler M, McKay RA, Popoff IJ, Gaarde WA, Witchell D, et al. (2002) Specific inhibition of PTEN expression reverses hyperglycemia in diabetic mice. Diabetes 51: 1028–1034.
20. Chiu YJ, Chung HH, Yeh CH, Cheng JT, Lo SH (2011) Improvement of Insulin Resistance by Chlorella in Fructose-rich Chow-fed Rats. Phytother Res 25: 1306–1312.
21. Wang X, Ge A, Cheng M, Guo F, Zhao M, et al. (2012) Increased hypothalamic inflammation associated with the susceptibility to obesity in rats exposed to high-fat diet. Exp Diabetes Res 2012: 847246.
22. Bu Z, Kuok K, Meng J, Wang R, Xu B, et al. (2012) The relationship between polycystic ovary syndrome, glucose tolerance status and serum preptin level. Reprod Biol Endocrinol 10: 10.
23. Su CH, Liu IM, Chung HH, Cheng JT (2009) Activation of I2-imidazoline receptors by agmatine improved insulin sensitivity through two mechanisms in type-2 diabetic rats. Neurosci Lett 457: 125–128.
24. Steele R (1959) Influences of glucose loading and of injected insulin on hepatic glucose output. Ann N Y Acad Sci 82: 420–430.
25. Wang SH, Kao MY, Wu SC, Lo DY, Wu JY, et al. (2011) Oral administration of Trapa taiwanensis Nakai fruit skin extracts conferring hepatoprotection from CCl4-caused injury. J Agric Food Chem 59: 3686–3692.
26. Alonso-Castro AJ, Zapata-Bustos R, Domínguez F, García-Carrancá A, Salazar-Olivo LA (2011) Magnolia dealbata Zucc and its active principles honokiol and magnolol stimulate glucose uptake in murine and human adipocytes using the insulin-signaling pathway. Phytomedicine 18: 926–933.
27. Zu L, Shen Z, Wesley J, Cai ZP (2011) PTEN inhibitors cause a negative inotropic and chronotropic effect in mice. Eur J Pharmacol 650: 298–302.
28. Wedin WK, Diaz-Gimenez L, Convit AJ (2012) Prediction of insulin resistance with anthropometric measures: lessons from a large adolescent population. Diabetes Metab Syndr Obes 5: 219–225.
29. Kamezaki F, Sonoda S, Nakata S, Kashiyama K, Muraoka Y, et al. (2012) Proposed cutoff level of waist circumference in Japanese men: evaluation by homeostasis model assessment of insulin resistance levels. Intern Med 51: 2119–2124.
30. Zhao D, McCully BH, Brooks VL (2012) Rosiglitazone improves insulin sensitivity and baroreflex gain in rats with diet-induced obesity. J Pharmacol Exp Ther 343: 206–213.
31. Zhang Z, Sheng S, Guo L, Li G, Zhang L, et al. (2012) Intracerebroventricular administration of galanin antagonist sustains insulin resistance in adipocytes of type 2 diabetic trained rats. Mol Cell Endocrinol 361: 213–218.
32. Nandhini AT, Thirunavukkarasu V, Ravichandran MK, Anuradha CV (2005) Effect of taurine on biomarkers of oxidative stress in tissues of fructose-fed insulin-resistant rats. Singapore Med J 46: 82–87.
33. Hawke RL, Schrieber SJ, Soule TA, Wen Z, Smith PC, et al. (2010) Silymarin ascending multiple oral dosing phase I study in noncirrhotic patients with chronic hepatitis C. J Clin Pharmacol 50: 434–449.
34. Schrieber SJ, Hawke RL, Wen Z, Smith PC, Reddy KR, et al. (2011) Differences in the disposition of silymarin between patients with nonalcoholic fatty liver disease and chronic hepatitis C. Drug Metab Dispos. 39: 2182–2190.
35. Leber HW, Knauff S (1976) Influence of silymarin on drug metabolizing enzymes in rat and man. Arzneimittelforschung. 26: 1603–1605.
36. Khan RA, Khan MR, Ahmed M, Sahreen S, Shah NA, et al. (2012) Hepatoprotection with a chloroform extract of Launaea procumbens against CCl4-induced injuries in rats. BMC Complement Altern Med 12: 114.
37. Tzeng JI, Chen MF, Chung HH, Cheng JT (2012) Silymarin Decreases Connective Tissue Growth Factor to Improve Liver Fibrosis in Rats Treated with Carbon Tetrachloride. Phytother Res 27: 1023–1028.
38. Vengerovskii AI, Khazanov VA, Eskina KA, Vasilyev KY (2007) Effects of silymarin (hepatoprotector) and succinic acid (bioenergy regulator) on metabolic disorders in experimental diabetes mellitus. Bull Exp Biol Med 144: 53–56.
39. Vessal G, Akmali M, Najafi P, Moein MR, Sagheb MM (2010) Silymarin and milk thistle extract may prevent the progression of diabetic nephropathy in streptozotocin-induced diabetic rats. Renal Fail 32: 733–739.
40. Ashkavand Z, Malekinejad H, Amniattalab A, Rezaei-Golmisheh A, Vishwanath BS (2012) Silymarin potentiates the anti-inflammatory effects of Celecoxib on chemically induced osteoarthritis in rats. Phytomedicine 19: 1200–1205.
41. Cecen E, Dost T, Culhaci N, Karul A, Ergur B, et al. (2011) Protective effects of silymarin against doxorubicin-induced toxicity. Asian Pac J Cancer Prev 12: 2697–2704.
42. Baluchnejadmojarad T, Roghani M, Khastehkhodaie Z (2010) Chronic treatment of silymarin improves hyperalgesia and motor nerve conduction velocity in diabetic neuropathic rat. Phytother Res 24: 1120–1125.
43. Malekinejad H, Rezabakhsh A, Rahmani F, Hobbenaghi R (2012) Silymarin regulates the cytochrome P450 3A2 and glutathione peroxides in the liver of streptozotocin-induced diabetic rats. Phytomedicine 19: 583–590.
44. Mak LH, Vilar R, Woscholski R (2010) Characterisation of the PTEN inhibitor VO-OHpic. J Chem Biol 3: 157–163.
45. Alexandrov IM, Ivshina M, Jung DY, Friedline R, Ko HJ, et al. (2012) Cytoplasmic polyadenylation element binding protein deficiency stimulates PTEN and Stat3 mRNA translation and induces hepatic insulin resistance. PLoS Genet 8: e1002457.
46. Lee SK, Lee JO, Kim JH, Kim SJ, You GY, et al. (2011) Metformin sensitizes insulin signaling through AMPK-mediated PTEN down-regulation in preadipocyte 3T3-L1 cells. J Cell Biochem 112: 1259–1267.
47. DeFronzo RA, Ferrannini E, Hendler R, Felig P, Wahren J (1983) Regulation of splanchnic and peripheral glucose uptake by insulin and hyperglycemia in man. Diabetes 32: 35–45.
48. Sarabia V, Lam L, Burdett E, Leiter LA, Klip A (1992) Glucose transport in human skeletal muscle cells in culture. Stimulation by insulin and metformin. J Clin Invest 90: 1386–1395.
49. Landau BR, Spring-Robinson CL, Muzic RF Jr, Rachdaoui N, Rubin D, et al. (2007) 6-Fluoro-6-deoxy-D-glucose as a tracer of glucose transport. Am J Physiol Endocrinol Metab 2007; 293: 237–245.
50. Blodgett AB, Kothinti RK, Kamyshko I, Petering DH, Kumar S, et al. (2011) A fluorescence method for measurement of glucose transport in kidney cells. Diabetes Technol Ther 13: 743–751.
51. Zou C, Wang Y, Shen Z (2005) 2-NBDG as a fluorescent indicator for direct glucose uptake measurement. J Biochem Biophys Methods 64: 207–215.
52. Louzao MC, Espiña B, Vieytes MR, Vega FV, Rubiolo JA, et al. (2008) "Fluorescent glycogen" formation with sensibility for in vivo and in vitro detection. Glycoconj J 25: 503–510.
53. Alonso-Castro AJ, Salazar-Olivo LA (2008) The anti-diabetic properties of Guazuma ulmifolia Lam are mediated by the stimulation of glucose uptake in normal and diabetic adipocytes without inducing adipogenesis. J Ethnopharmacol 118: 252–256.
54. Yu HC, Chen LJ, Cheng KC, Li YX, Yeh CH, et al. (2012) Silymarin inhibits cervical cancer cell through an increase of phosphatase and tensin homolog. Phytother Res 26: 709–715.

3

Association of Insulin Resistance Indexes to Carotid Intima–Media Thickness

Angela Sciacqua[1], Maria Adelaide Marini[2], Marta Letizia Hribal[1], Francesco Perticone[1], Giorgio Sesti[1]*

1 Department of Medical and Surgical Sciences, University "Magna Graecia" of Catanzaro, Catanzaro, Italy, **2** Department of Internal Medicine, University of Rome-Tor Vergata, Rome, Italy

Abstract

Objectives: Accumulating evidence suggests an association between insulin resistance (IR) and cardiovascular diseases The aim of this study was to examine the relationship between indexes of IR and common carotid intima–media thickness (IMT), an indicator of vascular damage.

Methods: In 847 non-diabetic Caucasians a 75 g oral glucose tolerance test was performed and surrogate indexes of IR were computed according to published formulas. IMT was measured by ultrasound method.

Results: The Stumvoll ISI_{OGTT} index was correlated with IMT more strongly than the other indexes of IR. The IR indexes correlated significantly ($P<0.0001$) with all cardiovascular risk factors examined. The Stumvoll ISI_{OGTT} index was correlated with waist circumference and high sensitivity C-reactive protein more strongly than the other indexes of IR. The area under the ROC curve (AUC), used to evaluate the accuracy of the IR indexes in identifying individuals with vascular damage defined as IMT >0.9 mm, for the Stumvoll ISI_{OGTT} index was significantly higher (0.710) as compared with the AUCs of Matsuda (0.642) ($P=0.0009$), OGIS (0.666) ($P=0.04$), HOMA (0.611) ($P<0.0001$) and Liver IR (0.648) ($P=0.0008$) indexes. In a logistic regression model adjusted for age and gender, subjects in the lowest tertile of the Stumvoll ISI_{OGTT} index had the highest risk of having vascular damage (OR 4.95, 95% CI 2.99–8.192) as compared to the corresponding tertiles of the other surrogate indexes.

Conclusion: The Stumvoll ISI_{OGTT} index correlated more strongly than other validated surrogates indexes of IR with carotid IMT, and, therefore, it might be a significant indicator of vascular damage.

Editor: Francesco Giorgino, University of Bari, Italy

Funding: The authors have no support or funding to report.

Competing Interests: The authors have declared that no competing interests exist.

* E-mail: sesti@unicz.it

Introduction

Cardiovascular disease is one of the major causes of mortality and morbidity in adult individuals. Insulin resistance (IR) is considered an important risk factor for both atherosclerotic cardiovascular disease [1,2] and type 2 diabetes [3], and a key determinant of cardiovascular risk factors, including visceral obesity, atherogenic dyslipidemia, and hypertension, clustering within the metabolic syndrome [4–6]. Accumulating evidence suggests an association between hyperinsulinemia and/or IR and cardiovascular diseases [7–10]. Importantly, it has been shown that IR, evaluated by the frequently sampled intravenous glucose tolerance test with minimal model analysis [11] or by the euglycemic hyperinsulinemic clamp [12], rather than hyperinsulinemia, was independently associated with early vascular atherosclerosis. However, methods to directly measure IR are complex, time-consuming, expensive, and unsuitable for large scale epidemiological studies. Therefore, surrogate indexes of insulin sensitivity have been developed using fasting insulin and/or glucose levels alone [13] or in combination with insulin and glucose levels during an oral glucose tolerance test (OGTT) [14] as well as with other metabolic variables [15–17]. Since IR occurs in multiple tissues, these indexes reflects predominantly either hepatic [13,17] or muscle IR [14–16].

Whether these IR indexes are differentially associated with vascular atherosclerosis is still undefined. Intima–media thickness (IMT) of common carotid artery is a well-recognized index of vascular damage, and is widely utilized as a surrogate marker for cardiovascular disease [18].

The aim of this study was to examine the relationship between different indexes of insulin resistance and common carotid IMT in a cohort of nondiabetic Caucasian individuals.

Materials and Methods

Ethics Statement

The Protocol was approved by the Ethical Committee "Comitato Etico Azienda Ospedaliera Universitaria Mater Domini". Informed written consent was obtained from all participants. All the investigations were performed in accordance with the principles of the Declaration of Helsinki.

Table 1. Anthropometric and metabolic characteristics of the study subjects.

Variables	Whole study group	Men	Women	*P*
Gender (M/F)	414/433	414	433	0.079
Age *(yrs)*	48.4±10.0	49.1±10.0	47.7±9.9	0.04
BMI *(kg/m^2)*	29.6±5.9	29.4±4.8	29.9±6.7	0.24
Waist circumference (*cm*)	98±13	101±11	96±14	<0.0001
Fat mass (%)	32.7±9.9	27.6±7.7	37.6±9.3	<0.0001
SBP *(mmHg)*	131±16	134±15	127±17	<0.0001
DBP *(mmHg)*	82±10	84±10	79±10	<0.0001
Fasting Glucose *(mgl/dl)*	94±12	97±11	92±11	<0.0001
90 min Glucose *(mgl/dl)*	140±43	147±44	134±41	<0.0001
2-h Glucose *(mgl/dl)*	124±34	127±35	121±33	0.003
Fasting Insulin *(μU/ml)*	13±8	13±9	12±7	0.02
2-h Insulin *(μU/ml)*	86±77	90±75	82±78	0.16
Total cholesterol *(mg/dl)*	203±36	203±35	203±37	0.97
HDL *(mg/dl)*	50±13	44±10	56±13	<0.0001
Triglycerides *(mg/dl)*	133±85	152±98	116±66	<0.0001
hsCRP *(mg/l)*	3.2±3.1	3.1±3.0	3.3±3.2	0.36
IMT (mm)	0.75±0.2	0.77±0.2	0.72±0.1	0.001
HOMA	3.0±2.1	3.3±2.3	2.8±1.9	0.001
Liver IR index	2.93±0.37	2.95±0.37	2.92±0.37	0.28
OGIS (ml×min^{-1}×m^{-2})	381±75	263±64	298±80	<0.0001
Matsuda	73±46	67±43	79±48	<0.0001
Matsuda2	71±45	65±43	77±47	<0.0001
Stumvoll ISI$_{OGTT}$ (μmol×kg^{-1}×min^{-1}×pM^{-1})	0.96±0.02	0.95±0.02	0.97±0.02	0.29
NGT,IFG, IGT, IFG/IGT n (%)	459/150/118/120 (54.2/17.7/13.9/14.2)	189/89/56/80 (45.7/21.5/13.5/19.3)	270/61/62/40 (62.4/14.1/14.3/9.2	<0.0001

Data are means ± SD. *P* values for differences of continuous variables between the two groups using unpaired Student's t. Categorical variables were compared by χ^2 test. M = male; F = female; BMI = body mass index; SBP = systolic blood pressure; DBP = diastolic blood pressure; HDL = high density lipoprotein; hsCRP = high sensitivity C reactive protein; IMT = intima-media thickness; HOMA = homeostasis model assessment; OGIS = oral glucose insulin sensitivity; ISI = Insulin sensitivity index; Matsuda2 = not including fasting glucose and insulin levels in mean values of glucose and insulin during OGTT; IFG = impaired fasting glucose; IGT = impaired glucose tolerance.

Subjects

847 non-diabetic Caucasian subjects, aged 30–70 years, consecutively recruited in the University of Rome and the University of Catanzaro areas participated to this cross-sectional study for assessment of cardio-metabolic risk factors as previously described [19,20]. Subjects were excluded if they had history of cardiovascular disease including peripheral atherosclerosis, chronic gastrointestinal diseases associated with malabsorption, chronic pancreatitis, history of any malignant disease, history of alcohol or drug abuse, positivity for antibodies to hepatitis C virus (HCV) or hepatitis B surface antigen (HBsAg), and liver or kidney failure. Subjects were excluded if they had diabetes mellitus, defined as ≥126 mg/dl or 2-h post-challenge plasma glucose ≥200 mg/dl. After a 12-h fasting, all subjects underwent anthropometrical evaluation including assessment of body mass index (BMI), and waist circumference, and readings of clinic blood pressure (BP) obtained in the left arm of the supine patients, after five minutes of quiet rest, with a sphygmomanometer. Values were calculated as the average of the last two of three consecutive measurements obtained at 3-mins intervals. A 75 g oral glucose tolerance test (OGTT) was performed with 0, 30, 60, 90 and 120 min sampling for plasma glucose and insulin determination.

IMT of the common carotid artery was measured by ATL HDI 3000 ultrasound system (Advanced Technology Laboratories, Bothell, WA) equipped with a 5 MHz linear array transducer as previously described [12]. Manual measurements were conducted in plaque-free portions of the 10-mm linear segment proximal to the carotid bulb. For each patient two measurements were performed bilaterally, and the values were averaged, to obtain the mean of IMT of the common carotid artery. Ultrasound studies were performed by an experienced examiner who was unaware of the subjects' clinical and laboratory findings. A value of IMT >0.9 mm was used as index of vascular damage according to the 2007 Guidelines for the management of arterial hypertension released by the Task Force for the Management of Arterial Hypertension of the European Society of Hypertension (ESH) and of the European Society of Cardiology (ESC) [21].

Analytical Determinations

Glucose, triglyceride, total and high density lipoprotein (HDL-C) cholesterol concentrations were determined by enzymatic methods (Roche, Basel, Switzerland) and plasma insulin concentration was assessed with a chemiluminescence-based assay (Immulite®, Siemens, Italy). High sensitivity C-reactive protein

Table 2. Age and gender adjusted univariate correlations between anthropometric and metabolic variables and IMT in the whole study group.

Variables	IMT	
	Pearson's correlation coefficient (*r*)	*P*
BMI *(kg/m^2)*	0.23	<0.0001
Waist circumference *(cm)*	0.16	<0.0001
Fat mass (%)	0.18	<0.0001
SBP *(mmHg)*	0.13	<0.0001
DBP *(mmHg)*	0.08	0.02
Fasting Glucose *(mgl/dl)*	0.11	0.002
90-min Glucose *(mgl/dl)*	0.14	0.001
2-h Glucose *(mgl/dl)*	0.09	0.01
Fasting Insulin *(µU/ml)*	0.14	<0.0001
2-h Insulin *(µU/ml)*	0.12	0.001
Total cholesterol *(mg/dl)*	0.03	0.41
HDL *(mg/dl)*	−0.10	0.008
Triglycerides *(mg/dl)*	0.05	0.13
hsCRP *(mg/l)*	0.12	0.001
HOMA	0.14	<0.0001
Liver IR index	0.18	<0.0001
OGIS (ml×min^{-1}×m^{-2})	−0.17	<0.0001
Matsuda	−0.14	<0.0001
Matsuda2	−0.14	<0.0001
Stumvoll ISI_{OGTT} (µmol×kg^{-1}×min^{-1}×pM^{-1})	−0.25	<0.0001

P values refer to results after analysis with adjustment for age and gender. IMT = intima-media thickness; HOMA = homeostasis model assessment; OGIS = oral glucose insulin sensitivity; Matsuda2 = not including fasting glucose and insulin levels in mean values of glucose and insulin during OGTT; ISI = Insulin sensitivity index.

(hsCRP) levels were measured by an automated instrument (CardioPhase® hsCRP, Siemens, Italy).

Calculations

The homeostasis model assessment (HOMA) index was calculated as fasting insulin×fasting glucose/22.5 [13]. The Matsuda index was calculated as 10,000/square root of [fasting glucose (mmol/L)×fasting insulin (mU/L)]×[mean glucose×mean insulin during OGTT] [14]; the Matsuda2 index was calculated as 10,000/square root of [fasting glucose (mmol/L)×fasting insulin (mU/L)]×[mean $glucose_{30-120}$×mean $insulin_{30-120}$ during OGTT] not including in the formula fasting glucose and insulin levels in mean values of glucose and insulin during OGTT; the Stumvoll Insulin Sensitivity Index $(ISI)_{OGTT}$ was calculated as $0.226 - 0.0032\times BMI - 0.0000645\times Insulin_{120} - 0.00375\times Glucose_{90}$ [15]; the oral glucose insulin sensitivity (OGIS) was calculated as previously described using a spreadsheet calculator downloaded from http://webmet.pd.cnr.it/ogis [16]; the liver IR index was calculated using the formula: −0.091+ (log insulin AUC 0–120 min×0.400)+(log fat mass %×0.346) - (log HDL Cholesterol×0.408)+(log BMI×0.435) [17]. The trapezoidal method was used to calculate glucose and insulin AUC during an OGTT.

Statistical Analysis

Triglycerides values were natural log transformed for statistical analysis due to their skewed distribution. Continuous data are expressed as means ± SD. Comparisons between two groups were performed using unpaired Student's t-test. Categorical variables were compared by χ^2 test. Relationships between variables were determined by Pearson's correlation coefficient (r). Partial correlation coefficients adjusted for age and gender were computed between variables. The ability of each index to detect subjects with vascular damage, defined as IMT >0.9 mm [21], was assessed by the area under the receiver operating characteristic (ROC) curve. The area under the ROC curve (AUC) was used as a measure of how well IR indexes identify vascular damage. An AUC of 1.0 indicates perfect classification of individuals with vascular damage, whereas 0.5 means that the classification is not better than chance. Statistical differences between the AUC under the ROC curves were determined by the method described by DeLong et al. [22]. A multiple regression analysis was performed to estimate the independent contribution of indexes of IR to carotid IMT. A multivariable logistic regression analysis was used to determine the association between vascular damage and the tertiles of IR indexes. A *P* value <0.05 was considered nominally significant. All analyses were performed using SPSS software programme Version 16.0 for Windows.

Results

Men were older, had more central adiposity, but lower fat mass than women (Table 1). Men also had higher BP, fasting, 90 min, and 2-h post-load plasma glucose concentration, fasting insulin levels, triglycerides, and carotid IMT, and lower HDL cholesterol. Men were more insulin resistant than women as they showed significantly higher values of HOMA and Liver IR indexes and lower values of Matsuda, Matsuda2 and OGIS indexes (Table 1).

Table 3. Age and gender adjusted univariate correlations between insulin resistance indexes and cardiovascular risk factors in the whole study group.

	HOMA		Liver IR index		OGIS		Matsuda		Stumvoll ISI_{OGTT}	
	Pearson's correlation coefficient (*r*)	*P*	Pearson's correlation coefficient (*r*)	*P*	Pearson's correlation coefficient (*r*)	*P*	Pearson's correlation coefficient (*r*)	*P*	Pearson's correlation coefficient (*r*)	*P*
Waist circumference (*cm*)	0.40	<0.0001	0.63	<0.0001	−0.41	<0.0001	−0.42	<0.0001	−0.75	<0.0001
SBP (*mmHg*)	0.11	0.001	0.20	<0.0001	−0.15	<0.0001	−0.17	<0.0001	−0.25	<0.0001
DBP (*mmHg*)	0.13	<0.0001	0.20	<0.0001	−0.18	<0.0001	−0.16	<0.0001	−0.23	<0.0001
total cholesterol (*mg/dl*)	0.01	0.99	0.03	0.40	−0.12	<0.0001	−0.07	0.03	−0.01	0.77
HDL (*mg/dl*)	−0.26	<0.0001	−0.45	<0.0001	0.20	<0.0001	0.24	<0.0001	0.24	<0.0001
Triglycerides (*mg/dl*)	0.19	<0.0001	0.27	<0.0001	−0.18	<0.0001	−0.21	<0.0001	−0.19	<0.0001
hsCRP (*mg/l*)	0.26	<0.0001	0.27	<0.0001	−0.22	<0.0001	−0.24	<0.0001	−0.34	<0.0001

P values refer to results after analysis with adjustment for age and gender. SBP = systolic blood pressure; DBP = diastolic blood pressure; HDL = high density lipoprotein hsCRP = high sensitivity C reactive protein; HOMA = homeostasis model assessment; OGIS = oral glucose insulin sensitivity; ISI = Insulin sensitivity index; OGTT = oral glucose tolerance test.

By contrast, no gender-dependent differences in Stumvoll ISI_{OGTT} values were observed probably due to the lack of differences between man and women in two variables considered in the index calculation i.e. BMI and $Insulin_{120}$.

Age and gender adjusted univariate correlations between anthropometric and metabolic variables and IMT in the whole study group are showed in Table 2. IMT was significantly correlated with BMI, waist circumference, fat mass, systolic blood pressure (SBP), diastolic blood pressure (DBP), triglycerides, HDL cholesterol, hsCRP, fasting glucose, 2-h glucose, fasting insulin, and 2-h insulin. Among these variables, BMI exhibited the strongest association ($r = 0.23$). The Stumvoll ISI_{OGTT} index was correlated with IMT more strongly than the other indexes of IR. The same degree of correlation was observed with the canonical Matsuda index and with the Matsuda2 index which does not average fasting glucose and insulin levels when computing mean values of glucose and insulin during OGTT.

Age and gender adjusted univariate correlations between IR indexes and cardiovascular risk factors in the whole study group are showed in Table 3. The IR indexes correlated significantly ($P<0.0001$) with all cardiovascular risk factors examined (Table 3). The Stumvoll ISI_{OGTT} index was correlated with waist circumference and hsCRP more strongly than the other indexes of IR (Table 3).

To estimate the independent contribution of indexes of IR to carotid IMT, we carried out a multiple regression analysis using carotid IMT as the dependent variable and including age, gender, BMI, SBP, DBP, diastolic blood pressure, triglycerides, total cholesterol, HDL cholesterol, hsCRP and indexes of IR as independent variables. As shown in Table 4, all indexes of IR remained significantly associated with carotid IMT with the Stumvoll ISI_{OGTT} index showing the strongest independent association. When BMI was entered into the regression model 1, the four indexes of IR that remained significantly associated with carotid IMT were Matsuda, OGIS, Liver IR, and Stumvoll ISI_{OGTT} with the latter index showing the strongest independent association (Table 5).

The area under the ROC curve (AUC) was used to evaluate the accuracy of the IR indexes in identifying individuals with vascular damage, defined as IMT >0.9 mm. The AUC for the Stumvoll ISI_{OGTT} index was significantly higher (0.710) as compared with the AUCs of Matsuda (0.642, $P = 0.0009$), OGIS (0.666, $P = 0.04$), HOMA (0.611, $P<0.0001$) and Liver IR (0.648, $P = 0.0008$) indexes (Figure 1).

Next, the subjects were stratified into tertiles according to the values of the IR indexes. In a logistic regression model adjusted for age and gender, SBP, DBP, triglycerides, total cholesterol, HDL cholesterol, hsCRP, subjects in the lowest tertile of the Stumvoll ISI_{OGTT} index had a 3.71-fold higher risk of having vascular damage as compared with those in the highest tertile (OR 3.71, 95% CI 2.07–6.61), subjects in the lowest tertile of Matsuda index had a 1.87-fold higher risk of having vascular damage as compared with those in the highest tertile (OR 1.87, 95% CI 1.09–3.21), subjects in the lowest tertile of OGIS index had a 2.21-fold higher risk of having vascular damage as compared with those in the highest tertile (OR 2.21, 95% CI 1.25–3.93), subjects in the highest tertile of HOMA index had a 2.05-fold higher risk of having vascular damage as compared with those in the lowest tertile (OR 2.05, 95% CI 1.20–3.51), and subjects in the highest tertile of Liver IR index had a 2.45-fold higher risk of having vascular damage as compared with those in the lowest tertile (OR 2.45, 95% CI 1.40–4.31).

Table 4. Multiple regression analysis testing the independent association between indexes of insulin resistance and carotid intima-media thickness (IMT) in a model including age, gender, systolic blood pressure, diastolic blood pressure, triglycerides, total cholesterol, HDL cholesterol, and hsCRP as independent variables (Model 1).

HOMA		Liver IR index		OGIS		Matsuda		Stumvoll ISI_{OGTT}	
β coefficient	*P*	β coefficient	*P*	β coefficient	*P*	β coefficient	*P*	β coefficient	*P*
0.13	<0.0001	0.15	<0.0001	−0.17	<0.0001	−0.13	<0.0001	−0.22	<0.0001

HOMA = homeostasis model assessment; OGIS = oral glucose insulin sensitivity; ISI = Insulin sensitivity index.

Discussion

IR is typically defined as a condition of diminished ability of target tissues to take up and metabolize glucose in response to insulin, and it plays a major role in the development of type 2 diabetes. IR is also a key feature of a spectrum of metabolic abnormalities such as obesity and glucose intolerance, and is associated with multiple cardiovascular risk factors (visceral adiposity, hypertension, atherogenic dyslipidemia), a clinical constellation that has been referred to as metabolic syndrome [4]. IR is a predictor of atherosclerotic cardiovascular disease [2], and this association has vast social implications, and calls for intensive investigation of the causes of the disease, to optimize its treatment and to possibly prevent its onset.

IR occurs in multiple tissues, particularly in the skeletal and cardiac muscle, adipose tissue and liver [23]. Although accurate methods have been developed to measure directly tissue-specific IR with the glucose clamp technique combined with tracers, these methods are impractical for large scale epidemiological studies since they are invasive, laborious, costly, and time-consuming. Therefore, simpler methods to measure IR have been developed using fasting insulin and/or glucose levels alone [13] or in combination with insulin and glucose levels during an OGTT [14–17], a widely employed test to assess glucose homeostasis in clinical practice. All surrogates indexes correlate reasonably well with insulin sensitivity measured by euglycemic-hyperinsulinemic clamp [13–17], although they differentially reflect the contribution of individual organs, e.g., liver and muscle, to insulin resistance. Indexes derived from measurements of fasting plasma glucose and insulin levels such HOMA [13] primarily reflect the basal measurement of hepatic glucose production (HGP) [24], while the liver IR index was specifically developed to measure hepatic IR [17]. Finally, the Matsuda and the Stumvoll ISI_{OGTT} indexes primarily reflect muscle insulin sensitivity [14,15,24], whereas the OGIS reflects the metabolic clearance rate of glucose [16].

In the present study, we documented that these IR indexes are differentially associated with vascular damage, as assessed by IMT of common carotid artery [18]. We found that the Stumvoll ISI_{OGTT} index correlates better with IMT than the four other surrogate indexes as indicated by the significantly higher value of the area under the ROC curve and by the increased risk of having vascular damage for subjects in the lowest tertile of the Stumvoll ISI_{OGTT} index as compared to the corresponding tertiles of the other surrogate indexes. To the best of our knowledge, this is the first study to investigate the associations between different surrogate indexes of IR and IMT in a large cohort of non-diabetic individuals.

The better association observed between the Stumvoll ISI_{OGTT} index and vascular damage may be partially explained by the fact that it takes into consideration BMI in addition to insulin and glucose concentrations during an OGTT. Consequently, this index may signal not only muscle IR but also other important domains for vascular damage such a visceral adiposity, and low-grade inflammation. In support of this notion, we found that, compared to the other surrogate indexes of IR, the Stumvoll ISI_{OGTT} index was more strongly correlated with waist circumference, and hsCRP circulating levels. Several adipokines released from adipocytes and adipose tissue-derived macrophages are risk factors for cardiovascular disease [25]. These adipokines can contribute to inflammation and to the increased synthesis of inflammatory proteins, such as CRP. CRP in turn may directly affect vasculature facilitating the development of atherosclerosis, and, eventually, cardiovascular diseases [26]. However, we cannot exclude that other variables employed in the Stumvoll ISI_{OGTT} index such as $Insulin_{120}$ and $Glucose_{90}$, which exhibited a significant association with carotid IMT, may account for the present results.

The strengths of the present study are the relatively large sample size, the homogeneous population, the carefully characterized phenotype of individuals with different degree of glucose tolerance, and the exclusion of confounding conditions such as previous cardiovascular disease, history of malignant disease, and liver or kidney failure. Nevertheless, the present study has some limitations. The cross-sectional nature of our study does not provide

Table 5. Multiple regression analysis testing the independent association between indexes of insulin resistance and carotid intima-media thickness (IMT) in a model including age, gender, BMI systolic blood pressure, diastolic blood pressure, triglycerides, total cholesterol, HDL cholesterol, and hsCRP as independent variables (Model 2).

HOMA		Liver IR index		OGIS		Matsuda		Stumvoll ISI_{OGTT}	
β coefficient	*P*	β coefficient	*P*	β coefficient	*P*	β coefficient	*P*	β coefficient	*P*
0.07	0.04	0.04	0.38	−0.13	0.001	−0.08	0.03	−0.21	0.001

HOMA = homeostasis model assessment; OGIS = oral glucose insulin sensitivity; ISI = Insulin sensitivity index.

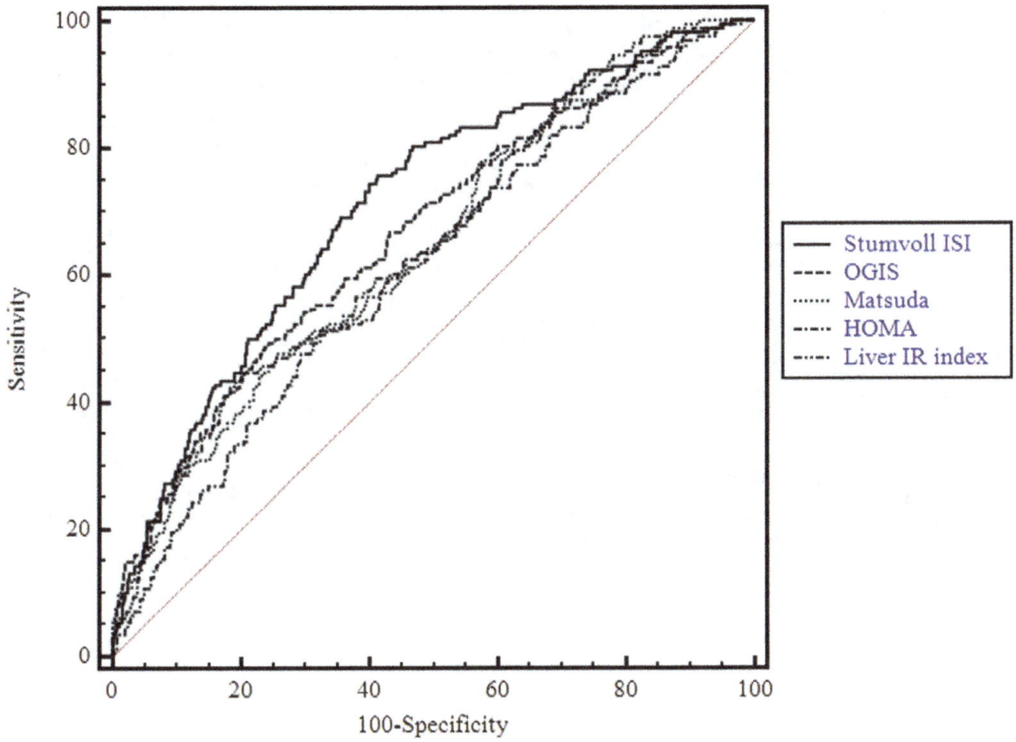

Figure 1. ROC curve analyses for detecting subjects with early atherosclerosis according to HOMA, Matsuda, OGIS, Stumvoll ISI_{OGTT}, and Liver IR indexes.

insight into the time course of atherosclerotic cardiovascular disease, and, therefore, no conclusions regarding cause-effect relationships can be made. In addition, the present findings are only based on Caucasian individuals, and results might vary as a function of ethnic group. Indeed, previous studies have shown differences in insulin sensitivity among different ethnic groups with Mexican Americans and African Americans being more insulin resistant than Caucasians [27,28], likely due to sociodemographic, lifestyle, anthropometric, and genetic characteristics. Finally, the study included only non-diabetic subjects, thus excluding from the analysis subjects at very high risk of cardiovascular disease such as patients with type 2 diabetes.

Conclusions

In conclusion, in the present study we demonstrated that, among the different validated surrogates indexes of IR, the Stumvoll ISI_{OGTT} index correlates better with vascular damage, as assessed by IMT of common carotid artery, in a large cohort of non-diabetic individuals. Thus, the Stumvoll ISI_{OGTT} index might be a significant indicator of vascular damage with an important clinical significance.

Author Contributions

Conceived and designed the experiments: AS FP GS. Performed the experiments: AS MAM MLH. Analyzed the data: AS MAM. Contributed reagents/materials/analysis tools: MLH. Wrote the paper: AS MAM GS.

References

1. Howard G, O'Leary DH, Zaccaro D, Haffner S, Rewers M, et al. (1996) Insulin sensitivity and atherosclerosis. The Insulin Resistance Atherosclerosis Study (IRAS) Investigators. Circulation 93: 1809–1817.
2. Rutter MK, Meigs JB, Sullivan LM, D'Agostino RB Sr, Wilson PW (2005) Insulin resistance, the metabolic syndrome, and incident cardiovascular events in the Framingham Offspring Study. Diabetes 54: 3252–3257.
3. Lorenzo C, Okoloise M, Williams K, Stern MP, Haffner SM, San Antonio Heart Study (2003) The metabolic syndrome as predictor of type 2 diabetes: the San Antonio heart study. Diabetes Care 26: 3153–3159.
4. Reaven G (1988) Role of insulin resistance in human disease. Diabetes; 37: 1595–607.
5. Alberti KG, Eckel RH, Grundy SM, Zimmet PZ, Cleeman JI, et al. (2009) Harmonizing the metabolic syndrome: a joint interim statement of the International Diabetes Federation Task Force on Epidemiology and Prevention; National Heart, Lung, and Blood Institute; American Heart Association; World Heart Federation; International Atherosclerosis Society; and International Association for the Study of Obesity. Circulation 120: 1640–1645.
6. Ford ES (2005) Risks for all-cause mortality, cardiovascular disease, and diabetes associated with the metabolic syndrome: a summary of the evidence. Diabetes Care 28: 1769–1778.
7. Yip J, Facchini FS, Reaven GM (1998) Resistance to insulin-mediated glucose disposal as a predictor of cardiovascular disease. J Clin Endocrinol Metab 83: 2773–2776.
8. Despres JP, Lamarche B, Mauriege P, Cantin B, Dagenais GR, et al. (1996) Hyperinsulinemia as an independent risk factor for ischemic heart disease. N Engl J Med 334: 952–957.
9. Hanley AJ, Williams K, Stern MP, Haffner SM (2002) Homeostasis model assessment of insulin resistance in relation to the incidence of cardiovascular disease: the San Antonio Heart Study. Diabetes Care 25: 1177–1184.
10. Hu G, Qiao Q, Tuomilehto J, Eliasson M, Feskens EJ, et al. (2004) DECODE Insulin Study Group: Plasma insulin and cardiovascular mortality in non-diabetic European men and women: a meta-analysis of data from eleven prospective studies. Diabetologia 47: 1245–1256.
11. Howard G, O'Leary DH, Zaccaro D, Haffner S, Rewers M, et al. (1996) Insulin sensitivity and atherosclerosis. Circulation 93: 1809–1817.
12. Cardellini M, Marini MA, Frontoni S, Hribal ML, Andreozzi F, et al. (2007) Carotid artery intima-media thickness is associated with insulin-mediated glucose disposal in nondiabetic normotensive offspring of type 2 diabetic patients. Am J Physiol Endocrinol Metab 292: E347–352.
13. Matthews DR, Hosker JP, Rudenski AS, Naylor BA, Treacher DF, et al. (1985) Homeostasis model assessment: insulin resistance and beta-cell function from

fasting plasma glucose and insulin concentrations in man. Diabetologia 28: 412–419.
14. Matsuda M, De Fronzo RA (1999) Insulin sensitivity indices obtained from oral glucose tolerance testing: comparison with the euglycemic insulin clamp. Diabetes Care 22: 1462–1470.
15. Stumvoll M, Mitrakou A, Pimenta W, Jenssen T, Yki-Järvinen H, et al. (2000) Use of the oral glucose tolerance test to assess insulin release and insulin sensitivity. Diabetes Care 23: 295–301.
16. Mari A, Pacini G, Murphy E, Ludvik B, Nolan JJ (2001 A Model-Based Method for Assessing Insulin Sensitivity from the Oral Glucose Tolerance Test. Diabetes Care 24: 539–548.
17. Vangipurapu J, Stančáková A, Kuulasmaa T, Paananen J, Kuusisto J, et al. (2011) A novel surrogate index for hepatic insulin resistance. Diabetologia 54: 540–543.
18. O'Leary DH, Polak JF, Kronmal RA, Manolio TA, Burke GL, et al (1999) Carotid artery intima and media thickness as a risk factor for myocardial infarction and stroke in older adults. N Engl J Med 340: 14–22.
19. Marini MA, Succurro E, Frontoni S, Hribal ML, Andreozzi F, et al. (2007) Metabolically healthy but obese women have an intermediate cardiovascular risk profile between healthy non-obese women and obese insulin resistant women. Diabetes Care 30: 2145–2147.
20. Succurro E, Marini MA, Arturi F, Grembiale A, Lugarà M, et al. (2009) Elevated one-hour post-load plasma glucose levels identifies subjects with normal glucose tolerance but early carotid atherosclerosis. Atherosclerosis 207: 245–249.
21. Mancia G, De Backer G, Dominiczak A, Cifkova R, Fagard R, et al. (2007) The task force for the management of arterial hypertension of the European Society of Hypertension, The task force for the management of arterial hypertension of the European Society of Cardiology. 2007 Guidelines for the management of arterial hypertension: The Task Force for the Management of Arterial Hypertension of the European Society of Hypertension (ESH) and of the European Society of Cardiology (ESC). Eur Heart J 28: 1462–1536.
22. DeLong ER, DeLong DM, Clarke-Pearson DL (1988) Comparing the areas under two or more correlated receiver operating characteristic curves: a nonparametric approach. Biometrics 44: 837–845.
23. Sesti G (2006) Pathophysiology of insulin resistance. Best Practice & Research Clinical Endocrinology & Metabolism 20: 665–679.
24. Abdul-Ghani MA, Matsuda M, Balas B, DeFronzo RA (2007) Muscle and liver insulin resistance indexes derived from the oral glucose tolerance test. Diabetes Care 30: 89–94.
25. Verma S, Wang CH, Li SH, Dumont AS, Fedak PW, et al. (2002) A self−fulfilling prophecy: C−reactive protein attenuates nitric oxide production and inhibits angiogenesis. Circulation 106: 913–919.
26. Osborn O, Olefsky JM (2012) The cellular and signaling networks linking the immune system and metabolism in disease. Nat Med 18: 363–374.
27. Haffner SM, D'Agostino R Jr, Saad MF, Rewers M, Mykkänen L, et al. (1996) Increased insulin resistance and insulin secretion in nondiabetic African-Americans and Hispanics compared with non-Hispanic whites: the Insulin Resistance Atherosclerosis Study. Diabetes 45: 742–748.
28. Haffner SM, Stern MP, Dunn J, Mobley M, Blackwell J, et al. (1990) Diminished insulin sensitivity and increased insulin response in nonobese, nondiabetic Mexican Americans. Metabolism 39: 842–847.

4

Reduction in Adiposity, β-Cell Function, Insulin Sensitivity, and Cardiovascular Risk Factors

Maki Goto[1,2,3], Akemi Morita[3,4], Atsushi Goto[1,2,3], Kijo Deura[5], Satoshi Sasaki[6], Naomi Aiba[7], Takuro Shimbo[8], Yasuo Terauchi[2], Motohiko Miyachi[3], Mitsuhiko Noda[1,9]*, Shaw Watanabe[3], for the SCOP Study Group

1 Department of Diabetes Research, Diabetes Research Center, National Center for Global Health and Medicine, Tokyo, Japan, **2** Department of Endocrinology and Metabolism, Yokohama City University Graduate School of Medicine, Yokohama, Japan, **3** National Institute of Health and Nutrition, Tokyo, Japan, **4** Department of Nutrition, College of Nutrition, Koshien University, Hyogo, Japan, **5** Saku Central Hospital, Nagano, Japan, **6** Department of Social and Preventive Epidemiology, School of Public Health, University of Tokyo, Tokyo, Japan, **7** Department of Nutrition and Life Science, Kanagawa Institute of Technology, Kanagawa, Japan, **8** Department of Clinical Research and Informatics, National Center for Global Health and Medicine, Tokyo, Japan, **9** Department of Diabetes and Metabolic Medicine, Center Hospital, National Center for Global Health and Medicine, Tokyo, Japan

Abstract

Background: A reduction in adiposity may be associated with an improvement in insulin sensitivity and β-cell function as well as cardiovascular disease (CVD) risk factors; however, few studies have investigated these associations in a longitudinal setting.

Methods: To investigate these associations over a 1-year period, we conducted an observational analysis of 196 Japanese subjects with obesity in the Saku Control Obesity Program. We investigated the relations between changes in adiposity (body mass index [BMI], waist circumference, subcutaneous fat area [SFAT], and visceral fat area [VFAT]) and changes in HbA1c, fasting plasma glucose (FPG), insulin sensitivity index (ISI), the homeostasis model assessment β cell function (HOMA-β), lipids, and blood pressure.

Results: All adiposity changes were positively associated with HbA1c and FPG changes. Reductions in BMI and VFAT were associated with HOMA-β reduction. Reductions in all adiposity measures were associated with an improvement in the ISI. Changes in most adiposity measures were positively associated with changes in blood pressure and lipid levels, except for LDL.

Conclusion: The present findings provide additional supportive evidence indicating that a reduction in adiposity may lead to an improvement in insulin sensitivity and the reduction of CVD risk factors in obese individuals.

Editor: Andrew Wolfe, John Hopkins University School of Medicine, United States of america

Funding: The authors have no support or funding to report.

Competing Interests: The authors have declared that no competing interests exist.

* E-mail: mnoda@hosp.ncgm.go.jp

Introduction

Since the identification of obesity as the a strong risk factor for various diseases, such as cardiovascular disease (CVD), stroke, and type 2 diabetes, lifestyle modification and weight loss have become major strategies for disease prevention. The development of CVD may be mediated through obesity, decreased insulin sensitivity, dyslipidemia, or high blood pressure [1-3]. Previous studies have investigated the associations between obesity and CVD risk factors [2,4-7], but few studies have examined the associations between changes in adiposity measures and changes in CVD risk factors [8,9]. Furthermore, simple adiposity assessments (e.g., body mass index [BMI], waist circumference, or waist-to-hip ratio) might underestimate the contribution of adiposity to the risk of CVD [10]. Therefore, the use of the visceral fat area (VFAT) and the subcutaneous fat area (SFAT) determined using computed tomography might detect important relations between changes in adiposity and changes in CVD risk factors [9].

In light of effective diabetes prevention, strategies for preserving β-cell function are of great importance. It has now been recognized that a compensatory period (i.e., a compensatory increase in insulin secretion secondary to insulin resistance with little change in the glucose levels) exists before the diagnosis of diabetes, and the insulin secretion decreases after the diagnosis of diabetes [11]. Insulin resistance is considered to be responsible for the increase in insulin levels during the compensatory period. Therefore, it is of great interest to investigate whether reduction in adiposity is associated with improvement in insulin secretion as well as insulin resistance. However, the relationship between the changes in adiposity and insulin resistance or β-cell function has not been well-understood.

Therefore, we investigated the associations between changes in adiposity, including SFAT and VFAT evaluated using computed tomography, and changes in insulin secretion and sensitivity as well as CVD risk factors in 196 Japanese participants with obesity over a 1-year period.

Materials and Methods

Ethics statement

This study was reviewed and approved by the Ethical Committee of the National Institute of Health and Nutrition and Saku Central Hospital. Participants received a precise explanation of the study and provided their written informed consent.

Subjects

This study is a secondary analysis of a randomized controlled trial, the Saku Control Obesity Program (SCOP), examining the effect of behavioral treatment and exercise at the Saku Central Hospital Human Dock Center. The details and design of the study have been previously described elsewhere [12 reatment at the Saku Health Dock Center. People who had undergone health checkups at the center were registered in the database, and 976 members between the ages of 40 and 64 years who did not have type 1 diabetes or severe diseases, such as stroke, cardiovascular disease, advanced cancer or significant renal or hepatic dysfunction, and had a body mass index (BMI) in the upper five percentile of all examinees (28.3 or above) were invited. A total of 237 people participated in the study and were randomly assigned to two groups: group A, who participated in a lifestyle intervention program during year 1; and group B, who participated in the same intervention program during year 2. The intervention group received individual-based counseling on diet and physical activity, and by 1 year, the intervention group had significantly lost more weight than the control group (−5.0 kg vs. 0.1 kg among men, $P < 0.01$; −2.9 kg vs. −0.2 kg among women, $P < 0.01$) [15].

In this study, we excluded 29 patients who had already been diagnosed as having diabetes and were receiving treatment at baseline or at 1 year (27 participants and 2 participants, respectively), 3 participants not in fasting states at the time of blood sampling, and 9 participants who did not complete the study. Finally, 196 participants were included in the analysis.

Anthropometric Measurements

The height (cm) and weight (kg) of the subjects were measured using an automatic scale (BF-220; Tanita, Tokyo, Japan), and the BMI was calculated as the weight (kg) divided by the squared height (m^2). The waist circumference was measured twice in a standing position at the umbilicus level using a fiber glass measuring tape, and the average was used for the analysis. Blood pressure was measured in a sitting position using a validated automated blood pressure monitor (HEM-907; Omron, Kyoto, Japan) [16].

The VFAT and SFAT were assessed based on a CT scan at the level of the umbilicus while the subject was in a supine position (Fat scan; N2 system Corp., Japan) [6]. Physical activity levels were obtained from a questionnaire that aimed to identify activity levels during the recent month as follows: light activity, approximately 1 hour of walking or 3 hours of standing per day; medium activity, approximately 2 hours of walking or 6 to 7 hours of standing per day; moderately-to-heavy activity, approximately 1 hour of intense activity plus 9 hours of walking or standing per day; heavy activity, approximately 2 hours of intense activity plus 9 hours of walking or standing per day.

Laboratory Procedures

Following an overnight fast, blood samples were collected at the time of each health checkup at the Saku Health Dock Center. Blood samples were collected in tubes containing EDTA and heparin for the measurement of fasting plasma glucose (FPG), insulin, and HbA1c and in serum gel separator tubes for the measurement of total cholesterol, high-density lipoprotein cholesterol (HDL), and triglyceride (TG) levels. Routine laboratory blood analyses were performed at the Saku Central Hospital. HbA1c levels were measured using a high-performance liquid chromatography method (TOSOH HLC-723 G8, Tosoh Corporation, Tokyo, Japan) with intra- and inter-assay coefficients of variation (CVs) ≤1.4%. The plasma glucose levels were analyzed using an enzymatic method (ECO glucose buffer; A&T Corporation, Kanagawa, Japan), with intra- and inter-assay CVs ≤0.8%. The plasma insulin levels were analyzed using an electrochemiluminescence immunoassay (Modular E170; Roche Diagnostics, Mannheim, Germany) with intra- and inter-assay CVs ≤3.6%. The serum total cholesterol, HDL, and TG concentrations were determined using enzymatic methods (Detaminar L TC II, Kyowa Medex, Tokyo, Japan; Cholestest N HDL, Sekisui Medical Co Ltd, Tokyo, Japan; and Mizuho TG-FR Type II, Mizuho Medi, Saga, Japan, respectively) and an autoanalyzer BM-2250 (Nihon Denshi, Tokyo, Japan) with intra- and inter-assay CVs of ≤2.3%. The HbA1c values were determined as Japan Diabetes Society (JDS) values and then converted to National Glycohemoglobin Standardization Program (NGSP) values using the following conversion formula: HbA1c (NGSP) = 1.02×HbA1c (JDS)+0.25% [17]. The low-density lipoprotein cholesterol levels (LDL) were calculated using the Friedewald equation: LDL = total cholesterol-(HDL + [TG/5]).

To evaluate insulin sensitivity, we used the homeostasis model assessment for insulin resistance (HOMA-IR)[18] and the insulin sensitivity index (ISI) with reduced time points [19]; to evaluate β cell function, we used the homeostasis model assessment β cell function (HOMA-β)[20] and the insulinogenic index[21,22] based on a 75 g oral glucose tolerance test (OGTT). The HOMA-IR was calculated as follows: fasting insulin (I_0) (μIU/ml) × fasting glucose (G_0) (mg/dL)/405 [18]. We calculated the ISI using reduced time points because of the absence of 90-minute glucose-load values from the OGTTs, with the measurement of the insulin and glucose levels at 0, 60 and 120 minutes as follows: ISI = 10,000/[square root of (G_0 × I_0 × mean OGTT glucose concentration × mean OGTT insulin concentration)] [23]. This index has been reported to be well correlated with the original composite index; we did not use G_{30} and I_{30} in our calculations because this time point was not recommended when using reduced time points to calculate the ISI [23]. The HOMA-β was calculated using the formula: 360 × I_0 (μIU/mL)/[G_0 (mg/dL) −63]. The insulinogenic index was calculated as follows: $(I_{30}-I_0)/(G_{30}-G_0)$ [24].

Data analysis

The characteristics of the study population are presented as the mean for continuous variables. We calculated the means (± SDs) and the proportions of the covariates. A visual inspection of the histograms did not reveal any violations of the assumption of normality; we conducted the analysis without the use of log transformation. To compare the characteristics of the participants at baseline and at 1 year, we used a paired *t* test (Table 1). Then, we investigated the associations of CVD risk factors and insulin secretion and sensitivity using adiposity measures (Tables 2, 3, 4). We used multiple linear regression models to estimate the point estimates, the 95% confidence intervals (95% CIs), and the *P*-values with adjustments for potential confounding factors including age, sex, baseline adiposity measures, baseline insulin related indexes, intervention group assignment, and physical activity level. In addition, we conducted the following sensitivity analyses: (i) stratification according to sex, (ii) stratification according to WHO diagnostic criteria for impaired glucose tolerance (IGT) and diabetes, and (iii) exclusion of participants with medications for hyperlipidemia. We also examined the associations with stratification according to the intervention assignment, but the direction and strength of the associations remained consistent across the subgroups. Thus, we focused primarily on the associations for the full sample (i.e., the product terms were not included in the models).

Two-sided *P* values <0.05 were considered to be statistically significant. Analyses were performed using Stata software (version 12; Stata Corp, College Station, TX).

Results

Among a total of 196 participants aged 40 to 64 years, the mean age was 53.8 years. At baseline, all the participants had obesity with relatively high average glucose levels accompanied by insulin resistance and hyperinsulinemia (Table 1). Over a 1-year period, reductions in all adiposity measures, HbA1c, insulin secretion, TG, and systolic blood pressure were observed, possibly because of the trial intervention (Table 1).

After adjustments for age, sex, physical activity, intervention assignment, baseline adiposity measures, and the baseline value of the outcome variable, reductions in all adiposity measures, including BMI, SFAT, VFAT, and waist circumference, were associated with reductions in the HbA1c and FPG levels (Table 2). The relations between the changes in adiposity and glucose levels were consistent with previous findings. In this study, we were able to further examine the associations of changes in adiposity with the changes in insulin secretion and resistance. As expected, reductions in BMI and VFAT were associated with an improvement in insulin sensitivity as measured using the HOMA-IR and ISI (Table 3). Furthermore, reductions in all adiposity measures were associated with an elevation in the ISI. Decreases in BMI and visceral fat area were related to reduced insulin secretion as measured using the HOMA-β. In contrast, changes in the insulinogenic index were not related to changes in any adiposity measure (Table 3).

Table 2. Associations between changes in adiposity measures and glucose indices from baseline to 1 year.

Outcome variables	Δ HbA1c (%)		Δ FPG (mg/dL)	
	Coef.	*P* value	Coef.	*P* value
Explanatory variables	(95% CL)		(95% CL)	
Δ BMI (kg/m^2)	0.09	<0.001	1.90	0.001
	(0.05, 0.12)		(0.79, 3.02)	
Δ Subcutaneous fat area (cm^2)	0.003	<0.001	0.07	0.003
	(0.002, 0.005)		(0.03, 0.12)	
Δ Visceral fat area (cm^2)	0.005	<0.001	0.08	0.01
	(0.003, 0.007)		(0.02, 0.14)	
Δ Waist circumference (cm)	0.03	<0.001	0.48	0.01
	(0.01, 0.04)		(0.11, 0.86)	

Abbreviations: BMI, body mass index; FPG, fasting plasma glucose; Coef., coefficient; CL, confidence limit.
A multiple linear regression model was used to adjust for potential confounding factors including age, sex, physical activity levels, intervention assignment, the baseline adiposity measure of interest, and the baseline value of the outcome variable.

Table 1. Baseline characteristics of participants.

	Baseline	1 year	P value*
N	196	196	
Male/Female (n)	96/100		
Age (years)	53.8 ± 6.4		
BMI (kg/m^2)	30.5 ± 3.1	29.6 ± 3.5	< 0.001
Subcutaneous fat area (cm^2)	294 ± 102	268 ± 94	< 0.001
Visceral fat area (cm^2)	139 ± 48	123 ± 47	< 0.001
Waist circumference (cm)	102 ± 8	100 ± 9	< 0.001
HbA1c (%)	6.0 ± 0.8	5.8 ± 0.5	< 0.001
Fasting plasma glucose (mg/dL)	106 ± 13	107 ± 14	0.21
Fasting insulin (μIU/mL)	11.3 ± 8.0	9.4 ± 10.0	0.01
HOMA-IR	3.0 ± 2.2	2.6 ± 3.3	0.14
HOMA-β	100 ± 72	77 ± 62	< 0.001
Insulin Sensitivity Index	4.8 ± 3.4	6.5 ± 4.2	< 0.001
Insulinogenic index	0.84 ± 0.90	0.91 ± 1.8	0.57
LDL (mg/dL)	126 ± 34	128 ± 30	0.37
HDL (mg/dL)	53 ± 12	52 ± 13	0.21
Triglyceride (mg/dL)	162 ± 106	142 ± 72	< 0.001
Systolic blood pressure (mmHg)	138 ± 19	132 ± 20	< 0.001
Diastolic blood pressure (mmHg)	85 ± 14	83 ± 14	0.07

Data are (*n*) or means ± SD. * *P* value for paired *t* test.
Abbreviations: BMI, body mass index; HOMA-IR, homeostasis model assessment ratio; HOMA-β, homeostasis model assessment β cell function.

Changes in any of the adiposity measures were not associated with the change in the LDL level, but a change in VFAT was inversely associated with a change in HDL while changes in the BMI, VFAT, and waist circumference were positively associated with a change in the TG level (Table 4). In addition, changes in the BMI, VFAT, and waist circumference were positively associated with changes in the systolic and diastolic blood pressure (Table 4).

A sensitivity analysis stratified according to sex did not substantially change the results; and furthermore, the exclusion of the participants with hyperlipidemia medications (n = 38) did not materially alter the results (data not shown). According to the WHO diagnostic criteria [25], there were 86 participants with normal glucose tolerance (NGT), 11 participants with impaired fasting glycemia (IFG), 76 participants with impaired glucose tolerance (IGT), and 23 participants with diabetes. The adiposity-HbA1c association was slightly stronger among the participants with IFG, IGT, and diabetes (n = 110), compared with those with NGT. After excluding participants with diabetes, the associations between the changes in HOMA-β and the changes in adiposity measures (e.g., VFAT) became stronger (coefficient, 0.62; 95%CI 0.31, 0.92).

Table 3. Associations between changes in adiposity measures and insulin related indexes from baseline to 1 year.

Outcome variables	Δ Insulin (μIU/mL)		Δ HOMA-IR		Δ ISI		Δ HOMA-β		Δ Insulinogenic index	
	Coef.	***P* value**	**Coef.**	***P* value**	**Coef.**	***P* value**	**Coef.**	***P* value**	**Coef.**	***P* value**
Explanatory variables	(95% CL)		(95% CL)		(95% CL)		(95% CL)		(95% CL)	
Δ BMI (kg/m^2)	1.09	0.02	0.32	0.045	-1.05	<0.001	7.43	0.007	0.14	0.12
	(0.16, 2.01)		(0.01, 0.64)		(-1.32, -0.78)		(2.02, 12.8)		(-0.04, 0.31)	
Δ Subcutaneous fat area (cm^2)	0.02	0.29	0.01	0.39	-0.03	<0.001	0.12	0.31	0.003	0.39
	(-0.02, 0.06)		(-0.01, 0.02)		(-0.04, -0.02)		(-0.11, 0.36)		(-0.004, 0.01)	
Δ Visceral fat area (cm^2)	0.06	0.01	0.02	0.048	-0.05	<0.001	0.50	0.001	-0.0005	0.92
	(0.01, 0.11)		(0.0001, 0.03)		(-0.06, -0.03)		(0.21, 0.79)		(-0.01, 0.009)	
Δ Waist circumference (cm)	0.25	0.10	0.07	0.18	-0.29	<0.001	1.80	0.053	0.04	0.15
	(-0.05, 0.56)		(-0.03, 0.18)		(-0.39, -0.20)		(-0.02, 3.62)		(-0.02, 0.10)	

Abbreviations: BMI, body mass index; HOMA-IR, homeostatic model assessment for insulin resistance; ISI, insulin sensitivity index; HOMA-β, homeostasis model assessment for β-cell function; Coef., coefficient; CL, confidence limit.
A multiple linear regression model was used to adjust for potential confounding factors including age, sex, physical activity levels, intervention assignment, the baseline adiposity measure of interest, and the baseline value of insulin related indices.

Discussion

In this prospective study, changes in all the examined adiposity measures were positively associated with changes in glycemia in 196 Japanese participants with obesity. Furthermore, we found that reductions in BMI, visceral fat area, and waist circumference were associated with a reduction in HOMA-β, while no association was observed for the insulinogenic index. Reductions in BMI and VFAT were also associated with an improvement in insulin sensitivity. In addition, changes in adiposity were related to changes in TG and blood pressure. These findings suggest that controlling adiposity among obese individuals may effectively improve CVD risk factors and insulin sensitivity.

These results were consistent with a preceding study among obese individuals with type 2 diabetes, in which weight loss was associated with an improvement in glycemia, blood pressure, TG, and HDL [8,9]. In the current study, we were able to assess VFAT and SFAT changes using computed tomography. We found that a reduction in visceral adiposity as well as the BMI was associated with an improvement in the CVD risk factors. Consistent with the previous study [8], the adiposity change was not associated with the LDL change in the current study. In another study reviewing weight loss effects and lipid outcomes [26], weight loss was reported to be associated with the LDL reduction. This dissociation may be because, in a previous review [26], studies with a large weight reduction (22 to 55 kg) as a result of surgical intervention were included. In the current study, the mean weight

Table 4. Associations between changes in adiposity measures and lipid levels and blood pressure from baseline to 1 year.

Outcome variables	Δ LDL		Δ HDL		Δ Triglyceride		Δ Systolic blood pressure		Δ Diastolic blood pressure	
	(mg/dL)		**(mg/dL)**		**(mg/dL)**		**(mmHg)**		**(mmHg)**	
	Coef.	***P* value**	**Coef.**	***P* value**	**Coef.**	***P* value**	**Coef.**	***P* value**	**Coef.**	***P* value**
Explanatory variables	(95% CL)		(95% CL)		(95% CL)		(95% CL)		(95% CL)	
Δ BMI (kg/m^2)	0.47	0.67	-0.63	0.06	9.37	<0.001	2.03	0.01	1.48	0.01
	(-1.71, 2.66)		(-1.28, 0.03)		(4.75, 14.0)		(0.47, 3.59)		(0.35, 2.62)	
Δ Subcutaneous fat area (cm^2)	0.04	0.39	-0.01	0.49	0.19	0.06	0.03	0.32	0.03	0.19
	(-0.05, 0.13)		(-0.04, 0.02)		(-0.01, 0.39)		(-0.03, 0.10)		(-0.02, 0.08)	
Δ Visceral fat area (cm^2)	-0.03	0.56	-0.05	0.01	0.48	<0.001	0.12	0.005	0.07	0.04
	(-0.15, 0.08)		(-0.08, -0.01)		(0.23, 0.72)		(0.04, 0.20)		(0.004, 0.13)	
Δ Waist circumference (cm)	0.33	0.36	-0.17	0.11	2.61	0.001	0.66	0.01	0.45	0.02
	(-0.38, 1.05)		(-0.39, 0.04)		(1.07, 4.15)		(0.15, 1.18)		(0.08, 0.82)	

Abbreviations: BMI, body mass index; LDL, low density cholesterol; HDL, high density cholesterol; Coef., coefficient; CL, confidence limit.
A multiple linear regression model was used to adjust for potential confounding factors including age, sex, physical activity levels, intervention assignment, the baseline adiposity measure of interest, and the baseline value of lipid levels.

reduction within 1 year was 2.4 kg (SD 4.3), so the amount of the weight reduction may have been insufficient to detect any changes.

Among adiposity measures, changes in BMI and VFAT were positively associated with changes in insulin and HOMA-IR and were inversely associated with changes in ISI. Indeed, the change in ISI was inversely associated with changes in all the adiposity measures. These findings indicate that a reduction in adiposity may lead to an improvement in insulin sensitivity. This finding is consistent with a preceding study showing that baseline adiposity measures were inversely associated with future insulin sensitivity indices [6]. Although changes in SFAT and the waist circumference were also related to some of the insulin related indices, our findings may suggest that BMI and VFAT may be better markers of adiposity in this obese population. This finding is consistent with the results of preceding studies among Japanese-Americans, which have shown that the baseline VFAT, but not the SFAT, was associated with future insulin resistance [6].

Reductions in BMI, VFAT, and waist circumference were associated with a decrease in HOMA-β. Importantly, a previous study has shown that HOMA β-cell function, another measure of β-cell function, is elevated 3–4 years before the diagnosis of diabetes, and then decreases until the time of diagnosis, indicating that a period of compensation for insulin resistance exists [27]. In our study, a reduction in adiposity was related to a reduction in insulin resistance, which was accompanied by a reduction in HOMA-β. Furthermore, the associations between the HOMA-β change and the adiposity changes became stronger after the exclusion of participants with diabetes (coefficient for ΔVFAT-ΔHOMA-β, 0.50 to 0.62). This finding may suggest that a compensatory period actually exists among obese individuals who did not develop diabetes_and the adiposity reduction may reduce the needs for compensatory hyperinsulinemia.

Preceding studies have also reported that a decrease in the early-phase insulin response to glucose is a major feature of glucose tolerance among Japanese [22,28,29]. However, the change in the insulinogenic index was not related to changes in any adiposity measures in our study. This finding may suggest that the insulinogenic index may not measure compensatory hyperinsulinemia observed during the compensatory period, but might instead evaluate residual β-cell function. Thus, the null association between the insulinogenic index change and the adiposity change suggests that a reduction in adiposity may be insufficient to improve residual β-cell function.

Some limitations of the present study need to be addressed. First, participants in this study were Japanese individuals with obesity, and the sample size was limited; thus generalizability may be a problem. Second, although smoking has been reported to be related to CVD and weight reduction [2], smoking data was not available, and the analysis could not be adjusted for smoking. Third, we did not have intermediate measurements. Finally, because the follow up period was relatively short, a longer period observation period is needed to confirm the results. The major strengths of this study were the high compliance of our study participants, which enabled us to assess CVD risk factors, and the observation of adiposity changes using computed tomography over a 1-year period with few participant dropouts.

Conclusions

Our findings suggest that the reduction of obesity, especially the BMI and visceral fat area, may be associated with an improvement in CVD risk factors. Furthermore, we found that reductions in BMI and visceral adiposity were associated with a reduced HOMA-β and HOMA-IR. These findings support the notion that controlling adiposity among obese individuals may effectively improve CVD risk factors and insulin resistance.

Acknowledgments

We would like to acknowledge all SCOP members and the study participants for their participation in this research. We thank Tomoko Yasuda for her assistance.

Author Contributions

Conceived and designed the experiments: MG AM AG MN SW. Performed the experiments: MG AM AG KD SS NA MM MN. Analyzed the data: MG AG TS. Contributed reagents/materials/analysis tools: MG AG MN. Wrote the paper: MG AG YT MN.

REFERENCES

1. Donahue RP, Abbott RD, Bloom E, Reed DM, Yano K (1987) Central obesity and coronary heart disease in men. Lancet 1: 821–824.
2. Fujimoto WY, Leonetti DL, Bergstrom RW, Shuman WP, Wahl PW (1990) Cigarette smoking, adiposity, non-insulin-dependent diabetes, and coronary heart disease in Japanese-American men. Am J Med 89: 761–771.
3. Look ARG, Wing RR (2010) Long-term effects of a lifestyle intervention on weight and cardiovascular risk factors in individuals with type 2 diabetes mellitus: four-year results of the Look AHEAD trial. Arch Intern Med 170: 1566–1575.
4. Carr DB, Utzschneider KM, Boyko EJ, Asberry PJ, Hull RL, et al. (2005) A reduced-fat diet and aerobic exercise in Japanese Americans with impaired glucose tolerance decreases intra-abdominal fat and improves insulin sensitivity but not beta-cell function. Diabetes 54: 340–347.
5. Pouliot MC, Despres JP, Nadeau A, Moorjani S, Prud'Homme D, et al. (1992) Visceral obesity in men. Associations with glucose tolerance, plasma insulin, and lipoprotein levels. Diabetes 41: 826–834.
6. Hayashi T, Boyko EJ, McNeely MJ, Leonetti DL, Kahn SE, et al. (2008) Visceral adiposity, not abdominal subcutaneous fat area, is associated with an increase in future insulin resistance in Japanese Americans. Diabetes 57: 1269–1275.
7. Albu JB, Murphy L, Frager DH, Johnson JA, Pi-Sunyer FX (1997) Visceral fat and race-dependent health risks in obese nondiabetic premenopausal women. Diabetes 46: 456–462.
8. Wing RR, Lang W, Wadden TA, Safford M, Knowler WC, et al. (2011) Benefits of modest weight loss in improving cardiovascular risk factors in overweight and obese individuals with type 2 diabetes. Diabetes Care 34: 1481–1486.
9. Matsushita Y, Nakagawa T, Yamamoto S, Takahashi Y, Yokoyama T, et al. (2012) Effect of longitudinal changes in visceral fat area and other anthropometric indices to the changes in metabolic risk factors in Japanese men: the Hitachi Health Study. Diabetes Care 35: 1139–1143.
10. Goncalves FB, Koek M, Verhagen HJ, Niessen WJ, Poldermans D (2011) Body-mass index, abdominal adiposity, and cardiovascular risk. Lancet 378: 227; author reply 228.
11. Tabák AG, Jokela M, Akbaraly TN, Brunner EJ, Kivimäki M, et al. Trajectories of glycaemia, insulin sensitivity, and insulin secretion before diagnosis of type 2 diabetes: an analysis from the Whitehall II study. The Lancet 373: 2215–2221.
12. Watanabe S, Morita A, Aiba N, Miyachi M, Sasaki S, et al. (2007) Study Design of the Saku Control Obesity Program (SCOP). Anti-Aging Medicine 4: 70–73.
13. Morita A, Ohmori Y, Suzuki N, Ide N, Morioka M, et al. (2008) Anthropometric and Clinical Findings in Obese Japanese: The Saku Control Obesity Program (SCOP). Anti-Aging Medicine 5: 13–16.
14. Tanaka T, Morita A, Kato M, Hirai T, Mizoue T, et al. (2011) Congener-specific polychlorinated biphenyls and the prevalence of diabetes in the Saku Control Obesity Program. Endocrine journal.
15. Nakade M, Aiba N, Suda N, Morita A, Miyachi M, et al. (2012) Behavioral change during weight loss program and one-year follow-up: Saku Control Obesity Program (SCOP) in Japan. Asia Pac J Clin Nutr 21: 22–34.
16. White WB, Anwar YA (2001) Evaluation of the overall efficacy of the Omron office digital blood pressure HEM-907 monitor in adults. Blood Press Monit 6: 107–110.
17. Kashiwagi A, Kasuga M, Araki E, Oka Y, Hanafusa T, et al. (2012) International clinical harmonization of glycated hemoglobin in Japan: From Japan Diabetes Society to National Glycohemoglobin Standardization Program values. Journal of Diabetes Investigation 3: 39–40.
18. Matthews DR, Hosker JP, Rudenski AS, Naylor BA, Treacher DF, et al. (1985) Homeostasis model assessment: insulin resistance and beta-cell function from

fasting plasma glucose and insulin concentrations in man. Diabetologia 28: 412–419.

19. DeFronzo RA, Matsuda M (2010) Reduced time points to calculate the composite index. Diabetes Care 33: e93.
20. Wallace TM, Levy JC, Matthews DR (2004) Use and abuse of HOMA modeling. Diabetes Care 27: 1487–1495.
21. Kosaka K, Hagura R, Kuzuya T (1977) Insulin responses in equivocal and definite diabetes, with special reference to subjects who had mild glucose intolerance but later developed definite diabetes. Diabetes 26: 944–952.
22. Yoneda H, Ikegami H, Yamamoto Y, Yamato E, Cha T, et al. (1992) Analysis of early-phase insulin responses in nonobese subjects with mild glucose intolerance. Diabetes Care 15: 1517–1521.
23. DeFronzo RA, Matsuda M (2010) Reduced time points to calculate the composite index. Diabetes Care 33: e93.
24. Wareham NJ, Phillips DI, Byrne CD, Hales CN (1995) The 30 minute insulin incremental response in an oral glucose tolerance test as a measure of insulin secretion. Diabet Med 12: 931.
25. Alberti KG, Zimmet PZ (1998) Definition, diagnosis and classification of diabetes mellitus and its complications. Part 1: diagnosis and classification of diabetes mellitus provisional report of a WHO consultation. Diabet Med 15: 539–553.
26. Poobalan A, Aucott L, Smith WC, Avenell A, Jung R, et al. (2004) Effects of weight loss in overweight/obese individuals and long-term lipid outcomes-a systematic review. Obes Rev 5: 43–50.
27. Tabak AG, Jokela M, Akbaraly TN, Brunner EJ, Kivimaki M, et al. (2009) Trajectories of glycaemia, insulin sensitivity, and insulin secretion before diagnosis of type 2 diabetes: an analysis from the Whitehall II study. Lancet 373: 2215–2221.
28. Kosaka K, Kuzuya T, Hagura R, Yoshinaga H (1996) Insulin response to oral glucose load is consistently decreased in established non-insulin-dependent diabetes mellitus: the usefulness of decreased early insulin response as a predictor of non-insulin-dependent diabetes mellitus. Diabet Med 13: S109–119.
29. Matsumoto K, Miyake S, Yano M, Ueki Y, Yamaguchi Y, et al. (1997) Glucose tolerance, insulin secretion, and insulin sensitivity in nonobese and obese Japanese subjects. Diabetes Care 20: 1562–1568.

5

Mifepristone Reduces Insulin Resistance in Patient Volunteers with Adrenal Incidentalomas that Secrete Low Levels of Cortisol

Miguel Debono[1], Rita Chadarevian[3], Richard Eastell[2], Richard J. Ross[1], John Newell-Price[1]*

1 Academic Unit of Diabetes, Endocrinology and Reproduction, Department of Human Metabolism, University of Sheffield, Sheffield, United Kingdom, **2** Academic Unit of Bone Metabolism, Department of Human Metabolism, University of Sheffield, Sheffield, United Kingdom, **3** HRA Pharma, Paris, France

Abstract

Background: Incidental adrenal masses are commonly detected during imaging for other pathologies. 10% of the elderly population has an 'adrenal incidentaloma', up to 20% of these show low-grade autonomous cortisol secretion and 60% of patients with autonomous cortisol secretion have insulin resistance. Cortisol excess is known to cause insulin resistance, an independent cardiovascular risk marker, however in patients with adrenal incidentalomas it is unknown whether their insulin resistance is secondary to the excess cortisol and therefore potentially reversible. In a proof of concept study we examined the short-term effects of glucocorticoid receptor (GR) antagonism in patients with an adrenal incidentaloma to determine whether their insulin resistance was reversible.

Methodology/Principal Findings: In a prospective open-label pilot study, six individuals with adrenal incidentalomas and autonomous cortisol secretion were treated with mifepristone (a GR antagonist) 200 mg twice daily and studied for 4 weeks on a Clinical Research Facility. Insulin resistance at four weeks was assessed by insulin resistance indices, lnHOMA-IR and lnMatsuda, and AUC insulin during a 2-hour glucose tolerance test. Biochemical evidence of GR blockade was shown in all individuals and across the group there was a significant reduction in insulin resistance: lnHOMA-IR (1.0vs0.6; $p=0.03$), lnHOMA-%beta (4.8vs4.3; $p=0.03$) and lnMatsuda (1.2vs1.6; $p=0.03$). Five out of six individuals showed a reduction in insulin AUC >7237 pmol/l.min, and in two patients this showed a clinically significant cardiovascular benefit (as defined by the Helsinki heart study).

Conclusions: Short-term GR antagonism is sufficient to reduce insulin resistance in some individuals with adrenal incidentalomas and mild cortisol excess. Further assessment is required to assess if the responses may be used to stratify therapy as adrenal incidentalomas may be a common remediable cause of increased cardiovascular risk.

Editor: Harpal Singh Randeva, University of Warwick – Medical School, United Kingdom

Funding: The study was funded in part by HRA Pharma grant number: R/123263. The funder had no role in data collection, analysis and decision to publish. The study design, and all ethical applications and associated administration, were conceived and written by JN-P and MD. The funder contributed to study design and the preparation of the manuscript.

Competing Interests: MD, RE and RJR have declared that no competing interests exist. RC is an employee of HRA Pharma. JN-P has received grant support and honoraria from HRA Pharma.

* E-mail: j.newellprice@sheffield.ac.uk

Introduction

Adrenal masses incidentally disclosed on computed tomography (CT) scans, 'adrenal incidentalomas' are common. Prevalence increases during life such that they are found in ten percent of the population aged 70 years or more [1,2]. Between five to twenty percent of these are associated with mild cortisol excess without the classical external features typically associated with Cushing's syndrome [3], often termed 'subclinical Cushing's syndrome', or 'subclinical hypercortisolism' [4]. One of cortisol's major functions is the regulation of glucose metabolism: it promotes gluconeogenesis by activation of phosphoenolpyruvate carboxykinase and glucose-6-phosphatase in the liver [5,6]; inhibits insulin release in the pancreas [7]; decreases insulin sensitivity in skeletal muscle and adipose tissue [8]. Consequently, an important complication of cortisol excess is insulin resistance (IR) [9], a major independent marker of cardiovascular risk [10], and this is reflected by the fact that over 60% of individuals with adrenal incidentalomas and low grade cortisol secretion have IR, impaired glucose tolerance or diabetes mellitus compared to age, sex and BMI-matched controls [11]. However, as IR is common in the general population it is unknown whether the IR in patients with adrenal incidentalomas is secondary to the low level cortisol secretion or other factors.

The GR antagonist mifepristone (11-[4-(Dimethylamino)phenyl]-17-hydroxy-17-[1-propynyl]-[11ß,17ß]-estra-4,9-dien-3-one) has been shown to improve glucose tolerance in patients with overt Cushing's syndrome [12]. We hypothesized that insulin resistance in individuals with adrenal incidentalomas and low-grade cortisol excess without the classical external features typically associated with Cushing's syndrome might also be improved by short-term GR blockade if in these individuals IR is driven by cortisol excess. Our findings showed, for the first time, that even short-term GR blockade in these individuals improved insulin resistance. These data could inform the design of a much awaited prospective interventional randomized controlled study aimed to identify whether such an approach could be used as a prediction tool to stratify an affected individual to surgery, medical therapy or observation [13].

Methods

Ethics Statement & Participants

The study protocol was approved by the North Sheffield Research Ethics committee, and the Medicines and Health Regulatory Authority, UK and was performed according to the requirements of the Declaration of Helsinki as revised in 2000. Written informed consent was obtained from all participants. The study is reported according to the Transparent Reporting of Evaluations with Nonrandomized Designs (TREND) [14]. These are guidelines for the reporting of nonrandomised trials to help improve the clarity of a report and to encourage more detailed description of the study design and the findings. The statement presents a checklist for investigators to follow and which are mainly directed towards intervention evaluation studies. The protocol for this trial and supporting TREND checklist are available as supporting information; see Checklist S1 and Protocol S1.

This prospective open-label pilot study was performed at the Clinical Research Facility, Sheffield Teaching Hospitals NHS Foundation Trust and The University of Sheffield, UK between January 2010 and March 2010 in six patients. Patients were identified by continuous sampling from referrals to the Endocrine Investigation Unit as part of an incidentaloma work-up protocol at the Royal Hallamshire Hospital, Sheffield. It was planned to perform the study over 8 weeks, but we analyzed at four weeks, focusing on IR. Metabolic outcome was achieved and all 6 patients had IR indices and BP measurements suitable for analysis. After ingestion of 200 mg of mifepristone, peak concentrations are reached within 1 to 2 hours, there is an initial redistribution phase of 6–10 h followed by a plateau for 24 h or more. The terminal half-life ($t_{1/2}$) is 30 hours. Dose-dependent antiglucocorticoid effects last for at least 24 hours after a single dose, hence significant effects would already be expected by a week [15,16]. Two patients had been withdrawn after four weeks. All subjects were known to have an adrenal incidentaloma, with benign characteristics as assessed on CT, lacking external clinical features classically associated with Cushing's [4,17,18], but having evidence of excess cortisol as shown by lack of suppression of serum cortisol to <50 nmol/L (1.8 ug/dL) on 1 mg over-night dexamethasone suppression and 2 mg/day 48 hour low-dose dexamethasone suppression testing [18]. All were on stable anti-hypertensive treatment for at least three months and none were on anti-diabetes medications. Although this was an exploratory human subject study to assess if insulin resistance could be reversed and not a formal outcome study *per se*, it was still registered at Clinical trials.gov: ID NCT00721201.

Study Design & End-points

The flow chart in Figure 1, as recommended by the TREND statement, describes the different phases and design of the study. One patient who was approached and screened did not meet the entry criteria, whilst one other declined to participate. Study visits occurred weekly up to week 4 and procedures at each visit are shown in Figure 2. The baseline glucose tolerance test was performed on the first day of treatment (treatment start) before the first dose of mifepristone whilst the baseline 24-hour ambulatory BP monitoring was performed between the first visit (screening) and second visit (treatment start). During each visit renal function, 0900 h and 2300 h salivary cortisol (representing free cortisol) and 0900 h plasma ACTH and serum cortisol (total cortisol) levels were assessed to confirm compliance and efficacy of GR blockade. All interventions were performed by the clinical research team on the Facility. Since mifepristone blocks the GR the expectation was a rise in plasma ACTH and serum and salivary cortisol by activation of the hypothalamo-pituitary-adrenal (HPA) axis, but with blockade of GR-mediated activity. Saliva samples were obtained using the Salivette tubes (cotton swab with citric acid preparation; Sarstedt, Numbrecht). Subjects were instructed to refrain from brushing their teeth, smoking, eating or drinking anything for at least 60 min prior to sampling. To provide a saliva sample, patients were asked to chew on the cotton swab for 1–2 min and then place it back in the plastic container. The bone formation marker serum osteocalcin was measured in a 0900 h fasting sample, and the second morning urine sample was used to measure the bone resorption marker urine N-telopeptide crosslinks of type 1 collagen (NTX). Full clinical assessment including resting BP, weight and temperature was made at each visit - monitoring for symptoms and signs for adrenal insufficiency can only be performed on a clinical, and not biochemical, basis when on mifepristone. The oral dose of mifepristone was kept the same at 200 mg twice a day at 0900 h and 2100 h, one hour before any food, throughout the study. Although once daily dosing might have sufficed, twice daily dosing was chosen in an effort to maintain as constant a GR blockade effect as possible.

To establish a normal 95% reference range for IR we analyzed data from the Helsinki Policemen study, a 22 year follow up investigating what level of IR, as reflected by insulin AUC on an OGTT, predicted cardiovascular events. By taking the mean±2SD of the values of those followed for 22 years (n = 755) and in whom no cardiovascular event was observed, we define the upper end of the 95% reference range of insulin AUC associated with no cardiovascular risk as 63420 pmol/l.min (26940±2SD pmol/l.min) [10]. In addition we took values <26940 pmol/l.min to represent definite normalization of AUC and only a decrease in insulin AUC greater than 7237 pmol/l.min, during a 2-hour OGTT, was considered significant as this exceeds biological variation [19]. The insulin AUC was appropriate for our group as in patients with fasting insulin levels less than 200 pmol/l the insulin AUC is reproducible [19]. We chose insulin AUC on OGTT as our primary estimate of IR as this allowed direct comparison to the seminal Helsinki heart study data examining the long term effects of IR on cardiovascular risk. Resting and 24-hour ambulatory blood pressure as measured using standard British Hypertension Society approved monitors were other primary end points.

Secondary end points were the means for fasting glucose, fasting insulin, the homeostasis model assessment of IR and beta cell function (HOMA-IR and HOMA-%beta) [20], and the Insulin Sensitivity Index (ISI) – Matsuda [21], as calculated from an oral glucose tolerance test. The difference in fasting lipids and bone turnover markers at study end were also measured.

Assays

Total serum cortisol was measured in a Siemens Advia Centaur Cortisol assay: analytical range 5.5–2069 nmol/l; inter-assay co-efficient of variation (CV), 6.2% at 134 nmol/l, 5.5% at

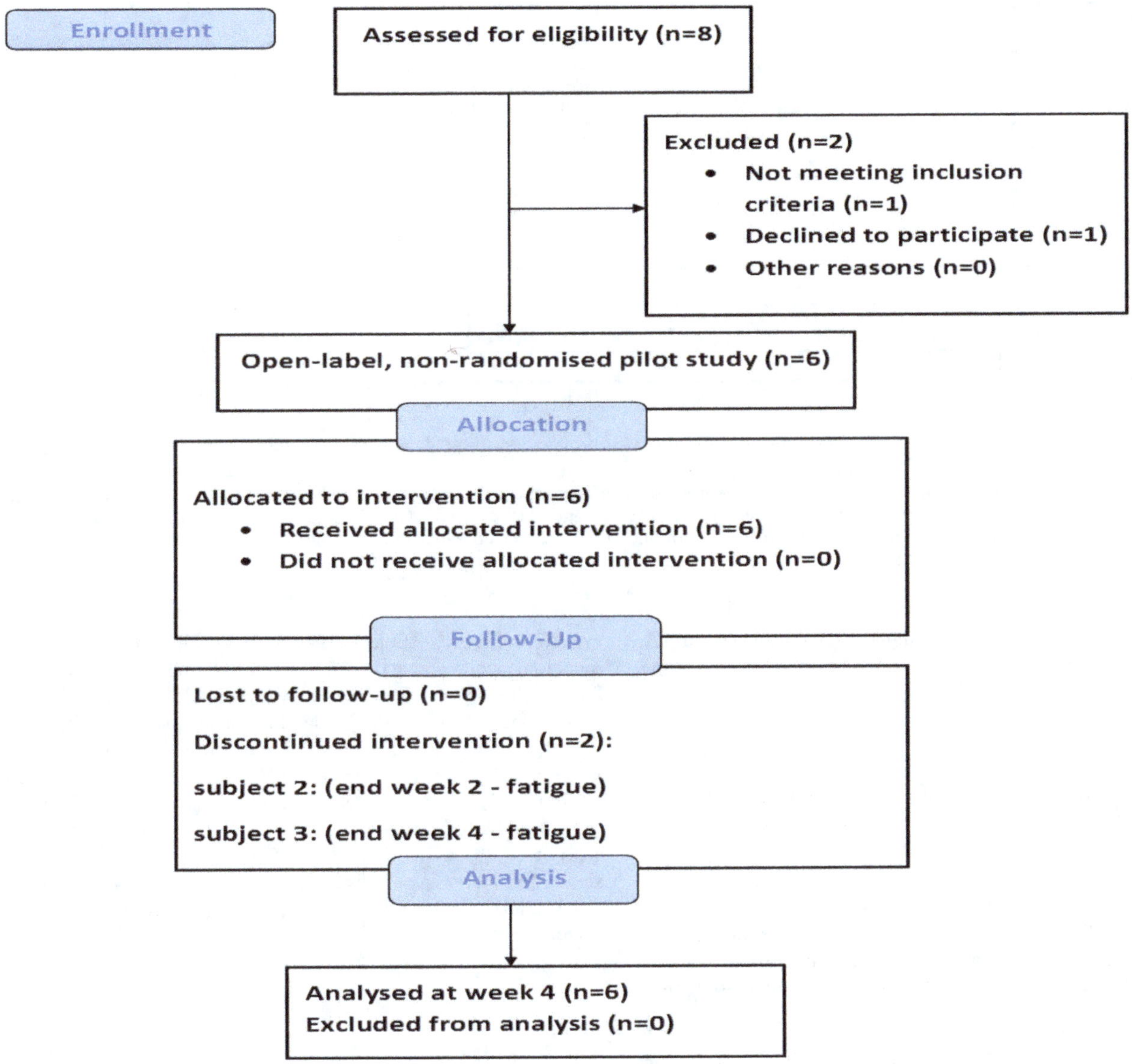

Figure 1. Flow chart indicating the different phases of the study to week four as recommended by the TREND statement [14]. Analysis performed at week four as all six patients had insulin resistance and blood pressure measurements suitable for analysis.

491 nmol/l and 6.0% at 836 nmol/l. Plasma ACTH was measured in a Siemens Immulite 2000 chemiluminescent assay: Analytical range 1.1–275 pmol/l; inter-assay CVs 6.4% at 7 pmol/l, 6.5% at 105 pmol/l. Salivary cortisol was measured by Liquid Chromatography Tandem Mass spectrometry (LC-MS/MS) as previously described [22]. Glucose was measured using the Hexokinase method, Beckman Coulter Inc, with CV 2.6% at 3.3 mmol/l and 2.1% at 20.3 mmol/l. Insulin was measured by Siemens Advia Centaur chemiluminescent immunometric assay with a CV of 5.3% at 222 pmol/l, 4.9% at 760.5 pmol/l and 5.8% at 1409 pmol/l. The analysis of serum osteocalcin and urine NTX was performed by Cobas e411 Autoanalyser (Roche Diagnostics) and the Ortho Clinical Vitros device respectively, with interassay CV's of 4.5% and 6.6% respectively. Urine NTX was expressed as a ratio to urinary creatinine. Standard biochemistry and hematological methods were used for renal, liver and thyroid function, lipid profiles and the full blood count.

Statistical Analysis

Statistical analyses were performed using SPSS version 16 (SPSS, Chicago, IL, USA) and Microsoft Office Excel 2010. Rates were calculated for categorical data, and means and 95% confidence intervals for continuous data. We used non-parametric Wilcoxon's signed rank test for repeated measures to analyze the effect of up to four weeks of mifepristone treatment on variables of glucose, insulin and insulin sensitivity, resting and 24 hour BP, bone markers, lipids, renal, liver and thyroid function. As the distribution of fasting insulin levels is usually skewed measures of insulin sensitivity were log-transformed [23]. As per protocol, any missing data from premature withdrawal was replaced by at least one post-baseline measured efficacy parameter that was carried forward. Efficacy evaluation was based on the intention to treat population (ITT), where all patients who received at least one dose of mifepristone and from whom at least one efficacy measurement is obtained after the study treatment start were analysed. All

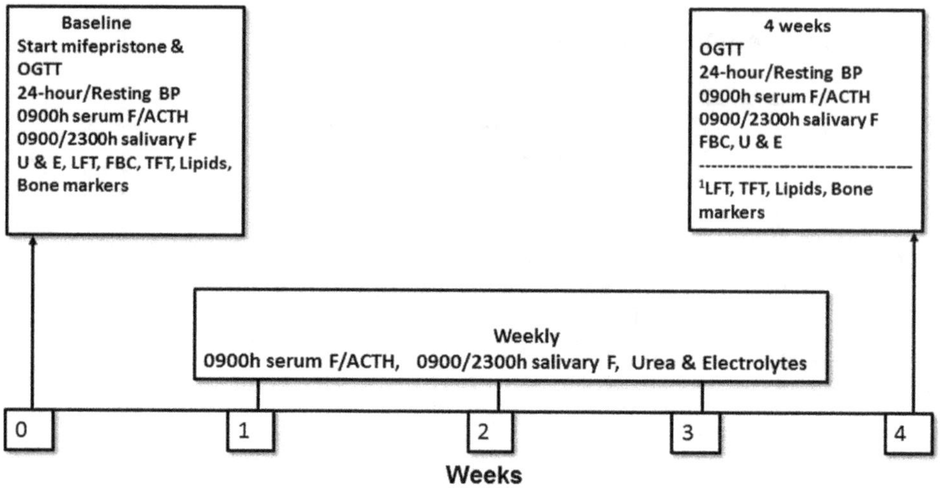

Figure 2. Study Design showing investigations and intervention performed on six patients from baseline to four weeks. One subject was withdrawn after end of second week. [1]variables measured at baseline and end of study. OGTT: Oral Glucose Tolerance Test - insulin & glucose at 0, 15, 30, 60, 90, 120 min, F: cortisol, ACTH: Adrenocorticotropic Hormone, U & E: urea, electrolytes and creatinine, LFT: Liver Function Tests, FBC: Full Blood Count, TFT: Thyroid Function Tests.

significances were two-sided and values of $p<0.05$ were regarded as statistically significant.

Results

Baseline Characteristics

Demographic data for each subject and means (±95%CI) are shown in Table 1. Baseline characteristics were similar to the target population of interest [24,25].

Hypothalamo-pituitary-adrenal axis analysis

Mifepristone blocked glucocorticoid action as evidenced by activation of the HPA axis. Baseline mean serum cortisol level was 372.5 nmol/l (95%CI 309.0–435.9 nmol/l), this increased progressively in each subject, such that at one week levels had increased significantly (1065 nmol/l 95% CI 636.0–1495.4 nmol/l; $p=0.03$) and further increased by 4 weeks (1551 nmol/l (95%CI 615–2486 nmol/l; $p=0.03$). Baseline mean plasma ACTH was low at 1.9 pmol/l (95%CI 0.7–3.1 pmol/l) whilst plasma ACTH levels at 4 weeks were 13.6 pmol/l (95%CI 4.4–22.9 pmol/l; $p=0.03$) (Figure 3a). Baseline mean salivary cortisol levels at 0900 h and 2300 h were 4.8 nmol/l (95%CI 3.4–6.2 nmol/l) and 1.3 nmol/l (95%CI 0.2–2.4 nmol/l), respectively. There was a significant increase in salivary cortisol over 4 weeks at 0900 h (99.3 nmol/l; $p=0.03$) and 2300 h (9.4 nmol/l; $p=0.03$) (Figure 3b).

Table 1. Demographic data – Subject Baseline Characteristics.

Subject	1	2	3	4	5	6	Mean (±95% CI)
Gender	M	F	F	F	M	M	
Age (yrs) (range)	72	58	74	56	64	75	67 (58–75)
Mean Weight (kg)	86.0	75.6	70.9	109.0	101.5	110.0	92.2 (74.3–110.0)
Mean BMI (kgm^2)	29.1	31.1	24.5	43.7	32.0	39.9	33.4 (26.9–40.5)
Serum Cortisol post ONDST (nmol/l)	67.9	104.0	83.9	88.8	59.9	73.9	79.7 (63.2–96.3)
Serum Cortisol post LDDST (nmol/l)	80.0	54.1	85.0	105.1	80.0	61.0	77.5 (58.2–96.8)
0900 h salivary cortisol (nmol/l)	4.7	6.8	5.2	3.4	5.3	3.4	4.8 (3.4–6.2)
2300 h salivary cortisol (nmol/l)	0.5	0.6	0.9	3.0	2.1	0.5	1.3 (0.2–2.4)
ACTH (pmol/l)	1.9	1.1	2.0	4.1	1.1	1.2	1.9 (0.9–2.9)
Side of adenoma	R	R	L	R	R	R	
Size of adenoma (cm)	3.8	2.5	3.6	3.5	2.7	2.0	3.02 (2.3–3.8)
24-hour blood pressure	136/91	143/75	149/86	150/86	138/81	147/77	
Fasting glucose (mmol/l)	4.8	6.3	4.7	4.9	5.1	6.5	5.4 (4.6–6.2)
Fasting insulin (pmol/l)	44.4	124.2	34.0	177.1	69.2	86.8	76.4 (39.9–146.4)[1]

ONDST: Overnight dexamethasone suppression test; LDDST: 48-hour 2 mg low dose dexamethasone suppression test; R = Right, L = Left;
[1]Geometric mean.

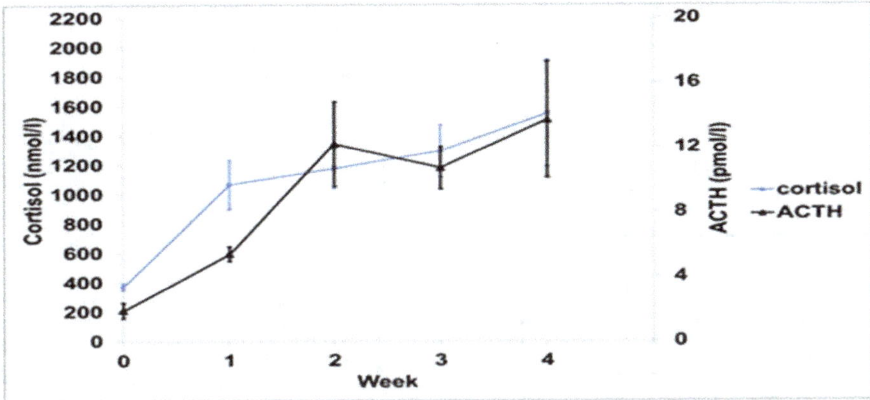

a

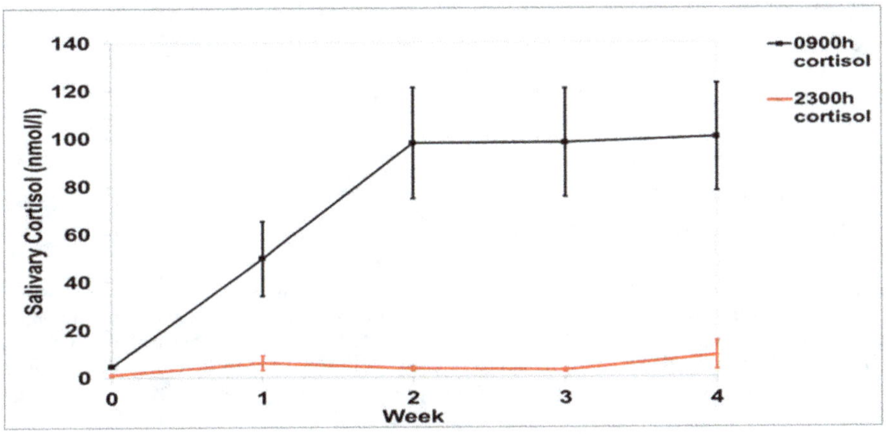

b

Figure 3. a: Graph showing mean ±SEM 0900 h serum cortisol and ACTH levels at baseline and 4 weeks. Activation of the HPA axis, that is a rise in serum cortisol and ACTH, is already evident one week after starting mifepristone. **b: Graph showing mean ±SEM 0900 h and 2300 h salivary cortisol levels at baseline and 4 weeks.** Circadian rhythm of cortisol is maintained evidenced by high levels at 0900 h and low levels at 2300 h, but amplified by the use of mifepristone 200 mg twice per day.

Changes in insulin resistance

As a group there were significant reductions in IR (lnHOMA-IR) and improvements in sensitivity (lnMatsuda index) compared to baseline following mifepristone treatment (Table 2). Five out of six individuals showed a reduction in insulin AUC (Figure 4). In subjects 2 and 5 there was a clinically significant reduction in insulin AUC from above the reference range into the upper half of the normal reference range. In subjects 1 and 6, insulin AUC fell by approximately 50% from the upper end of the reference range to the lower half of the reference range (<26940 pmol/l.min): patient 1: 51001 pmol/l.min to 25742 pmol/l.min; patient 6: 55972 pmol/l/min to 23668 pmol/l.min. In subject 3 insulin AUC fell, but this was within the lower half of the reference range at baseline. Subject 4 was highly insulin resistant and did not show any improvement in IR.

Changes in other metabolic markers

Subjects 2 and 5 improved their mean 24-hour BP from 143/75 to 135/67 and from 138/81 to 130/81, respectively. As a group there were no significant changes in resting or ambulatory blood pressure, serum osteocalcin and urine NTX/creat. There were no significant differences in the full lipid profile but interestingly there was a decrease in HDL in Subjects 2 and 5 from 0.93 mmol/l to 0.72 mmol/l and 0.84 mmol/l to 0.6 mmol/l respectively.

Safety analysis

Five subjects completed the study to week four. One (subject 2) developed clinical symptoms of lassitude and fatigue at end of week two whilst another developed similar symptoms at the end of week four (subject 3). Importantly, there was no hypotension, indicating the relative clinical safety of using mifepristone in this setting despite the vague symptoms in these individuals. Data collected for withdrawn subject after week 2 were considered suitable for analysis as a significant drug effect is achieved by this time [15]. Serum potassium levels for these subjects were to 3.2 and 3.1 mmol/l, respectively, at the second and fourth week. There was a significant reversible change in thyroid stimulating hormone (TSH) (1.45 vs 4.07 mU/l; $p = 0.03$).

Discussion

We have shown that short-term use of mifepristone can reduce IR in subjects with adrenal incidentalomas and low-grade autonomous cortisol secretion. To our knowledge, use of mifepristone in subjects with adrenal incidentalomas has never been tested. These data support recent findings in a study in patients with overt Cushing's syndrome where an improvement in insulin AUC and HOMA-IR was shown in the combined diabetes mellitus/impaired glucose tolerance and hypertension groups [12].

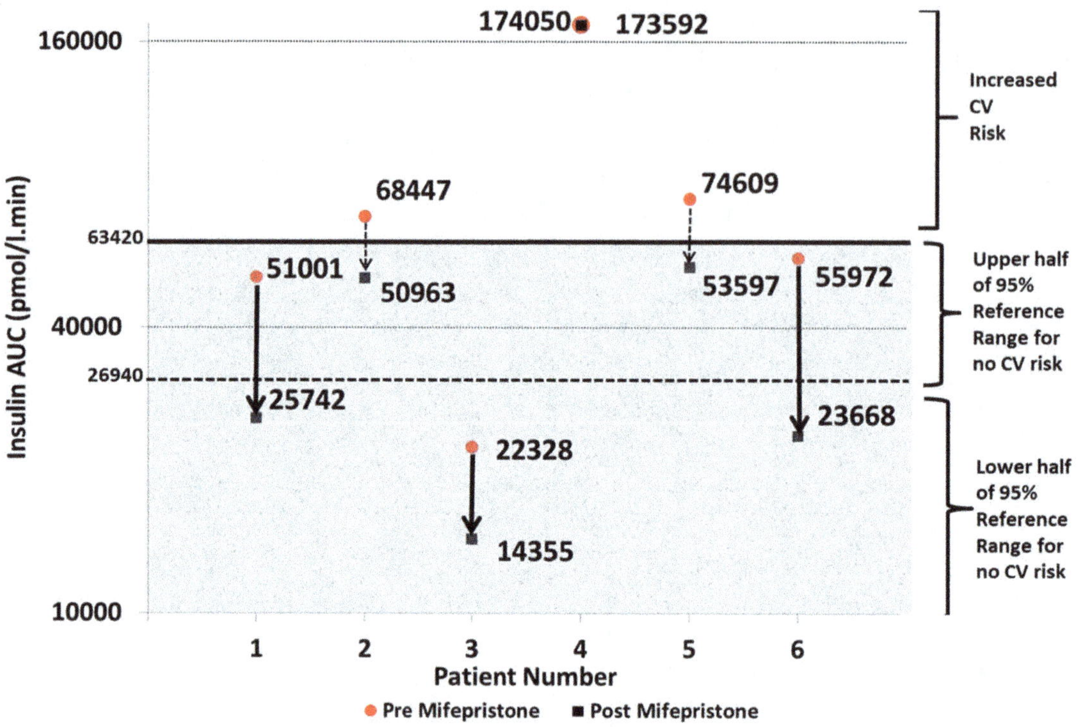

Figure 4. Graphs showing the changes in insulin AUC pre (red circle) and post (black square) mifepristone. The upper white area represents insulin AUC levels associated with increased risk for cardiovascular (CV) events. The grey shaded area represents the insulin AUC upper and lower 95% reference range (not associated with cardiovascular events). Mean: 26940 pmol/l.min; 2SD: 63420 pmol/l.min. Subjects 2 and 5 show a clinically significant improvement in their insulin AUC post mifepristone (dotted arrow). Subjects 1 and 6 both show a reduction in insulin AUC from the upper to the lower 95% reference range (solid arrow). Patient 4 remains at CV risk post mifepristone, indicating no clinical benefit. The insulin AUC is plotted on the y axis as a logarithmic scale to base 4.

As a group we showed a significant reduction in IR and five of our subjects had a decrease in insulin AUC greater than 7237 pmol/l.min, exceeding biological variation. In addition, to establish whether GR blockade might also be associated with cardiovascular benefit, we defined our cut-off for insulin AUC from data published from the Helsinki Policemen Study, which investigated the relationship between baseline IR and the risk for cardiovascular disease over 22 years [10]. In that study, on an OGTT a mean (±SD) insulin AUC of 26940±18240 pmol/l.min was found in those without a future cardiovascular event. We used, therefore, the mean insulin AUC (±2SD) as our 95% reference range. Using this method we identified two subjects (numbers 2, 5) who had IR above this level but in whom IR decreased into the normal range with GR antagonism, consistent with a likely clinical benefit. Two other subjects (numbers 1, 6) experienced a reduction of their insulin AUC to the lower half of the reference range, whilst subject 3 had an insulin AUC value at baseline in the lower half of the reference range that improved further. Conversely, subject 4 has insulin resistance, which despite GR blockade, was not reversed. It may be that in some cases insulin resistance is more

Table 2. Baseline and 4 week insulin sensitivity and glucose tolerance data after the use of mifepristone in 6 patients.

Variable (means ±95% CI)	Baseline	4 weeks	p value
Fasting glucose (mmol/l)	5.4 (4.6–6.2)	5.6 (5.0–6.1)	0.34
2-hour glucose (mmol/l)	10.2 (8.0–12.5)	11.4 (8.7–14.1)	0.21
AUC glucose (mmol/l.min)	1176 (1013–1339)	1187 (988–1384)	0.60
Geom Fasting insulin (pmol/l))	76.4 (39.9–146.4)	53.3 (25.8–109.9)	0.03
Geom 2-hour insulin (pmol/l)	628.5 (258.4–1528.3)	420.5 (159.4–1109.5)	0.20
Geom AUC insulin (pmol/l.min)	61973 (30889–124337)	40083 (16020–100289)	0.03
lnHOMA-IR	1.0 (0.2–1.7)	0.6 (−0.1–1.4)	0.03
lnHOMA-%β	4.8 (4.2–5.4)	4.3 (3.7–5.0)	0.03
lnMatsuda	1.2 (0.4–1.9)	1.6 (0.7–2.4)	0.03

Repeated measures effect analysed by non-parametric Wilcoxon's signed rank test.
AUC: Area under the curve HOMA - IR: Homeostatic Model Assessment of Insulin Resistance; HOMA - %β: Homeostatic Model Assessment of Beta Cell function.

'fixed' and less dependent on cortisol. We chose insulin AUC on OGTT as our primary estimate of IR as this allowed direct comparison to the seminal Helsinki heart study data examining the long term effects of IR on cardiovascular risk.

In addition to insulin AUC we used other estimates of insulin sensitivity. The Matsuda index of whole body insulin sensitivity, representing a composite of hepatic and peripheral tissues, and which considers insulin sensitivity in the basal state and after the ingestion of a glucose load, correlates strongly with estimates of insulin sensitivity from the 'gold standard' euglycemic insulin clamp ($r = 0.73$; $p<0.0001$) [21]. Although HOMA, or even stronger, log-transformed HOMA indices, correlate well with euglycemic clamps, they measure fasting steady state glucose and insulin concentrations and assume that hepatic and peripheral insulin sensitivity are equivalent [20,23]. Nonetheless all insulin sensitivity indices significantly improved. Our data give strong support to the notion that even mild cortisol excess may be deleterious on insulin sensitivity/resistance, and that short-term antagonism of GR may be one means of teasing out which subjects have potentially reversible IR.

There remains an open question as to whether individuals who have been identified with adrenal incidentaloma should undergo any intervention. A number of studies have been carried out in individuals with cortisol secreting incidentalomas who have been subjected to adrenalectomy [26,27] and improvements have been noted in weight, blood pressure, lipid profiles, fibrinogen levels, and glycemic control [11,28,29,30,31]. There is, however, no consensus on the criteria for the diagnosis of low-grade cortisol excess in patients with adrenal incidentalomas [13,27] creating a dilemma on whom should be referred to surgery. Recently, tests of the HPA axis associated with known metabolic consequences of hypercortisolemia in these individuals have been suggested [32], but benefit from adrenal surgery has been demonstrated in subjects without 'subclinical hypercortisolemia' [26]. Whilst one interpretation is that this argues against a direct role for cortisol in their phenotype [27], an alternative interpretation is that the definition of 'sub clinical' is not correct, with some of those undergoing surgery being labeled as 'normal' in fact having clinically significant excess cortisol. Here, we have used dexamethasone suppression tests with a serum cortisol cut-off of 50 nmol/l. Diagnosis was supported by a low mean baseline 0900 h ACTH of 1.9 pmol/l. Whilst in a general population this strategy runs the risk of including too many false positives, in an individual with adrenal incidentalomas there is a considerable *a priori* likelihood that there is *some* abnormality of cortisol secretion, and thus a positive screening raises the post-test probability of hypercortisolemia to approximately 99% [18,33]. It was for these reasons that we specifically focused on what would often be regarded as truly mild cases, to ask the question as to whether we would see any metabolic changes by antagonizing the GR without a pre-conceived definition 'subclinical Cushing's/hypercortisolemia'; other than a diagnostic strategy that is in keeping with Endocrine Society guidelines [18]. Although we did not measure plasma dexamethasone levels there does not appear to be an advantage to using the 8 mg DST [34], and thus we feel that it is unlikely that our patients tested false positive.

As a group no significant changes were detected in the other metabolic markers investigated. Interestingly the two patients with clinically significant decreases in insulin AUC (patients 2 and 5) showed improvements in average 24-hour ambulatory blood pressure. Meta-analysis of several large prospective studies has shown that a 5 to 6 mm Hg decrease in diastolic blood pressure is associated with a 38% reduction in risk for stroke and a 16% reduction in coronary heart disease events [35], whilst a 10 mmHg reduction in systolic blood pressure is associated with a reduction in risk of stroke by one third [36]. Cortisol-induced hypertension is mediated by several mechanisms including an increased vascular responsiveness to catecholamines [37], elevated circulating catecholamine levels [38], and potentially, through a mineralocorticoid effect, when cortisol occupies the mineralocorticoid receptor if in excessive amounts consequent to HPA axis activation. The latter effect could explain why we did not see a significant change in BP in the group. The decrease in HDL although on first glance may seem non beneficial, in patients on mifepristone this has previously been shown to be associated with an increased efflux capacity of serum HDL on a per particle basis, hence no proportional impairment in HDL function [39].

As expected with glucocorticoid receptor antagonism the HPA axis was rapidly activated with serum and salivary cortisol and plasma ACTH levels rising appropriately. Hence, monitoring of changes in serum or salivary cortisol can be used to confirm subject compliance and drug efficacy. Throughout the study as indicated by the 0900 h/2300 h salivary cortisol ratio the physiological circadian rhythm of cortisol was maintained but the amplitude widened with maximal effects of mifepristone occurring in the morning. Limitations of our pilot study include the open design, a small sample and two patients were withdrawn after 2 and 4 weeks of mifepristone treatment, respectively. All patients received 400 mg per day, in two divided doses of 200 mg. The two patients who were withdrawn and who developed some symptoms of adrenal insufficiency were lighter, and hence had the highest relative dose, followed by highest HPA axis activation. Importantly, however, there was no hypotension, indicating the relative clinical safety of using mifepristone in this setting despite the vague symptoms in these individuals. These data reinforce the dose-dependent effect of mifepristone, with a dose of around 5 mg/kg/day being most appropriate. The nature of our study precludes generalization without further studies being performed.

In summary, we have shown that a short period of GR antagonism for up to four weeks in individuals with mild cortisol excess resulted in significant improvements in insulin sensitivity, and potentially clinically significant improvements in two out of six. These effects can now be examined in randomized controlled studies to establish whether GR blockade or cortisol-lowering strategies, are a suitable means for the individualized stratification of individuals with adrenal incidentaloma to medical or surgical intervention, or observation.

Author Contributions

Conceived and designed the experiments: MD RE RJR JN-P. Performed the experiments: MD JN-P. Analyzed the data: MD JN-P. Contributed reagents/materials/analysis tools: JN-P. Wrote the paper: MD RJR JN-P.

References

1. Mansmann G, Lau J, Balk E, Rothberg M, Miyachi Y, et al. (2004) The clinically inapparent adrenal mass: update in diagnosis and management. Endocr Rev 25: 309–340.
2. Young WF Jr (2007) Clinical practice. The incidentally discovered adrenal mass. N Engl J Med 356: 601–610.

3. Terzolo M, Stigliano A, Chiodini I, Loli P, Furlani L, et al. (2011) AME position statement on adrenal incidentaloma. Eur J Endocrinol 164: 851–870.
4. Newell-Price J, Bertagna X, Grossman AB, Nieman LK (2006) Cushing's syndrome. Lancet 367: 1605–1617.
5. Friedman JE, Yun JS, Patel YM, McGrane MM, Hanson RW (1993) Glucocorticoids regulate the induction of phosphoenolpyruvate carboxykinase (GTP) gene transcription during diabetes. J Biol Chem 268: 12952–12957.
6. Vander Kooi BT, Onuma H, Oeser JK, Svitek CA, Allen SR, et al. (2005) The glucose-6-phosphatase catalytic subunit gene promoter contains both positive and negative glucocorticoid response elements. Mol Endocrinol 19: 3001–3022.
7. Davani B, Khan A, Hult M, Martensson E, Okret S, et al. (2000) Type 1 11beta -hydroxysteroid dehydrogenase mediates glucocorticoid activation and insulin release in pancreatic islets. J Biol Chem 275: 34841–34844.
8. Qi D, Rodrigues B (2007) Glucocorticoids produce whole body insulin resistance with changes in cardiac metabolism. Am J Physiol Endocrinol Metab 292: E654–667.
9. Nosadini R, Del Prato S, Tiengo A, Valerio A, Muggeo M, et al. (1983) Insulin resistance in Cushing's syndrome. J Clin Endocrinol Metab 57: 529–536.
10. Pyorala M, Miettinen H, Halonen P, Laakso M, Pyorala K (2000) Insulin resistance syndrome predicts the risk of coronary heart disease and stroke in healthy middle-aged men: the 22-year follow-up results of the Helsinki Policemen Study. Arterioscler Thromb Vasc Biol 20: 538–544.
11. Tauchmanova L, Rossi R, Biondi B, Pulcrano M, Nuzzo V, et al. (2002) Patients with subclinical Cushing's syndrome due to adrenal adenoma have increased cardiovascular risk. J Clin Endocrinol Metab 87: 4872–4878.
12. Fleseriu M, Biller BM, Findling JW, Molitch ME, Schteingart DE, et al. (2012) Mifepristone, a Glucocorticoid Receptor Antagonist, Produces Clinical and Metabolic Benefits in Patients with Cushing's Syndrome. J Clin Endocrinol Metab.
13. Chiodini I (2011) Clinical review: Diagnosis and treatment of subclinical hypercortisolism. J Clin Endocrinol Metab 96: 1223–1236.
14. Des Jarlais DC, Lyles C, Crepaz N (2004) Improving the reporting quality of nonrandomized evaluations of behavioral and public health interventions: the TREND statement. Am J Public Health 94: 361–366.
15. Kawai S, Nieman LK, Brandon DD, Udelsman R, Loriaux DL, et al. (1987) Pharmacokinetic properties of the antiglucocorticoid and antiprogesterone steroid RU 486 in man. J Pharmacol Exp Ther 241: 401–406.
16. Heikinheimo O (1997) Clinical pharmacokinetics of mifepristone. Clin Pharmacokinet 33: 7–17.
17. Newell-Price J, Trainer P, Besser M, Grossman A (1998) The diagnosis and differential diagnosis of Cushing's syndrome and pseudo-Cushing's states. Endocr Rev 19: 647–672.
18. Nieman LK, Biller BM, Findling JW, Newell-Price J, Savage MO, et al. (2008) The diagnosis of Cushing's syndrome: an Endocrine Society Clinical Practice Guideline. J Clin Endocrinol Metab 93: 1526–1540.
19. Gordon BA, Fraser SF, Bird SR, Benson AC (2011) Reproducibility of multiple repeated oral glucose tolerance tests. Diabetes Res Clin Pract 94: e78–82.
20. Matthews DR, Hosker JP, Rudenski AS, Naylor BA, Treacher DF, et al. (1985) Homeostasis model assessment: insulin resistance and beta-cell function from fasting plasma glucose and insulin concentrations in man. Diabetologia 28: 412–419.
21. Matsuda M, DeFronzo RA (1999) Insulin sensitivity indices obtained from oral glucose tolerance testing: comparison with the euglycemic insulin clamp. Diabetes Care 22: 1462–1470.
22. Perogamvros I, Owen LJ, Newell-Price J, Ray DW, Trainer PJ, et al. (2009) Simultaneous measurement of cortisol and cortisone in human saliva using liquid chromatography-tandem mass spectrometry: application in basal and stimulated conditions. J Chromatogr B Analyt Technol Biomed Life Sci 877: 3771–3775.
23. Muniyappa R, Lee S, Chen H, Quon MJ (2008) Current approaches for assessing insulin sensitivity and resistance in vivo: advantages, limitations, and appropriate usage. Am J Physiol Endocrinol Metab 294: E15–26.
24. Tsagarakis S, Roboti C, Kokkoris P, Vasiliou V, Alevizaki C, et al. (1998) Elevated post-dexamethasone suppression cortisol concentrations correlate with hormonal alterations of the hypothalamo-pituitary adrenal axis in patients with adrenal incidentalomas. Clin Endocrinol (Oxf) 49: 165–171.
25. Di Dalmazi G, Vicennati V, Rinaldi E, Morselli-Labate AM, Giampalma E, et al. (2012) Progressively increased patterns of subclinical cortisol hypersecretion in adrenal incidentalomas differently predict major metabolic and cardiovascular outcomes: a large cross-sectional study. Eur J Endocrinol 166: 669–677.
26. Chiodini I, Morelli V, Salcuni AS, Eller-Vainicher C, Torlontano M, et al. (2010) Beneficial metabolic effects of prompt surgical treatment in patients with an adrenal incidentaloma causing biochemical hypercortisolism. J Clin Endocrinol Metab 95: 2736–2745.
27. Stewart PM (2010) Is subclinical Cushing's syndrome an entity or a statistical fallout from diagnostic testing? Consensus surrounding the diagnosis is required before optimal treatment can be defined. J Clin Endocrinol Metab 95: 2618–2620.
28. Midorikawa S, Sanada H, Hashimoto S, Suzuki T, Watanabe T (2001) The improvement of insulin resistance in patients with adrenal incidentaloma by surgical resection. Clin Endocrinol (Oxf) 54: 797–804.
29. Rossi R, Tauchmanova L, Luciano A, Di Martino M, Battista C, et al. (2000) Subclinical Cushing's syndrome in patients with adrenal incidentaloma: clinical and biochemical features. J Clin Endocrinol Metab 85: 1440–1448.
30. Terzolo M, Pia A, Ali A, Osella G, Reimondo G, et al. (2002) Adrenal incidentaloma: a new cause of the metabolic syndrome? J Clin Endocrinol Metab 87: 998–1003.
31. Toniato A, Merante-Boschin I, Opocher G, Pelizzo MR, Schiavi F, et al. (2009) Surgical versus conservative management for subclinical Cushing syndrome in adrenal incidentalomas: a prospective randomized study. Ann Surg 249: 388–391.
32. Morelli V, Masserini B, Salcuni AS, Eller-Vainicher C, Savoca C, et al. (2010) Subclinical hypercortisolism: correlation between biochemical diagnostic criteria and clinical aspects. Clin Endocrinol (Oxf) 73: 161–166.
33. Elamin MB, Murad MH, Mullan R, Erickson D, Harris K, et al. (2008) Accuracy of diagnostic tests for Cushing's syndrome: a systematic review and metaanalyses. J Clin Endocrinol Metab 93: 1553–1562.
34. Reimondo G, Allasino B, Bovio S, Saba L, Ardito A, et al. (2011) Pros and cons of dexamethasone suppression test for screening of subclinical Cushing's syndrome in patients with adrenal incidentalomas. J Endocrinol Invest 34: e1–5.
35. Hebert PR, Moser M, Mayer J, Glynn RJ, Hennekens CH (1993) Recent evidence on drug therapy of mild to moderate hypertension and decreased risk of coronary heart disease. Arch Intern Med 153: 578–581.
36. Lawes CM, Bennett DA, Feigin VL, Rodgers A (2004) Blood pressure and stroke: an overview of published reviews. Stroke 35: 1024.
37. Whitworth JA, Brown MA, Kelly JJ, Williamson PM (1995) Mechanisms of cortisol-induced hypertension in humans. Steroids 60: 76–80.
38. Kumai T, Asoh K, Tateishi T, Tanaka M, Watanabe M, et al. (2000) Involvement of tyrosine hydroxylase up regulation in dexamethasone-induced hypertension of rats. Life Sci 67: 1993–1999.
39. Page ST, Krauss RM, Gross C, Ishida B, Heinecke JW, et al. (2012) Impact of mifepristone, a glucocorticoid/progesterone antagonist, on HDL cholesterol, HDL particle concentration, and HDL function. J Clin Endocrinol Metab 97: 1598–1605.

6

Post-Receptor Crosstalk between Growth Hormone and Insulin Signal in Rats Born Small for Gestational Age with Catch-Up Growth

Hong-Zhu Deng[1,3], Hong Deng[2]*, Chao-Qun Cen[1], Kai-Yun Chen[1], Min-Lian Du[3]

1 Department of Pediatrics, the Third Affiliated Hospital of Sun Yat-sen University, Guangzhou, China, **2** Department of Infectious diseases, the Third Affiliated Hospital of Sun Yat-sen University, Guangzhou, China, **3** Department of Pediatrics, the First Affiliated Hospital of Sun Yat-sen University, Guangzhou, China

Abstract

Objective: Insulin resistance has been observed in individuals born small for gestational age (SGA) with catch-up growth (CUG), yet the mechanisms involved remain unclear. This study examined the role of GH and insulin signaling crosstalk in insulin resistance of SGA rats with CUG.

Design and Methods: SGA rats were developed by dietary restriction in pregnant rats. GH receptor inhibition was performed on four-week old CUG-SGA and AGA rats. Phosphorylation of IRS-1, AKT, and ERK, and expression of SOCS3 in the skeletal muscle were determined via immunoblot analysis at baseline and after insulin stimulation in CUG-SGA, NCUG-SGA and AGA groups.

Results: Compared to AGA controls, phosphorylation of IRS-1 and AKT in response to insulin stimulation in CUG-SGA rats was significantly blunted ($P<0.05$), and phosphorylation of ERK at baseline was dramatically activated ($P<0.05$). SOCS3 expression was significantly increased in CUG-SGA compared to AGA ($P=0.001$) and NCUG-SGA ($P=0.006$) rats, and was significantly suppressed following *GHR* inhibition ($P<0.05$). Furthermore, phosphorylation of IRS-1 and AKT in response to insulin stimulation increased after *GHR* inhibition ($P<0.05$).

Conclusions: Insulin resistance in CUG-SGA rats is associated with impairment of IRS-1-PI3K-AKT signaling, which may result from GH signaling-induced up-regulation of SOCS3.

Editor: Victor Sanchez-Margalet, Virgen Macarena University Hospital, School of Medicine, University of Seville, Spain

Funding: The study was supported by the Natural Science Foundation of China (grant number 81100571) and the Natural Science Foundation of Guangdong Province (grant number S2011020005224). The funders had no role in study design, data collection and analysis, decision to publish, or preparation of the manuscript.

Competing Interests: The authors have declared that no competing interests exist.

* Email: denghong2@foxmail.com

Introduction

Accumulating evidence demonstrates that metabolic syndrome and associated obesity, dyslipidemia, hypertension, insulin resistance and diabetes in adults closely correlate with being born small for gestational age (SGA) [1–5]. Approximately 80% of the children born SGA demonstrate catch-up growth (CUG), which generally occurs in the first few years of postnatal life. Previous studies indicated that insulin resistance in children born SGA is associated with height and weight CUG [6]. The molecular mechanisms of insulin resistance in children born SGA with CUG, however, are still poorly understood.

The elevated levels of the growth hormone (GH)/insulin-like growth factor (IGF-1) axis had been found in SGA rats with CUG in our previous study [7]. GH promotes longitudinal growth and somatic maturation in children and adolescents and is also an important regulator of substrate metabolism and insulin sensitivity. In the post-absorptive phase, where endogenous GH secretion is stimulated, GH promotes lipolysis and oxidation of fatty acids at the expense of glucose [8]. The predominant GH signaling cascade comprises activation of the growth hormone receptor (*GHR*) dimer, phosphorylation of Janus kinase 2 (JAK2) and subsequently of signal transductor and activator of transcription 5 (STAT5). Insulin is also a key hormone regulating metabolism and growth. Insulin binding to the insulin receptor (*IR*) results in phosphorylation/activation of the *IR*, and activates the phosphatidylinositol 3-kinase (PI3K)/Akt and the extracellular signal-regulated kinase 1/2(ERK1/2) pathways. Insulin-stimulated glucose transport into skeletal muscle depends on the activation of a signaling cascade involving insulin receptor substrate 1 (IRS-1), PI3K and Akt. Due to their important roles in growth and metabolism, GH and insulin can functionally interact with each other, regulating cellular metabolism. In addition, recent animal and *in vitro* evidence suggest that GH and insulin can share post-receptor signaling pathways, and these pathways may contribute to GH-induced insulin resistance [9]. Convergence has been reported at the level of suppressor of cytokine signaling 3 (SOCS3) as well as on protein kinases comprising the insulin signaling pathway, including insulin receptor substrate-1/2 (IRS1/2), PI3K, Akt, and ERK1/2 [10,11]. However, the interaction by signaling cross-talk between GH and insulin signaling pathways has not been confirmed in SGA models *in vivo*. This may relate to the design of these studies.

Both GH resistance and insulin resistance are present in SGA subjects, which regulated by GH and insulin signals in metabolism and growth. Hence, we hypothesize that the post-receptor crosstalk of GH and insulin signaling would have an effect on CUG and insulin resistance in SGA. In the present study, we examine the insulin resistance in skeletal muscle tissue obtained from animals born SGA with CUG. We aim to confirm whether inhibiting *GHR* under baseline conditions can alter the post-receptor activity of GH and insulin signaling, and explore the possible mechanisms linking CUG and insulin resistance in SGA.

Methods and Procedures

Reagents

The sources of materials are as follows: short-acting insulin (Novolin, 400 IU/10 ml) produced by Novo Nordisk, Denmark, the *GHR* antagonist Somavert(Pegvisomant,10 mg/10 ml) from Pfizer Inc., USA, and the insulin radioimmunoassay from Pharmacia & Upjohn Diagnostics AB, Sweden. The following primary antibodies were purchased from Cell Signaling, USA: rabbit anti-rat IRS, anti-p-IRS, anti-AKT, anti-p-AKT (Ser473), anti-ERK, anti-p-ERK1/2 (Thr202/Tyr204) and anti-SOCS3 (L210). Rabbit anti-phosphorylation polyclonal antibody was purchased from Abcam, UK.

Animals and experimental assignment

All animal procedures conformed to the requirements of the Animal Welfare Act, and protocols were approved by the Institutional Animal Care and Use Committee of Sun Yat-sen University. The animals were housed under conditions approved by the Association for the Assessment and Accreditation of Laboratory Animal Care International.

A total of forty-five healthy female and twenty healthy male Sprague-Dawley rats weighing 230 to 280 g [animal license No. SYXK (Guangdong Province, China) 2007-0081] were obtained from the Animal Center, North Campus of Sun Yat-sen University in China. Standard rat fodder [license No. SCXK (Guangdong Province, China) 2003-0002; Guangdong supervison No. 2008D002] was provided by the Medical Laboratory Animal Center of Guangdong Province in China. Pregnant rats subjected to dietary restriction were utilized to establish the SGA rat model [17]. Rats were randomly housed in standard rat cages at a 2:1 female-to-male ratio. A vaginal smear examination under a standard optical microscope was performed daily, and the day on which sperm appeared in the smear was determined as day 1 (D1) of pregnancy.

Pregnant female rats were randomly divided into either the dietary restriction or the control group. Rats in the control group were fed 18–20 g/d, whereas rats in the dietary restriction group were fed only 8–9 g/d (approximately 50% of normal intake) after D1.

Offspring

All pups were weighed at birth and litter sizes were recorded. Litter size was adjusted to 8–10 pups per litter, with random pups excluded if the litter was over 10 pups in size. The pups of each litter in the SGA group were marked with 3% methyl violet after delivery and with 3% picric acid after two weeks. Post-delivery, the mother rats in the two groups were fed a standard control diet. The pups were fed by breastfeeding for the first 3 weeks, and thereafter they were housed in separate cages and fed the same diet as their mothers until the completion of the experiment. Food intakes of the maternal and young rats at 4 weeks of age in the different groups are shown in Table 1. No obvious difference in the food intakes was observed among the CUG-SGA, NCUG-SGA and AGA groups (Table 1). The weight and nose-anus length of all pups were recorded weekly.

Animal model of CUG

SGA infant rats were defined as having a birth weight and/or body length greater than two standard deviations (SDs) below the average birth weight and/or body length of the control group. Non-CUG-SGA (NCUG-SGA) animals were defined by a body weight and body length greater than two SDs below the average body weight and body length of the control group at four weeks of age. Criteria for CUG-SGA rats consisted of body weights and body lengths less than two SDs below the average body weight and body length of the control group at four weeks of age.

Insulin stimulation

According to body weight and length, all four-week old offspring rats in the three groups [CUG-SGA, NCUG-SGA and appropriate for gestational age (AGA)] were further separated into two sub-groups, namely control and insulin stimulation groups. The insulin stimulation group animals received intraperitoneal injection of 3.0 IU/100 g insulin (diluted to 2 mL with 0.9% saline) 30 min before sacrifice. Control group animals were given intraperitoneal injection of 2 mL saline 30 min prior to sacrifice.

GHR inhibition

Four-week old rats in either the CUG-SGA or AGA groups were further divided into three sub-groups, including control, insulin stimulation and insulin stimulation plus *GHR* inhibition. Control group animals were given intraperitoneal injection of 2 mL saline at 50 hr, 2 hr, and 30 min before sacrifice. Insulin stimulation group animals were administrated intraperitoneal injection of saline at 50 hr and 2 hr pre-sacrifice, followed by injection of 3.0 IU/100 g insulin 30 min before sacrifice. The insulin stimulation plus *GHR* inhibition group animals received 0.001 mg/g Somavert via intraperitoneal injection at 50 hr and 2 hr pre-sacrifice, followed by an injection of 3.0 IU/100 g insulin 30 min before sacrifice.

Measurements of biochemical parameters

Animals in each group were fasted for 12 hr and sacrificed by 10% chloralic hydras (0.3 mg/kg) injection. Blood and gastrocnemius specimens were extracted and stored at −70°C until laboratory assessment. Serum glucose was determined by a peroxidase method (Photometric Instrument 4010, Roche, Switzerland) (between-group variance <2.0%), and serum insulin was measured using an immunoradiometric assay (Pharmacia & Upjohn Diagnostics AB, Sweden) (between-group variance < 5.3%, within-group variance <7.6%). Homoeostasis Model Assessment for Insulin Resistance (HOMA-IR) was used to estimate insulin resistance according to the formula: fasting plasma insulin (μU/mL)*fasting plasma glucose (mmol/L)/22.5 [12].

Immunoblot analysis

A total of 100 mg of gastrocnemius muscle tissue was extracted from each group and rinsed with PBS 3 times, then homogenized in 1 unit pre-chilled histiocyte lysate consisting of 1 ml LysisBuffer, 5 μl phosphatase, 1 μl protease inhibitors, and 5 μl PMSF. The homogenates were centrifuged at 2000 rpm for 10 min at 4°C. The protein concentrations were measured using the BCA

Table 1. Food intakes of the maternal and young rats in different groups.

	Food intake, g/day		
	AGA	NCUG-SGA	CUG-SGA
Maternal rats	20.97±3.14	18.36±2.23	20.08±2.52
Young rats at 4 weeks of age			
Males(n = 31,36,and 34)	9.43±1.95	8.53±2.17	10.04±2.33
Females(n = 25,33,and 20)	8.75±1.81	8.24±1.96	9.27±2.15

The numbers of rats in the maternal appropriate for gestational age (AGA), small for gestational age with catch-up growth (CUG-SGA) and small for gestational age with no catch-up growth (NCUG-SGA) groups were 15, 20 and 20, respectively. Young rats at 4 weeks: n = 56 in AGA group, n = 54 in CUG-SGA group, n = 69 in NCUG-SGA group. There are not significant differences in AGA, CUG-SGA and NCUG-SGA groups. Food intakes of young male rats in different groups were comparable to those of females respectively.

method. Aliquots of protein samples were mixed with an equal volume of 2×SDS buffer solution and heated at 100°C for 5–10 min. Total protein 50 μg/well was resolved and subjected to sodium dodecyl sulfate-polyacrylimide gel electrophoresis (10% gels), and then proteins were electroblotted onto PVDF membranes. The membrane was blocked with 5% bovine serum albumin for 1 h at room temperature and subsequently incubated with primary antibody overnight at 4°C. After being washed in 1×TBST [50 mM Tris/HCl (pH 7.4), 150 mM NaCl and 0.2% Tween-20], the membranes were incubated with a horseradish peroxidase-conjugated anti-rabbit secondary IgG antibody (1: 1,000 dilution in 5%BSA). Signal was detected using an ECL kit (Pierce Biotechnology, USA) and quantified using the Bio-Rad GS-800 scanner (USA). Phosphoprotein content was determined relative to the total protein content (ratio p/T).

Statistical analysis

Data were analyzed using the Statistical Package for the Social Sciences (SPSS) 13.0 (SPSS Inc., USA). Insulin levels and HOMA-IR were not normally distributed; thus, these values were converted to logarithms and were presented as the geometrical mean ± standard error of the mean (SEM). Other data were presented as the arithmetic mean ± SD. Differences among groups were evaluated by analysis of variance (ANOVA) and interactions were analyzed by least significant difference (LSD). A P value<0.05 (two-tailed) was considered statistically significant.

Results

A total of 249 pups were born in the dietary restriction group, including 224 SGA pups (89.96%). One-hundred-and-twenty-three newborn SGA rats were recruited into the present study. Fifty-four (43.9%) of the 123 SGA rats demonstrated CUG with body weights and lengths less than 2 SDs below those of age- and sex-matched AGA controls at four weeks of age.

Physical characteristics of the offspring animals

Birth body weights and lengths of CUG-SGA and NCUG-SGA newborn rats were significantly lower than AGA animals (Table 2, $P<0.05$). Body weights and lengths of CUG-SGA rats demonstrated CUG as early as the first week post-delivery, and reached comparable measurements to those of the AGA group by the fourth week. Body weights and body lengths of the NCUG-SGA rats remained significantly lower than those in the AGA group by the fourth week, however (Table 2, $P<0.05$).

Insulin resistance index

No significant differences were observed in the levels of serum glucose among the three groups. The serum insulin and HOMA-IR values in the CUG-SGA and NCUG-SGA groups were significantly higher than those in the AGA group (serum insulin: $P<0.001$, $P=0.001$; HOMA-IR: $P<0.001$, $P<0.001$; respectively). Moreover, the serum insulin ($P=0.006$) and HOMA-IR ($P=0.002$) values in the CUG-SGA were higher than in the NCUG-SGA rats (Table 3).

Table 2. Anthropometric parameters of SGA and AGA groups.

	Body length(cm)			Body weight(g)		
	AGA	CUG-SGA	NCUG-SGA	AGA	CUG-SGA	NCUG-SGA
	(n = 56)	(n = 54)	(n = 69)	(n = 56)	(n = 54)	(n = 69)
0W	5.18±0.18	4.57±0.17*	4.41±0.15*	6.28±0.51	4.72±0.37*	4.67±0.35*
1W	6.80±0.15	6.66±0.35	6.20±0.46*#	14.56±0.58	14.72±2.06	12.93±2.51*#
2W	8.91±0.37	8.78±0.47	8.11±0.72*#	25.68±1.68	26.96±3.04	21.33±4.65*#
3W	10.67±0.29	10.71±0.50	9.50±0.53*#	39.96±2.91	43.93±6.56	32.55±4.62*#
4W	13.89±0.58	13.62±0.65	12.51±0.58*#	72.79±9.43	76.21±4.72	64.98±6.68*#

The ratioes of male to female in appropriate for gestational age (AGA), small for gestational age with catch-up growth (CUG-SGA) and small for gestational age with no catch-up growth (NCUG-SGA) groups were 26/30, 29/25 and 41/28. No significant differences were observed in the ratio of male to female among the three groups ($p>0.05$). *$P<0.05$ CUG-SGA or NCUG-SGA *vs* AGA; #$P<0.05$ CUG-SGA *vs* NCUG-SGA; Data are means±SD.

Table 3. Serum insulin levels and HOMA-IR values of CUG-SGA, NCUG-SGA rats and AGA rats.

Variable	AGA(n = 56)	CUG-SGA(n = 54)	NCUG-SGA(n = 69)
GLU(mmol/L)			
Males(n = 31,34,and 36)	4.52±0.17	5.37±0.12	4.97±0.08
Females(n = 25,20,and 33)	4.73±0.15	5.58±0.15	4.65±0.09
INS(mU/ml)			
Males	10.25±0.33	39.64±1.68*#	25.16±1.13*
Females	9.56±0.24	40.87±1.53*#	26.07±0.86*
HOMA-IR			
Males	2.05±0.29	10.06±0.65*#	5.79±0.69*
Females	1.97±0.31	10.85±0.57*#	5.41±0.58*

Appropriate for gestational age (AGA), small for gestational age with catch-up growth (CUG-SGA), small for gestational age with no catch-up growth (NCUG-SGA), homoeostasis model assessment for insulin resistance (HOMA-IR). *$P<0.05$ CUG-SGA or NCUG-SGA *vs* AGA; #$P<0.05$ CUG-SGA *vs* NCUG-SGA.

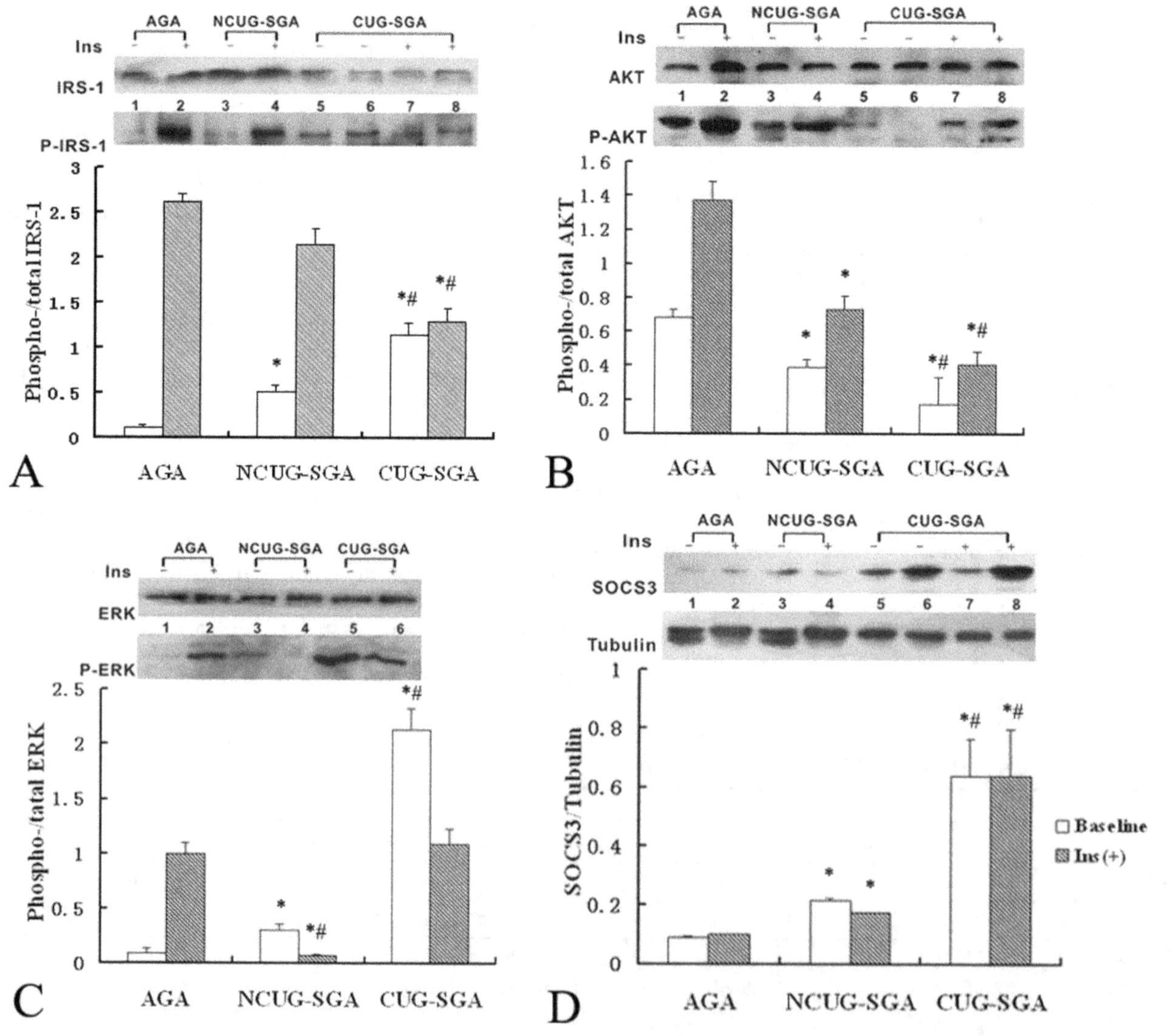

Figure 1. Immunoblot analysis of p-IRS-1, p-AKT, p-ERK and SOCS3 in skeletal muscle cell lysates from CUG-SGA, NCUG-SGA and AGA rats. Rats in appropriate for gestational age (AGA), small for gestational age with catch-up growth (CUG-SGA) and small for gestational age with no catch-up growth (NCUG-SGA) groups (n = 16 for each group) were either intraperitoneal injected intravenously with insulin (Ins) or saline (baseline control) at 4 weeks of age and the skeletal muscles were excised for examination of IRS-1, AKT, ERK, SOCS3 and the phosphorylation of IRS-1, AKT, ERK (p-IRS-1/p-AKT/p-ERK) via Immunoblot analysis. Activation of IRS-1, AKT and ERK were expressed as the ratio of p-IRS-1/p-AKT/p-ERK to total IRS-1, AKT and ERK, respectively. The level of SOCS3 was expressed as the ratio of SOCS3 to tubulin. Data were quantified from 16 samples and were presented as the mean ± SD. *$P<0.05$ CUG-SGA or NCUG-SGA *vs* AGA; #$P<0.05$ CUG-SGA *vs* NCUG-SGA.

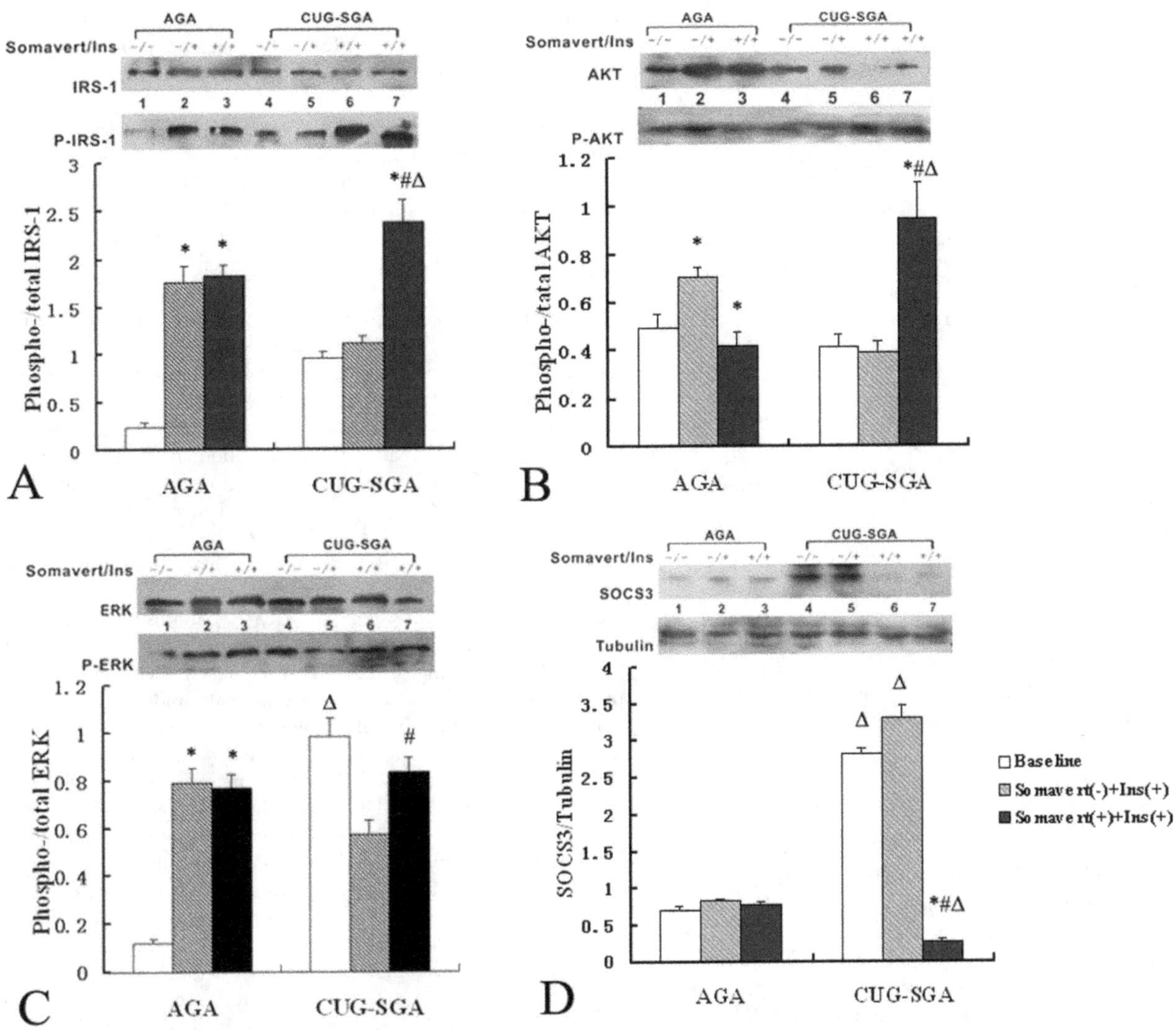

Figure 2. Immunoblot analysis of p-IRS-1, p-AKT, p-ERK and SOCS3 in skeletal muscle cell lysates from CUG-SGA and AGA rats before and after GHR inhibition. Rats in the appropriate for gestational age (AGA) and small for gestational age with catch-up growth (CUG-SGA) groups (n = 16 per group) were further separated into three sub-groups. At four weeks of age, sub-group one received intraperitoneal injection of saline (control), sub-group two received insulin (Ins) stimulation and sub-group three received the GHR inhibitor Somavert before insulin stimulation. The skeletal muscle was then excised for examination of IRS-1, AKT, ERK, SOCS3, and the phosphorylation of IRS-1, AKT, ERK (p-IRS-1/p-AKT/p-ERK) via Immunoblot analysis. Activation of IRS-1, AKT and ERK were expressed as the ratio of p-IRS-1/p-AKT/p-ERK to total IRS-1, AKT and ERK, respectively. The level of SOCS3 was expressed as the ratio of SOCS3 to tubulin. Data were quantified from 16 samples and presented as the mean ± SD. *$P<0.05$ Somavert(-)+Ins(+) or Somavert(+)+Ins(+) *vs* baseline; #$P<0.05$ Somavert(-)+Ins(+) *vs* Somavert(+) +Ins(+); Δ$P<0.05$ CUG-SGA *vs* AGA.

Expression of signaling molecules in muscle tissue

Immunoblot analysis was performed to test the activation of IRS/PI3K signaling in skeletal muscle tissue 30 min after insulin stimulation. The levels of p-IRS-1 significantly increased after insulin stimulation ($P<0.05$) in the NCUG-SGA and AGA control groups. In contrast, the levels of p-IRS-1 were significantly higher at baseline and did not increase significantly after insulin stimulation in the CUG-SGA group. The levels of p-ERK were also significantly higher at baseline in the CUG-SGA group and decreased to levels comparable to those observed in the AGA group (Figure 1).

The levels of p-AKT after insulin stimulation in the CUG-SGA and NCUG-SGA groups were significantly lower than those in the AGA group. Additionally, the levels of p-AKT in the CUG-SGA group were only 50% of those in the NCUG-SGA group (Figure 1).

Low levels of SOCS3 were observed in AGA control animals under baseline conditions, whereas SOCS3 expression was significantly higher in the CUG-SGA ($P=0.001$) and NCUG-SGA ($P=0.037$) rats. Furthermore, the expression of SOCS3 in the CUG-SGA group was significantly higher than that in the NCUG-SGA group ($P=0.006$). There were no statistically significant differences in the expression of SOCS3 within any group after insulin stimulation ($p>0.05$).

Expression of signaling molecules in the skeletal muscle of CUG-SGA rats after *GHR* inhibition

As shown in Figure 2, the level of SOCS3 did not significantly change after *GHR* inhibition in the AGA group. However, the expression of SOCS3 in CUG-SGA rats was significantly down-regulated after *GHR* inhibition ($P<0.001$). Likewise, no significant differences were detected in the expression of p-IRS-1 and p-AKT

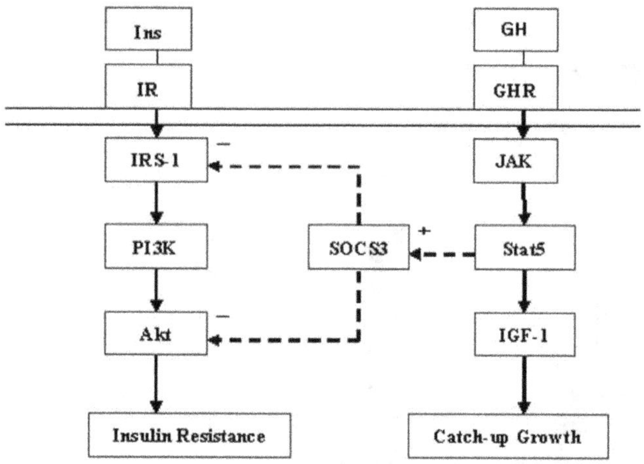

Figure 3. Crosstalk between insulin and GH signaling. GH signaling induces up-regulation of SOCS3 in SGA with Catch-up Growth. Higher SOCS3 levels result in impairment of IRS-1-PI3K-AKT signaling and it may have a role in insulin resistance.

after insulin stimulation in the AGA group after *GHR* inhibition, whereas p-IRS-1, p-AKT and p-ERK were all dramatically up-regulated in the CUG-SGA group after *GHR* inhibition ($P = 0.001$). The reduced levels of p-ERK after insulin stimulation alone were restored to basal levels in the CUG-SGA rats treated with the *GHR* inhibitor.

Discussion

In the present study, we demonstrate that 1) insulin resistance was observed in SGA rats with or without CUG, and rats with CUG show even greater insulin resistance; 2) insulin-stimulated IRS-1 and AKT phosphorylation was significantly blunted in CUG-SGA rats; 3) SOCS3 expression was upregulated in CUG-SGA rats; 4) *GHR* inhibition significantly suppressed SOCS3 but elevated the expression of p-IRS-1, p-AKT and p-ERK in insulin-stimulated CUG-SGA animals. This evidence suggests that insulin resistance in CUG-SGA rats is associated with impairment of IRS-1-PI3K-AKT signaling, which results from *GHR* signaling-induced upregulation of SOCS3 expression (Figure 3).

We found that insulin resistance indexes were much higher in the CUG-SGA group than in the NCUG-SGA and AGA groups. This indicates that SGA rats with CUG demonstrate more significant insulin resistance, which is in accordance with our previous clinical results [6]. Skeletal muscle was the most common and earliest affected tissue during CUG in individuals with SGA [13]. Hence, we next investigated the alteration of molecular pathways in the skeletal muscle of SGA rats with CUG.

IRS-1, a crucial upstream signaling molecule in the insulin signaling pathway, plays a critical role in skeletal muscle cells. Shirakami *et al.* found that knockout of the IRS-1 gene in mice induced profound insulin resistance, insulin-like growth factor resistance, and impaired glucose intolerance after intraperitoneal injection of glucose [14]. De Blasio *et al.* used placental restriction to establish the intrauterine growth restriction sheep model, and showed that placental restriction could decrease the expression of IRS-1 to 28% and AKT to 44% in skeletal muscle. In addition, this positively correlated with insulin resistance without altering insulin levels or related genes expressed in the liver [15]. In the present study, insulin-stimulated IRS-1 and AKT phosphorylation in skeletal muscle were significantly blunted in CUG-SGA rats, which is consistent with a previous report [16], and suggests that impairment of the IRS-1-PI3K-AKT signaling pathway may contribute to the insulin resistance observed in the CUG-SGA rats.

The p-ERK levels in the NCUG- and CUG-SGA groups were significantly increased (chronically stimulated) by 3-fold and 20-fold, respectively. Interestingly, the p-ERK level at baseline and its reaction to insulin stimulation in the CUG-SGA rats was the opposite of what was observed with p-AKT expression in these same animals. Thus, to a certain extent, insulin resistance accompanied with rapid CUG can be demonstrated in infancy. The impairment of the IRS-1-PI3K pathway, occurred in the subjects of CUG-SGA. The IRS-1-ERK pathway may be chronically activated under baseline conditions to promote CUG during early postnatal life in SGA children.

Additionally, no significant difference was found in the expression of p-IRS-1 after *GHR* inhibition in the AGA group, indicating that for AGA, IRS-1 may not respond to GH signaling. However, the levels of p-IRS-1 increased in response to insulin stimulation after inhibition of *GHR* in CUG-SGA group, indicating that abnormal GH signaling may contribute to the inhibition of insulin-IRS-1 signal transduction. Examination of AKT, the downstream signal of IRS-1, demonstrated that the levels of p-AKT decreased after *GHR* inhibition in the AGA group. These findings suggest that GH signaling could induce phosphorylation of AKT in AGA animals under physiological conditions. GH may regulate glucose metabolism, first by its insulin-like effect in acute phase, followed by its antagonistic effect [8]. The expression of p-AKT did not increase when IRS-1 was chronically activated in CUG-SGA, even upon insulin stimulation. The expression of p-AKT increased profoundly after *GHR* inhibition, suggesting that GH signaling may impede the signal transduction of the IRS-1-AKT pathway. Thus, we conclude that GH can affect IRS-1-AKT signal transduction in SGA with CUG. A previous study demonstrated that silencing of the *GHR* gene could ameliorate insulin sensitivity in mice fed high fat diets, decrease the content of triglyceride in muscle and liver, and increase IL-15 levels [17]. Our findings further confirm that GH signaling may impair the metabolic axis.

We investigated another signal pathway, MAPK-ERK, and did not find profound differences in the expression of p-ERK upon insulin stimulation before or after GH inhibition in the AGA group. These results demonstrate that ERK is activated mainly by insulin stimulation in AGA animals under physiological conditions, but not GH signaling. These observations are in accordance with a previous study which indicated that GH signaling could not activate the ERK pathway [18]. The activity of ERK in response to *GHR* inhibition in the CUG-SGA group was similar to that of p-IRS-1, implying the IRS-1-ERK axis may be only slightly influenced or not influenced by GH signaling. In summary, two signaling pathways were affected by *GHR* inhibition: 1) GH signaling may influence the signal transduction of IRS-1-AKT and 2) the MAPK-ERK pathway may be activated to promote growth by chronic insulin stimulation.

SOCS3, described as a suppressor of cytokine signaling, can be activated through the JAK-STAT pathway by GH, insulin or cytokines [19,20]. SOCS3 competitively inhibits the activation of signaling proteins and is degraded by ubiquitin-mediated proteasomal degradation *in vitro*, thus negatively regulating the insulin signaling pathway [21]. Therefore, high level of SOCS3 expression is closely associated with insulin resistance [22]. In our study, the expression of SOCS3 was significantly increased under baseline conditions in the CUG-SGA and NCUG-SGA groups. SOCS3 expression was greatly reduced after *GHR* inhibition in the

CUG-SGA group, and this was accompanied by enhanced activation of IRS-1 and AKT. This demonstrates that GH may inhibit the IRS-PI3K-AKT signaling pathway through up-regulation of SOCS3. In SOCS3-silenced hepatocytes, the expression of IRS-1 and PI3K were both elevated, suggesting an important role for SOCS3 in regulating the IRS-PI3K-AKT pathway [23]. The mice of SOCS3 specifically deleted (SOCS MKO) showed enhanced skeletal muscle insulin receptor substrate 1 (IRS-1) and AKT phosphorylation [24]. Our present study further confirms this hypothesis using *in vivo* tissue samples.

In conclusion, our current study demonstrates that SGA rats with CUG exhibit increased insulin resistance. Moreover, insulin resistance in CUG-SGA rats is associated with impairment of the IRS-1-PI3K-AKT signaling pathway, which results from GH signaling-induced upregulation of SOCS3 expression.

Acknowledgments

The authors thank Professor Ke Han, PhD for his expert advice in statistical analysis.

Author Contributions

Conceived and designed the experiments: HZD HD MLD. Performed the experiments: HZD HD. Analyzed the data: HZD HD MLD. Wrote the paper: HZD HD. Literature search: HD CQC KYC.

References

1. Rotteveel J, van Weissenbruch MM, Twisk JW, Delemarre-Van de Waal HA (2008) Infant and childhood growth patterns, insulin sensitivity, and blood pressure in prematurely born young adults. Pediatrics 122:313–321.
2. Varvarigou AA (2010) Intrauterine growth restriction as a potential risk factor for disease onset in adulthood. J Pediatr Endocrinol Metab 23:215–224.
3. Hofman PL, Regan F, Jackson WE, Jefferies C, Knight DB, et al. (2004) Premature birth and later insulin resistance. N Engl J Med 351:2179–2186.
4. Hovi P, Andersson S, Eriksson JG, Jarvenpaa AL, Strang-Karlsson S, et al. (2007) Glucose regulation in young adults with very low birth weight. N Engl J Med 356:2053–2063.
5. Irving RJ, Belton NR, Elton RA, Walker BR (2000) Adult cardiovascular risk factors in premature babies. Lancet 355:2135–2136.
6. Deng HZ, Li YH, Su Z, Ma HM, Huang YF, et al. (2011) Association between height and weight catch-up growth with insulin resistance in pre-pubertal Chinese children born small for gestational age at two different ages. Eur J Pediatr 170:75–80.
7. Deng HZ, Deng H, Ma HM, Shen ZY, Du ML (2011) Changes of somatotropin axis in catch-up growth rats born small for gestational age. Chinese Journal of Pathophysiology 27:1360–1365. (in Chinese)
8. Moller N, Jorgensen JO (2009) Effects of growth hormone on glucose, lipid, and protein metabolism in human subjects. Endocr Rev 30:152–177.
9. Xu J, Messina JL (2009) Crosstalk between growth hormone and insulin signaling. Vitam Horm 80:125–153.
10. Dominici FP, Argentino DP, Munoz MC, Miquet JG, Sotelo AI, et al. (2005) Influence of the crosstalk between growth hormone and insulin signalling on the modulation of insulin sensitivity. Growth Horm IGF Res 15:324–336.
11. Huang TT, Du M, Kuluz JW, Li Y, Ma H (2008) Postreceptor crosstalk on PI3K/Akt between GH and insulin in non-catch-up growth rats born small for gestational age. Horm Res 70:29–35.
12. Matthews DR, Hosker JP, Rudenski AS, Naylor BA, Treacher DF, et al. (1985) Homeostasis model assessment: insulin resistance and beta-cell function from fasting plasma glucose and insulin concentrations in man. Diabetologia 28:412–419.
13. Dulloo AG, Jacquet J, Montani JP (2002) Pathways from weight fluctuations to metabolic diseases: focus on maladaptive thermogenesis during catch-up fat. Int J Obes Relat Metab Disord 26 Suppl 2:S46–57.
14. Shirakami A, Toyonaga T, Tsuruzoe K, Shirotani T, Matsumoto K, et al. (2002) Heterozygous knockout of the IRS-1 gene in mice enhances obesity-linked insulin resistance: a possible model for the development of type 2 diabetes. J Endocrinol 174:309–319.
15. De Blasio MJ, Gatford KL, Harland ML, Robinson JS, Owens JA (2012) Placental restriction reduces insulin sensitivity and expression of insulin signaling and glucose transporter genes in skeletal muscle, but not liver, in young sheep. Endocrinology 153:2142–2151.
16. Vuguin P, Raab E, Liu B, Barzilai N, Simmons R (2004) Hepatic insulin resistance precedes the development of diabetes in a model of intrauterine growth retardation. Diabetes 53:2617–2622.
17. Vijayakumar A, Wu Y, Sun H, Li X, Jeddy Z, et al. (2012) Targeted loss of GHR signaling in mouse skeletal muscle protects against high-fat diet-induced metabolic deterioration. Diabetes 61:94–103.
18. Jorgensen JO, Jessen N, Pedersen SB, Vestergaard E, Gormsen L, et al. (2006) GH receptor signaling in skeletal muscle and adipose tissue in human subjects following exposure to an intravenous GH bolus. Am J Physiol Endocrinol Metab 291:E899–905.
19. Croker BA, Kiu H, Nicholson SE (2008) SOCS regulation of the JAK/STAT signalling pathway. Semin Cell Dev Biol 19:414–422.
20. Peraldi P, Filloux C, Emanuelli B, Hilton DJ, Van Obberghen E (2001) Insulin induces suppressor of cytokine signaling-3 tyrosine phosphorylation through janus-activated kinase. J Biol Chem 276:24614–24620.
21. Fasshauer M, Kralisch S, Klier M, Lossner U, Bluher M, et al. (2004) Insulin resistance-inducing cytokines differentially regulate SOCS mRNA expression via growth factor- and Jak/Stat-signaling pathways in 3T3-L1 adipocytes. J Endocrinol 181:129–138.
22. Emanuelli B, Peraldi P, Filloux C, Chavey C, Freidinger K, et al. (2001) SOCS-3 inhibits insulin signaling and is up-regulated in response to tumor necrosis factor-alpha in the adipose tissue of obese mice. J Biol Chem 276: 47944–47949.
23. Ye J, Zheng R, Wang Q, Liao L, Ying Y, et al. (2012) Downregulating SOCS3 with siRNA ameliorates insulin signaling and glucose metabolism in hepatocytes of IUGR rats with catch-up growth. Pediatr Res 72:550–559.
24. Jorgensen SB, O'Neill HM, Sylow L, Honeyman J, Hewitt KA, et al. (2013) Deletion of skeletal muscle SOCS3 prevents insulin resistance in obesity. Diabetes 62:56–64.

7

AT1 Receptor Blockade Attenuates Insulin Resistance and Myocardial Remodeling in Rats with Diet-Induced Obesity

Silvio A. Oliveira-Junior[1,2]*, Paula F. Martinez[1,2], Danielle M. Guizoni[1], Dijon H. S. Campos[1], Tiago Fernandes[3], Edilamar M. Oliveira[3], Marina P. Okoshi[1], Katashi Okoshi[1], Carlos R. Padovani[4], Antonio C. Cicogna[1]

1 Botucatu Medical School, São Paulo State University, Botucatu, Brazil, **2** School of Physiotherapy, Federal University of Mato Grosso do Sul, Campo Grande, Brazil, **3** School of Physical Education and Sport, University of São Paulo, São Paulo, Brazil, **4** Botucatu Biosciences Institute, São Paulo State University, Botucatu, Brazil

Abstract

Background: Although obesity has been associated with metabolic and cardiac disturbances, the carrier mechanisms for these responses are poorly understood. This study analyzed whether angiotensin II blockade attenuates metabolic and cardiovascular disorders in rats with diet-induced obesity.

Material and Methods: Wistar-Kyoto (n = 40) rats were subjected to control (C; 3.2 kcal/g) and hypercaloric diets (OB; 4.6 kcal/g) for 30 weeks. Subsequently, rats were distributed to four groups: C, CL, OB, and OBL. L groups received Losartan (30 mg/kg/day) for five weeks. After this period we performed in vivo glucose tolerance and insulin tolerance tests, and measured triacylglycerol, insulin, angiotensin-converting enzyme activity (ACE), and leptin levels. Cardiovascular analyzes included systolic blood pressure (SBP), echocardiography, myocardial morphometric study, myosin heavy chain composition, and measurements of myocardial protein levels of angiotensin, extracellular signal-regulated (ERK1/2), c-Jun amino-terminal kinases (JNK), insulin receptor subunit β (βIR), and phosphatidylinositol 3-kinase (PI3K) by Western Blot.

Results: Glucose metabolism, insulin, lipid, and ACE activity disorders observed with obesity were minimized by Losartan. Moreover, obesity was associated with increased SBP, myocardial hypertrophy, interstitial fibrosis and improved systolic performance; these effects were also minimized with Losartan. On a molecular level, OB exhibited higher ERK, *Tyr*-phosphorylated βIR, and PI3K expression, and reduced myocardial angiotensin and JNK expression. ERK and JNK expression were regulated in the presence of Losartan, while angiotensin, *Tyr-βR*I, total and *Tyr*-phosphorylated PI3K expression were elevated in the OBL group.

Conclusion: Angiotensin II blockade with Losartan attenuates obesity-induced metabolic and cardiovascular changes.

Editor: Michael Bader, Max-Delbrück Center for Molecular Medicine (MDC), Germany

Funding: Grant support: FAPESP (#08/55339-4) - www.fapesp.br. The funds were used to purchase consumables needed for research development. The funders had no role in study design, data collection and analysis, decision to publish, or preparation of the manuscript.

Competing Interests: The authors have declared that no competing interests exist.

* E-mail: oliveirajr.ufms@gmail.com

Introduction

Cardiac remodeling consists of many adaptive alterations to the heart aimed at maintaining myocardial performance in response to stress conditions, including mechanical and volumetric overload [1]. This process is particularly common in obesity [2] and is characterized by time-dependent evolution involving several adaptive changes which are clinically represented by changes in cardiac shape, size, and function [1,3]. Experimental evidence has shown that diet-induced obesity is associated with cardiac remodeling, substantiated by contractile disturbances [4–8], hypertrophy [4–9], interstitial fibrosis [5,7], and molecular expression changes in contractile proteins including myosin heavy chain (MyHC) β isoform synthesis [5,7], and endocrine disturbances such as insulin and glucose metabolism disorders [6–9].

Several molecular signaling pathways can mediate cardiac remodeling in obesity, including parietal deformation, cytokines, and growth factors [10]. As a result, differential mechanisms can interact in multiple points of the cytosol supporting the development of molecular *cross-talk* during the cardiac remodeling progress [10]. Recently, several studies have shown important forms of molecular interaction between the signal transmission pathways that mediate insulin and angiotensin II (ANG II) actions in the heart [11–14]. Insulin actions are highly regulated by many factors, including a large number of endocrine, inflammatory, neural, and cell-intrinsic agents, which have been shown to be dysregulated in obesity [14]. In general, regulatory mechanisms attenuate metabolic signaling from insulin stimuli by decreasing tyrosine-phosphorylation of proteins members from insulin pathway, including insulin receptor β subunit (Rβ) and phosphatidylinositol 3-kinase (PI3K) messenger [15]. Consequently, insulin resistance is a common pathological state in which target cells fail to respond to normal stimuli from circulating insulin [15–17]. Obesity-associated insulin resistance is a major risk factor for type 2 diabetes and cardiovascular disease [17].

ANG II actions are initiated through interaction with G-protein coupled receptors, especially, the ANG II type 1 receptor (AT1R) [14]. As well as coupling with the heterotrimeric G proteins, tyrosine kinase activation is intimately involved in AT1R receptor signaling [10,14]. Both non-receptor type tyrosine kinases [Src, Fyn, Yes, Pyk2, focal adhesion kinase, and Janus kinase 2] and receptor-type tyrosine kinases (epidermal growth factor and platelet-derived growth factor receptors) are activated by AT1R [11,14]. These tyrosine kinases regulate downstream signaling mechanisms, including mitogen-activated protein kinase (MAPK) cascades, with activation of MAPK subtypes *extracellular signal-regulated kinase* (ERK) and *c-Jun N-terminal kinase* (JNK), thereby playing a critical role in ANG II cardiac remodeling actions [18]. Parallel to its effects on cardiac muscle, AT1R activation also affects metabolic actions from insulin, such as protein degradation and/or inhibition of tyrosine-phosphorylation of Rβ, insulin receptor substrate (IRS), and PI3K messenger [14,16]. Therefore, activation states of the renin-angiotensin system contribute to AT1R stimulation and may support the occurrence of remodeling and insulin resistance in the heart [17].

As obesity is a metabolic condition characterized by chronic activation of the renin-angiotensin system [19–25], in this study we evaluated whether MAPK cascade activation by AT1R stimulation is associated with myocardial remodeling and has an inhibitory effect on tyrosine phosphorylation of insulin cascade proteins in hearts of obese rats. Although this possible cross-talk has not been clarified in studies with experimental diet-induced obesity models, our initial hypothesis is that obesity is associated with AT1R and MAPK activation and, as consequence, cardiac remodeling and insulin cascade inhibition due to tyrosine phosphorylation reduction of key insulin pathway messengers in the myocardium.

Materials and Methods

Experimental design, metabolic and biometry characterization

The experimental protocol was approved by the Ethics Committee on Experiments of Botucatu Medical School, Sao Paulo State University, in accordance with US National Institutes of Health "Guide for the Care and Use of Laboratory Animals" (NIH Publication No. 85–23, revised 1996) [26].

Male 60-day-old *Wistar-Kyoto* rats (n = 40) were randomly distributed into two groups: Control (C) and Obese (OB). Group C received commercial rat chow (RC Focus 1765) and OB received a palatable hypercaloric diet [4] for 30 weeks. After this period, animals were assigned to four groups: Control (C); Control with Losartan intervention (CL), Obese (OB), and Obese with Losartan intervention (OBL). In addition to their feeding program, CL and OBL groups received 30 mg/kg/day Losartan in their drinking water for an additional five weeks. Age matched animals from C and OB groups continued to receive respective dietary support for the corresponding period. Animals were individually housed under controlled conditions of 22–24°C, 50–70%RH, and time-controlled 12-hour light/dark cycles. All animals had free access to water and chow (50 g/d). Food consumption was measured daily and water intake and body weight (BW) were evaluated once a week. Weekly calorie intake was calculated: average weekly food consumption × diet energy density. Feed efficiency - the ability to convert calorie intake into BW - was determined by: mean BW gain (g)/total calorie intake (Kcal).

The hypercaloric diet model consisted of five different palatable diets (HD1, HD2, HD3, HD4, and HD5) which were prepared from a mixture of industrialized products and supplementary ingredients added to commercial rat chow. These diets were alternately administered, with each chow type offered for seven days. Dietary composition was analyzed by the Animal Nutrition and Improvement Laboratory, School of Agricultural Sciences, UNESP and was as detailed in a previous study [4].

Hypercaloric diets were isocaloric with ~30% more energetic content than the standard commercial rat chow (4.6 Kcal/g vs 3.2 Kcal/g); HD2 and HD4 were richer in lipids only, HD1 and HD5 also had an important carbohydrate content, especially sucrose. Although HD3 had similar energetic density (4.5 Kcal/g) to the other hypercaloric diets, its composition was mainly based on surplus sucrose from water solution. This diet model is similar to many other interventions used in studies on diet-induced obesity [4–8].

After the 35 week experimental period, GTT and ITT were realized in all animals.

To make the GTT, animals were maintained in 12–15h fasting. Subsequently, a blood sample was collected from the tip of the tail in a heparinized tube. Blood glycemia (basal condition) level for each animal was immediately determined using a handheld glucometer (Accuchek Advantage; Roche Diagnostics Co., Indianapolis, IN). Then, an injection of 2 g/kg glucose (Sigma-Aldrich1, St Louis, MO, USA) was given intraperitoneally. Blood glycemia levels were measured after 30, 60, 90, 120, 180, and 240 min [8].

For ITT, rats were fasted for 6 h before submission to insulin tolerance test. After determination of basal glycemia condition, 1.5 IU/kg insulin (Novolin® R, Novo Nordisk, Bagsvaerd, Denmark) was infused intraperitoneally and glucose measured 5, 10, 15, 20, 25, and 30 min thereafter [27].

After 12-15h fasting, animals were anesthetized with sodium pentobarbital (50 mg/kg) and euthanized by decapitation. Animals were thoracotomized and adipose depots (AD) from visceral, retroperitoneal, and epidydimal sites were measured. The adiposity index (%) was obtained from the sum of the weights of individual fat pads: $\Sigma AD \times 100/BW$ [28].

Trunk blood was collected and centrifuged at 3000 g for 15 min at 4°C. Serum was separated by centrifugation at 3000 g for 15 minutes at 48°C and stored at −80°C until further analysis. Serum fractions of glucose, cholesterol, and triacylglycerol were measured with an automatic enzymatic analyzer system (Technicon, RA-XT™ System, Global Medical Instrumentation, Minnesota, USA) and enzyme kits (Kovalent Diagnosis, Rio de Janeiro/RJ, Brazil). Serum concentrations of non-esterified fatty acid (NEFA) were determined as per Johnson and Peters [29] using colorimetric kits (WAKO, Wako Pure Chemical Industries, Osaka, Japan). Serum leptin and insulin concentrations were determined by ELISA using commercial kits (Linco Research Inc., St. Louis, MO, USA).

The insulin metabolism was studied using the homeostatic model assessment index (HOMA-IR) calculated by the following formula: HOMA-IR = ¼[fasting GL (mmol/l) fasting insulin (mU/ml)]/22.5 [30]. All rats ate normally and regained their body weight within 1 d after this regimen. ACE activity in rat serum and tissue extracts were determined using Abz-FRK(Dnp)P-OH derivatives as substrates by continuously measuring fluorescence according to previous studies [31,32].

Cardiovascular study

At the end of the experiment (35 weeks), systolic blood pressure (SBP) was measured by the non-invasive tail-cuff method with a Narco BioSystems® Electro-Sphygmomanometer (International Biomedical, Austin, TX, USA) [33]. The average of two readings was recorded for each animal. To analyze in vivo heart structure and performance, all animals were weighed and evaluated via transthoracic echocardiographic examination performed with a commercially available echocardiography machine (Sonos 5500, Philips, Andover, MA, USA) equipped with a 12-MHz phased array transducer. All measurements were obtained by the same observer using the method recommended by the American Society of Echocardiography [34].

For morphometric analysis, myocardial samples were fixed with a 10% formol solution for 48 h and then embedded in paraffin blocks. Histological sections (7 μm) stained with hematoxylin-eosin were used to measure cardiomyocyte cross-sectional area (CSA); determined for at least 100 myocytes per slide [35]. Major and minor nuclear diameters were also measured to determination nuclear volume [36]; fifty nuclei from each animal were measured. Nuclear volume (V) was estimated using the formula for a prolate ellipsoid: $V = \pi AB^2/6$; where A is the major diameter and B the minor diameter [36].

Collagen interstitial fraction was determined by Picrosirius red staining of myocardium sections, analyzed under polarized light. Histological images were obtained using a LEICA DM LS microscope at 40× magnification coupled to a computer equipped with *Image Pro-plus*, an image analysis program (Media Cybernetics, Silver Spring, Maryland, USA).

MyHC isoform analysis was performed in duplicate by sodium dodecyl sulfate polyacrylamide gel electrophoresis. Sample preparation methods and electrophoresis conditions are detailed in a previous study [4]. Myocardial tissue protein levels were analyzed by Western blot. Sample preparation methods and electrophoresis conditions are detailed in Martinez et al. [37]. Western blot analysis was performed using antibodies against angiotensin (sc-7419), ERK (sc-93), JNK (sc-137019), β subunit of insulin receptor (Rβ; sc-711), $Tyr^{1162/1163}$ phosphorylated Rβ (sc-25103), PI 3-kinase subunit p85α (sc-1637), and Tyr^{508} phosphorylated PI 3-kinase p85α (sc-12929), purchased from Santa Cruz Biotechnology, Inc. (Santa Cruz, CA). Protein levels were normalized to those of GAPDH (6C5, sc-32233, Santa Cruz Biotechnology).

Statistical analysis

Nutritional, metabolic, and cardiovascular variables were evaluated by two-way ANOVA. When significant differences were found ($p<0.05$), the *post hoc* Tukey's multiple comparisons test for parametric, or Dunn's test for non-parametric distributions was performed. Level of significance was considered to be 5%.

Results

Although nutritionally, obesity has been associated with low calorie intake, OB groups exhibited higher feed efficiency, BW, and adiposity values compared to their respective Controls ($p<0.01$). Moreover, obesity *per se*, was also accompanied by elevated cholesterol, insulin, and insulin resistance levels, and leptinaemia. Also, obesity was characterized by higher triacylglycerol, NEFA and ACE activity leptinaemia as well as impaired glycemic tolerance, as seen by larger glycemic response AUC's in OB (Table 1) and by increased GTT glucose levels (Figure 1A).

Although C and OB showed similar responses in ITT (Figure 1B), obesity was independently associated with higher AUC responses ($p=0.03$; Table 1). With the exception of enzymatic activity and ITT, CL and OBL groups did not present differences in relation to metabolic and hormonal variables. Specifically, NEFA and ACE activity sustained obesity and Losartan interaction ($p<0.05$) while OB animals exhibited higher NEFA and ACE glycemic responses than C; Losartan attenuated these effects in OBL. Losartan independently reduced insulin values and HOMA-IR at both comparison levels (CL versus C and OBL versus OB; Table 1).

Taking into account *in-vivo* cardiovascular parameters, diet-induced obesity has been associated with increased systolic blood pressure, as seen between the non-medicated groups ($p<0.05$). Also, echocardiographic analysis showed lower left ventricular end-systolic diameter (LVESd) values, accompanied by higher interventricular septum diastolic thickness (IVST), posterior wall diastolic thickness (PWT), and left ventricle relative thickness in OB compared to C. Importantly, SBP, heart rate, IVST, and PWT values were lower with the medication, although the morphological differences in IVST and PWT were maintained between CL and OBL. Left ventricle relative thickness was similar between L groups (Table 2).

With respect to heart performance, endocardial fractional shortening (EFS), ejection fraction, and posterior wall shortening velocity (PWSV) were higher in OB than C. With the exception of PWSV, these alterations were attenuated by the Losartan, as CL and OBL presented similar systolic function results. In regard to diastolic performance, obesity reduced left ventricle isovolumetric relaxation time (IVRT) in absolute values and in relation to heart rate R-R interval ($IVRT/R\text{-}R^{0.5}$). Losartan treatment reduced IVRT and E/A indexes in both L groups, maintaining similar results between CL and OBL groups (Table 2).

Post-mortem exam revealed a significant interaction between the condition and medication with respect to cardiomyocyte cross-sectional area ($p=0.034$) and nuclear volume ($p<0.001$). Obesity increased cardiomyocyte cross-sectional area (C 269±12; OB 332±23; CL 292±9; OBL 290±10 μm^2) and nuclear volume (C 6.56±0.54; OB 21.61±1.65; CL 7.26±0.70; OBL 9.32±0.81 μm^3), demonstrated by OB compared to C (Figure 2A and 2B). Losartan administration reduced cross-sectional area and nuclear volume in OBL compared to OB.

In relation to interstitial collagen volume fraction (C 2.89±0.81; OB 4.81±0.41; CL 1.89±0.61; OBL 4.46±0.73%), obesity, as an independent factor, promoted interstitial fibrosis ($p<0.001$), while losartan, independently, attenuated collagen deposition in both medicated groups ($p=0.002$; Figure 2C). Also, β/α MyHC ratio (C 0.49±0.08; OB 1.12±0.45; CL 0.73±0.12; OBL 1.16±0.32) and β MyHC content (C 33.0±3.5; OB 51.1±9.8; CL 41.8±3.8; OBL 52.8±7.9%) were higher in both obese groups ($p<0.001$; Figure 3A, B, and C). Also, AT1R blockade on its own reduced interstitial collagen fraction, but did not change β MHC content in the L groups.

In regard to molecular responses, total protein expression of angiotensin (C 1.00±0.09; OB 0.66±0.11AU; $p<0.05$) and JNK (C 1.00±0.07; OB 0.55±0.06AU; $p<0.05$) were lower and ERK (C 1.00±0.13; OB 1.73±0.05AU; $p<0.05$) was higher in OB than C. As an independent factor, Losartan reduced angiotensin expression in both L groups ($p<0.05$; CL 0.62±0.04; OBL 0.56±0.10AU). With respect to MAPK, Losartan normalized obesity effects, as ERK (CL 1.07±0.07; OBL 1.23±0.20AU) and JNK (CL 0.74±0.13; OBL 0.87±0.17AU) expression values were similar ($p<0.05$) in CL and OBL groups (Figure 4).

Also, although total Rβ expression was unchanged with obesity, OB exhibited higher Rβ expression in *Tyr*-phosphorylated form; importantly, Losartan increased *Tyr-phospho*-Rβ form expression in both L groups (C 1.00±0.15; OB 1.61±0.29; CL 1.87±0.23;

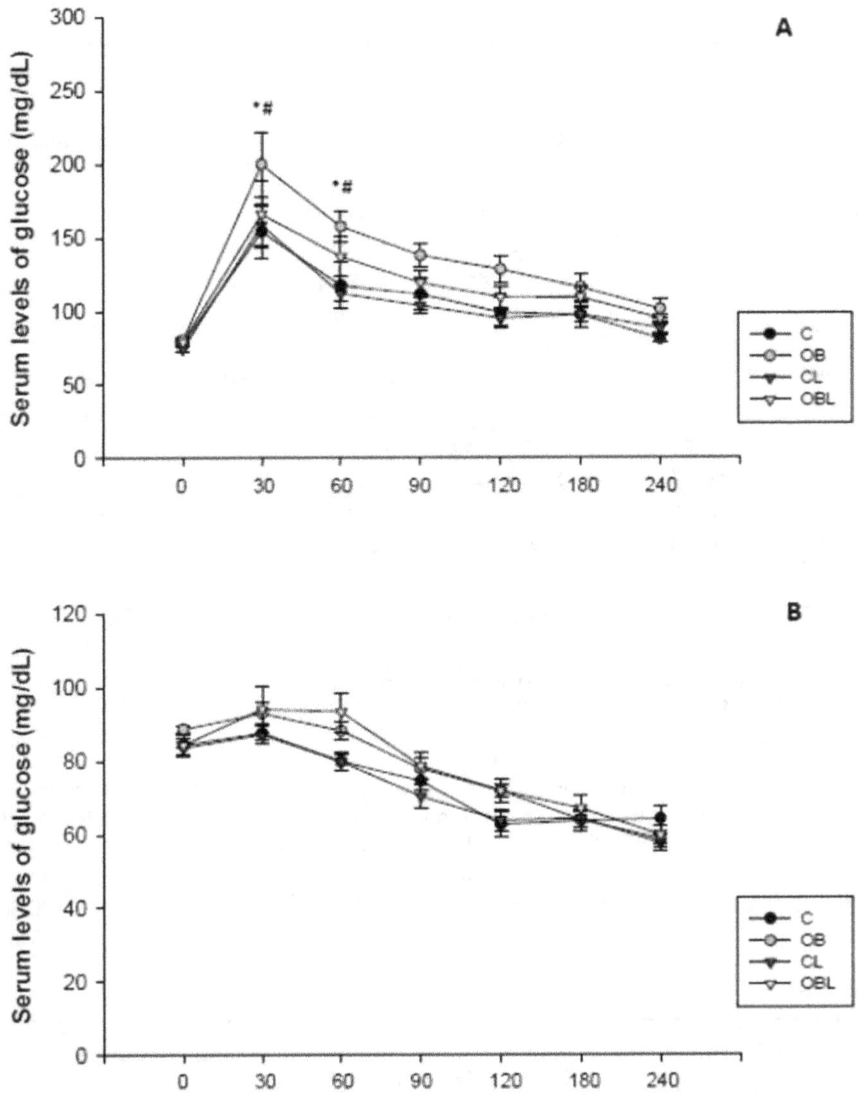

Figure 1. Serum glycemic levels following intraperitoneal glucose loads in (A) glucose tolerance test (GTT) and (B) insulin tolerance test; Data are expressed as means±SE; C: control group; CL: control group treated with losartan; OB: obese group; OBL: obese group treated with losartan; * p<0.05, OB vs. C group; #p<0.05, OB vs. OBL group; Repeated measures ANOVA and Bonferroni's test.

OBL 2.32±0.20AU; Figure 5). Obesity was also associated with higher total PI3-kinase expression (C 1.00±0.15; OB 1.23±0.06; CL 1.01±0.14; OBL 1.68±0.25AU); however *Tyr-phospho*-PI3-kinase expression remained unchanged with obesity (C 1.00±0.39; OB 0.90±0.07; CL 1.71±0.26; OBL 2.11±0.39AU). Losartan independently increased total PI3-kinase expression in OBL and improved *Tyr-phospho*-PI3-kinase expression in both medicated groups (Figure 6).

Discussion

Our initial hypothesis stated that obesity is associated with metabolic and cardiovascular disorders, including remodeling and insulin resistance in the heart. Our results confirmed the occurrence of several abnormalities including metabolic and endocrine disturbances as well as cardiovascular effects common to the present experimental model [4–8]. These effects were associated with MAPK activation and biochemical evidence of insulin resistance in the myocardium under the diet-induced obesity condition; importantly, a substantial part of these disorders were minimized with Losartan administration.

Obesity was induced by hypercaloric intervention with enhanced fatty acid content, including unsaturated and saturated lipids combined with sucrose overload, similar to a cafeteria diet [4]. Biometrically, both OB groups consisted of obese animals with higher body weight and adiposity values compared to their control counterparts. These effects were directly associated with improved feed efficiency in the OB groups although their calorie intake was lower (Table 1). Although this result is at variance with previous studies, the "hypophagia" observed with obesity may be due to the high serum leptin level (Table 1). Leptin, a hormone synthesized and secreted by adipose tissue, is mainly involved in the regulation of appetite and energy metabolism [38]. Particularly, the concept of selective leptin resistance might explain in part how hyperleptinemia could be accompanied by loss of appetite in the obese animals, despite body weight and adiposity levels in the OB

Table 1. Nutritional and endocrine evaluation.

	Groups				Factors (p-value)		
Variable	C	OB	CL	OBL	Condition	Medication	Interaction
Calorie intake(Kcal)	84.0±3.5	67.3±5.7**	84.2±5.2	68.6±8.7††	<0.001	0.687	0.772
Feed efficiency(mg/Kcal)	11.3±1.7	19.6±2.9**	11.3±1.8	19.1±3.3††	<0.001	0.783	0.718
Body weight(g)	557±44	645±45**	549±44	637±56††	<0.001	0.597	0.988
Adiposity(%)	5.9±1.0	12.0±2.3**	6.4±1.3	11.3±2.3††	<0.001	0.946	0.321
Cholesterol(mg/dl)	100.1±21.1	122.2±7.7**	113.3±10.9*	125.6±12.1†	<0.001	0.065	0.267
Triacylglycerol(mg/dl)	95±28	122±35*	96±19	102±17	0.050	0.278	0.211
NEFA(ng/dl)	0.32±0.03	0.44±0.08**	0.41±0.04**	0.39±0.07#	0.004	0.354	<0.001
Glucose(mg/dl)	126.8±21.3	139.9±15.9	145.3±22.6	102.3±16.6†#	0.128	0.020	<0.001
GTT(AUC)	26345±7530	34841±5073**	26519±3033	31300±6759	0.019	0.319	0.387
ITT(AUC)	2184±165	2341±144	2182±138	2383±292†	0.017	0.947	0.570
Insulin(ng/dL)	1.64±1.24	2.89±1.17**	1.03±0.67*	2.06±0.62†#	<0.001	0.024	0.722
HOMA-IR	10.2±8.4	18.8±8.4**	6.4±4.4	13.9±4.4†	<0.001	0.046	0.803
Leptin(ng/dL)	5.17±1.10	9.71±1.85**	5.29±1.25	10.27±2.38††	<0.001	0.539	0.683
ACE activity (UF·min^{-1}·mg^{-1}×1000)	90746±8544	101126±9162*	104094±13117*	94490±10252†	0.917	0.370	0.011

Values expressed as mean ± SD; NEFA: non-esterified fatty acid; AUC: area under curve from glucose tolerance test response; HOMA-IR: homeostatic model assessment index; * p<0.05, ** p<0.01 vs. Control (C) group; #p<0.05, ##p<0.01 vs. OB; † p<0.05, †† p<0.01 vs. CL; ANOVA and Tukey test.

groups. Actually, obesity is based on a disturbed energy balance, primarily through increased intake or decreased expenditure of energy [39].

Importantly, Losartan administration did not affect biometric and nutritional performance; comparatively, few studies [9,40–43] have shown the impact of AT1R blockade interventions on biometric profile in rats with diet-induced obesity. Only Rosseli et al. [42] showed that losartan promoted a significant decrease in body weight and adiposity in a 20 week dietary protocol. However, similar to our study, other investigators have shown

Table 2. Blood pressure and echocardiography study.

	Groups				Factors(p-value)		
Variable	C	OB	CL	OBL	Condition	Medication	Interaction
SBP(mmHg)	115±4	124±10*	109±8*	112±14	0.050	0.005	0.410
Heart rate(beats/min)	262±61	270±51	312±57*	306±42	0.925	0.015	0.672
LA(mm)	5.51±0.67	5.54±0.24	5.42±0.88	5.29±0.34	0.790	0.368	0.670
LVEDd(mm)	8.43±0.71	8.20±0.40	8.47±0.42	8.35±0.46	0.288	0.569	0.717
LVESd(mm)	4.58±0.46	4.10±0.48*	4.57±0.39	4.38±0.36	0.017	0.300	0.283
PWT(mm)	1.51±0.04	1.58±0.09*	1.46±0.06	1.5±0.08†	0.003	0.039	1.000
IVST(mm)	1.53±0.04	1.59±0.08*	1.47±0.06*	1.54±0.08#†	0.007	0.009	0.854
LV relative thickness	0.36±0.03	0.39±0.02*	0.35±0.02	0.37±0.03	0.010	0.071	0.857
EFS(%)	45.8±2.3	50.1±4.0*	46.0±4.1	47.4±4.2	0.018	0.300	0.223
Ejection Fraction(ml)	0.84±0.02	0.87±0.03*	0.84±0.03	0.85±0.03	0.022	0.281	0.268
PWSV(mm/s)	34.1±3.0	38.4±3.9*	33.6±2.8	37.9±4.3†	0.002	0.703	0.991
E/A	1.62±0.32	1.58±0.16	1.18±0.41*	1.39±0.32	0.408	0.004	0.213
DTE(ms)	49.5±4.2	50.7±8.5	55.5±2.1	48.4±8.1	0.378	0.581	0.223
IVRT(ms)	36.3±4.1	31.2±3.5**	31.5±4.1*	28.5±2.6 #	0.002	0.004	0.391
IVRT/R-R$^{0.5}$	75.3±12.9	65.8±8.7*	73.6±7.6	64.0±4.0†	0.004	0.577	0.985

Values expressed as mean ± standard deviation; SBP: systolic blood pressure; LA: left atrium diameter; LVEDd: left ventricular end-diastolic diameter; LVESd: left ventricular end-systolic diameter; PWT: posterior wall diastolic thickness of the left ventricle; IVST: interventricular septum diastolic thickness; LV relative thickness: relation between LV posterior wall systolic thickness and LVEDd; EFS: endocardium fraction shortening; PWSV: posterior wall shortening velocity; E/A: ratio between E and A waves evaluated in transmitral flow; DTE: E wave deceleration time; IVRT: LV isovolumetric relaxation time; IVRT/R-R0.5: ratio between IVRT and R-R heart rate interval; * p<0.05, ** p<0.01 vs. Control (C) group; #p<0.05, ##p<0.01 vs. OB; † p<0.05, †† p<0.01 vs. CL; ANOVA and Tukey test.

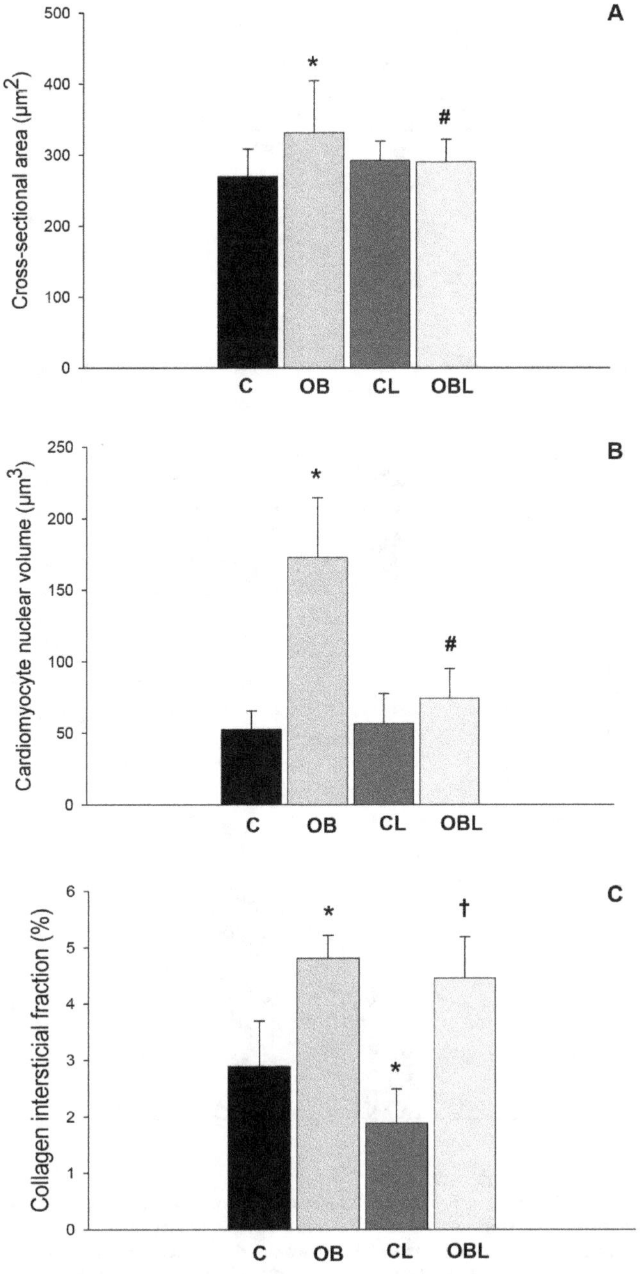

Figure 2. Morphometric analysis of the myocardial tissue; values presented as mean ± standard deviation. (A) Cardiomyocite cross-sectional area (μm^2); (B) cardiomyocyte nuclear volume (μm^3); (C) collagen interstitial fraction (%). C: control group; CL: control group treated with losartan; OB: obese group; OBL: obese group treated with losartan; * p<0.05 vs. C group; #p<0.05 vs. OB group; † p<0.05 vs. CL group; ANOVA and Tukey's test.

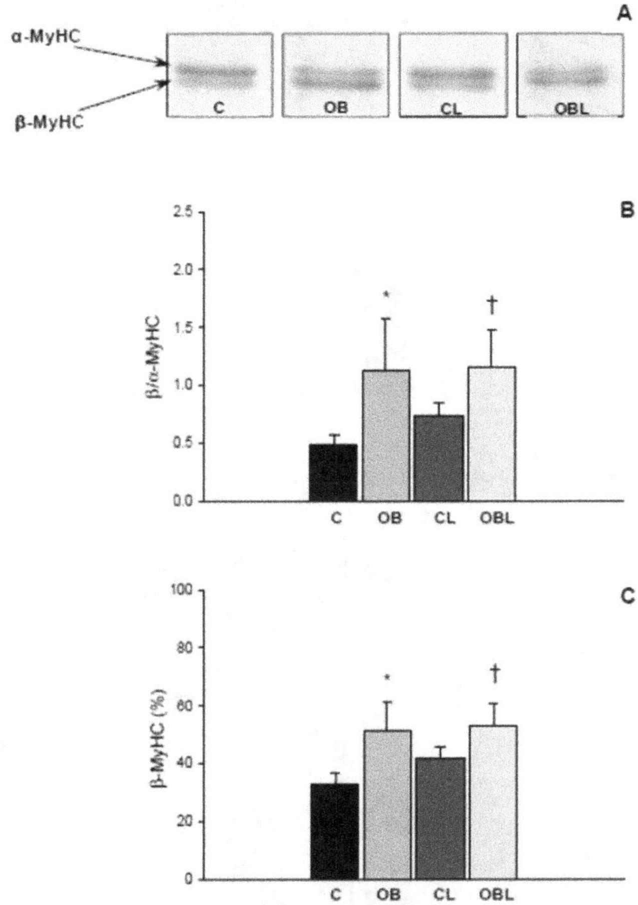

Figure 3. Myosin heavy chain (MyHC) expression in myocardial tissue; values presented as mean ± standard deviation. (A) β- and α-MyHC isoforms of the left ventricle; (B) relative contents (%) of β-MyHC; (C) ratio obtained from relationship between β- and α- MyHC expression. Electrophoresis conditions: sodium duodecyl sulfate polyacrylamide gel electrophoresis to 8%; running: 70 V, 20°C, 30-36 hours; sample concentrations: 10 μg/μl. Products were visualized with Coomassie brilliant blue staining. Band quantification was obtained by product densitometry analysis as integrated optical density. C: control group; CL: control group treated with losartan; OB: obese group; OBL: obese group treated with losartan; * p<0.05 vs. C group; #p<0.05 vs. OB group; † p<0.05 vs. CL group; ANOVA and Tukey's test.

that AT1R blockade at 10 mg/kg/day [40], 20 mg/kg/day [41,43], and 30 mg/kg/day [9] also did not affect nutritional behavior or biometric variables of rats submitted to 10 [41] or 16 week [9,40,43] protocols. In our study in particular, although absolute body weight and adiposity values were altered with AT1R blockade, calorie intake and feed efficiency between the 30th and 35th were reduced with medication. Possibly, the short intervention period (5 weeks) was not long enough to provoke more important modifications in nutritional and biometric profile, despite the substantial AT1R blockade dosage (30 mg/kg/day) used in this experiment.

Our results also showed that obesity, on its own, was associated with several metabolic and endocrine alterations, including dyslipidemia, hyperglycemia, insulin resistance, and hyperleptinaemia. These results and nutritional and biometric effects have been commonly seen in different experimental diet-induced obesity models [4–9,40]. Insulin signaling disorders are associated with metabolic alterations in macronutrients and after hyperinsulinemia [10,15]. Pharmacologically, losartan normalized the glycemia and insulin changes due to obesity, but OBL sustained superior HOMA values and impaired insulin sensitivity, as seen by ITT's AUC in relation to CL. These findings partially support the initial study hypothesis as ANG II configures a heterologous modulator of the insulin pathway [12,14]. Therefore, other agents common to obesity, such as neuroendocrine, inflammatory, and dietary factors [17] could be responsible for these metabolic disturbances in the OBL group.

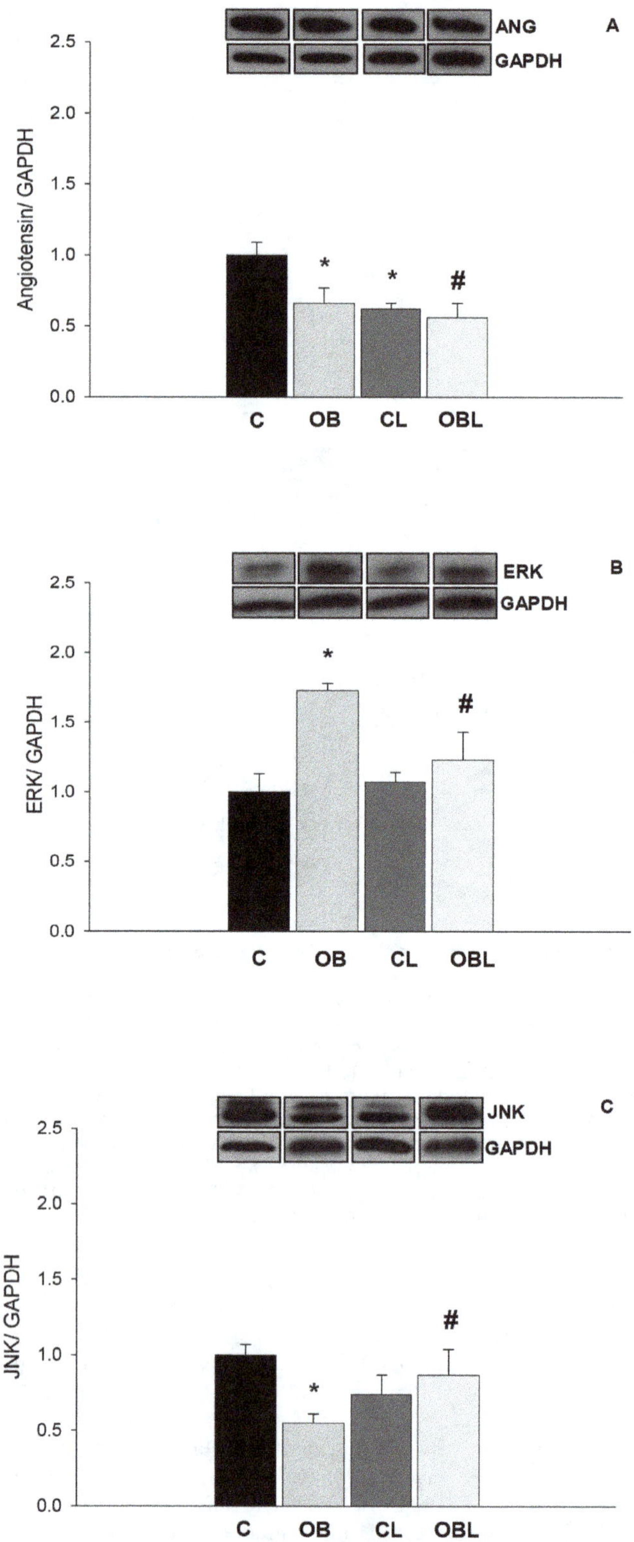

Figure 4. Protein levels of angiotensin and MAPK isoforms in myocardial tissue; values presented as mean ± standard deviation. Protein levels were normalized to GAPDH levels. (A) Angiotensin levels; (B) ERK levels; (C) JNK levels; C (n = 6): control group; CL (n = 6): control group treated with losartan; OB (n = 6): obese group; OBL (n = 6): obese group treated with losartan; * p<0.05 vs. C group; #p<0.05 vs. OB group; ANOVA and Tukey's test.

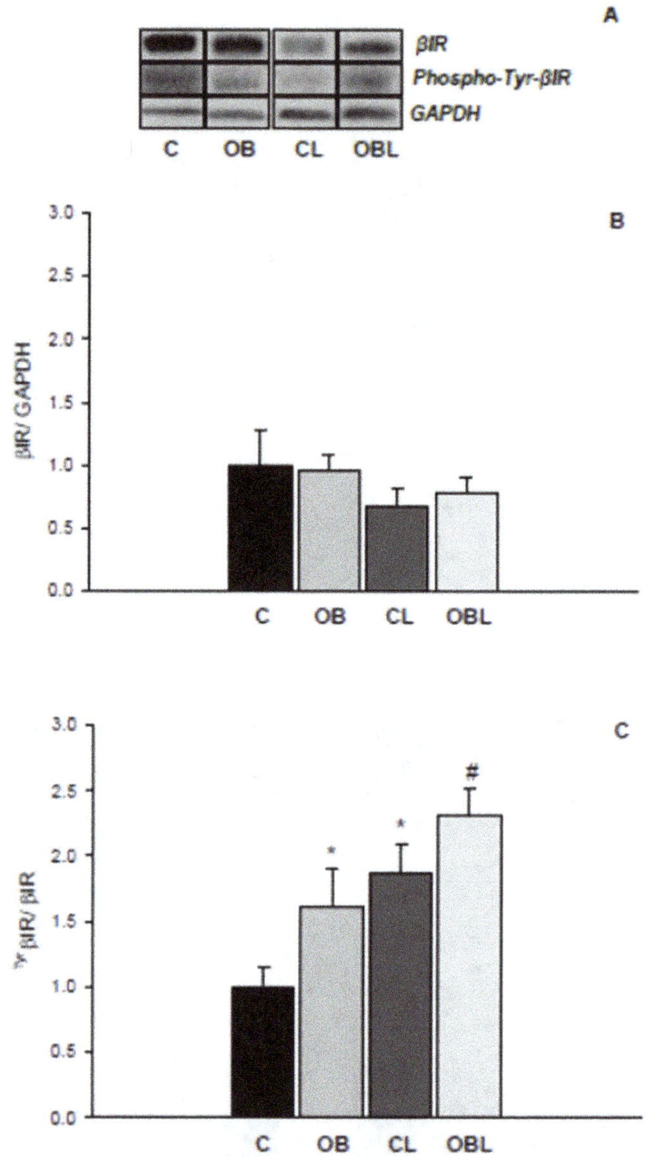

Figure 5. Protein levels of β-subunit of insulin receptor (βIR) in total and tyrosine phosphorylated forms in myocardial tissue; values presented as mean ± standard deviation. Total protein levels were normalized to GAPDH levels. (A) proteins bands for βIR, phosphor-Tyr-βIR and GAPDH; (B) βIR expression values; (C) phospho-Tyr-βIR expression values; C (n = 6): control group; CL (n = 6): control group treated with losartan; OB (n = 6): obese group; OBL (n = 6): obese group treated with losartan; * p<0.05 vs. C group; #p<0.05 vs. OB group; ANOVA and Tukey's test.

The occurrence of high serum cholesterol, triacylglycerol, and non-esterified fatty acid levels in the OB group can be explained by the chronic intake of lipids and sugar associated with renin-angiotensin system activation and insulin resistance in the obesity condition [15,17]. Since ACE activity also increased in obese animals and AT1R antagonism was shown to regulate lipidemic balance in OBL, it is possible to conclude that angiotensin II plays an important role in the occurrence of dyslipidemia in these obese animals. Similar results have been documented in genetic obesity models submitted to AT1R blockade interventions [22–24]. Specifically, in Du Toit et al. [9], AT1R blockade resulted in

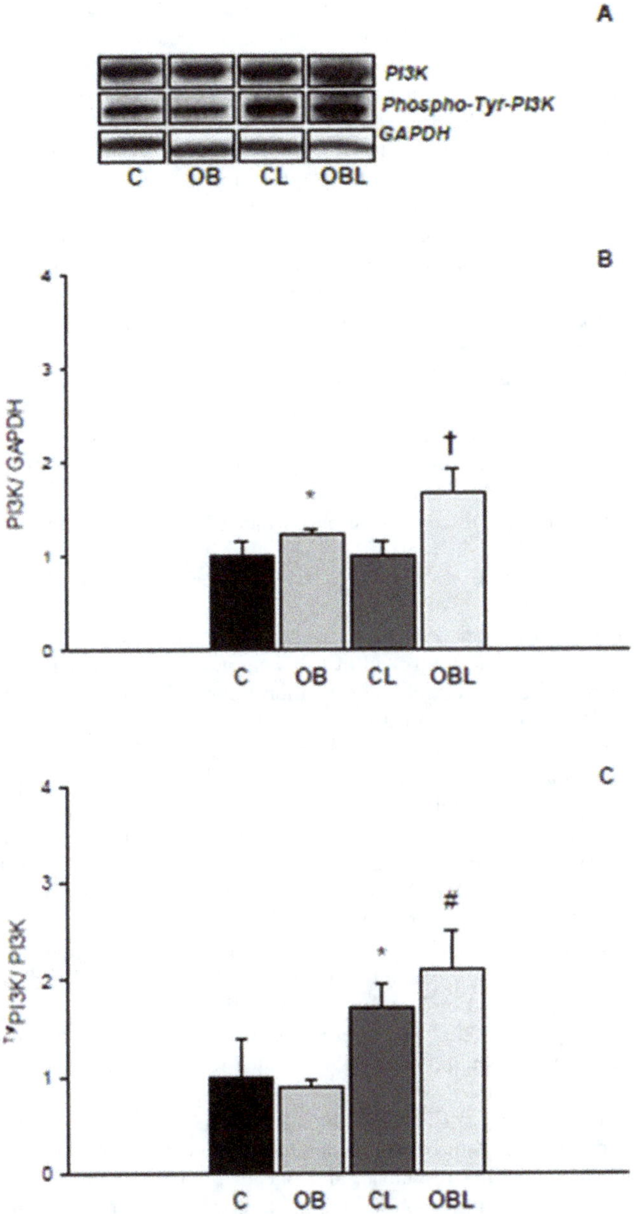

Figure 6. Protein levels of p85α subunit of PI 3-kinase (PI3K) in total and phosphorylated tyrosine forms in myocardial tissue; values presented as mean ± standard deviation. Total protein levels were normalized to GAPDH levels. (A) protein bands for PI3K, phosphor-Tyr-PI3K, and GAPDH; (B) PI3K expression values; (C) phospho-Tyr-PI3K expression values; C (n = 6): control group; CL (n = 6): control group treated with losartan; OB (n = 6): obese group; OBL (n = 6): obese group treated with losartan; * $p<0.05$ vs. C group; #$p<0.05$ vs. OB group; † $p<0.05$ vs. CL group; ANOVA and Tukey's test.

glucose level normalization although it did not change dyslipidemia in rats with cafeteria diet-induced obesity. Differently, cholesterol and leptin levels increased with obesity, but were not affected by losartan administration. Clinical [19,20] and experimental [44] studies have shown that cholesterol levels are generally determined by dietary concentration and are unaffected by AT1R blockade. Leptin is synthetized by adipose tissue and its concentration has been more correlated to the degree of body adiposity in experimental [45] and clinical [46] studies. ACE activity increased in the CL and decreased in OBL in relation to their control counterparts, supporting a significant interaction between obesity and losartan ($p<0.05$). The increased activity in CL could indicate an enzymatic feedback mechanism due to AT1 receptor blockade. However, losartan may be attenuating hepatic formation of angiotensinogen and/or rennin secretion in the kidneys of OBL animals which could reduce angiotensin I formation, and consequently ACE activity [47].

From the cardiovascular aspect, diet-induced obesity was associated with increased systolic blood pressure and some evidence of cardiac remodeling. Many studies have shown that dietary obesity is accompanied by vascular hyperactivity, an important mechanism in the installation of arterial hypertension [17]. Additionally, OB showed greater diastolic interventricular septal, left ventricular posterior diastolic wall, and relative thicknesses, as well as improved endocardium fraction shortening, ejection fraction, and posterior wall shortening velocity in relation to C (Table 2). Concerning contractile performance, systolic performance is related to factors such heart rate, contractility, preload, and afterload [48]. Although obesity did not have an impact on heart rate and LVEDd, increased wall thickness could be preserving or even decreasing cardiac preload; however, decreased preload would lead to reduced left ventricular ejection fraction [46], which was not found. Improved systolic function may therefore have resulted from modified afterload, but more probably from left ventricular hypertrophy. Afterload is a mechanical parameter directly influenced by ventricular pressure and diameter, and inversely related to wall thickness [1]. Persistently increased arterial pressure has been associated with greater afterload, parietal deformation, and cardiac hypertrophy [1,48]. In this context, all the *in vivo* morphological and morphometric evidence are consistent with left ventricular concentric hypertrophy [1,48]. Moreover, obese animals also showed higher collagen interstitial fraction levels and higher β-MyHC isoform expression than the C group. These effects have been associated with severe cardiac remodeling and could be indicative of diastolic dysfunction from a restrictive filling pattern [49]. However, with respect to ventricular performance, biometric condition did not alter diastolic function. A previous study revealed similar results after a 20 week experimental period [7].

Intriguingly, although β-MyHC composition did increase in obesity, left ventricular posterior wall shortening velocity was improved in the OB group. Generally, β-MyHC synthesis is associated with a reduction in myocardial contractile velocity and lower ATPase activity during the contractile cycle [50–52]. This dissociation between MyHC and functional performance results could be derived from factors such as variations in myocardial composition. In this context, previous studies [51,52] have revealed that β-MyHC level is irregular in the heart and is more concentrated in the anterior wall next to papillary muscles. Instead, echocardiographic analysis allows global assessment of cardiac morphology and function without detecting regional differences in contractile performance [53]. These peculiarities can explain the differences between the results of systolic performance and MyHC distribution.

Associated to these alterations, obese animals presented lower angiotensin and MAPK-JNK expression coupled with high MAPK-ERK expression in the myocardium (Figure 3). Reduced angiotensin expression could be indicating increased peptide degradation of protein precursors in cardiac tissue during obesity. This event has been associated with greater ACE-2 activity derived from AT1 stimulation [54]. ACE2 is a new homolog of ACE that favors the degradation of Ang II to Ang (1–7) [54], which is not preferentially detectable with polyclonal antibody (sc-7419). This could therefore possibly support the reduction of intracellular Ang

II levels; however this is only a supposition. Indeed, this process is a potential mechanism for extracellular conversion of the Ang II to Ang (1–7). Importantly, there was increased serum ACE activity in OB and CL groups. Generally, Ang (1–7) binds to Mas receptors and is considered a beneficial peptide of the RAS cascade in the cardiovascular system. ACE2 also cleaves Ang I to Ang (1–9), which is further converted by ACE into Ang (1–7). Acting on Mas receptors, Ang (1–7) might attenuate the actions of the ACE–Ang II–AT1R axis in cytosol [54]. Moreover, cardiac remodeling markers, such as myocardial hypertrophy and interstitial fibrosis, have been associated with elevated gene expression and increased ACE2 activity in the heart of nephrectomized [55] and infarcted rodents [56], and could be present in the OB group.

In relation to MAPK signaling, these proteins can be regulated by several and different molecular agents [18]. While ERK activation is more linked to growth factors and hormonal influence, JNK and p38K are particularly stimulated by mechanical deformation [10,18]. Moreover, when one MAPK subtype is activated, inhibitory mechanisms related to phosphatase action have been shown to modulate the other MAPK subtypes [57]. Therefore, the respective increase in ERK accompanied by reduced JNK expression in our study may be supported by specific activation and inhibition mechanisms of these two MAPK family members. In this aspect, ERK activation could result from cross-talk mechanisms linked to hyperinsulinaemia and AT1R stimulation [12–14,25] as postulated in the initial hypothesis. Growth and remodeling responses to insulin generally involve MAPK signaling pathways with *Shc* binding to the SH2 domain of Grb-2, which results in activation of the pre-associated GTP exchange factor Son of Sevenless (SOS) and GTP-binding protein *Ras*, which phosphorylate/activate MEK, and MAPK-ERK [12]. In support of this proposition, obesity was also related to greater expression of the phosphorylated form of the insulin receptor (Figure 4) and total PI3K (Figure 5), indicating that hyperinsulinaemia induced higher stimulation of the second messengers to insulin action. However, PI3K phosphorylation was not modified with these alterations, suggesting the occurrence of insulin resistance in the heart. Carvalheira et al. [25] documented similar responses the myocardial tissue of Zucker obese rats.

A large number of endocrine, inflammatory, neural, and cell-intrinsic pathways have been shown to be dysregulated in obesity. Although it is possible that one of these factors plays a dominant role, many are interdependent, and it is likely that their dynamic interplay underlies the pathophysiology of insulin resistance [17]. In our study, AT1R blockade administration promoted normalization of the metabolic and cardiovascular disturbances, including cardiac remodeling and insulin resistance, arising from hypercaloric diet-induced obesity. These findings support the occurrence of cross-talk between insulin and AT1R mechanisms from metabolic and cardiovascular perspectives and confirm our initial hypothesis. Cross-talk from heterologous receptor signaling pathways, such as AT1R, exert enhancing effects on these growth/remodeling signaling pathways whilst interfering with the metabolic signaling pathway [14,15].

AT1R activation induces several pleiotropic effects from angiotensin II, such as peripheral vasoconstriction, aldosterone secretion, sodium reabsorption, and arterial hypertension [12]. Therefore, AT1R blockade affects peripheral resistance, increasing blood irrigation in skeletal muscle and improving glycemic metabolism [20,21]. Similar beneficial responses have been described in rodents submitted to fructose overload [45] and cafeteria diet [9], which support the normalization of arterial pressure and glycemic metabolism seen in our OBL group. Moreover, acute or chronic reductions in systolic blood pressure have been associated with adaptive mechanisms destined to control arterial pressure [58]; in this context, heart rate elevation with the Losartan administration, *per se*, could be associated with sympathetic activation conjugated to parasympathetic inhibition through arterial baroreceptors, to compensate for decreased peripheral resistance. As a consequence, E/A, IVRT, and R-R interval were reduced with losartan in both medicated groups. These responses may be related to increased sarcolemmal influx of Ca^{2+} into cytosol and an increase in the rate of adenosine triphosphate (ATP) hydrolysis, with a positive inotropic effect on myocardial performance [48] designed to compensate for AT1R blockade with losartan.

With respect to contractile performance, since systolic function was normalized in the OBL group, it is acceptable that AT1R blockade attenuated the myocardial inotropic effect derived from the endocrine role of adipose tissue, with a consequent reduction in myofibril and sarcomere recruitment; actually, ventricular hypertrophy was controlled in OBL, as supported by macro and microscopic evidence. These morphological and functional findings have been directly associated with MAPK-ERK activation maintained by AT1R stimulation. Similarly, collagen interstitial fraction was reduced with losartan administration even though there are differences between CL and OBL due to the influence of obesity. Several studies have shown that AT1R activation is associated with interstitial fibrosis and that collagen accumulation is directly associated with ventricular hypertrophy [10]. These results support the fact that cardiac remodeling in our experimental model is strongly associated with angiotensin-aldosterone-rennin system activation, although MyHC effects were not affected by losartan administration. In this specific case, other agents, including hyperleptinaemia [17], dietary sucrose, and/or lipids could potentially be related to β-MyHC synthesis in the obese animals.

In conclusion, AT1R blockade attenuated several metabolic and cardiovascular disturbances, including dyslipidemia, glycemic alterations and insulin resistance, and phenotypical responses in myocardial tissue from obese animals. Cardiovascularly, losartan normalized arterial pressure disturbances and molecular mechanisms for manifestation of remodeling and insulin resistance in the heart.

Acknowledgments

The authors would like to thank Mr. José C Georgette, Mr. Mario B Bruno, Mr. Vítor M Souza for their technical assistance, and Colin E. Knaggs for English editing.

Author Contributions

Conceived and designed the experiments: SAOJ PFM MPO ACC. Performed the experiments: SAOJ PFM DMG TF DHSC KO. Analyzed the data: SAOJ CRP ACC. Contributed reagents/materials/analysis tools: EMO MPO KO ACC. Wrote the paper: SAOJ PFM MPO KO.

References

1. Cohn JN, Ferrari R, Sharpe N, Int Forum Cardiac R (2000) Cardiac remodeling-concepts and clinical implications: A consensus paper from an international forum on cardiac remodeling. J Am Coll Cardiol 35(3):569–582.
2. Abel ED, Litwin SE, Sweeney G (2008) Cardiac remodeling in obesity. Physiol Rev 88(2):389–419.
3. Swynghedauw B (2006) Phenotypic plasticity of adult myocardium: molecular mechanisms. J Exp Biol 209(12):2320–2327.

4. Oliveira Junior SA, Dal Pai-Silva M, Martinez PF, Campos DHS, Lima-Leopoldo AP, et al. (2010) Differential nutritional, endocrine, and cardiovascular effects in obesity-prone and obesity-resistant rats fed standard and hypercaloric diets. Med Sci Monit 16(7):BR208–217.
5. Oliveira Junior SA, Dal Pai-Silva M, Martinez PF, Lima-Leopoldo AP, Campos DHS, et al. (2010) Diet-induced obesity causes metabolic, endocrine and cardiac alterations in spontaneously hypertensive rats. Med Sci Monit 16(12):BR367–373.
6. Leopoldo AS, Sugizaki MM, Lima-Leopoldo AP, Nascimento AF, Luvizotto RAM, et al. (2010) Cardiac remodeling in a rat model of diet-induced obesity. Can J Cardiol 26(8):423–429.
7. Oliveira Junior SA, Padovani CR, Rodrigues SA, Silva NR, Martinez PF, et al. (2013) Extensive impact of saturated fatty acids on metabolic and cardiovascular profile in rats with diet-induced obesity: a canonical analysis. Cardiovasc Diabetol 12(1):65.
8. Lima-Leopoldo AP, Leopoldo AS, Sugizaki MM, Bruno A, Nascimento AF, et al. (2011) Myocardial dysfunction and abnormalities in intracellular calcium handling in obese rats. Arq Bras Cardiol 97(3):232–240.
9. Du Toit EF, Nabben M, Lochner A (2005) A potential role for angiotensin II in obesity induced cardiac hypertrophy and ischaemic/reperfusion injury. Basic Res Cardiol 100(4):346–354.
10. Barry S, Davidson S, Townsend P (2008) Molecular regulation of cardiac hypertrophy. Int J Biochem Cell 40(10):2023–2039.
11. Calegari VC, Alves M, Picardi PK, Inoue RY, Franchini KG, et al. (2005) Suppressor of cytokine signaling-3 provides a novel interface in the cross-talk between angiotensin II and insulin signaling systems. Endocrinology 146(2):579–588.
12. Cooper S, Whaley-Connell A, Habibi J, Wei Y, Lastra G, et al. (2007) Renin-angiotensin-aldosterone system and oxidative stress in cardiovascular insulin resistance. Am J Physiol-Heart Circ Physiol 293(4):H2009–H2023.
13. Maharsy WM, Kadi LN, Issa NG, Bitar KM, Der-Bogbossian AH, et al. (2007) Cross-talk related to insulin and angiotensin II binding on myocardial remodelling in diabetic rat hearts. J Renin Angiotensin Aldosterone Syst 8(2):59–65.
14. Olivares-Reyes J, Arellano-Plancarte A, Castillo-Hernandez J (2009) Angiotensin II and the development of insulin resistance: Implications for diabetes. Mol Cell Endocrinol 302(2):128–39.
15. Greenfield JR, Campbell LV (2004) Insulin resistance and obesity. Clin Dermatol 22(4):289–95.
16. Gual P, Le Marchand-Brustel Y, Tanti J (2005) Positive and negative regulation of insulin signaling through IRS-1 phosphorylation. Biochimie 87(1):99–109.
17. Qatanani M, Lazar M (2007) Mechanisms of obesity-associated insulin resistance: many choices on the menu. Genes & Development 21(12):1443–1455.
18. Rose BA, Force T, Wang Y (2010) Mitogen-activated protein kinase signaling in the heart: angels versus demons in a heart-breaking tale. Physiol Rev 90(4):1507–1546.
19. Feldman R (2000) ACE inhibitors versus AT(1) blockers in the treatment of hypertension and syndrome X. Can J Cardiol 16:E41–E44.
20. Fogari R, Derosa G, Zoppi A, Rinaldi A, Lazzari P, et al. (2005) Comparison of the effects of valsartan and felodipine on plasma leptin and insulin sensitivity in hypertensive obese patients. Hypertens Res 28(3):209–214.
21. Henriksen EJ, Jacob S, Kinnick TR, Teachey MK, Krekler M (2001) Selective angiotensin II receptor antagonism reduces insulin resistance in obese Zucker rats. Hypertension 38(4):884–890.
22. Duarte J, Martinez A, Bermejo A, Vera B, Gamez MJ, et al. (1999) Cardiovascular effects of captopril and enalapril in obese Zucker rats. Eur J Pharmacol 365(2–3):225–232.
23. Toblli JE, Cao G, De Rosa G, Forcada P (2005) Reduced cardiac expression of plasminogen activator inhibitor 1 and transforming growth factor beta(1) in obese Zucker rats by perindopril. Heart 91(1):80–86.
24. Ernsberger P, Johnson JL, Rosenthal T, Mirelman D, Koletsky RJ (2007) Therapeutic actions of allylmercaptocaptopril and captopril in a rat model of metabolic syndrome. Am J Hypertens 20(8):866–874.
25. Carvalheira JBC, Calegari VC, Zecchin HG, Nadruz W, Guimaraes RB, et al. (2003) The cross-talk between angiotensin and insulin differentially affects phosphatidylinositol 3-kinase- and mitogen-activated protein kinase-mediated signaling in rat heart: Implications for insulin resistance. Endocrinology 144(12):5604–5614.
26. National Research Council of the National Academies (2011) Committee for the Update of the Guide for the Care and Use of Laboratory Animals. Washington, D. C.: The National Academies Press. 220 p.
27. Yuan Q, Chen L, Liu C, Xu K, Mao X, et al. (2011) Postnatal pancreatic islet β cell function and insulin sensitivity at different stages of lifetime in rats born with intrauterine growth retardation. Plos One 6(10):e25167.
28. Leopoldo AS, Lima-Leopoldo AP, Sugizaki MM, Nascimento AF, Campos DHS, et al. (2011) Involvement of L-type calcium channel and serca2A in myocardial dysfunction induced by obesity. J Cell Physiol 226(11):2934–2942.
29. Johnson MM, Peters JP (1993) An improved method to quantify nonesterified fatty-acids in bovine plasma. J Anim Sci 71(2):753–756.
30. Matthews DR, Hosker JP, Rudenski AS, Naylor BA, Treacher DF, et al. (1985) Homeostasis model assessment: insulin resistance and β-cell function from fasting plasma glucose and insulin concentration in man. Diabetologia 28(7):412–419.
31. Alves MF, Araujo MC, Juliano MA, Oliveira EM, Krieger JE, et al. (2005) A continuous fluorescent assay for the determination of plasma and tissue angiotensin I-converting enzyme activity. Braz J Med Biol Res 38(6):861–868.
32. Barauna VG, Magalhães FC, Krieger JE, Oliveira EM (2008) AT1 receptor participates in the cardiac hypertrophy induced by resistance training in rats. Am J Physiol Regul Integr Comp Physiol 295(2):R381–R387.
33. Pfeffer JM, Pfeffer MA, Frohlich ED (1971) Validity of an indirect tail-cuff method for determining systolic arterial pressure in unanesthetized normotensive and spontaneously hypertensive rats. J Lab Clin Med 78:957–962.
34. Sahn DJ, De Maria A, Kisslo J, Weyman A (1978) Recommendations regarding quantitation in M-mode echocardiography: results of a survey of echocardiographic measurements. Circulation 58:1072–1083.
35. Matsubara LS, Matsubara BB, Okoshi MP, Cicogna AC (2000) Alterations in myocardial collagen content affect rat papillary muscle function. Am J Physiol Heart Circ Physiol 279:H1534–H1539.
36. Serra AJ, Higuchi ML, Ihara SSM, Antônio EL, Santos MH, et al. (2008) Exercise training prevents β-adrenergic hyperactivity-induced myocardial hypertrophy and lesions. Eur J Heart Fail 10(6):534–539.
37. Martinez PF, Okoshi K, Zornoff LAM, Carvalho RF, Oliveira Junior SA, et al. (2010) Chronic heart failure-induced skeletal muscle atrophy, necrosis, and changes in myogenic regulatory factors. Med Sci Monit 16(12):BR374–383.
38. Trayhurn P (2005) Endocrine and signalling role of adipose tissue: new perspectives on fat. Acta Physiol Scand 184(4):285–293.
39. Schrauwen P, Westerterp KR (2000) The role of high-fat diets and physical activity in the regulation of body weight. Br J Nutr 84(4):417–427.
40. Boustany C, Brown D, Randall D, Cassis L (2005) AT(1)-receptor antagonism reverses the blood pressure elevation associated with diet-induced obesity. Am J Physiol Regul Integr Comp Physiol 289(1):R181–R186.
41. Huisamen B, Perel S, Friedrich S, Salie R, Strijdom H, et al. (2011) ANG II type I receptor antagonism improved nitric oxide production and enhanced eNOS and PKB/Akt expression in hearts from a rat model of insulin resistance. Mol Cell Biochem 349(1–2):21–31.
42. Rosselli M, Burgueno A, Carabelli J, Schuman M, Pirola C, et al. (2009) Losartan reduces liver expression of plasminogen activator inhibitor-1 (PAI-1) in a high fat-induced rat nonalcoholic fatty liver disease model. Atherosclerosis 206(1):119–126.
43. Kong X, Zhang D, Wu H, Li F (2011) Losartan and Pioglitazone Ameliorate Nephropathy in Experimental Metabolic Syndrome Rats. Biol Pharm Bull 34(5):693–699.
44. Ran J, Hirano T, Adachi M (2004) Angiotensin II type 1 receptor blocker ameliorates overproduction and accumulation of triglyceride in the liver of Zucker fatty rats. Am J Physiol Endocrinol Metab 287(2):E227–E232.
45. Umeda M, Kanda T, Murakami M (2003) Effects of angiotensin II receptor antagonists on insulin resistance syndrome and leptin in sucrose-fed spontaneously hypertensive rats. Hypertens Res 26(6):485–492.
46. Masuo K, Mikami H, Ogihara T, Tuck M (2001) Weight reduction and pharmacologic treatment in obese hypertensives. Am J Hypertens 14(6):530–538.
47. Lu H, Boustany-Kari C, Daugherty A, Cassis L (2007) Angiotensin II increases adipose angiotensinogen expression. Am J Physiol Endocrinol Metab 292(5):E1280–E1287.
48. Okoshi K, Ribeiro HB, Okoshi MP, Matsubara BB, Gonçalves G, et al. (2004) Improved systolic ventricular function with normal myocardial mechanics in compensated cardiac hypertrophy. Jpn Heart J 45:647–656.
49. Zile MR, Brutsaert DL (2002) New concepts in diastolic dysfunction and diastolic heart failure: part II. Causal mechanisms and treatment. Circulation 105: 1503–1508.
50. Rundell VL, Manaves V, Martin AF, De Tombe PP (2005) Impact of beta-myosin heavy chain isoform expression on cross-bridge cycling kinetics. Am J Physiol Heart Circ Physiol 288(2):896–903.
51. Krenz M, Sadayappan S, Osinska HE, Henry JA, Beck S, et al. (2007) Distribution and structure-function relationship of myosin heavy chain isoforms in the adult mouse heart. J Biol Chem 282(33):24057:24064.
52. Carnes CA, Geisbuhler TP, Reiser PJ (2004) Age-dependent changes in contraction and regional myocardial myosin heavy chain isoform expression in rats. J Appl Physiol 97(1):446–453.
53. Litwin SE, Katz SE, Weinberg EO, Lorell HB, Aurigemma GP, et al. (1995) Serial echocardiographic-Doppler assessment of left ventricular geometry and function in rats with pressure overload hypertrophy chronic angiotensin-converting enzyme inhibition attenuates the transition to heart failure. Circulation 91:2642–2654.
54. Shi L, Mao C, Xu Z, Zhang L (2010) Angiotensin-converting enzymes and drug discovery in cardiovascular diseases. Drug Discov Today 15(9–10):332–341.353.
55. Burchill L, Velkoska E, Dean RG, Lew RA, Smith AI, et al. (2008) Acute kidney injury in the rat causes cardiac remodelling and increases angiotensin-converting enzyme 2 expression. Exp Physiol 93(5):622–630.
56. Burrell LM, Risvanis J, Kubota E, Dean RG, MacDonald PS, et al. (2005) Myocardial infarction increases ACE2 expression in rat and humans. Eur Heart J 26(4):369–375.
57. Kondoh K, Nishida E (2007) Regulation of MAP kinases by MAP kinase phosphatases. Biochim Biophys Acta 1773(8):1227–1237.
58. Sica DA (2006) Angiotensin receptor blockers: new considerations in their mechanisms of action. Curr Conc Pharm Hypertens 8(5):381–385.

8

Effect of Angiotensin II Type 2 Receptor-Interacting Protein on Adipose Tissue Function via Modulation of Macrophage Polarization

Fei Jing, Masaki Mogi, Li-Juan Min, Kousei Ohshima, Hirotomo Nakaoka, Kana Tsukuda, Xiaoli Wang, Jun Iwanami, Masatsugu Horiuchi*

Department of Molecular Cardiovascular Biology and Pharmacology, Ehime University Graduate School of Medicine, Ehime, Japan

Abstract

We demonstrated that angiotensin II type 2 (AT_2) receptor-interacting protein (ATIP) 1 ameliorates inflammation-mediated vascular remodeling independent of the AT_2 receptor, leading us to explore the possibility of whether ATIP1 could exert anti-inflammatory effects and play a role in other pathophysiological conditions. We examined the possible anti-inflammatory effects of ATIP1 in adipose tissue associated with amelioration of insulin resistance. In mice fed a high-cholesterol diet, adipose tissue macrophage (ATM) infiltration and M1-to-M2 ratio were decreased in ATIP1 transgenic mice (ATIP1-Tg) compared with wild-type mice (WT), with decreased expression of inflammatory cytokines such as tumor necrosis factor-α and monocyte chemoattractant protein-1 in white adipose tissue (WAT), but an increase in interleukin-10, an anti-inflammatory cytokine. Moreover, 2-[^{3}H]deoxy-d-glucose (2-[^{3}H]DG) uptake was significantly increased in ATIP1-Tg compared with WT. Next, we examined the roles of ATIP1 in BM-derived hematopoietic cells, employing chimeric mice produced by BM transplantation into irradiated type 2 diabetic mice with obesity, KKAy, as recipients. ATM infiltration and M1-to-M2 ratio were decreased in ATIP1 chimera (ATIP1-tg as BM donor), with improvement of insulin-mediated 2-[^{3}H]DG uptake and amelioration of inflammation in WAT. Moreover, serum adiponectin concentration in ATIP1 chimera was significantly higher than that in WT chimera (WT as BM donor) and KKAy chimera (KKAy as BM donor). These results indicate that ATIP1 could exert anti-inflammatory effects in adipose tissue via macrophage polarization associated with improvement of insulin resistance, and ATIP1 in hematopoietic cells may contribute to these beneficial effects on adipose tissue functions in type 2 diabetes.

Editor: Ryuichi Morishita, Osaka University Graduate School of Medicine, Japan

Funding: This study was supported by the Ministry of Education, Science, Sports, and Culture of Japan to MH and MM, and the Novartis Foundation for Gerontological Research to MM. The funders had no role in study design, data collection and analysis, decision to publish, or preparation of the manuscript.

Competing Interests: The authors have declared that no competing interests exist.

* E-mail: horiuchi@m.ehime-u.ac.jp

Introduction

Proteins interacting with G protein coupled receptors have been highlighted as factors regulating these receptors. Accordingly, we have cloned ATIP angiotensin type 2 (AT_2) receptor interacting protein (ATIP) [1], also known as AT_2 receptor binding protein (ATBP) [2], as a protein interacting with the C-terminal tail of this receptor, using a yeast two-hybrid system. ATIP1 was found to be identical to a ubiquitously expressed tumor suppressor protein localized in mitochondria [3]. ATIP is also named mitochondrial tumor suppressor gene 1 (MTUS1), which shows mutation or copy number variants in human malignant tumors [3,4,5]. We investigated the role of ATIP1 in vascular remodeling using ATIP1 transgenic mice (ATIP1-Tg) [6]. We demonstrated that neointimal formation following inflammation-associated vascular injury of the femoral artery, which was induced by polyethylene cuff placement around the artery, was significantly smaller, with decreased superoxide anion production and expression of proinflammatory cytokines compared to those in WT littermates. Interestingly, pretreatment with PD123319, an AT_2 receptor antagonist, could not prevent the reduction of neointimal formation, and superoxide anion production induced by not only angiotensin II but also thrombin was attenuated in vascular smooth muscle cells prepared from ATIP1-Tg [6]. These results suggest that ATIP1 plays an important role in pathological conditions via an AT_2 receptor-independent mechanism. These results led us to examine the possibility that ATIP1 could act as an AT_2 receptor-independent mechanism in other pathological conditions associated with inflammation.

A chronic low-grade inflammatory state in obesity plays a role in systemic metabolic dysfunction associated with obesity-linked disorders [7,8]. Inflammation in white adipose tissue (WAT) is known to contribute to the pathogenesis of insulin resistance and type 2 diabetes [9,10]. Although the detailed mechanisms are not fully understood, there is accumulating interest in the role of adipose tissue macrophages (ATM) as a player in inflammation in obesity [11,12]. ATM consist of at least two different phenotypes: classically activated M1 macrophages and alternatively activated M2 macrophages. Lumeng et al. reported that ATM isolated from lean animals expressed hallmarks of polarization toward M2 macrophages with IL-10 and arginase expression, whereas in obese animals with insulin resistance, monocyte chemoattractant protein-1 (MCP-1) released from obese WAT caused a shift to M1-polarized ATM with increased TNF-αα and inducible nitric oxide synthase (iNOS) [13]. Diet-induced obesity leads to a shift in the activation state of ATM from an M2-polarized state in lean animals to an M1-polarized state, resulting in insulin resistance [13]. Fujisaka et al. also demonstrated that increases in M1 polarization and M1-to-M2 ratio are closely associated with insulin resistance induced by a high-fat diet [14]. However, factors that trigger the phenotypic switch of macrophage polarization are not well known.

Variation in the cellular cholesterol level induces changes in the inflammatory status of macrophages, and accumulation of cholesterol in macrophages is central to foam cell formation and the development of atherosclerosis [15]. Recently, Subramanian et al. reported that the addition of 0.15% cholesterol in the diet resulted in a marked increase in accumulation of macrophages in WAT [16]. Furthermore, an overload of cholesterol enhanced macrophage infiltration into WAT, thereby giving rise to inflammation and resulting in impaired insulin sensitivity [17]. From these results, we investigated the possibility of whether ATIP1 could ameliorate inflammation and thereby improve insulin sensitivity in WAT, focusing on macrophage infiltration and polarization using ATIP1-Tg fed a high-cholesterol diet. We also examined the roles of ATIP1 in hematopoietic cells, focusing on inflammation in WAT, employing irradiated type 2 diabetic mice with obesity, KKAy, as recipients of bulk bone marrow cell (BMC) transplantation.

Materials and Methods

Animals and Treatment

This study was performed in accordance with the National Institutes of Health guidelines for the use of experimental animals. All animal studies were reviewed and approved by the Animal Studies Committee of Ehime University.

Adult male mice carrying the mouse ATIP1-myc (ATIP1-Tg) gene as described previously were used [6]. Moreover, adult male wild-type littermate mice (WT) and obese type 2 diabetic model mice, KKAy (CLEA, Tokyo, Japan), were used. Animals were kept in a room in which lighting was controlled (12 hours on, 12 hours off) and temperature was kept at 25°C. In experiment 1, ATIP1-Tg and WT were fed a high-cholesterol diet [HCD: 1.25% cholesterol and 10% coconut oil in MF (Oriental Yeast Co. Ltd., Tokyo, Japan)] from 10 weeks of age. All experiments using ATIP1-Tg and WT were performed at 28 weeks of age.

Quantitative RT-PCR

Expression of mRNA prepared from epididymal and retroperitoneal WAT was quantified by real-time RT-PCR with a SYBR Premix Ex Taq (Takara Bio Inc., Shiga, Japan) and primers as follows: 5′-CGAGTGACAAGCCTGTAGCC-3′ (forward) and 5′-GGTGAGGAGCACGATGTCG-3′ (reverse) for TNF-α, 5′-TTAACGCCCCACTCACCTGCTG-3′ (forward) and 5′-GCTTCTTTGGGACACCTGCTGC-3′ (reverse) for MCP-1, 5′-GCTCTTACTGACTGGCATGAG-3′ (forward) and 5′-CGCAGCTCTAGGAGCATGTG-3′ (reverse) for IL-10, and 5′-ATGTAGGCCATGAGGTCCAC-3′ (forward) and 5′-TGCGACTTCAACAGCAACTC-3′ (reverse) for glyceraldehyde-3-phosphate dehydrogenase (GAPDH).

Glucose Uptake in Adipose Tissue

Glucose uptake in WAT was measured as the rate constant of 2-[^{3}H]deoxy-d-glucose (2-[^{3}H]DG) uptake according to our previous report [18]. Epididymal and retroperitoneal WAT were rapidly dissected and weighed. The rate constant of adipose tissue uptake of 2-[^{3}H] DG was calculated as described previously [19].

Isolation of Stromal-vascular Fraction from Adipose Tissue

Epididymal WAT from mice was digested with collagenase (2 mg/ml) (Sigma-Aldrich, St. Louis, MO) with Krebs-Henseleit–HEPES buffer (Nacalai Tesque, Tokyo, Japan) supplemented with 20 mg/ml bovine serum albumin (Sigma-Aldrich) and 2 mmol/l glucose (Sigma-Aldrich) at 37°C with shaking for 20 min. Then, the samples were passed through a cell strainer (BD, Franklin Lakes, NJ) and fractionated by centrifugation at 1000 rpm as previously described [14]. Cells in the pallets were collected as the stromal-vascular fraction (SVF) for flow cytometric analysis.

Flow Cytometric Analysis

SVF were incubated with antibodies as follows: anti-mouse F4/80-FITC (eBioscience, San Diego, CA), CD11c-PE (eBioscience) and CD206-Alexa Fluor 647 (AbD Serotec, Oxford, UK) or the matching control isotypes (eBioscience) for 30 min at 4°C following incubation with 2.4G2 (BD) for 10 min. After incubation with 7-amino-actinomycin D (BD), the cells were analyzed with a Gallios (Beckman Coulter, Brea, CA). M1 macrophages were identified as F4/80-positive/CD11c-positive/CD206-negative and M2 macrophages as F4/80-positive/CD11c-negative/CD206-positive, according to a previous report [14].

Generation of Chimeric Mice

In experiment 2, to analyze the functional role of ATIP in hematopoietic cells, we generated chimeric mice as described previously with minor modification [20]. Briefly, 8-week-old male KKAy were exposed to a total dose of 8 Gy whole-body irradiation and used as recipients. Bone marrow cells (BMC) were isolated from six crushed bones (bilateral tibias, femurs, and iliac bones) from 8-week-old male KKAy, WT or ATIP1-Tg. Bulk BMC (1.0×10^6 cells) diluted in PBS (200 μL) were injected via the tail vein immediately after irradiation. Six weeks after transplantation, mice were used for the following experiments. To determine the chimerism, expression of ATIP1 in BMC was assessed by immunoblotting as shown in **Figure S1B**.

Serum Adiponectin and TNF-α Concentrations

Blood samples were obtained at 9 to 10 a.m. by the submandibular bleeding method using an animal bleeding lancet (Goldenrod, Medipoint, Inc., NY) from mice after fasting for 16 hours. Serum adiponectin and TNF-α were measured using a Mouse/Rat High Molecular Weight Adiponectin ELISA kit (AKMAN-011, Shibayagi Co. Ltd., Gunma, Japan) and Mouse TNF-α ELISA kit (AKMTN-011, Shibayagi Co. Ltd.) according to the manufacturer's protocol.

Immunohistochemical Staining

To assess localized macrophage clusters surrounding adipocytes, paraffin-embedded sections of epididymal WAT fixed with 10% formalin were immunostained with an antibody against F4/80. Briefly, endogenous peroxidase was blocked by incubation in 3% H_2O_2 for 15 min, and nonspecific protein binding was blocked by incubation for 10 min in Blocking Reagent (Nichirei Bioscience Inc., Tokyo, Japan). Then, the sections were incubated with monoclonal anti-F4/80 antibody (diluted 1:100) (BMA Biomedicals, August, Switzerland) followed by Histofine Simple Stain Max PO (Nichirei Bioscience Inc., Tokyo, Japan). Antibody binding was visualized with 3,3′-diaminobenzidine (DAB) using a detection kit (Nichirei Bioscience Inc., Tokyo, Japan), and all sections were counterstained with hematoxylin. Samples were examined with a Zeiss Axioskop2 microscope (Carl Zeiss, Oberkochen, Germany) equipped with a computer-based imaging system.

Statistical Analysis

All values are expressed as mean ± SEM in the text and figures. Data were evaluated by ANOVA followed by post hoc analysis for multiple comparisons. A difference with $P<0.05$ was considered significant.

Results

Decrease in WAT Weight and Adipocyte Hypertrophy in ATIP-1Tg

HCD was introduced at 10 weeks of age in ATIP1-Tg and WT. The ratio of abdominal WAT weight to body weight was more markedly increased by treatment with HCD from ND in WT (18.53±1.28% increase) than in ATIP-Tg (14.65±1.36% increase). Dietary intake did not differ between mice (2.8±0.2 g/day in ATIP1-Tg, 2.9±0.3 g/day in WT). The ratio of WAT weight to body weight both in epididymal and retroperitoneal tissue was significantly lower in ATIP1-Tg at 28 weeks of age compared with WT (**Figure 1A**). Histological examination of WAT showed that adipocyte size was smaller in ATIP1-Tg than in WT (**Figure 1B**). Accordingly, adipocyte number per field at ×100 magnification was markedly increased in ATIP1-Tg compared with WT (**Figure 1B**).

Decrease in Proinflammatory Cytokine Levels and Increase in Glucose Uptake in ATIP1-Tg

Next, we assessed mRNA levels of proinflammatory cytokines TNF-α and MCP-1, and an immunoregulatory cytokine IL-10 in epididymal and retroperitoneal WAT by RT-PCR. Expression of TNF-α and MCP-1 was markedly decreased in epididymal and retroperitoneal WAT of ATIP1-Tg treated with HCD compared with WT (**Figure 2A**). In contrast, IL-10 expression was significantly increased in ATIP1-Tg (**Figure 2A**). Insulin resistance is closely associated with chronic inflammation, so we examined glucose uptake in WAT using the rate constant of 2-[^{3}H]DG uptake. 2-[^{3}H]DG uptake was significantly increased in ATIP1-Tg compared with WT, both with and without insulin treatment (**Figure 2B**).

Reduction of Macrophage Infiltration and Ratio of M1 to M2 Fraction in WAT Macrophages in ATIP1-Tg

In WAT, accumulation of adipose tissue macrophages (ATM) is recognized as an important contributor to the pathogenesis of insulin resistance [11,21]. Moreover, we observed that mRNA expression of IL-10, an M2-polarized macrophage marker, was increased in WAT in ATIP-Tg, as shown in **Figure 2A**, and therefore we examined the macrophage fractions in WAT. M1 and M2-polarized macrophages were clearly separated by flow cytometry. The macrophage fraction in SVF evaluated by F4/80 staining was significantly smaller in ATIP1-Tg compared with that in WT (16.12%±1.64% in ATIP1-Tg, 24.58±2.96% in WT)

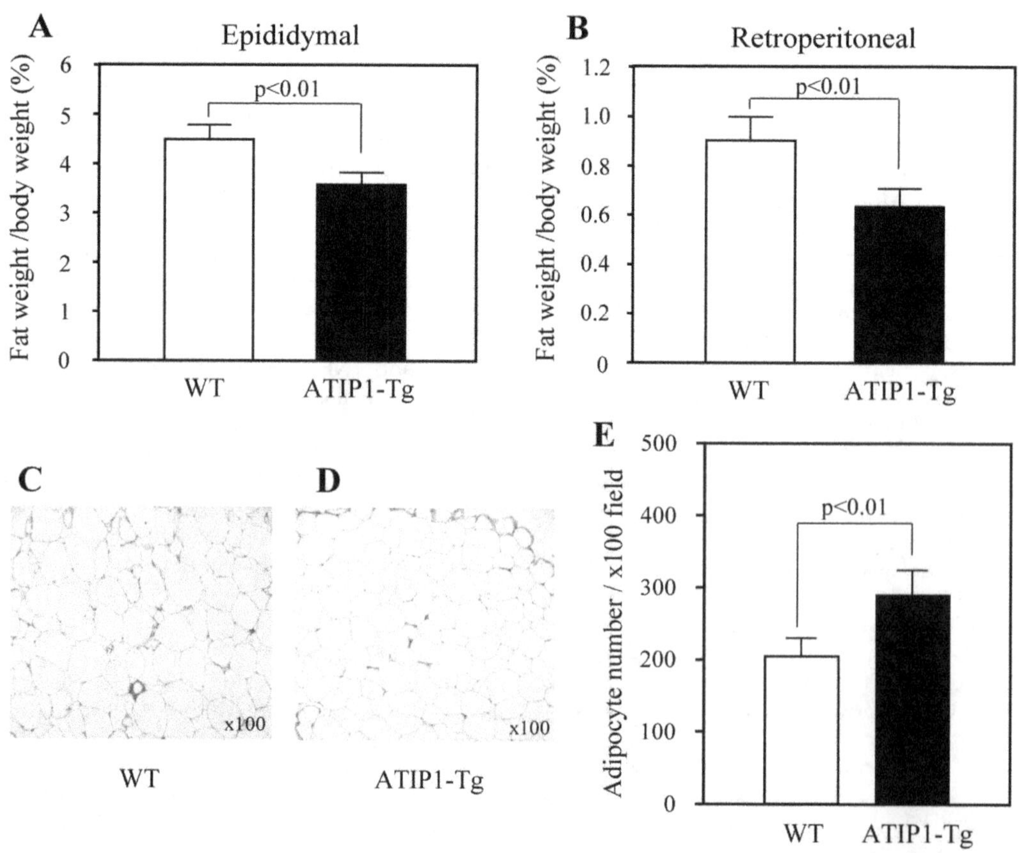

Figure 1. WAT in ATIP1-Tg and WT after treatment with high-cholesterol diet for 18 weeks. (**A**) Ratio of WAT weight to body weight in epididymal and retroperitoneal tissue. (**B**) Morphological comparison of epididymal WAT. Representative photomicrographs at ×100 magnification and histogram of adipocyte number per field. n = 7–8 for each group.

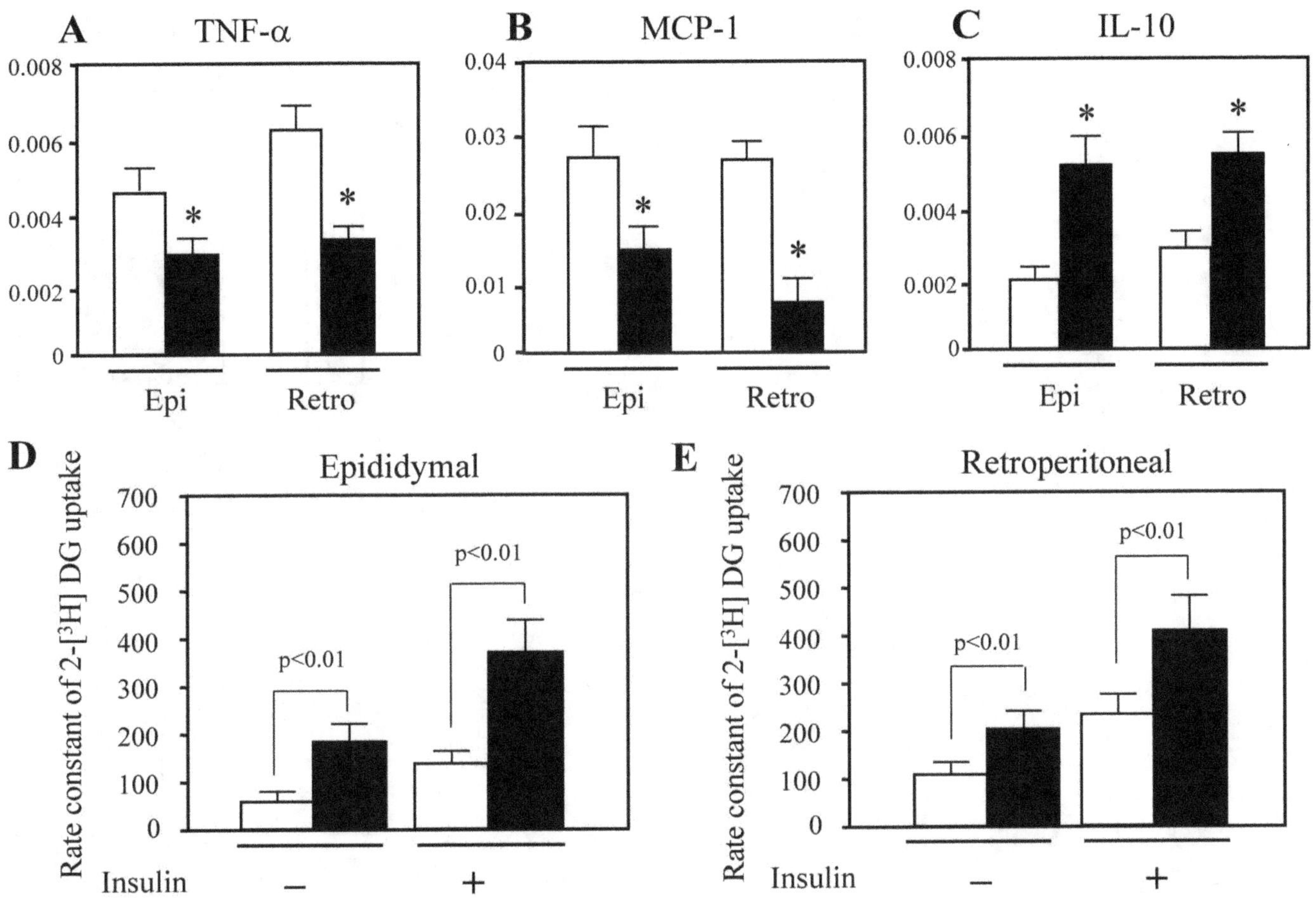

Figure 2. Cytokine levels and glucose uptake in WAT of ATIP1-Tg and WT after treatment with high-cholesterol diet. (**A**) Expression of TNF-α, MCP-1 and IL-10 in epididymal (Epi) and retroperitoneal (Retro) WAT. Open squares; WT, closed squares; ATIP1-Tg. n = 7–8 for each group. *$p<0.05$ vs. WT. (**B**) Rate constant of 2-[^{3}H] DG uptake in epididymal and retroperitoneal WAT was determined with and without insulin (1.0 U/kg) injection. Open squares; WT, closed squares; ATIP1-Tg. n = 6 for each group.

(**Figure 3B**). Moreover, ATIP1-Tg exhibited a lower ratio of M1 fraction and a higher ratio of M2 fraction compared to WT (**Figure 3C**).

Amelioration of Glucose Uptake, Inflammation and Adipocytokine Dysregulation in Type 2 Diabetic Mice Repopulated with BMC Prepared from ATIP1-Tg

ATM are known to be bone marrow-derived [9] and we observed that ATIP1 were highly expressed in BMC isolated from ATIP1-Tg (**Figure S1A**). Therefore, we examined the roles of ATIP1 in hematopoietic cells, focusing on inflammation and glucose uptake of WAT. For this purpose, we generated chimeric mice, ATIP1 chimera (BMC donor; ATIP1-Tg), WT chimera (BMC donor; WT) and KKAy chimera (BMC donor; KKAy), by bulk BMC transplantation using irradiated KKAy as recipients. ATIP1 chimera showed an increase in ATIP1 expression in BMC (**Figure S1B**), indicating successful reconstitution by BMC transplantation.

The rate constant of 2-[^{3}H]DG uptake in the basal condition was similar in both epididymal and retroperitoneal WAT among these three groups of chimera, whereas that in response to insulin was significantly greater in ATIP1 chimera than in other chimeras (**Figure 4A**). Moreover, mRNA expression of MCP-1 and TNF-α was markedly decreased in epididymal and retroperitoneal WAT of ATIP1 chimera compared with other chimeras (**Figure 4B**). In contrast, IL-10 expression was significantly increased in ATIP1 chimera (**Figure 4B**). Although KKAy exhibit a higher level of TNF-α and lower level of adiponectin in serum [22,23], TNF-α level was decreased and adiponectin level was increased in serum of ATIP1 chimera (**Figure 4C**).

Reduction of Macrophage Infiltration and Ratio of M1 and M2 Fraction in WAT Macrophages in Type 2 Diabetic Mice Repopulated with BMC Prepared from ATIP1-Tg

To examine whether the reduced inflammation in WAT of ATIP1 chimera was correlated with ATM, we also performed flow cytometry to detect M1 and M2 macrophages in F4-80-positive cells from the isolated SVF (**Figure 5A**). ATIP1 chimera displayed a smaller F4/80-positive cell fraction in SVF (32.40±2.46%) than that in WT chimera (44.18% ±4.08%) and KKAy chimera (47.92% ±3.15%) (**Figure 5B**). Moreover, in F4/80-positive cells isolated from SVF, M1-polarized macrophages were decreased and M2-polarized macrophages were increased in ATIP1 chimera compared with other chimeric mice (**Figure 5C**). Immunohistochemical staining of F4/80 in epididymal fat pads showed localized macrophage clusters surrounding adipocytes (**Figure 5D**). Consistent with the results of flow cytometry, the number of F4/80-positive macrophages per field at ×100 magnification was significantly decreased in ATIP1 chimera (**Figure 5D**).

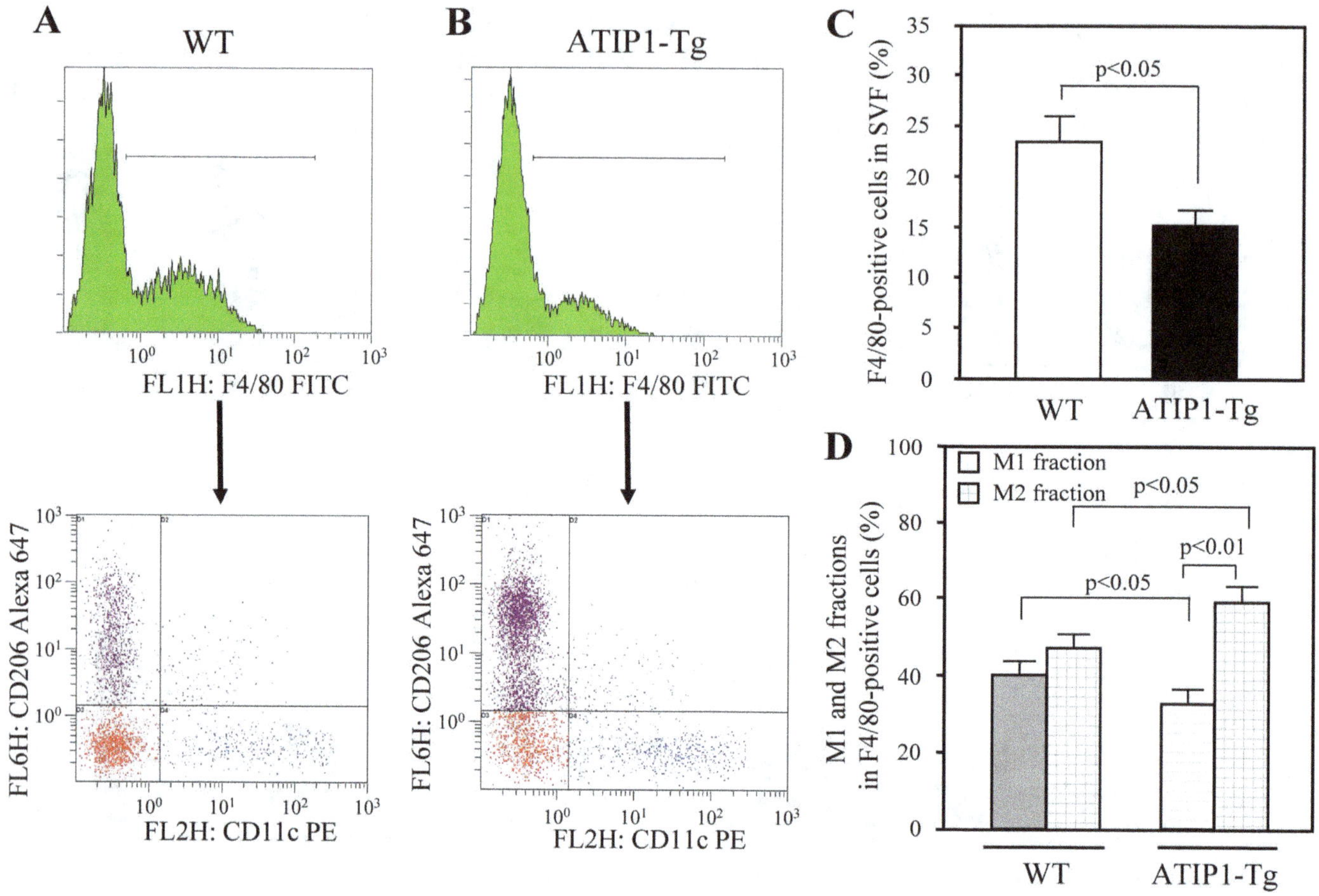

Figure 3. Macrophage infiltration and polarization in ATIP1-Tg and WT after treatment with high-cholesterol diet. Cells in the stromal vascular fraction (SVF) of the epididymal fat pad from each mouse were analyzed by flow cytometry as described in "Methods". (**A**) Representative results of flow cytometry. F4/80-positive cells were further analyzed with anti-CD11c and anti-CD206 antibodies. Blue dots show M1 macrophages and purple dots show M2 macrophages. Red dots represent both CD11c- and CD206-negative fraction evaluated using isotype controls. (**B**) Percentage of F4/80-positive cells in SVF. n = 5 for each group. (**C**) Ratio of M1 to M2 fraction in F4/80-positive cells. Light gray squares; M1 fraction, dark gray squares; M2 fraction. n = 5 for each group.

Discussion

The present study demonstrated that ATIP1 could play an important role in HCD-induced inflammation and insulin resistance in WAT through the attenuation of macrophage infiltration and M1 polarization, leading us to further explore the roles of ATIP1 in hematopoietic cells in the pathogenesis of insulin resistance, focusing on WAT. Accordingly, we observed that transplantation of ATIP1-overexpressing BMC improved inflammation and consequently ameliorated insulin resistance in WAT of type 2 diabetic and obese KKAy as the recipient. Macrophage accumulation in epididymal WAT and polarization toward an M1 state were reduced in ATIP1 chimeric mice. These findings suggest that ATIP1 in hematopoietic cells has a crucial role in amelioration of inflammation in WAT via macrophage infiltration and polarization.

Obesity is an early step in the progression of metabolic syndrome and type 2 diabetes [24]. Moreover, increasing evidence has suggested that low-grade inflammation with infiltration of inflammatory cells in WAT is closely associated with obesity [25], resulting in insulin resistance in WAT, which plays an important role in the onset and progression of type 2 diabetes [25,26]. Although the precise cell types and detailed mechanisms involved in this process are not fully understood, ATM are known to be an important contributor to inflammation followed by insulin resistance [27,28]. M1 ATM express proinflammatory cytokines such as TNF-α and IL-6, while M2 ATM are reported to express the chitinase family member Ym1, the anti-inflammatory cytokine IL-10, arginase and surface lectins Mgl1 and Mgl2 [29,30]. According to previous reports, ATM isolated from WAT of lean animals expressed hallmarks of polarization toward an M2 state, suggesting a potentially beneficial function of these cells, whereas in diet-induced obese animals, the number of M1 macrophages and the ratio of M1 to M2 macrophages were increased in WAT [13,14,31]. TNF-α, secreted from enlarged adipocytes, stimulates preadipocytes and endothelial cells to produce MCP-1 [32], then the increased MCP-1 recruits monocytes into the adipose tissue and stimulates M1 ATM differentiation [13,28]. Once macrophage activation and infiltration are initiated, they secrete numerous cytokines and chemokines to further activate themselves [12]. These feedback loops increasingly impair insulin signaling in adipocytes, eventually leading to massive adipocyte lipolysis, necrosis and systemic insulin resistance [11]. Based on our results, we speculate that ATIP1 may inhibit such feedback loops via attenuation of HCD- or obesity-induced inflammation.

Based on analysis of annotated functions of genes correlated with body mass, transcripts characteristic of macrophages were

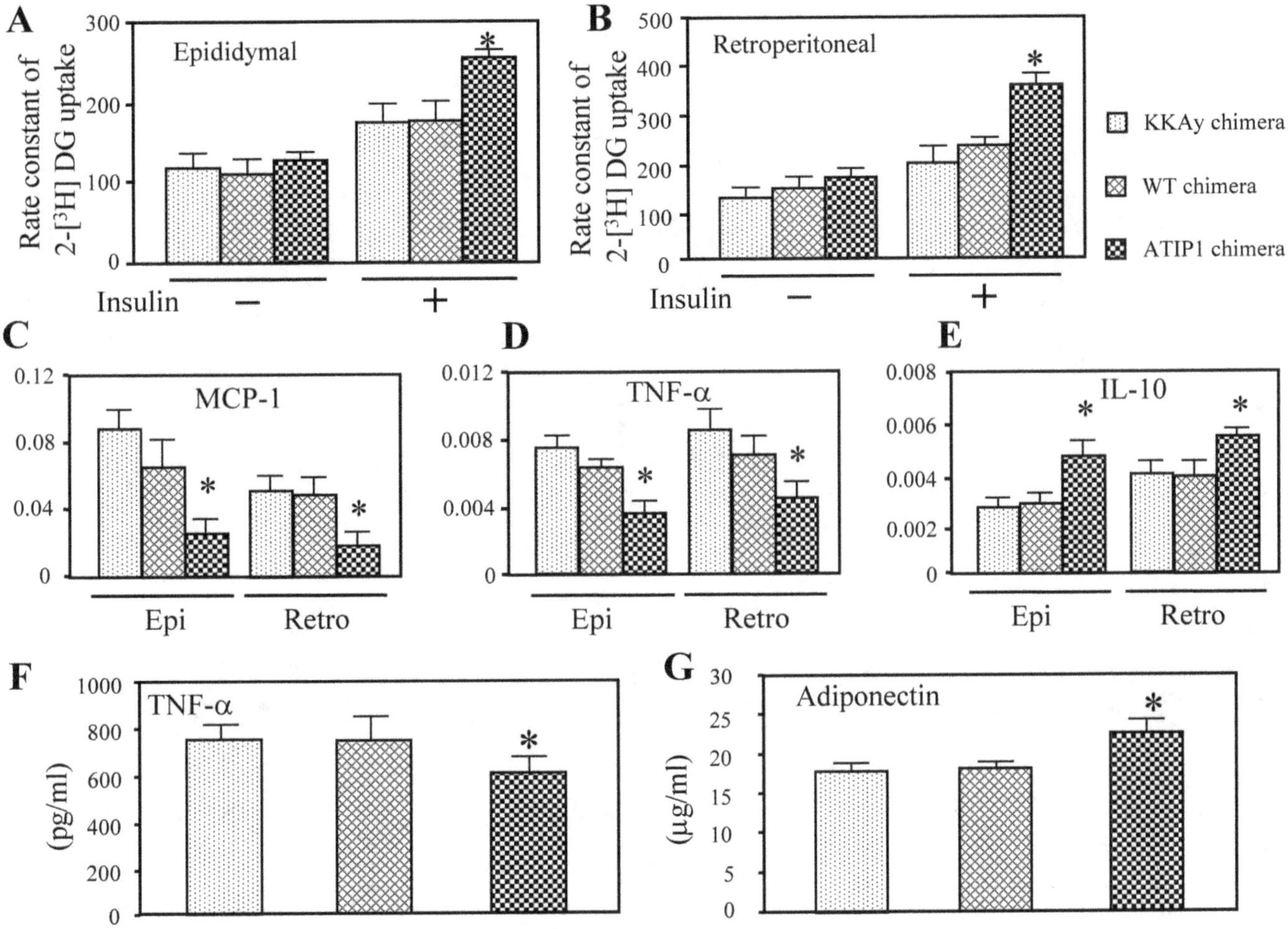

Figure 4. Glucose uptake and cytokines levels in white adipose tissue and serum levels of TNF-α and adiponectin in each chimeric mouse. (A) Rate constant of 2-[^{3}H] DG uptake in epididymal (Epi) and retroperitoneal (Retro) WAT were determined with and without insulin (1.0 U/kg) injection. n = 6 for each group. (B) Expression of TNF-α, MCP-1 and IL-10 in epididymal and retroperitoneal WAT. n = 6 for each group. (C) Serum TNF-α and adiponectin concentrations measured by ELISA. n = 8–10 for each group. *$p<0.05$ vs. KKAy chimera and WT chimera.

observed to be coordinately upregulated in direct proportion to body weight in several models of obesity [33,34]. This observation shows that macrophage infiltration in adipose tissue might be positively correlated with adiposity. In ATIP1-Tg mice with HCD, WAT weight and adipocyte size were decreased compared with those in WT controls (**Figure 1A and 1B**). Moreover, HCD-induced ATM infiltration and M1 differentiation were ameliorated in ATIP1-Tg mice (**Figure 3B**), with suppressed inflammation in WAT, supporting the possibility that ATM are activated in an adipocyte-dependent manner.

Weisberg et al. demonstrated that ATM were derived from bone marrow precursors that migrate from the peripheral circulation [9]. We observed that ATIP1 were highly expressed in BMC isolated from ATIP1-Tg mice (**Figure S1A**). The BMC transplantation approach has been expected to be a crucial technique in approaching the pathogenesis of metabolic disorders [35]. Saberi et al. showed that hematopoietic cell-specific deletion of Toll-like receptor 4 ameliorates adipose tissue insulin resistance in HCD-fed mice, using BMC-transplanted chimeric mice [36]. Cudejko et al. demonstrated that p16INK4a deficiency modulates macrophage polarization, using BMC chimeric mice [37]. Accordingly, we performed bone marrow transplantation of ATIP1-Tg using KKAy mice as recipients. Interestingly, ATIP1 chimera showed reduced ATM infiltration and M1 polarization, associated with amelioration of inflammation and improvement of insulin sensitivity in WAT (**Figures 4 and 5**). These observations support the idea that ATIP1-overexpressing ATM are less activated in obese mice and type 2 diabetic mice, which, in turn, could attenuate inflammation and enhance insulin sensitivity in WAT. Therefore, we speculate that the amelioration of ATM activation in ATIP1-Tg mice is at least in part due to the overexpression of ATIP1 in ATM.

Macrophages are mononuclear phagocytes and ATM migrate from circulating monocytes. MCP-1 and its receptor C-C motif chemokine receptor 2 (CCR2) are known to play an important role in monocyte migration to peripheral tissues [38,39]. Mouse monocytes can be divided into two subsets: CX3CR1^{high}CCR2^{-}Ly-6C^{low} (CCR2^{-}) monocytes and CX3CR1^{low}CCR2^{+}Ly-6C^{high} (CCR2^{+}) monocytes [40,41]. CCR2^{-} monocytes accumulate in noninflamed tissues and are termed "resident", while CCR2^{+} monocytes are potent inflammatory mediators with higher capacity for migration into inflamed tissues [42,43]. Consistent with this theory, Lumeng et al. demonstrated that in lean WAT, resident ATM are polarized toward an M2 state derived from CCR2^{-} monocytes, whereas obesity leads to an increase in circulating CCR2^{+} monocytes,

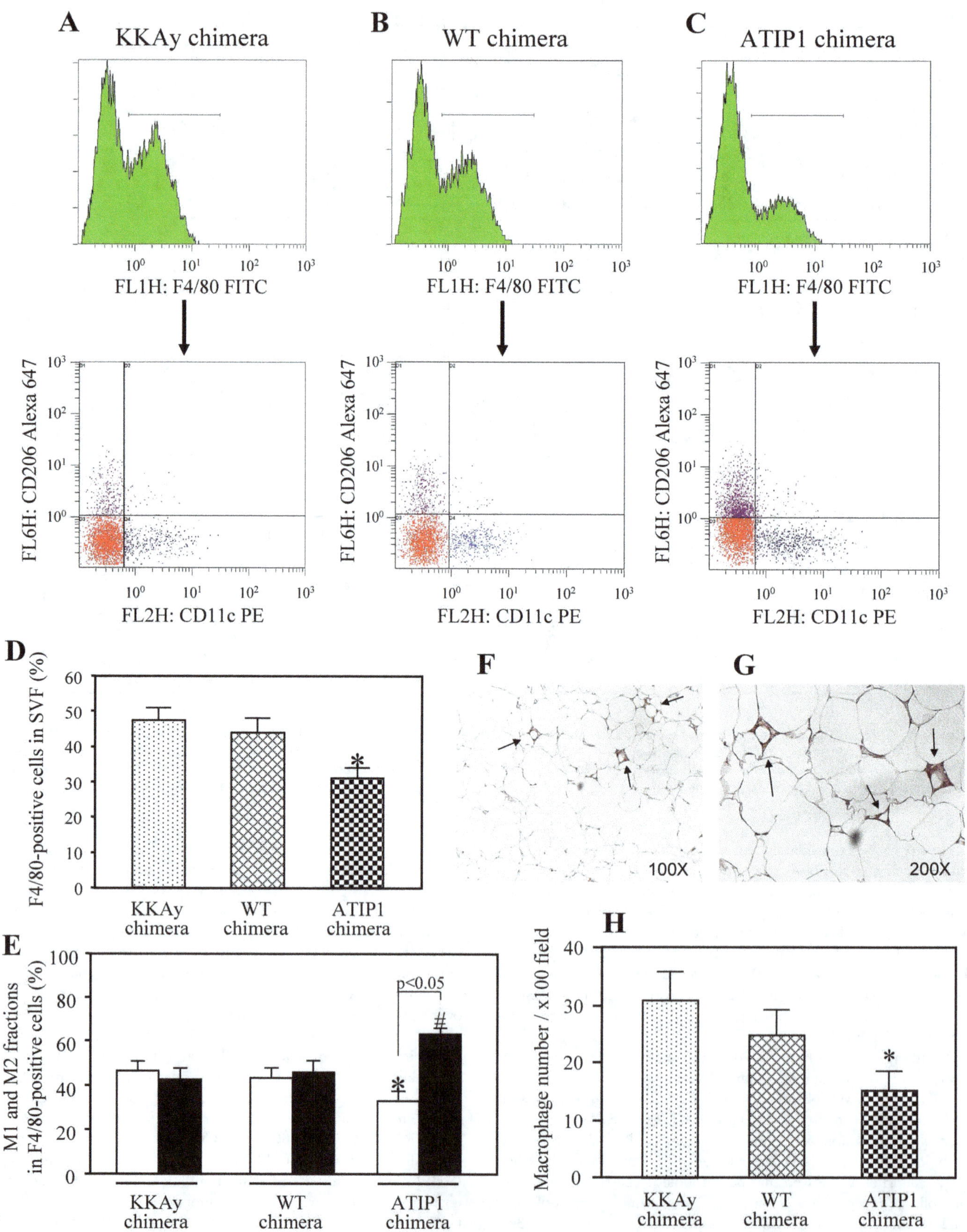

Figure 5. Comparison of macrophage infiltration and polarization in epididymal WAT of chimeric mice. Cells in the stromal vascular fraction (SVF) of the epididymal fat pad from each mouse were analyzed by flow cytometry as described in "Methods". (**A**) Representative results of flow cytometry. F4/80-positive cells were further analyzed with anti-CD11c and anti-CD206 antibodies. Blue dots show M1 macrophages and purple

dots show M2 macrophages. Red dots represent both CD11c- and CD206-negative fraction evaluated using isotype controls. (**B**) Percentage of F4/80-positive cells in SVF. n = 5 for each group. *p<0.05 vs. KKAy chimera and WT chimera. (**C**) Ratio of M1 and M2 fraction in F4/80-positive cells. Open squares; M1 fraction, closed squares; M2 fraction. *p<0.05 vs. M1 fraction in KKAy chimera and WT chimera, #p<0.05 vs. M2 fraction in KKAy chimera and WT chimera. n = 5 for each group. (**D**) Immunohistochemical staining of F4/80 in epididymal WAT at low (×100) and high (×200) magnification. Sections from epididymal fat pads of chimeric mice were stained with anti-F4/80 antibodies, followed by DAB staining. F4/80-positive cells are observed as localized macrophage clusters (arrow). Histogram of macrophage number per field at ×100 magnification is shown in the lower panel. n = 6 for each group. *p<0.05 vs. KKAy chimera and WT chimera.

which are the source of the infiltrating M1 macrophages in obese WAT [13]. In our study, HCD-induced M1 polarization was reduced in ATIP1-Tg mice (**Figure 3**); however, there was no significant difference in ATM content between ATIP1-Tg and WT when they were fed a normal diet (**Figure S2A, S2B and S2C**). Therefore, we assumed that ATIP1 would not have significant effects on resident CCR2^{-} monocytes/M2 ATM, but would suppress the increase in CCR2^{+} monocytes/M1 ATM related to the MCP-1/CCR2 axis. Further studies will be needed to elucidate the mechanisms by which ATIP1 regulates the MCP-1/CCR2 signaling cascade.

Transcriptional regulation of macrophage polarization has been extensively studied. For example, M1 macrophage polarization involves the activation of a set of transcription factors, such as NF-κB, AP-1, C/EBPb, PU.1 and IFN-regulatory factors (IRFs) [44,45]. On the other hand, M2 macrophage polarization involves the activation of a set of transcription factors, such as STAT6 and peroxisome proliferator-activated receptor (PPAR) γ [29,46]. Moreover, recent studies have revealed that epigenetic regulation also plays an important role in macrophage polarization [47]. In the present study, we have not investigated the detailed mechanism of ATIP1-induced M2 macrophage polarization; however, our recent study demonstrated that AT_2 receptor stimulation ameliorated insulin resistance in diabetic mice, associated with PPARγ activation [48], and there are relations between IRFs and the AT_2 receptor [49,50]. Therefore, we are investigating whether ATIP1-induced transcriptional regulation such as PPARγ activation would be involved in this mechanism. ATIP1 is known to localize in either the mitochondria [3] or Golgi [2], as well as the cell membrane; therefore, ATIP1 is considered to be a microtubule-associated protein [51]. Although the functions of ATIP associated with microtubules are totally unknown, microtubule-targeting agents including PPARγ inhibitors such as GW9662 are a very successful class of anti-cancer drugs with therapeutic benefits in both hematopoietic and solid tumors [52,53]. Potential roles of microtubule-associated protein in macrophage polarization still remain an enigma; however, non-binding of ATIP with the AT_2 receptor around microtubules could act in transcriptional regulation involving PPARγ etc.

Sica et al. reviewed the recent research on macrophage polarization in pathological conditions [54]. M2 macrophages play mainly a beneficial role in obesity, metabolism, inflammation and tissue repair; however, allergy is associated with M2 polarization of macrophages [55]. Moreover, tumor progression is associated with a phenotype switch from M1 to M2 at least in some models of carcinogenesis in the mouse [56]. ATIP1 is a mitochondrial protein that acts as a tumor suppressor [57]. ATIP1-induced M2 macrophage polarization may be a contradictory function in tumor pathogenesis. We speculate that an abnormal switch from M1 to M2 would inhibit M1 macrophage-induced antitumor activity of T cell-mediated elimination and equilibrium phases during tumor progression induced by cancer-related inflammation; however, originally ATIP1 could prevent progression of cancer itself. Further investigation is needed to assess the functional effect of ATIP1 on these balances between cancer cell progression and anti-tumor effects by the recruited cells surrounding the tumor.

We previously reported that over-expression of ATIP1 improves vascular remodeling independent of the AT_2 receptor in inflammation-induced vascular injury [6]. We cannot exclude the involvement of AT_2 receptor activation in the decrease of inflammation and improvement of insulin resistance in WAT. We tried to generate "AT_2 receptor-deleted chimeric mice" (BM donor: AT_2 receptor-deficient mice); however, this chimeric mouse was lethal and we could not analyze the effect of the AT_2 receptor in this set of experiments. Moreover, using an AT_2 receptor antagonist such as PD123319 is not appropriate in this study, because PD123319 has a short half-life, and its permeability and the appropriate concentration for adipose tissue are totally unknown. We speculate that deletion of the AT_2 receptor reduced BM engraftment due to less differentiation activity, since the AT_2 receptor is known to play an important role in cellular differentiation [58,59,60]. Therefore, we are not able to conclude whether the effect of ATIP on macrophage differentiation is dependent or independent of AT_2 receptor signaling. To address the involvement of the AT_2 receptor in ATIP-induced modulation of macrophage polarization, more detailed analysis should be performed in the future. It is also possible that the metabolic difference of adipose tissue between ATIP1-Tg and WT might result from differences of ATIP1 expression in adipose tissue and other organs, also independent of inflammation. This issue remains to be addressed.

In summary, we expect ATIP1 could be a novel therapeutic target to prevent and treat metabolic disorders via innate immunity, with a reduction in macrophage infiltration and a change in the ratio of M1 to M2 macrophages in WAT. Moreover, further elucidation of the functional regulation of ATIP1, including investigating phosphorylation and dephosphorylation and transcriptional control, and finding possible ligands should be performed.

Supporting Information

Figure S1 ATIP1 protein level in BMC. BMC were isolated from bilateral tibias, femurs and iliac bones, and protein level was measured by immunoblotting with an antibody against ATIP1. (**A**) ATIP1 protein level in BMC of ATIP1-Tg and WT. (**B**) ATIP1 protein level in BMC of KKAy chimera, WT chimera and ATIP1 chimera. Total protein was prepared from BMC isolated from six crushed bones (bilateral tibias, femurs, and iliac bones). Immunoblot analysis was performed using rabbit anti-mouse ATIP1 polyclonal antibody (kindly provided by Dr. C. Nahmias, Inserm, U1016, France) and a secondary anti-rabbit antibody (Cell Signaling Technology, Inc, Danvers, MA).

Figure S2 Comparison of macrophage polarization in epididymal WAT of ATIP1-Tg and WT fed normal diet (ND). Cells in the stromal vascular fraction (SVF) of the epididymal fat pad from mice fed ND for 18 weeks were analyzed by flow cytometry as described in "Methods". (**A**) Representative results of flow cytometry. F4/80-positive cells were further analyzed with anti-CD11c and anti-CD206 antibodies. Blue dots show M1 macrophages and purple dots show M2 macrophages. Red dots represent both CD11c- and CD206-negative fraction evaluated using isotype controls. (**B**) Percentage of F4/80-positive cells in SVF. n = 5 for each group. (**C**) Ratio of M1 to M2 fraction in F4/80-positive cells. Light gray squares; M1 fraction, dark gray squares; M2 fraction. n = 5 for each group.

Author Contributions

Conceived and designed the experiments: MM MH. Performed the experiments: FJ KO LJM HN KT XW JI. Analyzed the data: FJ KO. Contributed reagents/materials/analysis tools: FJ KO HN JI. Wrote the paper: FJ MM MH.

References

1. Nouet S, Amzallag N, Li JM, Louis S, Seitz I, et al. (2004) Trans-inactivation of receptor tyrosine kinases by novel angiotensin II AT2 receptor-interacting protein, ATIP. J Biol Chem 279: 28989–28997.
2. Wruck CJ, Funke-Kaiser H, Pufe T, Kusserow H, Menk M, et al. (2005) Regulation of transport of the angiotensin AT2 receptor by a novel membrane-associated Golgi protein. Arterioscler Thromb Vasc Biol 25: 57–64.
3. Seibold S, Rudroff C, Weber M, Galle J, Wanner C, et al. (2003) Identification of a new tumor suppressor gene located at chromosome 8p21.3–22. FASEB J 17: 1180–1182.
4. Di Benedetto M, Pineau P, Nouet S, Berhouet S, Seitz I, et al. (2006) Mutation analysis of the 8p22 candidate tumor suppressor gene ATIP/MTUS1 in hepatocellular carcinoma. Mol Cell Endocrinol 252: 207–215.
5. Frank B, Bermejo JL, Hemminki K, Sutter C, Wappenschmidt B, et al. (2007) Copy number variant in the candidate tumor suppressor gene MTUS1 and familial breast cancer risk. Carcinogenesis 28: 1442–1445.
6. Fujita T, Mogi M, Min LJ, Iwanami J, Tsukuda K, et al. (2009) Attenuation of cuff-induced neointimal formation by overexpression of angiotensin II type 2 receptor-interacting protein 1. Hypertension 53: 688–693.
7. Ouchi N, Parker JL, Lugus JJ, Walsh K (2011) Adipokines in inflammation and metabolic disease. Nat Rev Immunol 11: 85–97.
8. Romeo GR, Lee J, Shoelson SE (2012) Metabolic syndrome, insulin resistance, and roles of inflammation–mechanisms and therapeutic targets. Arterioscler Thromb Vasc Biol 32: 1771–1776.
9. Weisberg SP, McCann D, Desai M, Rosenbaum M, Leibel RL, et al. (2003) Obesity is associated with macrophage accumulation in adipose tissue. J Clin Invest 112: 1796–1808.
10. Qatanani M, Lazar MA (2007) Mechanisms of obesity-associated insulin resistance: many choices on the menu. Genes Dev 21: 1443–1455.
11. Xu H, Barnes GT, Yang Q, Tan G, Yang D, et al. (2003) Chronic inflammation in fat plays a crucial role in the development of obesity-related insulin resistance. J Clin Invest 112: 1821–1830.
12. Hotamisligil GS (2006) Inflammation and metabolic disorders. Nature 444: 860–867.
13. Lumeng CN, Bodzin JL, Saltiel AR (2007) Obesity induces a phenotypic switch in adipose tissue macrophage polarization. J Clin Invest 117: 175–184.
14. Fujisaka S, Usui I, Bukhari A, Ikutani M, Oya T, et al. (2009) Regulatory mechanisms for adipose tissue M1 and M2 macrophages in diet-induced obese mice. Diabetes 58: 2574–2582.
15. Levine DM, Parker TS, Donnelly TM, Walsh A, Rubin AL (1993) In vivo protection against endotoxin by plasma high density lipoprotein. Proc Natl Acad Sci U S A 90: 12040–12044.
16. Subramanian S, Han CY, Chiba T, McMillen TS, Wang SA, et al. (2008) Dietary cholesterol worsens adipose tissue macrophage accumulation and atherosclerosis in obese LDL receptor-deficient mice. Arterioscler Thromb Vasc Biol 28: 685–691.
17. Bie J, Zhao B, Song J, Ghosh S (2010) Improved insulin sensitivity in high fat- and high cholesterol-fed Ldlr−/− mice with macrophage-specific transgenic expression of cholesteryl ester hydrolase: role of macrophage inflammation and infiltration into adipose tissue. J Biol Chem 285: 13630–13637.
18. Shiuchi T, Nakagami H, Iwai M, Takeda Y, Cui T, et al. (2001) Involvement of bradykinin and nitric oxide in leptin-mediated glucose uptake in skeletal muscle. Endocrinology 142: 608–612.
19. Sudo M, Minokoshi Y, Shimazu T (1991) Ventromedial hypothalamic stimulation enhances peripheral glucose uptake in anesthetized rats. Am J Physiol 261: E298–303.
20. Iwanami J, Mogi M, Tsukuda K, Min LJ, Sakata A, et al. (2011) Effect of angiotensin II type 2 receptor deletion in hematopoietic cells on brain ischemia-reperfusion injury. Hypertension 58: 404–409.
21. Greenberg AS, Obin MS (2006) Obesity and the role of adipose tissue in inflammation and metabolism. Am J Clin Nutr 83: 461S–465S.
22. Ohashi K, Kihara S, Ouchi N, Kumada M, Fujita K, et al. (2006) Adiponectin replenishment ameliorates obesity-related hypertension. Hypertension 47: 1108–1116.
23. Hotamisligil GS, Shargill NS, Spiegelman BM (1993) Adipose expression of tumor necrosis factor-alpha: direct role in obesity-linked insulin resistance. Science 259: 87–91.
24. Alberti KG, Zimmet P, Shaw J (2005) The metabolic syndrome–a new worldwide definition. Lancet 366: 1059–1062.
25. Shoelson SE, Lee J, Goldfine AB (2006) Inflammation and insulin resistance. J Clin Invest 116: 1793–1801.
26. de Luca C, Olefsky JM (2008) Inflammation and insulin resistance. FEBS Lett 582: 97–105.
27. Neels JG, Olefsky JM (2006) Inflamed fat: what starts the fire? J Clin Invest 116: 33–35.
28. Kanda H, Tateya S, Tamori Y, Kotani K, Hiasa K, et al. (2006) MCP-1 contributes to macrophage infiltration into adipose tissue, insulin resistance, and hepatic steatosis in obesity. J Clin Invest 116: 1494–1505.
29. Gordon S (2003) Alternative activation of macrophages. Nat Rev Immunol 3: 23–35.
30. Raes G, Brys L, Dahal BK, Brandt J, Grooten J, et al. (2005) Macrophage galactose-type C-type lectins as novel markers for alternatively activated macrophages elicited by parasitic infections and allergic airway inflammation. J Leukoc Biol 77: 321–327.
31. Mantovani A, Sozzani S, Locati M, Allavena P, Sica A (2002) Macrophage polarization: tumor-associated macrophages as a paradigm for polarized M2 mononuclear phagocytes. Trends Immunol 23: 549–555.
32. Wellen KE, Hotamisligil GS (2003) Obesity-induced inflammatory changes in adipose tissue. J Clin Invest 112: 1785–1788.
33. Kullo IJ, Hensrud DD, Allison TG (2002) Comparison of numbers of circulating blood monocytes in men grouped by body mass index (<25, 25 to <30,>or = 30). Am J Cardiol 89: 1441–1443.
34. Soukas A, Cohen P, Socci ND, Friedman JM (2000) Leptin-specific patterns of gene expression in white adipose tissue. Genes Dev 14: 963–980.
35. Aparicio-Vergara M, Shiri-Sverdlov R, de Haan G, Hofker MH (2010) Bone marrow transplantation in mice as a tool for studying the role of hematopoietic cells in metabolic and cardiovascular diseases. Atherosclerosis 213: 335–344.
36. Saberi M, Woods NB, de Luca C, Schenk S, Lu JC, et al. (2009) Hematopoietic cell-specific deletion of toll-like receptor 4 ameliorates hepatic and adipose tissue insulin resistance in high-fat-fed mice. Cell Metab 10: 419–429.
37. Cudejko C, Wouters K, Fuentes L, Hannou SA, Paquet C, et al. (2011) p16INK4a deficiency promotes IL-4-induced polarization and inhibits proinflammatory signaling in macrophages. Blood 118: 2556–2566.
38. Dawson J, Miltz W, Mir AK, Wiessner C (2003) Targeting monocyte chemoattractant protein-1 signalling in disease. Expert Opin Ther Targets 7: 35–48.
39. Deshmane SL, Kremlev S, Amini S, Sawaya BE (2009) Monocyte chemoattractant protein-1 (MCP-1): an overview. J Interferon Cytokine Res 29: 313–326.
40. Geissmann F, Jung S, Littman DR (2003) Blood monocytes consist of two principal subsets with distinct migratory properties. Immunity 19: 71–82.
41. Nahrendorf M, Pittet MJ, Swirski FK (2010) Monocytes: protagonists of infarct inflammation and repair after myocardial infarction. Circulation 121: 2437–2445.
42. Gordon S, Taylor PR (2005) Monocyte and macrophage heterogeneity. Nat Rev Immunol 5: 953–964.
43. Sunderkotter C, Nikolic T, Dillon MJ, Van Rooijen N, Stehling M, et al. (2004) Subpopulations of mouse blood monocytes differ in maturation stage and inflammatory response. J Immunol 172: 4410–4417.
44. Takeuchi O, Akira S (2010) Pattern recognition receptors and inflammation. Cell 140: 805–820.
45. Medzhitov R, Horng T (2009) Transcriptional control of the inflammatory response. Nat Rev Immunol 9: 692–703.
46. Charo IF (2007) Macrophage polarization and insulin resistance: PPARgamma in control. Cell Metab 6: 96–98.
47. Satoh T, Takeuchi O, Vandenbon A, Yasuda K, Tanaka Y, et al. (2010) The Jmjd3-Irf4 axis regulates M2 macrophage polarization and host responses against helminth infection. Nat Immunol 11: 936–944.
48. Ohshima K, Mogi M, Jing F, Iwanami J, Tsukuda K, et al. (2012) Direct angiotensin II type 2 receptor stimulation ameliorates insulin resistance in type 2 diabetes mice with PPARgamma activation. PLoS One 7: e48387.
49. Horiuchi M, Yamada T, Hayashida W, Dzau VJ (1997) Interferon regulatory factor-1 up-regulates angiotensin II type 2 receptor and induces apoptosis. J Biol Chem 272: 11952–11958.
50. Horiuchi M, Koike G, Yamada T, Mukoyama M, Nakajima M, et al. (1995) The growth-dependent expression of angiotensin II type 2 receptor is regulated by transcription factors interferon regulatory factor-1 and -2. J Biol Chem 270: 20225–20230.
51. Rodrigues-Ferreira S, Nahmias C (2010) An ATIPical family of angiotensin II AT2 receptor-interacting proteins. Trends Endocrinol Metab 21: 684–690.

52. Schaefer KL (2008) PPARgamma inhibitors as novel tubulin-targeting agents. PPAR Res 2008: 785405.
53. Schaefer KL, Takahashi H, Morales VM, Harris G, Barton S, et al. (2007) PPARgamma inhibitors reduce tubulin protein levels by a PPARgamma, PPARdelta and proteasome-independent mechanism, resulting in cell cycle arrest, apoptosis and reduced metastasis of colorectal carcinoma cells. Int J Cancer 120: 702–713.
54. Sica A, Mantovani A (2012) Macrophage plasticity and polarization: in vivo veritas. J Clin Invest 122: 787–795.
55. Zaynagetdinov R, Sherrill TP, Polosukhin VV, Han W, Ausborn JA, et al. (2011) A critical role for macrophages in promotion of urethane-induced lung carcinogenesis. J Immunol 187: 5703–5711.
56. Kim HY, DeKruyff RH, Umetsu DT (2010) The many paths to asthma: phenotype shaped by innate and adaptive immunity. Nat Immunol 11: 577–584.
57. Di Benedetto M, Bieche I, Deshayes F, Vacher S, Nouet S, et al. (2006) Structural organization and expression of human MTUS1, a candidate 8p22 tumor suppressor gene encoding a family of angiotensin II AT2 receptor-interacting proteins, ATIP. Gene 380: 127–136.
58. Li JM, Mogi M, Tsukuda K, Tomochika H, Iwanami J, et al. (2007) Angiotensin II-induced neural differentiation via angiotensin II type 2 (AT2) receptor-MMS2 cascade involving interaction between AT2 receptor-interacting protein and Src homology 2 domain-containing protein-tyrosine phosphatase 1. Mol Endocrinol 21: 499–511.
59. Nahmod KA, Vermeulen ME, Raiden S, Salamone G, Gamberale R, et al. (2003) Control of dendritic cell differentiation by angiotensin II. FASEB J 17: 491–493.
60. Yamada H, Akishita M, Ito M, Tamura K, Daviet L, et al. (1999) AT2 receptor and vascular smooth muscle cell differentiation in vascular development. Hypertension 33: 1414–1419.

9

Effects of Growth Hormone (GH) Therapy Withdrawal on Glucose Metabolism in not Confirmed GH Deficient Adolescents at Final Height

Flavia Prodam[1,2,3*], Silvia Savastio[1], Giulia Genoni[1], Deepak Babu[4], Mara Giordano[3,4], Roberta Ricotti[1], Gianluca Aimaretti[2], Gianni Bona[1,3], Simonetta Bellone[1,2,3]

1 Division of Pediatrics, Department of Health Sciences, University of "Piemonte Orientale Amedeo Avogadro", Novara, Italy, **2** Endocrinology, Department of Clinical and Experimental Medicine, University of Piemonte Orientale, Novara, Italy, **3** I.C.O.S. (Interdisciplinary Center for Obesity Study), Novara, Italy, **4** Laboratory of Human Genetics, Department of Health Sciences, University of Piemonte Orientale, Novara, Italy

Abstract

Context, objective: Growth hormone deficiency (GHD) is associated with insulin resistance and diabetes, in particular after treatment in children and adults with pre-existing metabolic risk factors. Our aims were. i) to evaluate the effect on glucose metabolism of rhGH treatment and withdrawal in not confirmed GHD adolescents at the achievement of adult height; ii) to investigate the impact of GH receptor gene genomic deletion of exon 3 (d3GHR).

Design, setting: We performed a longitudinal study (1 year) in a tertiary care center.

Methods: 23 GHD adolescent were followed in the last year of rhGH treatment (T0), 6 (T6) and 12 (T12) months after rhGH withdrawal with fasting and post-OGTT evaluations. 40 healthy adolescents were used as controls. HOMA-IR, HOMA%β, insulinogenic (INS) and disposition (DI) indexes were calculated. GHR genotypes were determined by multiplex PCR.

Results: In the group as a whole, fasting insulin ($p<0.05$), HOMA-IR ($p<0.05$), insulin and glucose levels during OGTT ($p<0.01$) progressively decreased from T0 to T12 becoming similar to controls. During rhGH, a compensatory insulin secretion with a stable DI was recorded, and, then, HOMAβ and INS decreased at T6 and T12 ($p<0.05$). By evaluating the GHR genotype, nDel GHD showed a decrease from T0 to T12 in HOMA-IR, HOMAβ, INS ($p<0.05$) and DI. Del GHD showed a gradual increase in DI ($p<0.05$) and INS with a stable HOMA-IR and higher HDL-cholesterol ($p<0.01$).

Conclusions: In not confirmed GHD adolescents the fasting deterioration in glucose homeostasis during rhGH is efficaciously coupled with a compensatory insulin secretion and activity at OGTT. The presence of at least one d3GHR allele is associated with lower glucose levels and higher HOMA-β and DI after rhGH withdrawal. Screening for the d3GHR in the pediatric age may help physicians to follow and phenotype GHD patients also by a metabolic point of view.

Editor: Marta Letizia Hribal, University of Catanzaro Magna Graecia, Italy

Funding: This study was supported by Regione Piemonte (grant n° 2827, 2008), Università del Piemonte Orientale "A. Avogadro", Ministero dell'Università e della Ricerca Scientifica (MIUR, grant n° 20082P8CCE, 2008). The funders had no role in study design, data collection and analysis, decision to publish, or preparation of the manuscript.

Competing Interests: The authors have declared that no competing interests exist.

* E-mail: flavia.prodam@med.unipmn.it

Introduction

Growth hormone (GH) has pleiotropic functions in humans. GH/insulin-like growth factor-1 (IGF-I) axis is the main regulator of post-natal growth, but it has other main metabolic actions such as the regulation of body composition, muscle and bone metabolism. Furthermore, in the post-absorptive state, GH mainly acts on stimulating lipolysis and lipid oxidation in order to switch metabolism from glucose and protein to lipid utilization. At present, it is reported that GH administration is followed by lipolysis but also by insulin resistance and relatively sustained hyperglycemia [1–3]. GH-induced lipolysis appears as the most important determinant of GH anti-insulin actions, by inhibiting insulin-stimulated glucose uptake especially in muscles [4,5]. Whether the impairment in peripheral insulin sensitivity is mainly located in muscle and mostly due to higher disposable free fatty acids, GH is also able to reduce hepatic insulin sensitivity in healthy humans and to counterbalance the anti-lipolytic actions of hyperinsulinemia [1,6]. Some of these effects are direct actions, whereas others are IGF-I mediated [1].

Other mechanisms may be implicated on the metabolic effects of GH, as the interaction of GH with the insulin receptor [7,8] and the presence of several polymorphisms including the GH receptor (GHR) exon 3 deletion (d3GHR) which seems to play a role in glucose homeostasis in GHD subjects [9] and in general population [10,11].

Several studies in adults have determined the effects of GH replacement therapy on insulin sensitivity. Short-term rhGH therapy deteriorates insulin sensitivity with an improvement on long-term in the majority but not in all studies. These conflicting data are probably due to differences in sample size, methods of evaluation of insulin sensitivity and doses of rhGH [1,12–15]. There are suggestions that rhGH therapy increases the risk of type 2 and/or secondary diabetes in GHD adults with pre-existing metabolic risk factors [16]. Similarly, in children data from registries show a slower increase in the incidence of diabetes due to GH treatment in those patients with pre-existing risk factors [17,18]. Despite this, a few data describe insulin secretion at final height in the "so called" transition phase. Evidence to date suggests an increase in insulin sensitivity after cessation of GH treatment [19–21], but more studies are needed to clarify. In particular, no attention has been paid on those subjects which were not reconfirmed as GHD after stopping therapy.

Euglycemic hyper-insulinemic clamp is considered as the "gold standard" for quantifying insulin sensitivity in vivo, but this method is not applicable on a great population in daily clinical practice. Insulinogenic index (INS) and disposition index (DI) are new indirect methods for measure beta-cell function, using oral glucose tolerance test (OGTT) -derived measures, and are early markers of inadequate beta-cell or peripheral compensation. They allow the investigation of a larger number of patients [22]. Recent data indicate INS and DI as the best predictors of future type 2 diabetes in adults [23–25].

In order to understand the metabolic effects of rhGH therapy in adolescents with unconfirmed GHD at the achievement of adult height, we evaluated glucose metabolism in the last year of rhGH replacement and in first year after rhGH discontinuation compared with a healthy counterpart. Because some polymorphisms of the GHR could have a role in glucose metabolism and insulin resistance, we also evaluated whether the d3GHR deletion has a role on glucose homoeostasis during and after rhGH withdrawal.

Methods

This was a single-center longitudinal study conducted at Division of Pediatrics, University of Piemonte Orientale (Novara, Italy). We consecutively recruited 35 GH-deficient (GHD) adolescents at the end of puberty and in the last year of rhGH therapy and 45 healthy age and sex matched adolescents. The recruitment was opened from September 2006 to December 2011 The study was approved by the Ethics Committee of Maggiore della Carità Hospital (Novara) and informed written consent was obtained from all subjects and their parents before study. Patients were eligible if they had an idiopathic isolated GHD at diagnosis, had completed puberty (Tanner stage 4 and 5), the adult height was almost achieved with a bone age similar to the chronologic age and growth velocity near to 2 cm/year, and GHD was not confirmed at retesting (GD, group 1). Patients with coexistent other chronic or endocrine diseases, syndromes, diabetes, tumors or drugs interfering with glucose metabolism were excluded. Healthy control adolescents (CS, group 2) were eligible if they were at the end of puberty, normal-weight, with no history of organic or psychiatric diseases in particular no neurological, endocrine, liver, and kidney abnormalities.

Study Design and Assays

GHD adolescents were evaluated at fasting for IGF-1, total- (T-c), HDL- (HDL-c) cholesterol, triglycerides (TG), C-peptide and with an OGTT (1.75 g of glucose solution per kg, maximum 75 gr) in the last year of rhGH therapy (T0), and at 6 (T6) and 12 months (T12) after therapy withdrawal. In the year after GH discontinuation the retesting was performed with the GHRH plus arginine test with the adoption of the transition cut-offs [26]. In healthy adolescents the OGTT was performed at baseline.

Impaired fasting glucose (IFG) and impaired glucose tolerance (IGT) were defined according to American Diabetes Association classifications as fasting plasma glucose of ≥100 to 125 mg/dl nmol/l, and as 2-h post-OGTT glucose of ≥140 to 199 mg/dl, respectively. Also the definition of diabetes was performed according to the criteria of the American Diabetes Association [27].

Blood samples during OGTT were drawn for the determination of glucose and insulin every 30 min from 0′ to 120′ min. The area under curve (AUC) for plasma glucose and insulin were calculated by the trapezoidal rule.

Insulin resistance was estimated, in the basal state, by use of the homeostasis model assessment (HOMA-IR) = fasting glucose × fasting insulin/22.5; beta-cell function at fasting was calculated using the formula of HOMA-β = (20 × fasting insulin)/(fasting glucose −3.5). Insulin sensitivity was calculated from the Matsuda [10,000/$\sqrt{}$(fasting glucose × fasting insulin) × (Gm×Im)] and QUICKI (1/$\log_{10}$ fasting insulin+$\log_{10}$ fasting glucose) indexes [28].

The area under the curve (AUC) for parameters after OGTT was calculated according to the trapezoidal rule. Delta glucose (ΔG_{30-0}) and insulin (ΔI_{30-0}) were evaluated as the change in glucose and insulin concentrations from 0 to 30 min. The stimulus for insulin secretion in the increment in plasma glucose as insulinogenic index was calculated as the ratio of the changes in insulin and glucose concentration from 0 to 30 min (INS). *B*eta-cell compensatory capacity was evaluated by the disposition index defined as the product of the Matsuda Index and INS (DI) [29]. In addition, each subgroup and all subjects together were divided into four groups according to the 2-h glucose levels,: 1) less than 100 mg/dL, 2) 100–119 mg/dL, 3) 120–139 mg/dL 4) above 140 mg/dL according to the risk to have a lower DI [30].

Plasma glucose levels (mg/dl; 1 mg/dl:0,05551 mMol/liter) were measured by the gluco-oxidase colorimetric method (GLUCOFIX, by Menarini Diagnostici, Florence, Italy). Insulin (µUI/ml; 1 µUI/ml = 7.175 pmol/l) was measured by chemiluminescent enzyme-labelled immunometric assay (Diagnostic Products Corporation, Los Angeles, CA). Sensitivity: 2 µUI/ml. Intra- and inter-assay CV ranges: 2.5–8.3 and 4.4–8.6%.

HbA1c levels were measured by the high-performance liquid chromatography (HPLC), using a Variant machine (Biorad, Hercules, CA); intra- and inter-assay coefficients of variation are respectively lower than 0.6 and 1.6%. Linearity is excellent from 3.2% (11 mmol/mol) to 18.3% (177 mmol/mol).

T-c (mg/dl; 1 mg/dl: 0.0259 mMol/l), HDL-c (mg/dl; 1 mg/dl: 0.0259 mMol/l), TG (mg/dl; 1 mg/dl: 0.0113 mMol/l), and C-peptide (ng/ml) were evaluated using standardized methods in the hospital's chemistry laboratory. Plasma T-c concentration was measured by esterase and oxidase conversion (Advia 1650, Bayer Diagnostics, Newbury, UK); coefficient of variation (CV) 1.9%. Plasma TG and HDL-c concentrations were measured by enzymatic determination (Advia 1650, Bayer Diagnostics, Newbury, UK); CV 1.7%. LDL-c was calculated by Friedwald mathematical for individuals with TG<150 mg/dl.

Serum IGF-I was measured by Liason automated chemiluminescence analyzer supplied by DiaSorin with a measurement range of 3–1500 ng/ml. Age and gender-reference ranges were used to calculate an IGF1 SDS for each patient.

Anthropometric Measurements

Height was measured by the Harpenden stadiometer and weight by using electronic scale. Body mass index (BMI) was calculated as body weight divided by squared height (kg/m^2). Height, weight and BMI were stratified according to Italian growth charts [31]. Height velocity (HV) was calculated from the difference of mean heights obtained from 2 consecutive visits, divided by time between visits, and adjusted to a 12-month interval. Waist circumference was measured with a soft tape, midway between the lowest rib margin and the iliac crest, in the standing position. Hip circumference was measured over the widest part of the gluteal region, and the waist-to-hip ratio was calculated. Systolic (SBP) and diastolic (DBP) blood pressure were measured three times at the left arms by using a standard mercury sphygmomanometer and the mean value was recorded and stratified according to paediatric percentiles of National High Blood Pressure Education Program Working Group on High Blood Pressure in Children and Adolescents [32].

DNA Extraction and Genetic Analysis

At the end of the clinical protocol, after T12, genomic DNA was isolated from peripheral blood leukocytes by standard methods. The d3GHR polymorphism was detected as described previously [33] based on a multiplex PCR assay with a combination of 3 primers (G1, G2 and G3) that specifically amplify the wild type (935 base pairs bp) and the deleted (532 bp) alleles. Amplification products were visualized by electrophoresis on a 1.5% agarose gel stained with ethidium bromide (Figure S1).

Subjects with at least one copy of the exon-3 deleted GHR (d3/d3 and fl/d3; Del) were grouped together for comparison with full-length homozygote subjects (fl/fl; nDel).

Statistical Analysis

Data are expressed as mean±SEM. For continuous variables, the variation between groups was compared by means on nonparametric Wilcoxon, Mann-Whitney U, or chi-square tests, where appropriate. Trends were assessed by nonparametric Friedman test. A correlation analysis was performed using the Pearson's correlation test with a logarithmic transformation when necessary.

Statistical significance was assumed for $p<0.05$. All statistical analyses were performed with SPSS for Windows version 17.0 (SPSS INC; Chicago, IL, USA).

Results

GHD before and after GH Discontinuation

Of the 35 GHD enrolled subjects, 23 performed two OGTTs and completed the study. Of the 45 CS, 5 subjects had discomfort during OGTT and were excluded.

Clinical characteristics of CS and GHD at T0 and T12 are reported in Table 1 and 2. GHD subjects had received GH replacement therapy for 7.3±2.0 years. The last dose of GH was 12.0±0.5 mg/week. The GH peak at the Arginine+GHRH test was of 72.0±5.6 ng/ml.

One GHD subject showed IFG at T0 and T6 and two subjects IGT at T0. No glucose alterations were found at T12. The distribution of post-OGTT 2hrs glucose levels at each time point was reported in Table 2. HbA1c levels were 5.3±0.1% (34.0±1.0 mmol/mol) in the last year of therapy. No differences in waist, waist/hip ratio, BMI, SBP, DBP, LDL-c and TG were shown in GHD among visits. T-c and HDL-c levels were lower at T6 than T0, and HDL-c levels also at T12 than T0 in GHD although the trend among visits was not significant (Table 2).

Table 1. Clinical parameters of growth hormone deficient (GHD, group 1) children at the end (T0) of rhGH therapy (T0), after 12 months rhGH withdrawal (T12) and of control subjects (CS, group 2).

	GHD (group 1) T0	GHD (group 1) T12	CS (group 2)
N°	23	23	40
M/F	12/11	12/11	22/18
IFG/IGT	1/2	0/0	0/0
Age (yr)	15.9±0.2	17.9±0.2	15.4±0.2
Weight (kg)	55.4±1.8	58.6±2.1	61.3±1.4
Centile weight	23±2.1	25±2.1	27±1.5
Height (cm)	163.5±1.7[a]	166.1±1.2[c]	173.7±1.2[a,c]
SDS height	−0.9±0.1[a]	−1±0.2[c]	1.1±0,1[a,c]
BMI (kg/m^2)	20.9±0.5	21.2±0.5	20.4±0.2
HV (cm/yr)	1.5±0.4	1.0±0.1	-
Waist (cm)	72.8±1.2[a]	77.4±1.4	79±0.8[a]
SBP (mmHg)	119.7±2.1[b]	119.4±3	124.4±1.3[b]
DBP (mmHg)	77.2±1.4	78.0±2.6	79.8±1.2

Abbreviations. BMI, body mass index; HV, height velocity; IFG, impaired fasting glucose; IGT, impaired glucose tolerance; SBP: systolic blood pressure; DBP: diastolic blood pressure, SDS: standard deviation score.
Data are expressed as mean±SEM. a: $p<0.0001$ GHD T0 vs CS; b: $p<0.05$ GHD T0 vs CS; c: $p<0.0001$ GHD T12 vs CS.

Basal glucose levels were similar among the 3 times. Fasting insulin ($p<0.05$), HOMA-IR ($p<0.05$) insulin and glucose levels at each time point after OGTT ($p<0.01$), ΔG_{0-30} ($p<0.05$) and ΔI_{0-30}, insulin mean and insulin AUC ($p<0.01$) progressively decreased from T0 to T12. Conversely, C-peptide ($p<0.0001$), Matsuda and QUICKI indexes increased from T0 to T12 ($p<0.05$). Despite higher insulin resistance during the last year of GH treatment, a compensatory insulin secretion was recorded: HOMA-β and INS were higher at T0, and progressively decreased at T6 and T12 ($p<0.05$), with a stable DI. Also IGF1 levels and IGF-I SDS decreased from T0 to T12 ($p<0.0001$) (Table 2).

A trend to decrease in DI across 2 h glucose groups (<100; 100–119; 120–139; >140 mg/dl) was observed and maintained at each time point in GHD subjects; T0 (8.7±1.4; 7.2±1.1; 5.2±1.4; 3.2±0.8, respectively; $p<0.01$; χ^2 12.156), T6 (7.5±1; 7.0±0.9; 5.6±0.1, respectively; $p<0.05$; χ^2 6.695) and T12 (8.7±1.4; 7.6±1.7; 3.6±1.3, respectively; $p<0.05$; χ^2 6.593).

HOMA-IR ($p<0.03$), HOMA-β ($p<0.002$), QUICKI ($p<0.03$), Matsuda indexes ($p<0.002$), fasting ($p<0.05$) and at 120 min glucose ($p<0.01$) were worse in GHD subjects at T0 than in CS. No differences in metabolic parameters were shown between CS and GHD at T12 (Table 1).

GHD before and after GH Discontinuation According to GHR Genotype

By analysing the GHD group as a whole, we observed a huge dispersion in INS and DI as mean±SD. Indeed, we addressed to understand whether d3GHR has a role, according to some literature suggestions (9,10). All the GHD subjects were analysed for the GHR genotype, meanwhile 5 out of 40 CS withdrawn the consent to perform this analysis.

Table 2. Glucometabolic parameters of growth hormone deficient (GHD, group 1) children at the end of rhGH therapy (T0) and 6 (T6) and 12 (T12) months after rhGH withdrawal.

	T0	T6	T12	$p^{for\ trend}$
Fasting glucose (mg/dl)	83.6±1.7	84.5±1.8	84.1±1.8	NS
30-min plasma glucose (mg/dl)	145.5±5.7	138.3±5.4	127.2±5.9	<0.05
2-h plasma glucose (mg/dl)	110.1±4.2	98.6±3	92.5±5	<0.01
AUC Glucose 0-120 min	11592.4±521	11273.4±381	10691.8±613	NS
Mean Glucose (mg/dl)	114.7±4.2	111.1±3	105.4±4.9	NS
ΔG_{30-0}	59.9±4.8	53.2±4.9	42.9±5.5	<0.05
Fasting insulin (μUI/ml)	10.5±1.1	8±0.7	7.7±0.6	<0.05
30-min plasma insulin (μUI/ml)	99.4±12	80.6±11.6	59.8±9	<0.01
2-h plasma insulin (μUI/ml)	59.6±6.8	40.9±5.4	34.2±4.8	<0.01
AUC Insulin 0–120 min	7875.6±915	6554.4±864	4882.1±591	<0.01
Mean Insulin (μUI/ml)	66±7.2	53.3±6.4	40.6±4.3	<0.01
ΔI_{30-0}	88.8±11.2	72.5±11	52.2±8.6	<0.01
HOMA-IR	2.2±0.2	1.7±0.1	1.6±0.1	<0.05
HOMA%β	205.2±23.8	148.5±15.9	148.3±16.2	<0.05
INS	1.6±0.2	1.3±0.1	1.2±0.2	<0.05
DI	6.8±0.7	7.2±0.6	7.9±1.0	NS
C-peptide (ng/ml)	0.21±0.05	0.19±0.04	0.36±0.05	P<0.01
T-c (mg/dl)	141.6±4.6	136.2±4.5	136.8±6.9	NS
HDL-c (mg/dl)	52.2±2.0	46.2±1.7	48.2±2.6	NS
LDL-c (mg/dl)	76.1±3.6	77.5±3.2	76.6±5.7	NS
TG (mg/dl)	60.7±4.1	62.7±6.2	59.2±5.3	NS
IGF-1 (ng/ml)	629.6±38	356.8±17	332.6±25	<0.0001
IGF-1 SDS	1.21±0.19	-0.01±0.06	-0.15±0.17	<0.0001

Abbreviations. DI, disposition index; INS, insulinogenic index; AUC, area under the curve; ΔG0-30: delta glucose;; ΔI0-30: delta insulin; HDL-c, HDL-cholesterol; LDL-c, LDL-cholesterol; T-c, total-cholesterol; TG, triglycerides. Data are expressed as mean±SEM. The significance among the three measures (T0, T6 and T12) was calculated by Friedman test.

The frequencies of the tree genotypes, d3/d3, fl/d3 and fl/fl were respectively 9% [2], 35% [8], 56% [13] in GHD. Allele frequencies were not different from those observed in the 35 CS (Figure S1). Because frequency, the participants were therefore divided into two groups, those homozygote for the fl/fl alleles (Del) and those hetero- and homozygote for the deleted isoform combined (nDel).

Del and nDel GHD had similar anthropometric and metabolic parameters at T0 with exception of HDL-c which was higher in Del GHD (56.5±1.9 vs 49.1±3.0 mg/dl, $p<0.01$).

At T6, Del GHD showed lower glucose levels at baseline and after OGTT than nDel GHD (fasting glucose: 78.7±1.8 vs 87.5±2.9 mg/dl, $p<0.01$; T120 glucose: 90.7±4.6 vs 101.0±3.5 mg/dl, $p<0.01$; AUC 9703.0±476.6 vs 12316.7±447.7 mg/dl*h, $p<0.01$ and mean glucose 97.1±3.6 vs 118.5±2.8 mg/dl, $p<0.0001$). DI was higher in Del than nDel GHD (10.4±1.0 vs 5.4±0.4; $p<0.01$) without differences in INS, HOMA-IR and HOMA-β.

At T12, Del GHD showed lower glucose AUC (9449.0±552.4 vs 11771.0±1068.6 mg/dl*h; $p<0.05$) and ΔG_{30-0} (29.5±4.5 vs 53.0±9.0 mg/dl; $p<0.05$), and higher fasting insulin (9.0±0.8 vs 6.4±0.8 μUI/ml; $p<0.05$),HOMA-IR (1.8±0.1 vs 1.3±0.2; $p<0.05$) and C-peptide (0.39±0.09 vs 0.24±0.03 ng/ml; $p<0.04$) than nDel GHD. Moreover, Del GHD had INS (1.8±0.5 vs 0.7±0.1; $p<0.01$) and DI (10.7±1.8 vs 5.0±1.0; $p<0.01$) higher than nDel GHD. nDel GHD showed a progressively decrease from T0 to T12 in HOMA-IR, HOMA-β, INS ($p<0.05$) and DI (not significant) with stable C-peptide levels. Conversely, Del GHD showed a gradual increase in DI ($p<0.05$), INS (not significant), and C-peptide (0.20±0.08 vs 0.39±0.09; $p<0.01$) with a HOMA-IR decreasing from T0 to T6 with a slight increase to T12 ($p<0.01$ for trend) (Figure 1).

Del GHD presented stable higher HDL-c levels than nDel GHD at any time point, whereas T-c, LDL-c and TG remained similar. T-c levels decreased from T0 to T12 in nDel GHD (141.0±7.4 at T0; 137.2±7.5 mg/dl at T6, 133.5±8.4 mg/dl at T12; $p<0.0001$).

At T12, Del GHD presented lower fasting glucose (83.5±2.2 vs 88.0±2.2 mg/dl $p<0.03$), and higher fasting insulin (9.0±0.8 vs 6.8±0.6 μUI/ml; $p<0.03$), HOMA-β (167.7±20.1 vs 96.9±10.1; $p<0.003$), and DI (10.7±1.8 vs 9.1±1.0 $p<0.05$) than Del CS. Conversely, at T12 nDel GHD presented lower HOMA-IR (1.3±0.2 vs 1.8±0.1 $p<0.03$), INS (0.7±0.1 vs 1.2±0.1 $p<0.04$), and DI (5.0±1.0 vs 8.1±1.2 $p<0.04$) than nDel CS. Del and nDel CS had higher C-peptide levels with respect to their GHD counterpart ($p<0.001$).

Correlations

In GHD subjects during GH therapy, both INS and DI were correlated with GH weekly dose (r: −0.399; $p<0.05$ and r: −0.529; $p<0.01$, respectively). Correlation was maintained when

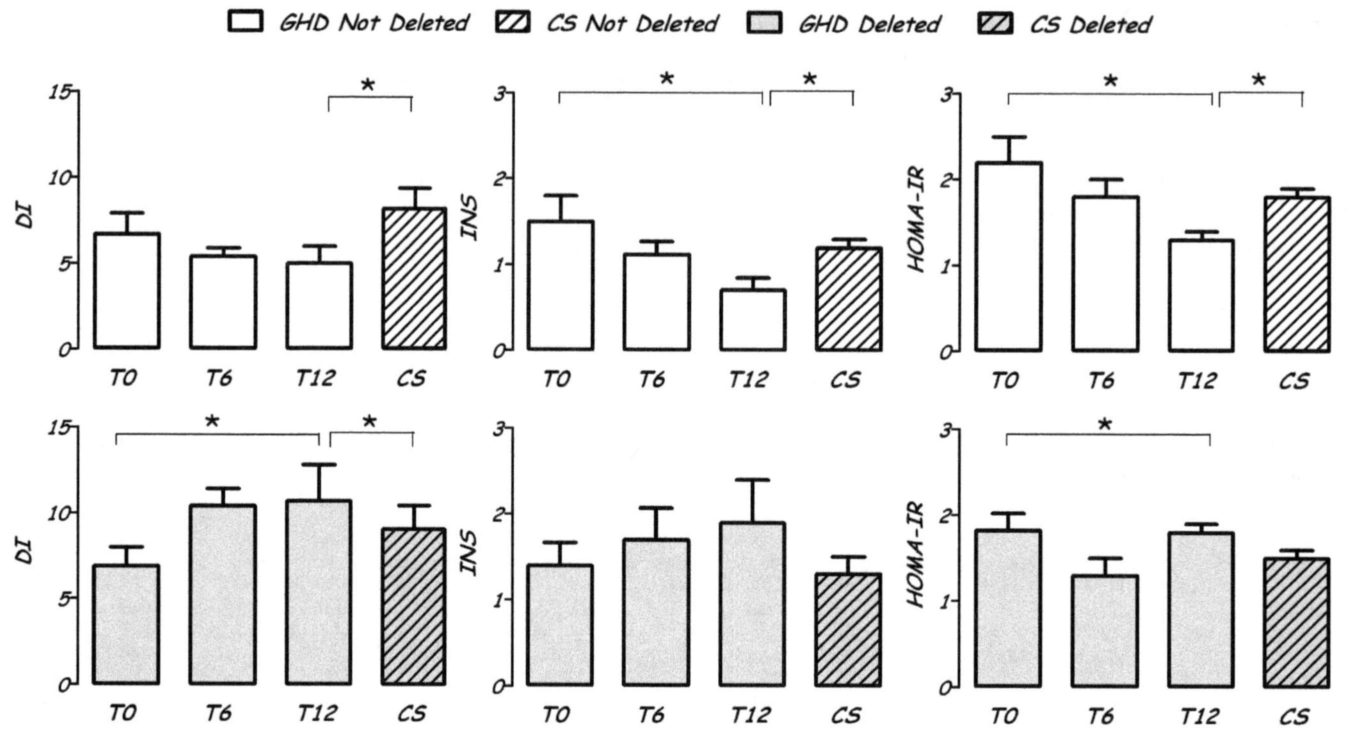

Figure 1. HOMA-IR, Insulinogenic (INS) and disposition (DI) index in GH deficient (GHD, group 1) and healthy (CS, group 2) adolescents with (Del, 27 subjects) and without (nDel, 31 subjects) the GH receptor (GHR) exon 3 deletion (d3GHR). GHD adolescents are evaluated in the last year of therapy (T0) and after six (T6) and twelve (T12) rhGH withdrawal. Data are expressed as mean±SEM. The significance among the three measures (T0, T6 and T12) was calculated by Friedman test. The significance between GHD and CS was calculated by Mann-Whitney U test. *p<0.05.

correcting for IGF-1 (INS r: −0.392, p<0.05; DI r: −0.526, p<0.01p<0.01) or IGF-SDS (INS r: −0.398, p<0.05; DI r: −0.531, p<0.01) which also weights for age and gender. No correlations were recorded after GH discontinuation.

IGF-1 levels and IGF-SDS were correlated with HOMA-IR at T6 (r: 0.518 and r: 0.514, p<0.01) and T12 (r: 0.518 and r: 0.518, p<0.01), and also with QUICKY and Matsuda indexes at T6 (QUICKI, r: −0.495 and r: −0.476, p<0.03; Matsuda index, −0.443 and r: 0.302; p<0.05) and T12 (QUICKI, r: −0.611 and r: 0.–609, p<0.02; Matsuda index, −0.543 and −0.359; p<0.05).

Discussion

A large number of studies have addressed the metabolic consequences of adult GHD, in contrast studies investigating glucose and insulin metabolism at the end of GH therapy in not confirmed GHD adolescents during the transition phase are lacking. The lack of published data reflects the clinical practice of stopping the follow up in adolescents at the achievement of adult height and with not confirmed GHD at reevaluation. This practice makes a gap in the understanding of GH biology and of long-term safety of rhGH treatment. In the present study, we observed that after 1 year of rhGH withdrawal metabolic parameters are similar between not confirmed GHD and matched control subjects. Moreover, during GH treatment, higher insulin-resistance at fasting and lower insulin-sensitivity during OGTT are associated with higher HOMA-β and insulinogenic index and a stable DI in the group as a whole. The d3GHR deletion may have a role on the metabolic risk with a more pronounced reduction of HOMA-IR and compensatory insulin secretion in nDel GHD, and with lower glucose levels and a higher increase in DI and fasting C-peptide in Del GHD at the end of the treatment.

First of all, we showed that whether glucose impairment and/or insulin resistance occurred during the treatment with rhGH, these are transient and quickly restored also in not confirmed GHD adolescents, as already demonstrated in literature in adolescents with persistent GHD [19,34]. Although puberty is ongoing, insulin resistance at fasting and insulin sensitivity during OGTT progressively return to similar levels to age, puberty, and weight matched healthy adolescents. On the other hand, it is interesting that GHD treated adolescents have the well-known higher insulin resistance at fasting [35,36] but it is coupled with a compensatory insulin secretion both at fasting, measured as HOMA-β, and during OGTT, measured as INS with also a stable DI. Indexes of insulin sensitivity (Matsuda index) and early insulin responses to oral glucose (INS) that were derived from baseline and follow-up OGTTs did not appear to be significant predictors for the development of type 2 diabetes. In contrast, the baseline DI, which significantly assesses beta-cell function in the context of insulin sensitivity, predicts the risk of deteriorating glucose tolerance in youths [30]. Thus, insulin secretion can be truly evaluated only in relation to the degree of insulin sensitivity. Indeed, our data on DI suggest that whether the treatment with GH has a detrimental role on insulin resistance because it stimulates lipolysis, in youths pancreas maintains a beta-cell compensatory capacity and is able to answer to a relative hyperglycemia with a higher insulin secretion which counterbalances the GH inhibited insulin-stimulated glucose uptake in the muscles without impact on future type 2 diabetes risk in those healthy [4,5]. Similarly, although M values at euglycemic hyperinsulinemic clamp were higher after a short rhGH withdrawal, in GHD treated young adults M values were similar than matched controls [36]. Also in small for gestational age GH treated adolescents, insulin sensitivity decreased but DI remained stable at puberty [37]. We could hypothesize that the preserved beta-cell function at early age protects from type 2 diabetes and that when DI progressively decreases with age and obesity a sustained glucose impairment arises more likely as in adults. A direct role of GH on insulin antagonism is supported by the negative correlation between GH weekly dose and INS and DI, suggesting that the pancreas compensation we observed is secondary to the peripheral detrimental action of GH.

Studies conducted in adults and children suggest that insulin resistance and glucose alteration are more frequent in GH treated subjects with risk factors like age, obesity, an adverse metabolic profile before therapy, syndromes or history of tumors [16]. Genomic profiles, like GHR polymorphisms could be inserted in this list. The d3GHR deletion is the most investigated polymorphism of GHR in both healthy subjects and patients with GHD or other diseases such as acromegaly or type 2 diabetes [38]. The d3GHR variant consisting of genomic exon 3 deletion has been linked with increased receptor activity due to an enhanced signal transduction. Its biological role on glucose metabolism is still controversial. Data derived by the Stockholm Diabetes Prevention Program suggest the homozygosity for the d3GHR allele as preventive of type 2 diabetes in adults. However, when other factors cause overt type 2 diabetes, the d3GHR allele confers a phenotype indicative of risk for metabolic disorders [10]. In Chinese obese children fasting insulin, HOMA-IR, and lipid profile were significantly lower in the homozygous and heterozygous d3GHR group than in the full-length GHR group [39]. Moreover, the presence of at least one d3GHR allele was associated with higher insulin secretion for a given degree of insulin sensitivity and with a higher disposition index in healthy normal weight children and adolescents during puberty in the COPENHAGEN puberty study [11].

All these data are in agreement with our observation that glucose levels are lower and DI, fasting C-peptide and nearly to significance INS, were higher in Del GHD adolescents after stopping therapy, suggesting that GHR exon 3 deletion gene polymorphism may play a role in modulating insulin secretion to a glucose challenge and peripheral insulin activity at least during periods of high endogenous GH secretion like puberty. Higher fasting C-peptide in subjects with at least one copy of the exon-3 deleted GHR than those with the full length one were also demonstrated in adults [10]. However, the changes are apparent after rhGH withdrawal in our population. This result is in line with that of Giavoli *et al.* who recorded a higher prevalence of impaired glucose tolerance after both 1 and 5 years of rhGH therapy in GHD adults positive for the d3GHR [9]. The enhanced activity of the d3GHR isoform may mediate the metabolic effects of rhGH on glucose homeostasis. We can speculate that a more pronounced GH activity has a strong lipolytic effect and insulin antagonism. As a consequence, a worse glucose homeostasis in adults and, more likely, a partial deterioration in peripheral insulin activity, reflected by DI, in adolescents become apparent. This hypothesis is fully in agreement with the fact that in healthy people when other factors cause overt type 2 diabetes, the d3GHR allele is not protective but confers a more impaired metabolic phenotype [10]. Because normal adolescents with d3GHR have higher DI during puberty and GHD unconfirmed subjects present an increase in DI after rhGH withdrawal, a threshold for the metabolic GH activity is suggested, in agreement with studies which failed to record alterations in glucose metabolism for treatments with rhGH very low doses [40].

GH plays an important role in the regulation of lipoprotein metabolism. In patients with d3GHR we also observed higher HDL-cholesterol levels during rhGH treatment and after rhGH withdrawal. These findings are in line with data in healthy and hypertensive adults [41] and support the idea that sequence variations in the GHR may have important effects on metabolic phenotype as a whole. Accordingly, other polymorphisms in the GHR have been shown to modify HDL cholesterol concentration also in hyperlipidaemic patients [42].

It has to note that our subjects progressively decreased IGF-I levels after rhGH withdrawal but remained in the middle part of the normal range. Higher IGF-I levels in the last year of rhGH treatment were due to the treatment and, in absence of a confirmed GHD during the transition phase, their levels quickly restored in the middle of normality. Interestingly, insulin resistance and sensitivity negatively correlated with them only after the withdrawal of the therapy. This is adequate with previous study that attest the U shape relation of IGF-I with the risk of diabetes is evident in a healthy population when confounders are removed [43].

There are limitations in the present study. First is that we did not perform an intravenous glucose tolerance test (IVGTT). The IVGTT is validated and more reproducible than the OGTT, because independent by confounding factors as the incretin effect is. However, the IVGTT only describes an experimental model and is far to be used in clinical practice. We decided to use the OGTT instead of IVGTT because OGTT describes the post-meal dynamics which is of interest for the GH physiology being GH a hormone that principally acts in the post-absorptive phase [1]. Moreover, we chose the OGTT-derived indices of insulin sensitivity and secretion because they correlate well with clamp measures in children [44,45], are easily calculated in epidemiological or intervention studies, and DI calculated by the OGTT has been demonstrated to predict diabetes development in adults [24]. Furthermore, the OGTT is the test that is classically performed in the clinical practice during rhGH treatment being simpler and cheaper than IVGTT. Moreover, we did not evaluate C-peptide during the test but only at fasting. The second limitation is that we were unable to demonstrate a gene dosage effect with respect to the d3GHR allele because the group of homozygous subjects was too small to analyse them separately. A study in a wider cohort could address this question. However, many published studies on the d3GHR also in wider populations [9–11] grouped together subjects bearing at least one copy of the exon-3 deleted GHR according to the hypothesis of the dominant model [46].

On the whole, in not confirmed GHD adolescents the fasting deterioration in glucose homeostasis is efficaciously coupled with a compensatory insulin secretion and activity for the degree of insulin-sensitivity at glucose challenge also in puberty. In adolescents during puberty, the presence of at least one d3GHR allele, despite a slightly higher fasting insulin resistance, is associated with lower glucose levels and higher HOMA-β, fasting C-peptide, HDL-cholesterol and DI at OGTT after rhGH withdrawal. Because a more pronounced activity of the d3GHR isoform, a major risk to develop an impairment in glucose homeostasis during the treatment could be hypothesized and future studies should address this question. OGTT should be routinely performed in clinical practice to better stratified GHD subjects during the treatment. Screening for the d3GHR in GHD treated subjects, also in childhood may help physicians to follow and phenotype patients during the treatment.

Supporting Information

Figure S1 Analysis of the GHR exon 3 polymorphism. a) Schematic representation of the multiplex PCR assay used to detect the GHR exon 3 polymorphism. One forward (G1) and two reverse primers (G2 and G3) were used. Primers G1 and G3 (this located within exon 3) are designed to detect the GHR-fl allele by the amplification of a 935 bp fragment (the 3248 bp fragment is non amplified under the conditions used); primers G1 and G2 allow the amplification of the GHR-d3 by producing a 532 bp fragment. b) Genotyping of the GHR exon 3 polymorphism. The presence of a 935 bp band indicates the genotypes homozygous for GHR-fl (#1,2,3,6,8,10,11,12) the presence of a band of 532 bp indicates the genotype homozygous for GHR-d3 (#4) and the presence of both the bands indicates the herozygotes (#5,7,9,13). A 100 bp ladder is used as a molecular weight marker. c) Distribution of the genotype in GHD and control (CS) subjects. Five out of 40 CS did not give the consent to perform the genetic analysis.

Acknowledgments

The authors wish to thank Caterina Balossini, Enza Giglione, Silvia Parlamento, and Stefania Moia for their technical assistance.

Author Contributions

Conceived and designed the experiments: FP GA GB MG SB. Performed the experiments: SS DB RR MG. Analyzed the data: FP SS GG MG SB. Contributed reagents/materials/analysis tools: DB RR MG. Wrote the paper: FP GA MG GB SB.

References

1. Møller N, Jørgensen JO (2009) Effects of growth hormone on glucose, lipid, and protein metabolism in human subjects. Endocr Rev 30: 152–177.
2. LeRoith D, Yakar S (2007) Mechanisms of disease: metabolic effects of growth hormone and insulin-like growth factor 1. Nat Clin Pract Endocrinol Metab 3: 302–310.
3. Oliveira CR, Meneguz-Moreno RA, Aguiar-Oliveira MH, Barreto-Filho JA (2011) Emerging role of the GH/IGF-I on cardiometabolic control. Arq Bras Cardiol 97: 434–439.
4. Segerlantz M, Bramnert M, Manhem P, Laurila E, Groop LC (2011) Inhibition of the rise in FFA by Acipimox partially prevents GH-induced insulin resistance in GH-deficient adults. J Clin Endocrinol Metab 86: 5813–5818.
5. Bramnert M, Segerlantz M, Laurila E, Daugaard JR, Manhem P et al. (2003) Growth hormone replacement therapy induces insulin resistance by activating the glucose-fatty acid cycle. J Clin Endocrinol Metab 88: 1455–1463.
6. Møller N, Butler PC, Antsiferov MA, Alberti KG (1989) Effects of growth hormone on insulin sensitivity and forearm metabolism in normal man. Diabetologia 32: 105–110.
7. Smith TR, Elmendorf JS, David TS, Turinsky J (1997) Growth hormone-induced insulin resistance: role of the insulin receptor, IRS-1, GLUT-1 and GLUT-4. Am J Physiol 272: 1071–1079.
8. Dominici FP, Turyn D (2002) Growth hormone-induced alterations in the insulin-signaling system. Exp Biol Med (Maywood) 227: 149–157.
9. Giavoli C, Ferrante E, Profka E, Olgiati L, Bergamaschi S, et al. (2010) Influence of the d3GH receptor polymorphism on the metabolic and biochemical phenotype of GH-deficient adults at baseline and during short- and long-term recombinant human GH replacement therapy. Eur J Endocrinol 163: 361–368.
10. Strawbridge RJ, Kärvestedt L, Li C, Efendic S, Ostenson CG, et al. (2007) GHR exon 3 polymorphism: association with type 2 diabetes mellitus and metabolic disorder. Growth Horm IGF Res 17: 392–398.
11. Sørensen K, Aksglaede L, Munch-Andersen T, Aachmann-Andersen NJ, Leffers H, et al. (2009) Impact of the growth hormone receptor exon 3 deletion gene polymorphism on glucose metabolism, lipids, and insulin-like growth factor-I levels during puberty. J Clin Endocrinol Metab 94: 2966–2969.
12. Rosenfalck AM, Maghsoudi S, Fisker S, Jørgensen JO, Christiansen JS, et al. (2000) The effect of 30 months of low-dose replacement therapy with recombinant human growth hormone (rhGH) on insulin and C-peptide kinetics, insulin secretion, insulin sensitivity, glucose effectiveness, and body composition in GH-deficient adults. J Clin Endocrinol Metab 85: 4173–4181.
13. Hoffman AR, Kuntze JE, Baptista J, Baum HB, Baumann GP, et al. (2004) Growth hormone (GH) replacement therapy in adult-onset GH deficiency: effects on body composition in men and women in a double-blind, randomized, placebo-controlled trial. J Clin Endocrinol Metab 89: 2048–2056.
14. Svensson J, Fowelin J, Landin K, Bengtsson BA, Johansson JO (2002) Effects of seven years of GH-replacement therapy on insulin sensitivity in GH-deficient adults. J Clin Endocrinol Metab 87: 2121–2127.
15. Bülow B, Erfurth EM (1999) A low individualized GH dose in young patients with childhood onset GH deficiency normalized serum IGF-I without significant deterioration in glucose tolerance. Clin Endocrinol (Oxf) 50: 45–55.
16. Appelman-Dijkstra NM, Claessen KM, Roelfsema F, Pereira AM, Biermasz NR (2013) Therapy of Endocrine disease: Long-term effects of recombinant human GH replacement in adults with GH deficiency: a systematic review. Eur J Endocrinol 169: R1–R14.
17. Cutfield WS, Wilton P, Bennmarker H, Albertsson-Wikland K, Chatelain P, et al. (2000) Incidence of diabetes mellitus and impaired glucose tolerance in children and adolescents receiving growth-hormone treatment. Lancet 355: 610–613.
18. Child CJ, Zimmermann AG, Scott RS, Cutler GB Jr, Battelino T, et al. (2011) Prevalence and incidence of diabetes mellitus in GH-treated children and adolescents: analysis from the GeNeSIS observational research program. J Clin Endocrinol Metab 96: E1025–E1033.
19. Nørrelund H, Vahl N, Juul A, Møller N, Alberti KG, et al. (2000) Continuation of growth hormone (GH) therapy in GH-deficient patients during transition from childhood to adulthood: impact on insulin sensitivity and substrate metabolism. J Clin Endocrinol Metab 85: 1912–1917.
20. Carroll PV, Drake WM, Maher KT, Metcalfe K, Shaw NJ, et al. (2004) Comparison of continuation or cessation of growth hormone (GH) therapy on body composition and metabolic status in adolescents with severe GH deficiency at completion of linear growth. J Clin Endocrinol Metab 89: 3890–3895.
21. Heptulla RA, Boulware SD, Caprio S, Silver D, Sherwin RS et al. (1997) Decreased insulin sensitivity and compensatory hyperinsulinemia after hormone treatment in children with short stature. J Clin Endocrinol Metab 82: 3234–3238.
22. Wallace TM, Levy JC, Matthews DR (2004) Use and abuse of HOMA modeling. Diabetes Care 27: 1467–1495.
23. Kahn SE (2003) The relative contributions of insulin resistance and beta-cell dysfunction to the pathophysiology of type 2 diabetes. Diabetologia 46: 3–19.
24. Utzschneider KM, Prigeon RL, Faulenbach MV, Tong J, Carr DB, et al. (2009) Oral disposition index predicts the development of future diabetes above and beyond fasting and 2-h glucose levels. Diabetes Care 32: 335–41.
25. Abdul-Ghani MA, Williams K, DeFronzo RA, Stern M (2007) What is the best predictor of future type 2 diabetes? Diabetes Care 2007 30: 1544–1548.
26. Corneli G, Di Somma C, Prodam F, Bellone J, Bellone S, et al. (2007) Cut-off limits of the GH response to GHRH plus arginine test and IGF-I levels for the diagnosis of GH deficiency in late adolescents and young adults. Eur J Endocrinol 157: 701–708.
27. American Diabetes Association (2013) Diagnosis and Classification of Diabetes Mellitus. Diabetes Care 36(Suppl.): 67–74.
28. Matsuda M, DeFronzo R (1999) Insulin sensitivity indices obtained from oral glucose tolerance testing: comparison with the euglycemic insulin clamp. Diabetes Care 22: 1462–1470.
29. Kahn SE, Prigeon RL, McCulloch DK, Boyko EJ, Bergman RN, et al. (1993) Quantification of the relationship between insulin sensitivity and beta-cell function in human subjects. Evidence for a hyperbolic function. Diabetes 42: 1663–1672.
30. Giannini C, Weiss R, Cali A, Bonadonna R, Santoro N, et al. (2012) Evidence for early defects in insulin sensitivity and secretion before the onset of glucose dysregulation in obese youths: a longitudinal study. Diabetes 61: 606–614.
31. Cacciari E, Milani S, Balsamo A, Spada E, Bona G, et al. (2006) Italian cross-sectional growth charts for height, weight and BMI (2 to 20 yr). J Endocrinol Invest 29: 581–593.
32. National High Blood Pressure Education Program Working Group on High Blood Pressure in Children and Adolescents (2004) The fourth report on the diagnosis, evaluation, and treatment of high blood pressure in children and adolescents. Pediatrics 114: 555–576.
33. Pantel J, Machinis K, Sobrier ML, Duquesnoy P, Goossens M, et al. (2000) Species-specific alternative splice mimicry at the growth hormone receptor locus revealed by the lineage of retro elements during primate evolution. J Biol Chem 23: 275: 18664–18669.
34. Seminara S, Merello G, Masi S, Filpo A, La Cauza F, et al. (1998) Effect of long-term growth hormone treatment on carbohydrate metabolism in children with growth hormone deficiency. Clin Endocrinol (Oxf) 49: 125–130.
35. Radetti G, Pasquino B, Gottardi E, Contadin IB, Rigon F, et al. (2004) Insulin sensitivity in growth hormone-deficient children: influence of replacement treatment. Clin Endocrinol (Oxf) 61: 473–477.
36. Jørgensen JO, Møller J, Alberti KG, Schmitz O, Christiansen JS, et al. (1993) Marked effects of sustained low growth hormone (GH) levels on day-to-day fuel metabolism: studies in GH-deficient patients and healthy untreated subjects. J Clin Endocrinol Metab 77: 1589–1596.

37. Van der Kaay D, Bakker B, van der Hulst F, Mul D, Mulder J, et al. (2010) Randomized GH trial with two different dosages in combination with a GnRH analogue in short small for gestational age children: effects on metabolic profile and serum GH, IGF1, and IGFBP3 levels. Eur J Endocrinol 162: 887–895.
38. Filopanti M, Giavoli C, Grottoli S, Bianchi A, De Marinis L, et al. (2011) The exon 3-deleted growth hormone receptor: molecular and functional characterization and impact on GH/IGF-I axis in physiological and pathological conditions. J Endocrinol Invest 34: 861–868.
39. Gao L, Zheng Z, Cao L, Shen S, Yang Y, et al. (2011) The growth hormone receptor (GHR) exon 3 polymorphism and its correlation with metabolic profiles in obese Chinese children. Pediatr Diabetes 12: 429–434.
40. Arafat AM, Möhlig M, Weickert MO, Schöfl C, Spranger J, et al. (2010) Improved insulin sensitivity, preserved beta cell function and improved whole-body glucose metabolism after low-dose growth hormone replacement therapy in adults with severe growth hormone deficiency: a pilot study. Diabetologia 53: 1304–1313.
41. Horan M, Newsway V, Yasmin, Lewis MD, Easter TE, et al. (2006) Genetic variation at the growth hormone (GH1) and growth hormone receptor (GHR) loci as a risk factor for hypertension and stroke. Hum Genet 119: 527–540.
42. Takada D, Ezura Y, Ono S, Iino Y, Katayama Y, et al. (2003) Growth hormone receptor variant (L526I) modifies plasma HDL cholesterol phenotype in familial hypercholesterolemia: intra-familial association study in an eight-generation hyperlipidemic kindred. Am J Med Genet A 121A: 136–140.
43. Schneider HJ, Friedrich N, Klotsche J, Schipf S, Nauck M, et al. (2011) Prediction of incident diabetes mellitus by baseline IGF1 levels. Eur J Endocrinol 64: 223–229.
44. Gungor N, Arslanian S (2004) Progressive beta cell failure in type 2 diabetes mellitus of youth. J Pediatr 144: 656–659.
45. Lee S, Bacha F, Gungor N, Arslanian S (2008) Comparison of different definitions of pediatric metabolic syndrome: relation to abdominal adiposity, insulin resistance, adiponectin, and inflammatory biomarkers. J Pediatr 152: 177–184.
46. Dos Santos C, Essioux L, Teinturier C, Tauber M, Goffin V, et al. (2004) A common polymorphism of the growth hormone receptor is associated with increased responsiveness to growth hormone. Nat Genet 36: 720–724.

Expression of Fibroblast Growth Factor-21 in Muscle is Associated with Lipodystrophy, Insulin Resistance and Lipid Disturbances in Patients with HIV

Birgitte Lindegaard[1,2,3*], Thine Hvid[1,2], Thomas Grøndahl[1,2], Christian Frosig[2,4], Jan Gerstoft[3], Pernille Hojman[1,2,3], Bente Klarlund Pedersen[1,2,3]

1 Centre of Inflammation and Metabolism, Department of Infectious Diseases, Rigshospitalet, Copenhagen, Denmark, **2** Copenhagen Muscle Research Centre, Rigshospitalet, Copenhagen, Denmark, **3** Department of Infectious Diseases, Rigshospitalet, Copenhagen, Denmark, **4** Institute of Exercise and Sport Sciences, Department of Human Physiology, Copenhagen, Denmark

Abstract

Background: Fibroblast growth factor (FGF)-21 is a novel regulator of glucose and lipid metabolism. Recently, increased FGF-21 mRNA expression in muscle was found in patients with type 2 diabetes, but the role for FGF-21 in muscle is not well understood. Patients with HIV-infection and lipodystrophy are characterised by various degree of lipid-driven insulin resistance. We hypothesized that muscle FGF-21 mRNA would be altered in HIV patients with lipodystrophy.

Design: Twenty-five HIV-infected men with lipodystrophy (LD) and 15 age-matched healthy controls, received an oral glucose tolerance test and a euglycemic-hyperinsulinemic clamp (50 mU/m2/min) combined with 6,6-H_2 glucose infusion. Muscle biopsies were obtained and FGF-21 mRNA and glycogen synthase (GS) activity were measured.

Results: Subjects with HIV were insulin resistant compared with non-HIV subjects. Compared to controls, HIV subjects demonstrated a twofold increase of plasma FGF-21 from 70.4±56.8 pg/ml vs 109.1±71.8 pg/ml, respectively ($p = 0.04$) and an eight-fold increase in muscular FGF-21 mRNA expression ($p = 0.001$). Muscle FGF-21 mRNA correlated inversely with the rate of disappearance of glucose during insulin clamp ($r = -0.54$, $p = 0.0009$), and the GS fractional velocity in muscle ($r = -0.39$, $p = 0.03$), and directly with fasting insulin ($r = 0.50$, $p = 0.0022$), HOMA-IR ($r = 0.47$, $p = 0.004$), triglycerides ($r = 0.60$. $P = 0.0001$), waist-to-hip ratio ($r = 0.51$, $p = 0.0001$) and limb fat mass (-0.46, $p = 0.004$), but not to plasma FGF-21.

Conclusion: FGF-21 mRNA is increased in skeletal muscle in HIV patients and correlates to whole-body (primarily reflecting muscle) insulin resistance, but not to plasma FGF-21. Those findings add to the evidence that FGF-21 is a myokine and may suggest that muscle FGF-21 is working in a local manner.

Editor: Michael Müller, Wageningen University, The Netherlands

Funding: The Centre of Inflammation and Metabolism (CIM) is supported by a grant from the Danish National Research Foundation (# 02-512-55). This study was further supported by the Danish Medical Research Council (# 22-04-0588), the Commission of the European Communities (Grant Agreement no. 223576 - MYOAGE), the Lundbeck Foundation, the Danish AIDS Foundation, the Novo Nordisk Foundation, Direktør Emil Hertz og Hustru Inger Hertz' Fond, Direktør Jacob Madsen og Hustru Olga Madsens Fond, Fonden for Lægevidenskabens fremme. CIM is part of the UNIK Project: Food, Fitness and Pharma for Health and Disease, supported by the Danish Ministry of Science, Technology and Innovation. CIM is a member of DD2 - the Danish Center for Strategic Research in Type 2 Diabetes (the Danish Council for Strategic Research, grant no. 09-067009 and 09-075724). The Copenhagen Muscle Research Centre is supported by a grant from the Capital Region of Denmark. The funders had no role in study design, data collection and analysis, decision to publish, or preparation of the manuscript.

Competing Interests: The authors have declared that no competing interests exist.

* E-mail: blm@rh.dk

Introduction

Fibroblast growth factor (FGF)-21 is a circulating hormone-like cytokine and has received much attention as a regulator for glucose and lipid metabolism in liver under fasting and ketotic conditions[1].

The majority of studies investigating the role of FGF-21 are based on animal studies. In rodents FGF-21 is produced mainly by the liver and adipose tissue. In murine models, FGF-21 is reducing plasma glucose, insulin, triglycerides, LDL and HDL cholesterol [2,3]. Furthermore, in diet-induced obesity in mice, FGF-21 is enhancing insulin-mediated suppression of endogenous glucose production and enhancing insulin-mediated glucose uptake in skeletal muscle [3]. In lipid metabolism, FGF-21 induces ketogenesis during starvation [4], promotes fatty acid oxidation [5] and lipolysis in adipose tissue [6] in rodents.

Paradoxically, circulating FGF-21 is increased in obese nondiabetic subjects [7] and in newly diagnosed type 2 diabetes, where it correlates positively with adiposity and fasting insulin [8]. One human study has shown that plasma FGF-21 concentrations correlate with both hepatic as well as with whole-body (muscle) insulin resistance [9].

Recently, FGF-21 was identified as a novel myokine in humans [10]. An elevated muscular expression of FGF-21 was found in patients with type 2 diabetes [11] and insulin was identified as a stimulator of muscle-FGF-21 in two separate studies [10,12]. However, little information is available on FGF-21 in muscle and its role in metabolism

A syndrome of lipodystrophy, characterised by subcutaneous fat loss, and a relative increase in central fat accumulation, develops in a subgroup of HIV patients, when treated with highly active combination antiretroviral therapy (HAART) that includes thymidine nucleoside analogues (NA) [13]. Lipodystrophy is associated with severe metabolic side effects, including dyslipidemia, hepatic insulin resistance, and lipid-driven impaired insulin-stimulated glucose uptake in muscle [14–16]. Recently, circulating FGF-21 was observed in HIV-infected patients, and especially those with lipodystrophy (11). This increase was, furthermore, closely associated with insulin resistance.

Since HIV patients with lipodystrophy share the same metabolic disturbances as subjects with type 2 diabetes we aimed to determine whether muscle FGF-21 mRNA is altered in these patients. The second aim of the study was to investigate the possible association of muscle FGF21 mRNA with other measures of adiposity and insulin resistance, including peripheral insulin resistance by using an insulin clamp combined with stable isotopes.

Patients and Methods

Patients

Twenty-three HIV-infected men were recruited from the outpatient clinic of the Department of Infectious Disease, Rigshospitalet in Copenhagen. LD was defined clinically by physical examination of peripheral lipoatrophy (defined by the presence of peripheral lipoatrophy with at least one moderate sign of fat loss in face, arms, buttocks, or legs based on a physical examination by a single investigator (BL) using a validated questionnaire developed by Carr et al. [17]. Some of the subjects have been included in a former study [18]. All patients were on a stable and effective nucleoside analogue based HAART with no changes in antiretroviral therapy during the preceding 8 weeks. Fifteen age-matched HIV-negative healthy men served as controls. Demographic data were collected for each patient: age, duration of HIV infection, duration and types of all antiretroviral therapy, weight, height, CD4 count, HIV-RNA copies. Inclusion criteria were: no signs of ongoing infections; fasting glucose under 7 mmol/L and 120 min glucose after an OGTT below 11.1 mmol/L, no dyslipidemia (triglycerides >1.7 mmol/L and/ or HDL-cholesterol <0.9 mmol/L); suppressed viral load (<20 copies/mL). Exclusion criteria were: Severe cardiovascular diseases; arthritis; severe neuropathy; opportunistic infections that required hospitalisation within the last 6 weeks; diabetes (fasting glucose ≥7 mmol/L or 2-hrs. glucose >11 mmol/L after an OGTT); hepatitis C; concurrent therapy with antidiabetic agents, anticoagulant or any hormones. Fifteen age- and VO_{2max} - matched HIV-seronegative healthy men served as controls. The control subjects have been included in a former a study [18].

Written informed consent was obtained from all subjects according to the requirements from the local ethical committee and the Helsinki Declaration II, and the approval from the local ethical committee (The Ethics Committee of Copenhagen and Frederiksberg) was obtained.

Biochemical measurements

Peripheral blood samples were obtained after an overnight fasting at 8 A.M.. Measurements of total cholesterol (mmol/L), HDL-cholesterol (mmol/L), LDL-cholesterol (mmol/L), triglycerids (mmol/L), plasma glucose (mmol/L), insulin (pmol/L), were determined immediately using routine methods.

CD4 cell counts were calculated by flowcytometry and HIV-RNA copies were measured by the Amplicor HIV Monitor (Roche Molecular Systems, Branchburg, NJ) (lower limit of dectection: 20 copies/ml).

FGF-21 was measured in plasma. Ethylenediaminetetraacetate (EDTA) was used as an anticoagulant. Plasma samples were stored at −80 C until analysed. FGF-21 was determined by enzyme-linked immunosorbent assay (ELISA) kits (Biovendor, Germany). The detection limits were 15 pg/ml and the interassay coefficient of variation was 3.9%. All samples and standards were run as duplicates and the mean of duplicates was used in the statistical analyses.

RNA analysis and quantitative PCR analysis

RNA was extracted from 20–30 mg of skeletal muscle biopsies using TriZol (Invitrogen, Carlsbad, CA) and reverse transcribed using random hexamer primers (TaqMan reverse transcription reagents; Applied Biosystems). Real-time PCR was performed on an ABI PRISM 7900 Sequence Detection System (PE Biosystems) using TaqMan reagents (Applied Biosystems). Sequence-specific FGF-21 primer/probe sets were used for FGF-21 amplification, while predeveloped household TaqMan primer/probe sets (Applied Biosystems) were used for 18S detection. The relative expression of FGF-21 was normalized to the endogenous control and expressed as FGF-21 expression per 18S expression. The levels of 18S in the skeletal muscle were not different between groups (data not shown).

Body composition analysis

Fat and fat-free tissue masses for the whole body, trunk and extremities were measured using dual-energy X-ray absorptiometry (DXA) scanner (Lunar Prodigy, GE Medical Systems Wisconsin, USA, version 8.8) [17]. Whole-body and regional fat measurements (trunk and extremity) were determined as previously described [18].

Insulin sensitivity

Insulin resistance was assessed from several measurements: fasting plasma insulin, homeostasis model (HOMA-IR) [19] and area under the curve (AUC) for the insulin concentration during an 75-g oral glucose tolerance test (OGTT)

Euglycemic-hyperinsulinemic clamp combined with stable isotope infusion. Diet was registered two days before the clamp and participants were advised to ingest the same diet at the end-of-study visit. Subjects were admitted at 0800 h to the laboratory after an overnight fast (including HAART). An euglycemic-hyperinsulinemic clamp combined with glucose stable isotope technique was undertaken as described previously [20]. In brief, after obtaining baseline blood samples to determine background glucose enrichment a primed 16 µmol/kg constant infusion (0.22 µmol/kg/min) of [6,6-$^2H_2$]-glucose (Cambridge Isotopes Laboratories, Inc., MA, USA) was maintained for 5 hrs to determine glucose kinetics. The clamp was initiated 2.5 hrs after the start of the isotope infusion (basal condition) and continued for 2.5 hrs, adapted after [21]. Insulin (Actrapid, Novo Nordisk Insulin), 100 IU/ml was infused at a rate of 50 mU/m^2/min (initiated with a two-step priming dose of 200 mU/m^2/min for 5 min followed by 100 mU/m^2/min for 5 min). Blood glucose was maintained at 5.5 mmol/L by infusion of 20% glucose enriched to 2.5% with [6,6-$^2H_2$]-glucose [22]. The infusion of [6,6-$^2H_2$]-glucose was decreased by 75% of basal infusion rate during insulin-stimulated condition to steadily maintain the plasma glucose enrichment by accounting for the expected decline in hepatic glucose production. In the morning, the hand was wrapped in a heating blanket to obtain arterialised blood samples every 10 min during the last 30 min of the basal and insulin-stimulated conditions to determine plasma glucose concentrations and tracer-to-tracee ratio.

Glycogen synthesis activity

GS activity was measured in muscle homogenates by using a Unifilter 350 microtiter plate assay (Whatman; Frisenette, Ebeltoft, Denmark) as described by Thomas et al.[23]. Glycogen synthase activity is expressed as fractional velocity (%FV) corresponding to GS activity at a subsaturating (0.17 mM) G-6-P concentration divided by GS activity at a saturating (8 mM) concentration of G-6-P.

Calculations

A physiological and isotopic steady state was achieved during the last 30 minutes of the basal and the insulin-stimulated conditions, so the rates of endogenous glucose appearance (R_a) and disappearance of glucose (R_d) were calculated as the tracer infusion rate divided by the tracer to-tracee ratio as previously described [20]. Glucose R_a and R_d are expressed per kg body weight ($\mu mol \cdot kg\ bwt^{-1} \cdot min^{-}$).

Statistical analysis

Statistical calculations were performed using SAS 9.1 (USA). Data are presented as means +/− SD. $P<0.05$ was considered significant in all analyses. Rd and Ra, Insulin, triglycerides, FFA, HDL-cholesterol, LDL-cholesterol, and FGF-21 were natural log-transformed to achieve an approximate normal distribution and equal variance. Parameters between HIV-infected patients and healthy controls were compared with unpaired t-test. Pearson's correlations were used to examine the relationship between muscle FGF-21 or plasma FGF-21 levels and markers of insulin sensitivity, as well as with anthropometric parameters.

Results

Baseline characteristics

Demographic, body composition and biochemical data appear from Table 1. The healthy men and the HIV-infected patients were matched on age and physical activity. All subjects were categorised as sedentary-normal active. HIV-infected patients displayed a redistribution of body fat as the percentage of fat on the limb were lower and the percentage of fat in the trunk was higher compared to control subjects. The patients also had disturbances in their lipid metabolism as fasting triglycerides and total-cholesterol levels were higher, and HDL-cholesterol level was lower. In addition, compared to controls, the HIV-infected patients were characterized by peripheral insulin resistance as whole-body insulin-stimulated glucose uptake (R_d) and incremental glucose uptake (R_d basal – R_d clamp) were decreased. Furthermore, the HIV subjects had higher basal endogenous glucose production, lower insulin-mediated suppression of endogenous glucose production (R_a), but no difference in the incremental suppression of endogenous glucose production during the clamp (R_a basal – R_a clamp) as compared to control subjects.

Plasma FGF-21 and FGF-21mRNA in muscle

Plasma FGF-21 was elevated in the HIV-group compared to healthy controls (70.4±56.8 pg/ml vs 109.1±71.8 pg/ml, respectively) ($P = 0.04$) (Figure 1A).

FGF-21 mRNA expression in skeletal muscle was increased 8-fold in patients with HIV relative to healthy individuals ($P<0.0001$, parametric statistics, and $p = 0.0002$ for non-parametric statistics) (Figure 1B). The association between plasma FGF-21 and muscle FGF-21 did not reach statistical significance ($r = 0.32$; $p = 0.056$).

Relationships between FGF-21 mRNA, plasma FGF-21 and insulin resistance

Muscle FGF-21 mRNA correlated positively to all markers of insulin resistance: fasting insulin ($r = 0.57$, $p = 0.0008$), homeostasis model assessment (HOMA) score ($r = 0.55$, $p = 0.001$), and $insulin_{AUC}$ ($r = 0.38$, $p = 0.02$) (Fig. 1 C–F).

To test whether the association between insulin and FGF-21 mRNA in muscle reflect an association with peripheral or hepatic insulin resistance, we performed a euglycemic-hyperinsulinemic clamp with stable isotopes. We found that muscle FGF-21 mRNA was negatively associated with the insulin-mediated glucose-uptake (Figure 1G), but not with hepatic insulin resistance (data not shown).

We did not find any association between plasma FGF-21 and parameters of insulin resistance (fasting insulin, plasma glucose, HOMA-IR, glucose $_{AUC}$, Insulin $_{AUC}$, R_a or R_d). However, when investigating by group, plasma FGF-21 correlated positive with insulin stimulated glucose-uptake in healthy subjects but not in the HIV patients ($r = 0.51$, $p = 0.049$) (data not shown).

Previous studies have demonstrated that insulin resistance in patients with HIV-LD are associated with decreased insulin-stimulated glycogen synthase (GS) activity [24]. Therefore, we measured GS activity. The GS fractional velocity of % total GS activity was lower in HIV patients compared with healthy controls (28±1.3; 35±1.6, respectively) in the basal stage. GS fractional velocity is known to correlate positively with the glucose R_d [25]. As high FGF-21 mRNA in muscle is associated with low rate of disappearance of glucose, this could be linked to low GS fractional velocity in muscle. In accordance with this hypothesis, we found that high levels of FGF-21 mRNA in muscle were associated with decreased GS fractional velocity in muscle (Fig. 1H).

Relationships between muscle FGF-21 mRNA, and fat distribution and lipids

We found a strong negative association between muscle FGF-21 mRNA and the amount of subcutaneous fat (limb fat mass) ($r = -0.46$; $p = 0.0038$) and positive association with trunk-limb-fat-ratio ($r = 0.51$; $p = 0.001$) and triglycerides ($r = 0.56$; $p = 0.0003$). FGF-21 mRNA was not associated with total fat mass or total trunk fat (data not shown).

Discussion

The novelty and the major findings of our study is that we demonstrate for the first time that FGF-21 mRNA expression is increased in skeletal muscle in patients with HIV-LD compared to healthy age-matched men and that muscle FGF-21 mRNA correlates negatively with the rate of insulin-stimulated glucose disappearance (primarily reflecting muscle). Furthermore, increased FGF-21 mRNA expression in muscle is associated with decreased limb fat mass, increased waist-to-hip ratio and increased triglycerides.

Only three studies are published on expression of FGF-21 in muscle in humans [10,12,26] and very little is known about the function of muscle FGF-21. Our result is in agreement with a previous study, in which FGF-21 mRNA was found to be increased in muscle from subjects with type 2 diabetes and the expression was increased by hyperinsulinemia [10]. However, this study did not distinguish between hepatic and peripheral insulin sensitivity as we do in the present study. Vienberg *et al.* [12] also

Table 1. Baseline characteristics of patients and healthy controls.

	HIV patients (n = 23)	Healthy controls (n = 15)
Age (years)	47.9 (9.5)	47.5 (6.1)
Duration of HIV infection (years)	15.6 (9.6)	
Duration of antiretroviral therapy (years)	10.3 (4.3)	
CD4+ cell (cells/μl)	558 (208)	
LogHIV-RNA (copies/ml)	1.33 (0.12)	
Antiretroviral use		
NNRTI-based HAART, PI-based HAART, NNRTI-,PI-based HAART regime, No.	12/14/2	
Current Thymidine-NRTI use, No. (%)	11 (47.8)	
Current PI use, No. (%)	13 (56.7)	
Current NNRTI use, No. (%)	11 (47.8)	
Physical activity parameters		
VO_{2max} (LO_2/min)	2.3 (0.5)	2.5 (0.6)
Body composition		
Body-mass index (kg/m^2)	23.7 (2.9)	23.7 (1.9)
Weight (kg)	73.6 (11.2)	76.9 (7.4)
Waist (cm)	93.6 (6.4)	90 (5.7)
Waist-to.hip ratio	1.01 (0.04)	0.94 (0.03)
Fat mass (kg)	13.8 (5.3)	15.7 (4.4)
Trunk fat mass (kg)	9.8 (3.9)	8.9 (3.0)
Trunk fat percentage (%)	71.2 (6.2) ****	56.1(5.2)
Limb fat mass (kg)	3.5 (1.6)****	6.2 (1.5)
Limb fat percentage (%)	25.1 (6.1) ****	40.2 (4.9)
Trunk-to-limb fat ratio	3.09 (1.17)*	1.4 (0.29)
Lean mass (kg)	57.0 (6.8)	58.2 (5.2)
Metabolic parameters		
Total-cholesterol (mmol/L)	5.5 (0.9)**	4.63 (0.64)
HDL-C (mmol/L)	1.23 (0.52)*	1.51 (0.32)
LDL-C (mmol/L)	3.7 (0.9)	3.3 (0.6)
Triglycerides (mmol/L)	2.55(1.43)****	0.76 (0.24)
Glucose (mmol/L)	5.4 (0.6)	5.2 (0.3)
Insulin (pmol/L)	52 (25)****	25 (8.9)
HOMA-IR	2.2 (1.4)****	0.99 (0.37)
Insulin sensitivity		
Rate of appearance (μmol glucose/kg/min)		
Basal	14.2 (0.49)***	11.8 (2.0)
Clamp	6.4 (1.8)**	4.0 (2.5)
Delta†	7.8 (2.1)	7.8 (1.9)
Rate of disappearance (μmol glucose/kg/min)		
Basal	14.2 (0.49)***	11.8 (2.0)
Clamp	40.2 (9.9)**	48.6 (8.4)
Delta†	26.02 (10.1)**	36.81 (7.14)
Glucose tolerance		
Glucose area under the curve (mmol/Lmin)	826 (200)*	670 (126)
Insulin area under the curve (pmol/Lmin)	52360 (31017)**	23505 (10598)

Data are presented as mean (SD).

†Delta, differences between clamp and basal values. HAART, highly active antiretroviral therapy; PI, protease inhibitor; NRTI, nucleoside reverse transcriptase inhibitor; NNRTI, non- nucleoside reverse transcriptase inhibitor. HOMA-IR, homeostatic model assessment for insulin resistance, Rate of appearance and disappearance, Rate of appearance and disappearance of glucose during a euglycemic-hyperinsulinemic clamp performed in both HIV patients and healthy controls.

*$P<0.05$;

**$P<0.01$;

***$P<0.001$,

****$P<0.0001$ by *t*-test.

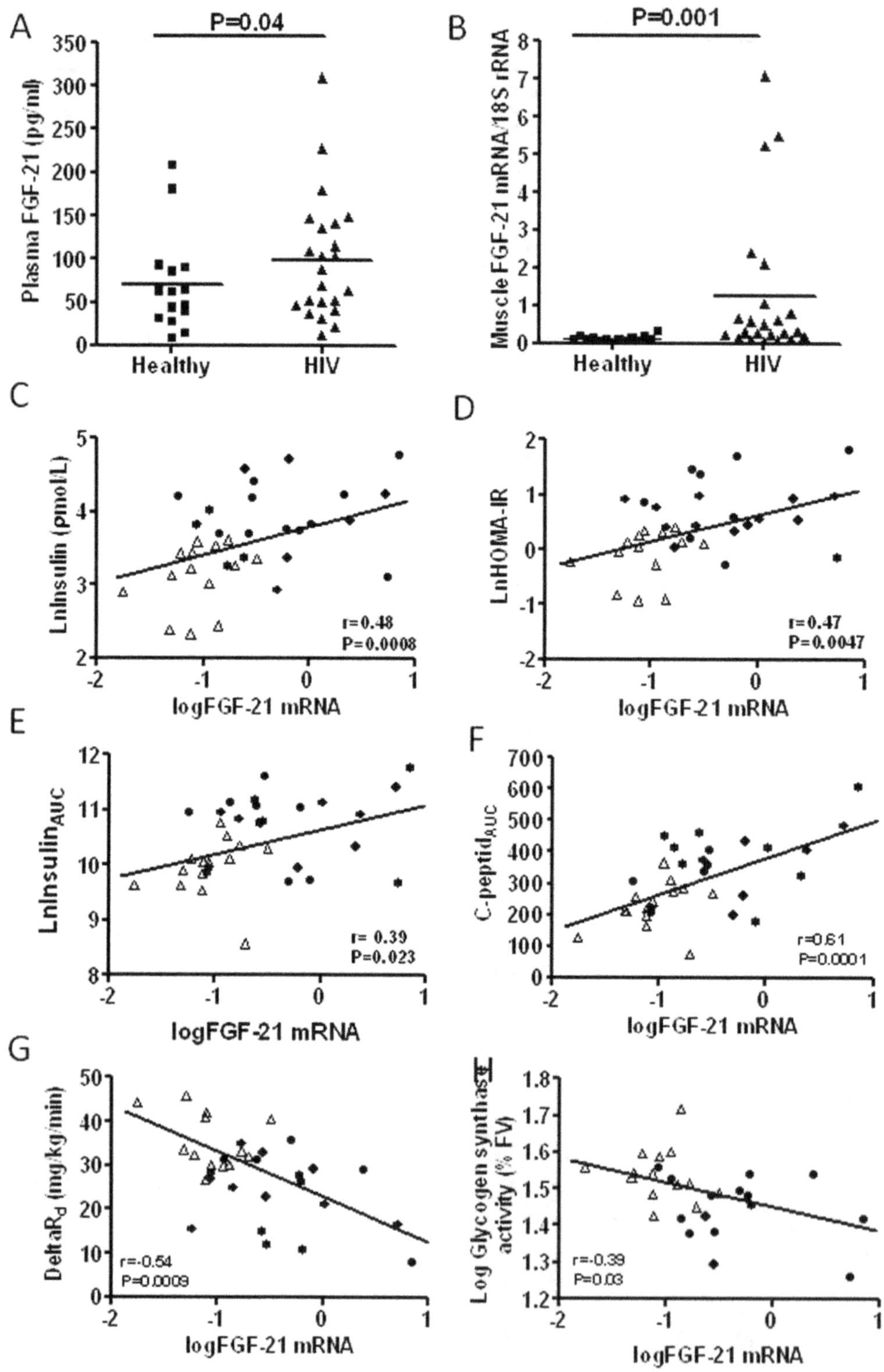

Figure 1. FGF-21 mRNA are increased in muscle from subjects with HIV-lipodystrophy and correlates to several measurement of insulin resistance. (A) Fasting plasma levels of fibroblast growth factor (FGF) 21 are increased 2-fold in HIV subjects with lipodystrophy compared to healthy men; (B) mRNA expression of FGF-21 are increased 8-fold in muscle biopsies from HIV subjects with lipodystrophy compared to healthy men; (C–F) Plots of FGF-21 mRNA in muscle versus several measurements of insulin resistance: FGF-21 mRNA in muscle are positively correlated to fasting insulin (C), HOMA-IR (D), Area under the curve for insulin during an oral glucose tolerance test (E), Area under the curve for C-peptide during an oral glucose tolerance test (F), and negatively correlated to the incremental rate of disappearance of glucose (G), and fractionel velocity of glycogen synthesis (H) in healthy (◇) and HIV subjects with lipodystrophy (●). In the dot plots data for each subjects are given and the line represent means. * $P<0.05$ and *** $P<0.001$ for healthy vs HIV-lipodystrophy patients. For plots, linear regression lines, correlations coefficient, and significance levels are given for all subjects.

find that FGF-21 mRNA was expressed in muscle, but they find no activation of muscle FGF-21 mRNA by a short term high fat overfeeding. In the study by Mashili *et al.* [26], FGF-21 mRNA was expressed in skeletal muscle, but no difference was found between obese subjects with normal glucose tolerance and obese subjects with Type 2 diabetes. However, in this study no healthy non-obese subjects were included.

A body of evidence show that in murine models FGF-21 lowers blood glucose, insulin, triglycerides, fat mass and increases insulin sensitivity [2,3]. In humans, circulating FGF-21 is increased in obesity and in subjects with type 2 diabetes [7,8]. Therefore, increased levels of circulating FGF-21 have been suggested to be a compensatory mechanism due to insulin resistance or a sign of FGF-21 resistance. In murine models, chronic administration of FGF-21 increases insulin-mediated glucose uptake in muscle, but only in diet induced obesity [3]. Furthermore, triglycerides deposit in muscle by FGF-21 administration is attenuated. Therefore, it has been suggested that the effect of FGF-21 on muscle is secondary to other events e.g. lipid toxicity in muscle.

Besides the strong correlation between insulin-mediated glucose uptake and FGF-21 mRNA in muscle, FGF-21 mRNA was also tightly correlated to triglycerides. Patients with HIV lipodystrophy have increased lipolysis and high triglycerides as wells as an increased amount of intra myocellular lipid accumulation [27]. We have previously shown that HIV patients display lipid driven insulin resistance [20]. Therefore, increased FGF-21 in muscle may be a compensatory mechanism to offset the lipid-induced insulin resistance in muscle. This explanation is supported by *in vitro* models, where FGF-21 is found to protect human myotubes from palmitate-induced insulin resistance [28], and to increase basal and insulin-stimulated glucose uptake in human myotubes [26].

In rodents, FGF21 has emerged as a hormone involved in energy homeostasis in the liver. We found lower fractional glycogen synthase activity in muscle in the patients indicating reduced capacity for deposition of glucose into glycogen in the muscle during basal condition. Furthermore, FGF-21 mRNA was associated with low fractional glycogen synthase activity in muscle. Therefore, in accordance to the role of FGF-21 in the liver in rodent, muscular FGF-21 in humans may be a marker of the substrate and energy levels in the muscle. Since our observations are cross-sectional in nature it is not possible to establish cause-and-effect relationship.

In line with FGF-21 as an energy sensor, the increased FGF-21 mRNA in muscle may be speculated to be related to mitochondrial dysfunction. Mice with late-onset mitochondrial myopathy show induction of FGF-21 in their muscles, which is closely related to the number of COX-negative muscle fibres [29], suggesting that mitochondria deficiency in skeletal muscle induces FGF21 expression. In skeletal muscle, HIV patients treated with NRTI have a reduced mitochondrial/nucleus DNA ratio, more frequent mtDNA deletions and possibly more COX-deficient muscle fibres than HIV-negative controls [30]. In addition, mitochondrial aging was recently found to be accelerated by anti-retroviral therapy through the clonal expansion of mtDNA mutations [31]. Therefore, the increase in FGF-21 could also be related to mitochondrial changes in the muscle.

Very little information on FGF receptors in humans exists. FGF21 acts through the interaction with specific FGF receptors and a cofactor called β-Klotho [32]. FGFR1 in adipose tissue has been suggested as the main receptor/tissue to serve to mediate the effect of FGF21 *in vivo* in rodents [33]. A very recent paper has shown a dramatically reduction of β-klotho mRNA in adipose tissue in HIV-patients with and without lipodystrophy [33], supporting the hypothesis that the increase in muscle FGF-21 mRNA may in part be a compensatory mechanism to the reduced FGF-21 signalling in adipose tissue and that adipose tissue may be target tissue for FGF21 in HIV-patients. A FGF-21 receptor in muscle has not yet been defined. As mentioned, FGF21 has direct effects in enhancing skeletal muscle glucose uptake in both rodents and human myocytes [3,26] and protects human myotubes from palmitate-induced insulin resistance [28], demonstrating that FGF-21 signals directly in muscle.

In agreement with Domingo *et al.* [34], we found increased circulating FGF-21 in HIV patients with lipodystrophy. However, in contrast to their study we did not find a correlation between plasma FGF-21 and measures of insulin resistance (fasting insulin, HOMA-IR, area under the curve for insulin during an OGTT and rate of glucose disappearance during an euglycemic-hyperinsulinemic clamp combined with stable isotopes). The explanation for this discrepancy is difficult to understand. The subjects in the study by Domingo *et al.* included naive, HAART- treated patients with or withour lipodystophy and a control group. The HIV study groups were comparable with regards to the range of circulating FGF-21, age, CD4 count and BMI. The HIV-patients in our study were more insulin resistant (HOMA 2.2 vs 1,7 in the study by Domingo *et al.*), had a higher trunk-to-limb ratio (3.09 vs 2.42), and had more hyperlipidemia (TC 5.5 vs 5.07, Triglyceriedes 2.55 vs 5.00) than the HIV subjects with lipodystrophy in the study by Domingo *et al.* In our study no patients were co-infected with hepatitis C or had chronic hepatitis B virus infection, whereas this was the case for 7.6% and 8.9% , respectively in the patients in the study by Domingo *et al.* In the study by Domingo *et al,* circulating FGF-21 was tightly correlated with markers of liver function such as AST, ALT and GGT. We did not measure AST, ALT or GGT and can therefore not speculate whether this could explain the discrepancy between the studies.

We did not find a significant correlation between high levels of circulating FGF-21 levels and FGF-21 mRNA in muscle, indicating that muscle is not the major source of circulating FGF-21. As previously suggested some evidence exists that liver may be the primary source of circulating FGF-21. The lack of association between circulating and muscle-expressed FGF-21 also suggests that muscle FGF-21 primarily works in a local manner regulating glucose metabolism in the muscle and/or signals to the adipose tissue in close contact to the muscle.

Our study has some limitations. The number of subjects is small and some correlations could have been significant with greater statistical power. Another aspect is that protein levels of FGF-21 were not determined in the muscles extracts, consequently we cannot be sure the increase in FGF-21 mRNA is followed by increased protein expression.

In conclusion, we show that FGF-21 mRNA is increased in skeletal muscle in HIV patients and that FGF-21 mRNA in muscle correlates to whole-body (primarily reflecting muscle) insulin resistance. These findings add to the evidence that FGF-21 is a myokine and that muscle FGF-21 might primarily work in an autocrine manner.

Acknowledgments

We thank the subjects for their participation in this study. Ruth Rousing, Hanne Willumsen, Carsten Nielsen and Flemming Jessen are thanked for excellent technical help. The Danish HIV-Cohort is thanked for providing us HIV-related data.

Author Contributions

Conceived and designed the experiments: BL BKP JG. Performed the experiments: BL TH TG CF PH. Analyzed the data: BL CF PH. Contributed reagents/materials/analysis tools: BL. Wrote the paper: BL.

References

1. Kharitonenkov A, Shiyanova TL, Koester A, Ford AM, Micanovic R, et al. (2005) FGF-21 as a novel metabolic regulator. J Clin Invest 115: 1627–1635.
2. Coskun T, Bina HA, Schneider MA, Dunbar JD, Hu CC, et al. (2008) Fibroblast growth factor 21 corrects obesity in mice. Endocrinology 149: 6018–6027.
3. Xu J, Lloyd DJ, Hale C, Stanislaus S, Chen M, et al. (2009) Fibroblast growth factor 21 reverses hepatic steatosis, increases energy expenditure, and improves insulin sensitivity in diet-induced obese mice. Diabetes 58: 250–259.
4. Inagaki T, Dutchak P, Zhao G, Ding X, Gautron L, et al. (2007) Endocrine regulation of the fasting response by PPARalpha-mediated induction of fibroblast growth factor 21. Cell Metab 5: 415–425.
5. Potthoff MJ, Inagaki T, Satapati S, Ding X, He T, et al. (2009) FGF21 induces PGC-1alpha and regulates carbohydrate and fatty acid metabolism during the adaptive starvation response. Proc Natl Acad Sci U S A 106: 10853–10858.
6. Badman MK, Pissios P, Kennedy AR, Koukos G, Flier JS, et al. (2007) Hepatic fibroblast growth factor 21 is regulated by PPARalpha and is a key mediator of hepatic lipid metabolism in ketotic states. Cell Metab 5: 426–437.
7. Zhang X, Yeung DC, Karpisek M, Stejskal D, Zhou ZG, et al. (2008) Serum FGF21 levels are increased in obesity and are independently associated with the metabolic syndrome in humans. Diabetes 57: 1246–1253.
8. Chen WW, Li L, Yang GY, Li K, Qi XY, et al. (2008) Circulating FGF-21 levels in normal subjects and in newly diagnose patients with Type 2 diabetes mellitus. Exp Clin Endocrinol Diabetes 116: 65–68.
9. Chavez AO, Molina-Carrion M, Abdul-Ghani MA, Folli F, DeFronzo RA, et al. (2009) Circulating fibroblast growth factor-21 is elevated in impaired glucose tolerance and type 2 diabetes and correlates with muscle and hepatic insulin resistance. Diabetes Care 32: 1542–1546.
10. Hojman P, Pedersen M, Nielsen AR, Krogh-Madsen R, Yfanti C, et al. (2009) Fibroblast growth factor-21 is induced in human skeletal muscles by hyperinsulinemia. Diabetes 58: 2797–2801.
11. Izumiya Y, Bina HA, Ouchi N, Akasaki Y, Kharitonenkov A, et al. (2008) FGF21 is an Akt-regulated myokine. FEBS Lett 582: 3805–3810.
12. Vienberg SG, Brons C, Nilsson E, Astrup A, Vaag A, et al. (2012) Impact of short-term high-fat feeding and insulin-stimulated FGF21 levels in subjects with low birth weight and controls. Eur J Endocrinol 167: 49–57.
13. Carr A, Samaras K, Burton S, Law M, Freund J, et al. (1998) A syndrome of peripheral lipodystrophy, hyperlipidaemia and insulin resistance in patients receiving HIV protease inhibitors. AIDS 12: F51–F58.
14. Haugaard SB, Andersen O, Dela F, Holst JJ, Storgaard H et al. (2005) Defective glucose and lipid metabolism in human immunodeficiency virus-infected patients with lipodystrophy involve liver, muscle tissue and pancreatic beta-cells. Eur J Endocrinol 152: 103–112.
15. Reeds DN, Yarasheski KE, Fontana L, Cade WT, Laciny E, et al. (2006) Alterations in liver, muscle, and adipose tissue insulin sensitivity in men with HIV infection and dyslipidemia. Am J Physiol Endocrinol Metab 290: E47–E53.
16. Meininger G, Hadigan C, Laposata M, Brown J, Rabe J, et al. (2002) Elevated concentrations of free fatty acids are associated with increased insulin response to standard glucose challenge in human immunodeficiency virus-infected subjects with fat redistribution. Metabolism 51: 260–266.
17. Carr A, Emery S, Law M, Puls R, Lundgren JD, et al. (2003) An objective case definition of lipodystrophy in HIV-infected adults: a case-control study. Lancet 361: 726–735.
18. Lindegaard B, Hansen T, Hvid T, van HG, Plomgaard P, et al. (2008) The effect of strength and endurance training on insulin sensitivity and fat distribution in human immunodeficiency virus-infected patients with lipodystrophy. J Clin Endocrinol Metab 93: 3860–3869.
19. Matthews DR, Hosker JP, Rudenski AS, Naylor BA, Treacher DF, et al. (1985) Homeostasis model assessment: insulin resistance and beta-cell function from fasting plasma glucose and insulin concentrations in man. Diabetologia 28: 412–419.
20. Lindegaard B, Frosig C, Petersen AM, Plomgaard P, Ditlevsen S, et al. (2007) Inhibition of lipolysis stimulates peripheral glucose uptake but has no effect on endogenous glucose production in HIV lipodystrophy. Diabetes 56: 2070–2077.
21. DeFronzo RA, Tobin JD, Andres R (1979) Glucose clamp technique: a method for quantifying insulin secretion and resistance. Am J Physiol 237: E214–E223.
22. Plomgaard P, Bouzakri K, Krogh-Madsen R, Mittendorfer B, Zierath JR, et al. (2005) Tumor necrosis factor-alpha induces skeletal muscle insulin resistance in healthy human subjects via inhibition of Akt substrate 160 phosphorylation. Diabetes 54: 2939–2945.
23. Thomas JA, Schlender KK, Larner J (1968) A rapid filter paper assay for UDPglucose-glycogen glucosyltransferase, including an improved biosynthesis of UDP-14C-glucose. Anal Biochem 25: 486–499.
24. Haugaard SB, Andersen O, Madsbad S, Frosig C, Iversen J, et al. (2005) Skeletal Muscle Insulin Signaling Defects Downstream of Phosphatidylinositol 3-Kinase at the Level of Akt Are Associated With Impaired Nonoxidative Glucose Disposal in HIV Lipodystrophy. Diabetes 54: 3474–3483.
25. Boden G, Jadali F, White J, Liang Y, Mozzoli M, et al. (1991) Effects of fat on insulin-stimulated carbohydrate metabolism in normal men. J Clin Invest 88: 960–966.
26. Mashili FL, Austin RL, Deshmukh AS, Fritz T, Caidahl K, et al. (2011) Direct effects of FGF21 on glucose uptake in human skeletal muscle: implications for type 2 diabetes and obesity. Diabetes Metab Res Rev 27: 286–297.
27. Torriani M, Thomas BJ, Barlow RB, Librizzi J, Dolan S, et al. (2006) Increased intramyocellular lipid accumulation in HIV-infected women with fat redistribution. J Appl Physiol 100: 609–614.
28. Lee MS, Choi SE, Ha ES, An SY, Kim TH, et al. (2012) Fibroblast growth factor-21 protects human skeletal muscle myotubes from palmitate-induced insulin resistance by inhibiting stress kinase and NF-kappaB. Metabolism .
29. Tyynismaa H, Carroll CJ, Raimundo N, Ahola-Erkkila S, Wenz T, et al. (2010) Mitochondrial myopathy induces a starvation-like response. Hum Mol Genet 19: 3948–3958.
30. Maagaard A, Holberg-Petersen M, Kollberg G, Oldfors A, Sandvik L, et al. (2006) Mitochondrial (mt)DNA changes in tissue may not be reflected by depletion of mtDNA in peripheral blood mononuclear cells in HIV-infected patients. Antivir Ther 11: 601–608.
31. Payne BA, Wilson IJ, Hateley CA, Horvath R, Santibanez-Koref M, et al. (2011) Mitochondrial aging is accelerated by anti-retroviral therapy through the clonal expansion of mtDNA mutations. Nat Genet 43: 806–810.
32. Kliewer SA, Mangelsdorf DJ (2010) Fibroblast growth factor 21: from pharmacology to physiology. Am J Clin Nutr 91: 254S–257S.
33. Gallego-Escuredo JM, Domingo P, Gutierrez MD, Mateo MG, Cabeza MC, et al. (2012) Reduced Levels of Serum FGF19 and Impaired Expression of Receptors for Endocrine FGFs in Adipose Tissue From HIV-Infected Patients. J Acquir Immune Defic Syndr 61: 527–534.
34. Domingo P, Gallego-Escuredo JM, Domingo JC, Gutierrez MM, Mateo MG, et al. (2010) Serum FGF21 levels are elevated in association with lipodystrophy, insulin resistance and biomarkers of liver injury in HIV-1-infected patients. AIDS 24: 2629–2637.

11

The Effect of Lithospermic Acid, an Antioxidant, on Development of Diabetic Retinopathy in Spontaneously Obese Diabetic Rats

Cheng Ji Jin[1,4], Sung Hoon Yu[1,5], Xiao-Mei Wang[4], Se Joon Woo[2], Hyo Jin Park[3], Hyun Chul Lee[6], Sung Hee Choi[1], Kyoung Min Kim[1], Jung Hee Kim[7], Kyong Soo Park[7], Hak Chul Jang[1], Soo Lim[1]*

1 Department of Internal Medicine, Seoul National University College of Medicine and Seoul National University Bundang Hospital, Seongnam, Korea, **2** Department of Ophthalmology, Seoul National University College of Medicine and Seoul National University Bundang Hospital, Seongnam, Korea, **3** Department of Pathology, Seoul National University College of Medicine and Seoul National University Bundang Hospital, Seongnam, Korea, **4** Department of Endocrinology, The ZhongShan Hospital, DaLian University, Dalian, China, **5** Department of Internal Medicine, Hallym University Hangang Sacred Hospital, Seoul, Korea, **6** Department of Internal Medicine, Yonsei University College of Medicine, Seoul, Korea, **7** Department of Internal Medicine, Seoul National University College of Medicine, Seoul, Korea

Abstract

Background: Lithospermic acid B (LAB), an active component isolated from *Salvia miltiorrhiza radix*, has been reported to have antioxidant effects. We examined the effects of LAB on the prevention of diabetic retinopathy in Otsuka Long-Evans Tokushima Fatty (OLETF) rats, an animal model of type 2 diabetes.

Methods and Findings: LAB (10 or 20 mg/kg) or normal saline were given orally once daily to 24-week-old male OLETF rats for 52 weeks. At the end of treatment, fundoscopic findings, vascular endothelial growth factor (VEGF) expression in the eyeball, VEGF levels in the ocular fluid, and any structural abnormalities in the retina were assessed. Glucose metabolism, serum levels of high-sensitivity C-reactive protein (hsCRP), monocyte chemotactic protein-1 (MCP1), and tumor necrosis factor-alpha (TNFα) and urinary 8-hydroxy-2′-deoxyguanosine (8-OHdG) levels were also measured. Treatment with LAB prevented vascular leakage and basement membrane thickening in retinal capillaries in a dose-dependent manner. Insulin resistance and glucose intolerance were significantly improved by LAB treatment. The levels of serum hsCRP, MCP1, TNFα, and urinary 8-OHdG were lower in the LAB-treated OLETF rats than in the controls.

Conclusions: Treatment with LAB had a preventive effect on the development of diabetic retinopathy in this animal model, probably because of its antioxidative effects and anti-inflammatory effects.

Editor: Ramani Ramchandran, Medical College of Wisconsin, United States of America

Funding: This work was supported by the Korean Diabetes Association (2009). The funders had no role in study design, data collection and analysis, decision to publish, or preparation of the manuscript.

Competing Interests: The authors have declared that no competing interests exist.

* E-mail: limsoo@snu.ac.kr

These authors contributed equally to this work.

Introduction

Diabetes mellitus has shown an exponential rise of late, causing serious economic, social and health repercussions. However, the causes of these problems and therapeutic options have yet not been fully uncovered. Among the side effects, diabetic retinopathy is the most common microvascular complication of individuals with both type 1 and type 2 diabetes, with nearly all patients with type 1 diabetes and more than 60% with type 2 diabetes being estimated to develop diabetic retinopathy 20 years after onset [1,2]. Proliferative diabetic retinopathy, the advanced stage of diabetic retinopathy, is characterized by the extensive formation of new blood vessels in the retina and invasion towards the vitreous body, followed by vitreous hemorrhaging and tractional retinal detachment, leading to visual impairment and irreversible blindness [3,4]. Although strict glycemic control has been shown to reduce the incidence of retinopathy considerably, it is not easily achieved or maintained. Its efficacy has also not been completely confirmed, given that 12% of patients with diabetes under intensive treatment develop retinopathy [1,5].

While laser treatment at best permits preservation of visual acuity in cases of diabetic retinopathy, many agents such as fenofibrate, ruboxistaurin, renin-angiotensin system blockers, and peroxisome proliferator-activated receptor gamma agonists have been used in attempts to delay or prevent diabetic retinopathy [6]. A recent reanalysis of two major randomized controlled trials – the Fenofibrate Intervention and Event Lowering in Diabetes (FIELD) and the Action to Control Cardiovascular Risk in Diabetes (ACCORD) studies – revealed that fibrate has a robust beneficial effect on diabetic retinopathy [7]. Recently, a new approach to inhibit angiogenesis in cases of diabetic retinopathy has been studied. Several clinical trials indicate that vision can improve with repeated injections of bevacizumab [8], ranibizumab [9] and pegaptanib [10]. One study also showed that the intravitreal

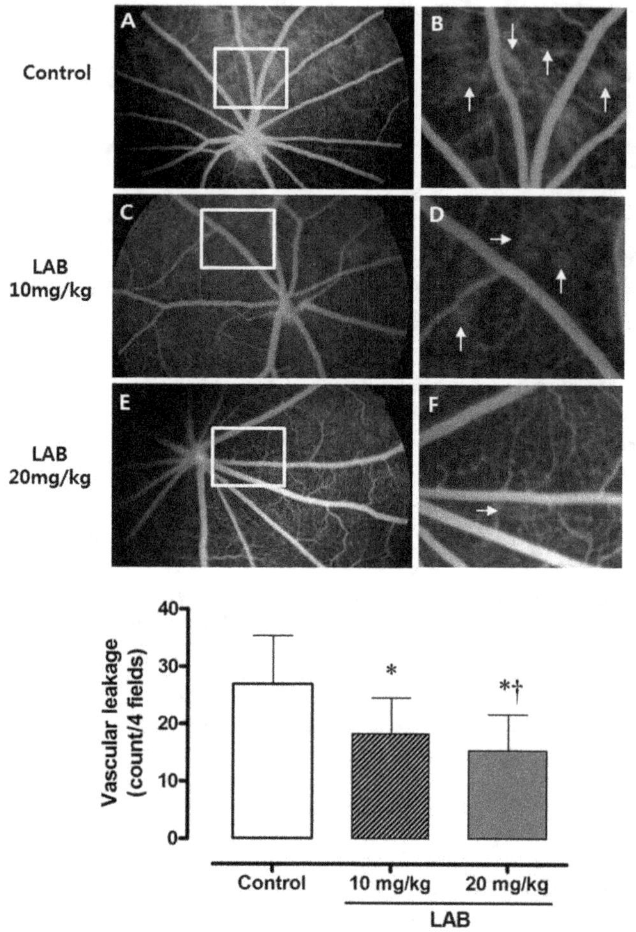

Figure 1. Vascular leakage in fluorescein angiography in study animals. *A, B*: Control group. *C, D*: 10 mg/kg LAB group. *E, F*: 20 mg/kg LAB group. Arrows indicate vascular leakage. *G:* Comparison of vascular leakage among three groups. *$P<0.05$ vs. control group, †$P<0.05$ vs. 10 mg/kg LAB-treated group.

injection of bevacizumab inhibited VEGF expression in the retina and that bevacizumab-chitosan nanoparticles had a longer duration of action [11].

It is currently believed that retinopathy is an inflammatory process, because various studies have shown that the circulating leukocytes activated in diabetic patients play an important role in the increased adhesion of leukocytes, macrophages and vascular adhesion molecules, and in the process of vascular occlusion and retinal ischemia [12–14]. Oxidative stress in the retina is also fundamental for angiogenic stimulation, which is mediated by growth factors, including vascular endothelial growth factor (VEGF) [15,16].

Today, antioxidants are known to be effective against microvascular complication such as diabetic nephropathy as well as macrovascular complications of diabetes such as myocardial infarction, atherosclerosis and stroke [17,18]. However, its potential efficacy against diabetic retinopathy, a microvascular complication of diabetes, has not been adequately explored or proven.

Salvia miltiorrhiza radix is a traditional Chinese herbal medicine that has been used for many years in East Asia for the treatment of diabetic complications. Lithospermic acid B (LAB), a recently isolated component of *S. miltiorrhiza*, is known to have multiple pharmacological actions such as antihypertensive [19] and antioxidant effects [20]. Interestingly, a recent study has shown that LAB protects pancreas beta cells against cytokine-induced apoptosis [21].

Treatment with LAB showed protective effects against micro- and macrovascular complications of diabetes [22–24]. Moreover, treatment with LAB prevented both injury-induced neointimal formation *in vivo* and platelet-derived growth factor-induced vascular smooth muscle cell proliferation and migration *in vitro* [23]. LAB treatment prevented diabetic nephropathy by inhibiting reactive oxygen species generation, protein kinase C (PKC) activation, and transforming growth factor (TGF)-β1 and fibronectin expression [22]. Considering similar phenomena are involved in the pathogenesis of diabetic retinopathy [25,26], LAB treatment might serve as a potential preventive therapeutic measure for diabetic retinopathy.

Reactive oxygen species have been reported to be associated with microvascular complications in patients with diabetes [27]. The DNA adduct 8-hydroxy-2′-deoxyguanosine (8-OHdG) is an indicator of oxidative stress damage [28]. A number of recent reports suggest that a low concentration of 8-OHdG following antioxidant therapy might reflect a reduced risk of diabetic complications [29,30]. These findings raise the possibility that LAB treatment might reduce the risk of retinopathy and that reduced levels of oxidative stress markers such as 8-OHdG might be associated with such efficacy. Based on the assumption, we investigated the effects of LAB on the occurrence of retinopathy and aimed to identify the mechanisms involved using an animal model of spontaneous diabetes.

Methods

Animals

All animals were handled in compliance with the Guide for Experimental Animal Research of the Laboratory, Seoul National University Bundang Hospital. Seoul National University Hospital Ethics Committee for Animal Study approved this study (63-2010-020). Thirty five-week-old male Otsuka Long-Evans Tokushima Fatty (OLETF) rats, an obese animal model of insulin resistance, were donated by the Otsuka Pharmaceutical Co. (Tokushima, Japan). They were allowed to grow to 24 weeks of age, when obesity and insulin resistance develop. The OLETF rats were held in the Preclinical Laboratory of Seoul National University Bundang Hospital, South Korea, for the duration of the study.

We divided the rats into three groups (n = 10 each). Controls received 5 mL normal saline per day and the experimental rats were given 10 mg/kg or 20 mg/kg of LAB per day. Rats were administered with LAB or normal saline using an oral Zonde needle (Natsume, Tokyo, Japan) at 9–10 am for 52 weeks. All rats were fed a regular chow diet and had free access to water; they were maintained in plastic cages in an air-conditioned room at 22±2°C and 55±10% humidity.

Isolation and purification of lithospermate B

Lithospermate B was isolated from 80% MeOH extract of *Salviae miltiorrhizae* Radix, and subsequently purified by normal silica gel column chromatography with polar-eluent (isopropyl alcohol/H_2O/ethyl acetate = 3/1/3) to give a 1.01% yield. Acidification of magnesium lithospermate B with 0.5 N-HCl afforded lithospermic acid B at an 84% yield [31].

Fundus photography and fluorescein angiography

Fundus photography on both eyes of each animal was performed by an experienced technician using a 45° fundus

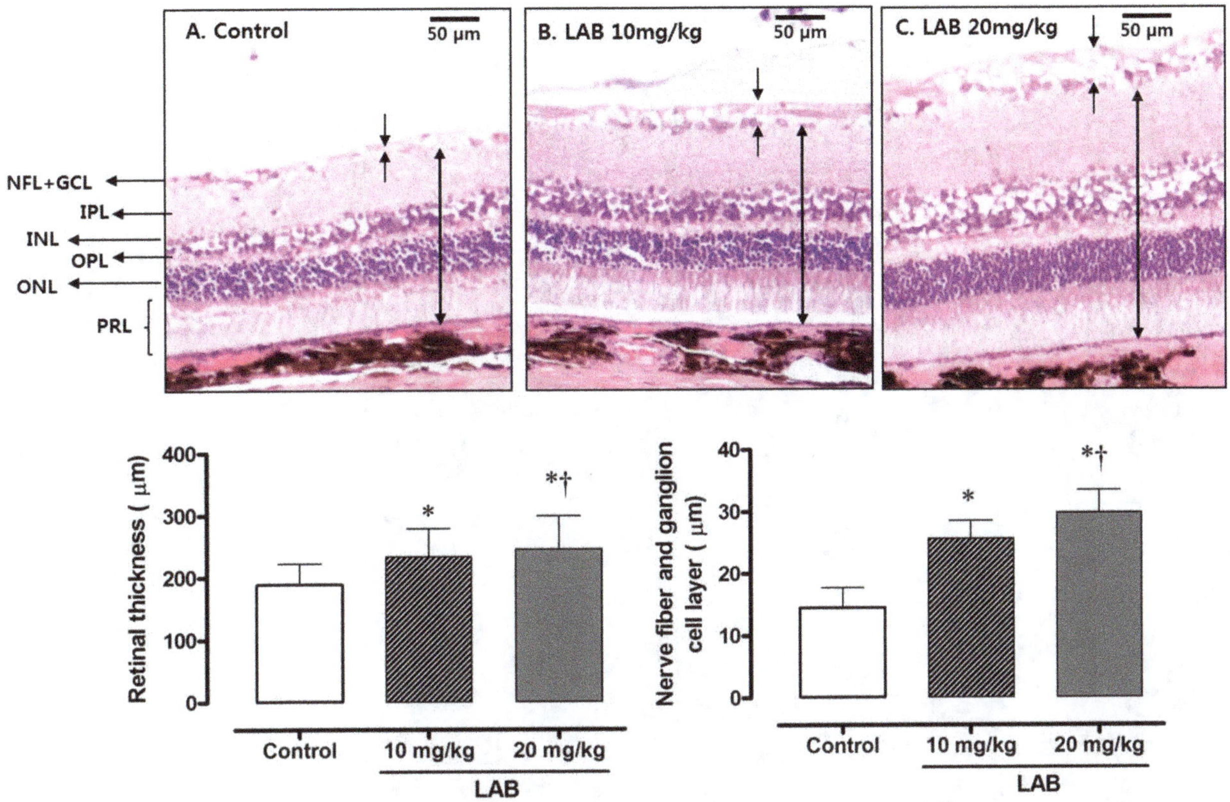

Figure 2. Histology of the rat retina using H&E staining. *A*: Control retina. *B*: 10 mg/kg LAB-treated retina. *C*: 20 mg/kg LAB-treated retina. Key: NFL, nerve fiber layer, GCL; ganglion cell layer; IPL, inner plexiform layer; INL, inner nuclear layer; OPL, outer plexiform layer; ONL, outer nuclear layer; PRL, photoreceptor layer.

camera (Retinal Camera CR6-45NM; Canon Inc., Tokyo, Japan) at week 0, 12, 24, 36, and 52 of the dosing phase. Fundus fluorescein angiography was performed on both eyes at 52 weeks. All retinal photographs and fluorescein angiography images were independently reviewed twice by one ophthalmologist (SJW), and the retinal vascular caliber was measured in each blood vessel 1 mm distant from the optic disc and averaged for each eye.

Eyeball extraction and histological analysis

Eyeballs were enucleated from rats (both control and LAB groups) after euthanasia with a lethal dose of pentobarbital and fixed in 10% neutral buffered formalin solution. They were embedded in paraffin wax. Sections (4 μm thickness) perpendicular to the optic disc were stained with hematoxylin and eosin (H&E) for light microscopy. Digital images were obtained using a high-resolution digital camera system (C3040-AD6, Olympus, Tokyo, Japan) linked to a microscope (CH30, Olympus, Tokyo, Japan) and desktop computer. For all eyes, retinal images were obtained at the same distance (1500 μm) from the optic nerve.

Immunohistochemistry

Sections were deparaffinized in xylene, rehydrated in a graded ethanol series, and stained using a BenchMark XT automated immunostainer (Ventana, Tucson, AZ, USA). Immunohistochemistry was performed using an anti-VEGF antibody (Clone C1, 1:500 dilution, Santa Cruz Biotechnology, Santa Cruz, CA, USA). Sections were washed with phosphate buffered saline (PBS) and incubated with a secondary antibody (anti-mouse IgG, istostain-Plus Bulk Kits; Zymed, San Francisco, CA, USA), prepared in PBS containing 1% horse serum, 1% bovine serum albumin and 0.3% Triton X-100, for 1 h at room temperature. Slides were washed with PBS.

VEGF levels in ocular fluid

Immediately after the rats were euthanized, the VEGF concentration was measured in ocular fluid–a mixture of the aqueous humor and vitreous fluid–by puncturing the ocular globe using disposable 1 mL syringes and 30 gauge needles. Samples were stored at −70°C until assayed. The VEGF concentration was measured with a rat VEGF-specific polyclonal antibody using a commercial enzyme-linked immunosorbent assay (ELISA) (Quantikine ELISA, R&D Systems, Minneapolis, MN, USA). The detection limit of the method was 31.2–2000 pg/mL, based on a standard curve from the manufacturers. All measurements were carried out in duplicate. The coefficients of variation in intra- and interassay variations were 7.2% (79.4±5.7 pg/mL) and 9.4% (87.6±8.2 pg/mL), respectively.

Assessment of retinal capillary basement membrane thickness

Electron microscopy was performed to determine the retinal basement membrane thickness. The eyes were enucleated, opened at the equator, fixed in 3.5% glutaraldehyde in 0.1 M cacodylate buffer (pH 7.4) for 1 h, and then postfixed in 2% osmium tetroxide. They were then dehydrated in ethanol series, and embedded in epoxy resin. Semithin sections (1 μm) were stained with toluidine blue for orientation and identification of the capillaries. Thin sections (60 nm) were cut with a diamond knife,

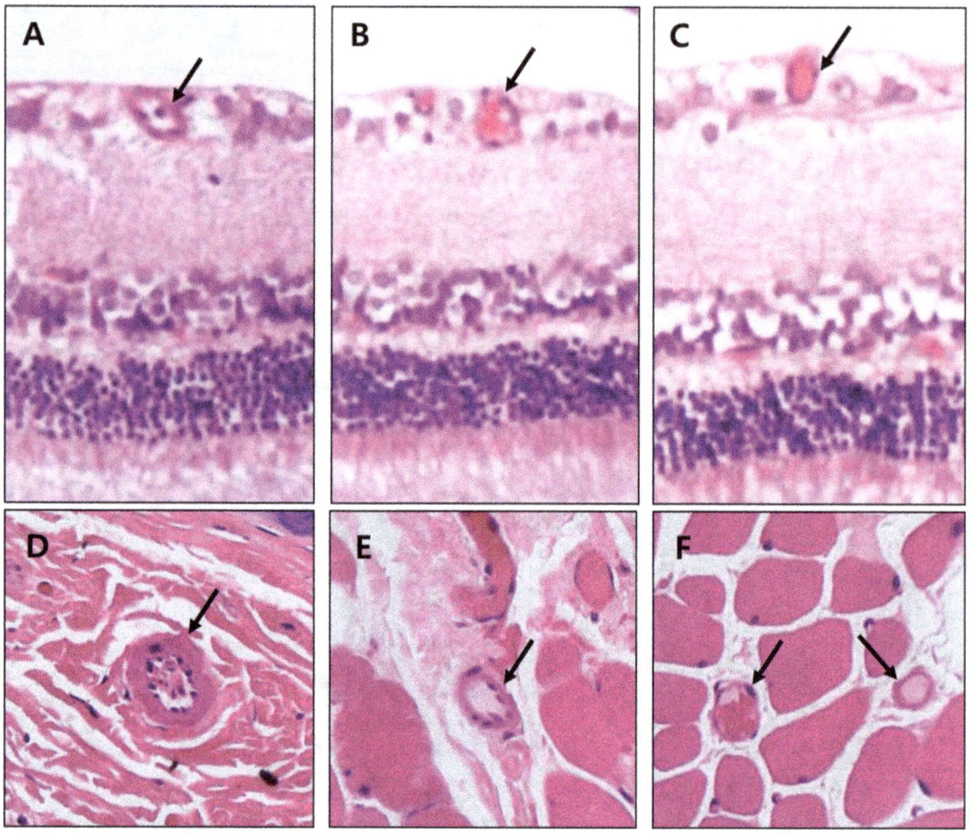

Figure 3. Capillaries in rat retinas and in surrounding connective tissues (× 200). *A, D*: Control. *B, E*: 10 mg/kg LAB treatment. *C, F*: 20 m/kg LAB treatment. Arrows indicate capillaries.

placed on 300-mesh copper grids, and stained with uranyl acetate and lead citrate. The sections were viewed and photographed using a JEOL JEM-100SX transmission electron microscope (JEOL, Tokyo, Japan). Each micrograph was analyzed using a commercial image analysis program (Image Pro 4.5, Media Cybernetics, Inc., Rockville, MD, USA). Basement membrane thickness was measured on four distinct capillaries for each eye and five measurements were taken per capillary with 10 independent measurements from each eye. One researcher (SJW) examined all eyes in the study and was blinded to the treatment groups.

Western blot analysis for quantification of VEGF in the retina

Tissue samples were homogenized in lysis buffer, and the protein concentration was determined using a protein assay kit (Pierce Biotechnology, Rockford, IL, USA). Extracted retinal tissues were lysed in RIPA buffer (25 mM Tris-HCl pH 7.6, 150 mM NaCl, 1% NP-40, 1% sodium deoxycholate, 0.1% SDS), and the proteins (10 mg/sample) were immediately heated at 100°C for 3 min. Total cell lysates were subjected to sodium dodecyl sulfate–polyacrylamide gel electrophoresis on gels containing 15% (wt/vol) acrylamide with each lane receiving 20 μg of the sample. After electrophoresis, proteins were transferred onto a nitrocellulose membrane for 2 h. The membrane was blocked by treatment with 5% skim milk in Tris-buffered saline (TBS) supplemented with 0.1% Tween-20 (TBST) for 1 h. It was then incubated with a primary polyclonal antibody (rabbit polyclonal to VEGF, Abcam Inc., Cambridge, MA, USA) at a final dilution of 1:1000, overnight in TBST. After three washes in TBST, the membrane was incubated with peroxidase-conjugated secondary antibody (final dilution, 1:3000) in TBS for 1 h and subsequently washed. An enhanced chemiluminescence reaction agent was reacted with the membrane for 3 min. Band density was quantified using a densitometer (Bio Image analyzer, CN-115, ETX-20MX, Marne-la-Vallée, France).

Serum levels of LAB in study animals

Levels of LAB were measured using a liquid chromatography-tandem mass spectrometry (LC-MS/MS) system from plasma samples collected at the end of the study. The standard curve was linear ($r^2 = 0.994$) over the concentration range of 1.0–1,000 μg/mL. The intra- and interassay coefficients of variation were 6.2% and 2.7%, respectively. The mean serum concentrations of LAB were 12.3±2.4 and 17.1±3.1 μg/mL in the rats treated with 10 and 20 mg/kg of LAB, respectively. LAB was not detected in the control rats.

Glucose metabolism, and inflammatory and prothrombotic markers

Possible relevant factors affecting the degree of diabetic retinopathy, such as glucose homeostasis, cytokines, and inflammatory status were evaluated. For glucose homeostasis, postprandial glucose concentrations were measured 2 h after refeeding on every other week from weeks 26 to 50. An intraperitoneal glucose tolerance test (IPGTT) was done at baseline and after 24 and 52 weeks of LAB treatment. After the 12 h fasting glucose concentration had been measured, each animal was injected

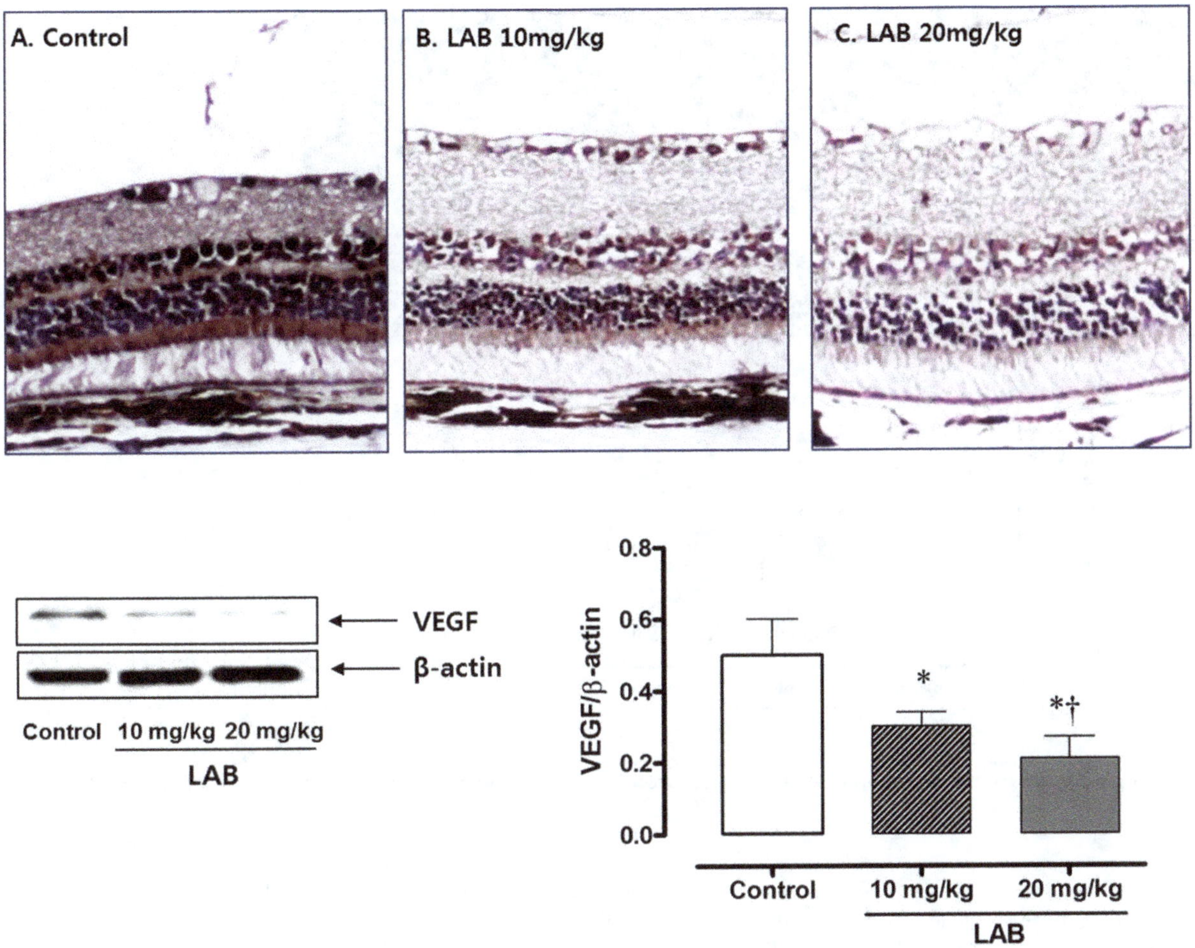

Figure 4. Immunohistochemistry for VEGF and western blot analysis of VEGF expression in the retina. *A*: Control group. *B*: 10 mg/kg LAB-treated group. *C*: 20 mg/kg LAB-treated group. *$P<0.05$ vs. control group, †$P<0.05$ vs. 10 mg/kg LAB-treated group.

intraperitoneally with 1.5 g/kg of a 50 M glucose solution. Blood samples (about 10 μL) were collected from an incision in the tail at 30, 60, 90 and 120 min after the glucose load. Plasma glucose concentration was measured using reagent strips read in a glucose meter (YSI 2300-STAT, Yellow Springs, OH, USA). Insulin was measured in duplicate using a commercial liquid phase radioimmunoassay kit (Linco Research, St Louis, MO, USA). The homeostasis model assessment of the insulin resistance (HOMA-IR) was calculated using fasting insulin and glucose levels. In addition, the area under the curve for glucose ($AUC_{glucose}$) was calculated using the trapezoid rule for glucose data from 0 to 120 min. High sensitivity C-reactive protein (hsCRP) was measured using ELISA kits developed by BD Biosciences Pharmingen (Heidelberg, Germany). Monocyte chemotactic protein-1 (MCP1), tumor necrosis factor-alpha (TNFα), and plasminogen activator inhibitor-1 (PAI1) activity were also measured using a multiplex kit (RADPK-81K, Linco, Billerica, MA, USA).

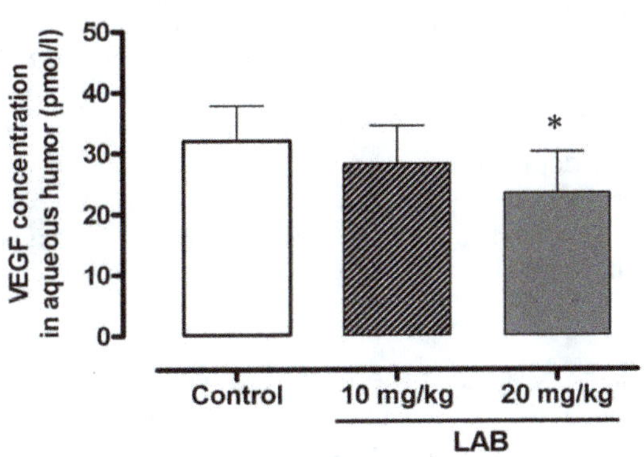

Figure 5. VEGF concentrations in ocular fluid among three groups. Each column represents mean ± SE (n = 5–6). *$P<0.05$ vs. control group.

Measurement of 8-hydroxy-2′-deoxyguanosine (8-OHdG), an oxidative stress marker, in urine

After 52 weeks of treatment of LAB or control, urine samples were collected directly from the urinary bladder with a 10 mL syringe on the day of euthanasia after fasting the rats overnight. The oxidative DNA damage marker, 8-OHdG was measured in the urine samples using an established high performance liquid chromatographic method based on anion exchange chromatography, fraction collection, and electrochemical detection [28]. The measurement of 8-OHdG (in micrograms) was normalized to urine creatinine (in grams).

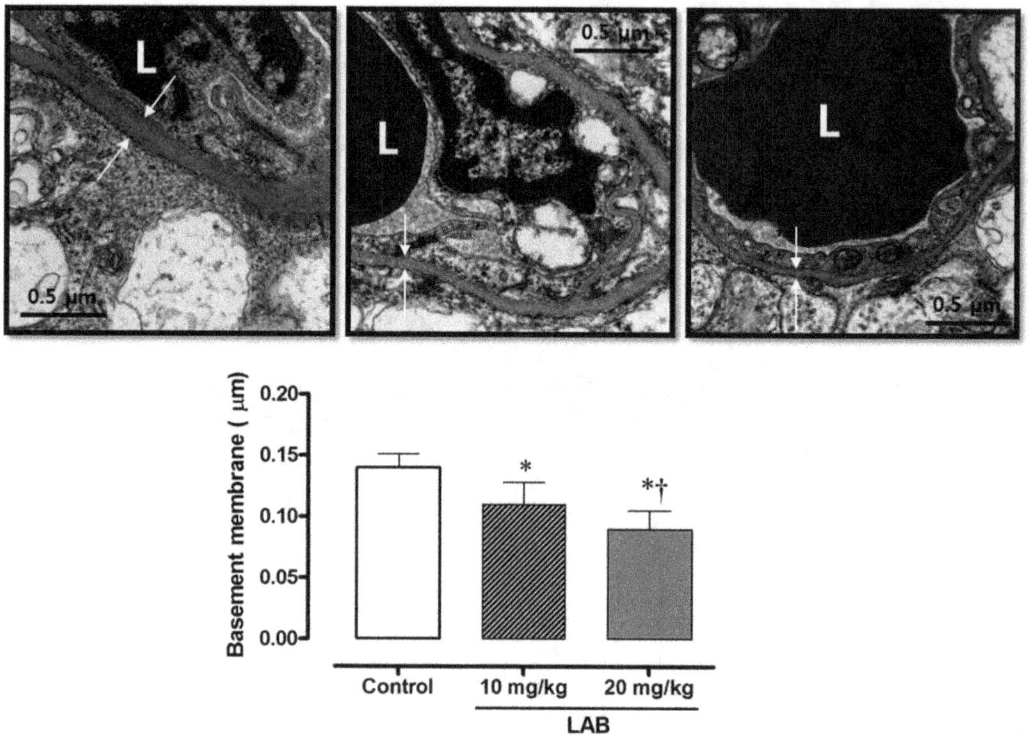

Figure 6. Retinal capillary basement membrane thickness assessed by electron microscopy. $^*P<0.05$ vs. control group, $^\dagger P<0.05$ vs. 10 mg/kg LAB group.

Statistical analysis

Results are reported as the mean ± standard error (SE). Mean values were compared for the LAB-treated groups and control group by analysis of variance (ANOVA) with Tukey's b *post hoc* test, and P values <0.05 were considered statistically significant. Analysis was done using SPSS for Windows (version 17.0; IBM Corp., Armonk, NY, USA).

Results

Fundus images and microvasculature

Images of the fundus from the control group showed dilated retinal vasculature compared with the LAB-treated groups, but this was not significant: 67±6.9 μm in controls; 58.3±7.8 μm in the 10 mg/kg LAB group, 53.2±8.8 μm in the 20 mg/kg LAB group (**Figure S1 in File S1**). Fluorescein angiography allowed more precise quantitative analysis of diabetes-induced microvascular dysfunction. At the end of treatment, the diabetic rats (control group) showed multiple diffuse leakages from retinal capillaries in the late phase of angiography (**Fig. 1*A, B***). The LAB-treated retinal angiograms showed a significantly lesser degree of vascular leakage compared with untreated control rats (**Fig. 1*C, D*** for the 10 mg/kg LAB group and **Fig. 1*E, F*** for the 20 mg/kg LAB group; Comparison among groups was shown in **Fig. 1*G***).

Retinal H&E staining and retinal thickness

After 52 weeks of treatment of LAB, microscopic examination of H&E-stained retinas showed no gross morphological abnormalities in study animals (**Fig. 2**). However, the retinas of the control group were slightly but significantly thinner than LAB-treated groups. Further, LAB-treated rats showed thicker nerve fiber and ganglion cell layers than did control rats, in a dose-dependent manner.

Vessels in the retina and in the surrounding connective tissues

As shown in **Fig. 3**, retinal capillaries in the control rats showed atherosclerotic changes including wall thickening and dilatation. Such atherosclerotic changes were not apparent in the LAB-treated rats.

Western blot results for VEGF expression in the retina

Immunohistochemical staining showed greater VEGF expression in the control diabetic rats than in the LAB-treated rats (**Fig. 4**). In the western blot analysis, the levels of VEGF were decreased in the LAB-treated groups compared with the control group ($P<0.05$). The high dose (20 mg/kg) LAB-treated group showed lower VEGF expression than did the low dose group ($P<0.05$).

VEGF levels in ocular fluid

Ocular fluid was obtained from five control, six 10 mg/kg LAB-treated, and five 20 mg/kg LAB-treated rats. The concentration of VEGF in the high dose treated group was significantly lower than in control rats **(Fig. 5).**

Retinal capillary basement membrane thickness

Retinal capillary basement membrane thickness was assessed by electron microscopy. For each animal, a minimum of 40 separate measurements of the basement membrane thickness was obtained. A representative micrograph of the basement membrane from each of the three groups is shown in **Fig. 6**. The basement membrane in control diabetic rats was thicker than in the LAB-

Table 1. Weight, biochemical parameters, insulin resistance index and inflammatory markers in an obese rat model of type 2 diabetes after 52 weeks of treatment with lithospermic acid B or with saline as control.

	Control (n = 10)		10 mg/kg LAB (n = 10)		20 mg/kg LAB (n = 10)		*P* value with *post hoc*†
	Mean	SD	Mean	SD	Mean	SD	
Weight, g	609.1	34.8	613.7	35.5	621.3	45.2	
Fasting glucose, mg/dL	128.6	19.6	121.2	9.9	118.8	12.8	
30 m postload glucose, mg/dL	405.2	13.3	385.5	16.1	371.2	16.1	
60 m postload glucose, mg/dL	459.4	20.8	443.6	17.0	435.1	22.6	
90 m postload glucose, mg/dL	372.7	34.0	354.6	24.7	311.5	21.2	$<0.05^{A,B}$
2 h postload glucose, mg/dL	236.3	56.2	201.8	46.1	189.4	29.8	$<0.05^{A,B}$
$AUC_{glucose}$	709.9	53.0	672.6	42.9	636.0	40.6	$<0.05^{A,B}$
Fasting insulin, pg/mL	156.2	78.2	145.1	69.3	128.7	59.2	
HOMA-IR	44.2	19.2	40.1	16.1	37.8	11.1	$<0.05^{B}$
Total cholesterol, mg/dL	82.6	15.3	81.9	12.9	77.6	9.9	
Triglycerides, mg/dL	78.1	24.4	63.4	21.8	60.2	15.8	
HDL-cholesterol, mg/dL	21.4	5.6	22.8	6.1	28.1	2.9	
LDL-cholesterol, mg/dL	49.0	13.1	42.6	11.9	43.1	7.1	
HsCRP, mg/L	0.16	0.03	0.12	0.01	0.10	0.01	$<0.05^{A,B}$
TNFα, pg/mL	9.9	2.9	7.6	3.8	5.9	4.1	$<0.05^{B}$
MCP1, pg/mL	156.2	57.2	123.9	43.4	107.2	35.2	$<0.05^{A,B}$
PAI1, pg/mL	512.5	182.5	422.8	103.9	456.8	128.4	
8-OHdG/creatinine, mg/g	8.2	2.6	6.2	1.8	5.1	0.9	$<0.05^{A,B}$

Key: $AUC_{glucose}$, Area under the curve of glucose; HDL, high-density lipoprotein; HsCRP, high-sensitivity C-reactive protein; HOMA-IR, homeostasis model assessment of insulin resistance; LDL, low-density lipoprotein; MCP1, monocyte chemotactic protein-1; PAI1, plasminogen activator inhibitor-1; TNFα, tumor necrosis factor-alpha; 8-OHdG, 8-hydroxy-2′-deoxyguanosine. †ANOVA with *post hoc* test (Tukey's b) was used. A, B and C superscripts indicate significant differences between pairs of groups: A, Control vs. 10 mg/kg LAB group; B, Control vs. 10 mg/kg LAB group; C, 10 mg/kg LAB vs. 20 mg/kg LAB groups; $P<0.05$ for all cases.

treated rats and there was a dose-dependent relationship for the measures: 0.14±0.01 μm in the control group, 0.11±0.2 μm in the 10 mg/kg LAB group, and 0.09±0.02 μm in the 20 mg/kg LAB group, $P<0.05$ among groups).

Effects of LAB treatment on glucose metabolism and biochemical parameters including markers associated with inflammatory processes, prothrombotic status, and oxidative stress

Postprandial 2 h glucose concentrations from weeks 24 to 50 (**Figure S2 in File S1**) revealed that control rats had higher glucose concentrations at weeks 46 and 48 than did the LAB-treated rats. There was no difference in glucose excursion for the IPGTTs performed at week 24 among the three groups (**Figure S3 in File S1**). After 52 weeks of LAB treatment, the 90 min and 2 h postload glucose concentrations and the $AUC_{glucose}$ during the IPGTT decreased significantly compared with that of the controls ($P<0.05$; **Table 1** and **Figure S4 in File S1**).

A tendency towards improved insulin resistance was observed, as indicated by a reduction in the HOMA-IR. Treatment with LAB significantly decreased the serum levels of hsCRP and MCP1, well-known inflammatory markers. The levels of TNFα, also involved in inflammatory processes, also tended to decrease after LAB treatment, although the difference between the control and the 10 mg/kg LAB group was not significant. LAB treatment also reduced the level of 8-OHdG, an oxidative stress marker, in a dose-dependent manner (**Table 1**).

Discussion

In this OLETF rat model of type 2 diabetes, treatments with LAB (10 and 20 mg/kg) for 52 weeks alleviated the development of diabetic retinopathy. Systemic LAB treatment prevented vascular leaking, reduced the expression and concentration of VEGF, and attenuated the disruption of the neurovascular units in the retina. The antioxidative and anti-inflammatory properties of LAB seem to account for this protective role. A significant improvement in postload glucose excursion with LAB treatment can be considered to contribute to this beneficial effect on the development of retinopathy.

Diabetic retinopathy is one of the biggest causes of blindness worldwide. Diabetic retinal capillary obstruction and resultant ischemic damage to the retinal neurons is irreversible, thus treatments to prevent the progression of diabetic retinopathy in the early stage should play a critical role in salvaging vision among patients with diabetes mellitus. In this sense, LAB has the potential to prevent the development and progression of diabetic retinopathy and related visual impairment.

The pathogenic mechanism in the development of diabetic retinopathy is complicated and has not been fully elucidated [32]. High serum and tissue levels of VEGF are the main culprit in the initiation and progression of retinal changes in patients with diabetes mellitus [33–35]. Oxidative stress and low grade inflammation as well as glycemic dysregulation increases the production of VEGF, which induces neovascularization, vascular leakage, and macular edema in the retina [34,36]. Indeed, VEGF is known as a vascular permeability factor, based on its ability to induce microvascular leakage [16,35]. In addition, VEGF plays an angiogenic and mitogenic role in vascular endothelial cells [37].

The mechanism of LAB in ameliorating the hyperglycemia-induced retinal vascular changes in OLETF rats seems to be associated with decreased VEGF expression in retina, as evidenced by reduced VEGF concentration in the retina and ocular fluid. PKC expression is also associated with VEGF-induced intraocular vascular permeability increases and neovascularization [38,39]. Activation of PKC isoforms is responsible for pathologies in patients with diabetic retinopathy by modulating Na^+-K^+-ATPase [40]. Moreover, treatment with LAB inhibits PKC activation and reduces TGF-β1 and fibronectin levels in renal mesangial cells [22]. Considering the interrelationship between VEGF and PKC and their contribution to diabetic retinopathy, LAB might be a possible therapeutic option for the treatment of diabetic retinopathy *per se* or as an adjunct to anti-VEGF agents [41].

In our study, total retinal thickness and the combined nerve fiber and ganglion cell layers were maintained in the LAB-treated rats compared with the control diabetic rats. This finding is consistent with previous studies showing neurodegeneration and microangiopathic changes involved in diabetic retinopathy [42,43]. In the milieu of diabetes mellitus, impaired insulin receptor signaling and loss of neurotrophic signals deteriorate cell survival and cell–cell interactions at synapses [44]. This can lead to an increase in apoptosis in the neural retina, and cause a breakdown of the blood–retinal barrier. Loss of this barrier integrity might also lead to compositional changes of the extracellular fluid in the retina, resulting in neuronal cell loss, especially in the ganglion cell layer. Atherosclerotic changes including wall thickening and dilatation were apparent in the retinal capillaries of control rats whereas treatment with LAB mitigated these changes. Collectively, it is conceivable that LAB maintains retinal thickness by attenuating the disruption of the neurovascular units of the retina.

Compared with the control diabetic rats, the basement membranes of retinal vessels were also maintained in the LAB-treated rats. Thickening of such basement membranes is a maladaptive response to impairment of glucose homeostasis and activation of various pathways associated with diabetic microvascular complications such as advanced glycation and increased PKC expression [32]. In a hyperglycemic milieu, synthesis of the basement membrane increases resulting in a thickened basement membrane caused by the accumulation of extracellular matrix [45]. Increased levels of VEGF, a growth factor and TNFα, an inflammatory cytokine contribute to thickening of the basement membrane [46].

Oxidative stress is also involved in the pathogenesis of diabetic retinopathy via activating angiogenesis and glial dysregulation [33]. In the present study, LAB treatment lowered urine 8-OHdG levels compared with control. This is a major marker of free radical-induced oxidative damage, and has therefore been used widely as an oxidative stress marker [47]. Taken together, the antioxidative and VEGF-reducing properties of LAB might be linked to neuroprotection and to maintenance of the integrity of the retinal basement membrane.

In this study, the LAB treatment reduced circulating MCP1 concentrations in a dose-dependent manner. MCP1 is a strong activator of monocytes and macrophages, suggesting that it is involved in the pathogenesis of diabetic retinopathy [48]. We also found that circulating levels of hsCRP and TNFα were significantly lower in the LAB-treated rats than in the untreated diabetic controls. In a large cohort study, the prevalence of retinopathy was positively associated with CRP levels in patients with diabetes [49]. Another study showed that patients with proliferative diabetic retinopathy had significantly higher serum TNFα levels compared with those with a milder form of retinopathy [50]. Moreover, the serum and vitreous humor levels of the soluble TNF receptor were elevated in patients with diabetic retinopathy [51]. Impairment of the blood–retinal barrier also leads to macrophage migration into the retina and accumulation of inflammatory mediators in the vitreous cavity, and vice versa. These findings suggest a potential role for LAB treatment in reducing oxidative stress and inflammatory responses in the pathogenesis of diabetic retinopathy.

In this study, we used OLETF rats, a rat model of obese type 2 diabetes with insulin resistance. Many investigators have used these rats as a model of diabetic retinopathy [43,52,53]. Thus, ganglion cell death was increased significantly in retinas from 35-week-old OLETF rats, and Akt phosphorylation was decreased compared with retinas from control LETO rats [53]. A recent study has shown that retinal neurodegeneration occurs in OLETF rats aged 36 weeks [43]. In another study with OLETF rats at the age of 40 weeks, VEGF expression extended into the outer plexiform layer, but expression was limited to the ganglion cell layer in control rats [52]. Thus, many studies have proven that alterations in retinal ultrastructure in OLETF rats are similar to those seen in human diabetic retinopathy, suggesting that the OLETF rat might be a useful animal model for the study of ocular complications in humans [54].

Although anti-VEGF therapy has been introduced for treating diabetic retinopathy, several limitations exist such as the need for intraocular injections, no clear rationale of use for preventive purposes, and the potential for aggravation upon discontinuing treatment, leading to a justification for the investigation of other therapies. A few studies suggest potential role of antioxidants in the prevention of diabetic retinopathy in human. L-carnitine, which facilitates the transport of long chain fatty acids into mitochondria, improves insulin sensitivity in insulin-resistant patients, suggesting a possible beneficial effect on the progression of diabetic retinopathy [55]. Recently, a preliminary human study suggested that α-lipoic acid treatment improved the electroretinogram results in patients with diabetic retinopathy [56]. However, the treatment period was only 4 weeks so the study could not reveal long-term results.

The present study had some limitations. First, the results of animal study cannot be extrapolated directly to humans with the same disease, although many studies have proven that the OLETF rat is a useful animal model for the study of human diabetic retinopathy. Second, we could not measure relevant biomarkers in ocular fluid because of its very small volume. Third, VEGF levels in ocular fluid were measured in limited numbers of animals because of difficulty in obtaining optimal volumes for the measurement.

In conclusion, our data demonstrate that LAB, an antioxidant, had preventive effects on the development of diabetic retinopathy in this obese type 2 diabetes rat model. These effects were probably mediated by its antioxidative effects and by reductions in inflammatory processes. Thus, LAB treatment might protect against the microvascular complications of diabetes, but further clinical studies are required to confirm this.

Supporting Information

Checklist S1

File S1 Supporting Figures. Figure a, Fundoscopic findings in 76-week-old OLETF rats after 52 weeks of treatment with LAB. *A*: Control group. *B*: 10 mg/kg LAB group. *C*: 20 mg/kg LAB group. **Figure b,** Postprandial 2 h glucose concentrations from weeks 26 to 50 in the LAB-treated and control rats. **Figure c,** Glucose concentrations from the intraperitoneal glucose tolerance test (IPGTT) at week 24 in the LAB-treated and control rats. **Figure d,** Glucose concentrations from the intraperitoneal glucose tolerance test (IPGTT) at week 52 in the LAB-treated and control rats.

Author Contributions

Conceived and designed the experiments: CJJ SHY SL. Performed the experiments: CJJ SHY SL. Analyzed the data: XW JHK SHC KMK KSP HCJ. Contributed reagents/materials/analysis tools: CJJ SHY SJW HJP HCL. Wrote the paper: CJJ SHY SL. Designed the software used in analysis: SL.

References

1. Clark CM Jr, Lee DA (1995) Prevention and treatment of the complications of diabetes mellitus. N Engl J Med 332: 1210–7.
2. Klein R, Klein BE, Moss SE (1989) The Wisconsin epidemiological study of diabetic retinopathy: a review. Diabetes Metab Rev 5: 559–70.
3. Imesch PD, Bindley CD, Wallow IH (1997) Clinicopathologic correlation of intraretinal microvascular abnormalities. Retina 17: 321–9.
4. Ishibashi T, Inomata H (1993) Ultrastructure of retinal vessels in diabetic patients. Br J Ophthalmol 77: 574–8.
5. The Diabetes Control and Complications Trial Research Group (1993) The effect of intensive treatment of diabetes on the development and progression of long-term complications in insulin-dependent diabetes mellitus. The Diabetes Control and Complications Trial Research Group. N Engl J Med 329: 977–86.
6. Porta M, Maldari P, Mazzaglia F (2011) New approaches to the treatment of diabetic retinopathy. Diabetes Obes Metab 13: 784–90.
7. Wong TY, Simo R, Mitchell P (2012) Fenofibrate – a potential systemic treatment for diabetic retinopathy? Am J Ophthalmol 154: 6–12.
8. Michaelides M, Kaines A, Hamilton RD, Fraser-Bell S, Rajendram R, et al. (2010) A prospective randomized trial of intravitreal bevacizumab or laser therapy in the management of diabetic macular edema (BOLT study) 12-month data: report 2. Ophthalmology 117: 1078–86.
9. Massin P, Bandello F, Garweg JG, Hansen LL, Harding SP, et al. (2010) Safety and efficacy of ranibizumab in diabetic macular edema (RESOLVE Study): a 12-month, randomized, controlled, double-masked, multicenter phase II study. Diabetes Care 33: 2399–405.
10. Cunningham ET Jr, Adamis AP, Altaweel M, Aiello LP, Bressler NM, et al. (2005) A phase II randomized double-masked trial of pegaptanib, an anti-vascular endothelial growth factor aptamer, for diabetic macular edema. Ophthalmology 112: 1747–57.
11. Lu Y, Zhou N, Huang X, Cheng JW, Li FQ, et al. (2014) Effect of intravitreal injection of bevacizumab-chitosan nanoparticles on retina of diabetic rats. Int J Ophthalmol 7: 1–7.
12. Barouch FC, Miyamoto K, Allport JR, Fujita K, Bursell SE, et al. (2000) Integrin-mediated neutrophil adhesion and retinal leukostasis in diabetes. Invest Ophthalmol Vis Sci 41: 1153–8.
13. Miyamoto K, Khosrof S, Bursell SE, Rohan R, Murata T, et al. (1999) Prevention of leukostasis and vascular leakage in streptozotocin-induced diabetic retinopathy via intercellular adhesion molecule-1 inhibition. Proc Natl Acad Sci U S A 96: 10836–41.
14. Woo SJ, Ahn SJ, Ahn J, Park KH, Lee K (2011) Elevated systemic neutrophil count in diabetic retinopathy and diabetes: a hospital-based cross-sectional study of 30,793 Korean subjects. Invest Ophthalmol Vis Sci 52: 7697–703.
15. Aiello LP, Pierce EA, Foley ED, Takagi H, Chen H, et al. (1995) Suppression of retinal neovascularization in vivo by inhibition of vascular endothelial growth factor (VEGF) using soluble VEGF-receptor chimeric proteins. Proc Natl Acad Sci U S A 92: 10457–61.
16. Tanaka Y, Katoh S, Hori S, Miura M, Yamashita H (1997) Vascular endothelial growth factor in diabetic retinopathy. Lancet 349: 1520.
17. Rask-Madsen C, King GL (2013) Vascular complications of diabetes: mechanisms of injury and protective factors. Cell Metab 17: 20–33.
18. Kaliora AC, Dedoussis GV, Schmidt H (2006) Dietary antioxidants in preventing atherogenesis. Atherosclerosis 187: 1–17.
19. Kamata K, Noguchi M, Nagai M (1994) Hypotensive effects of lithospermic acid B isolated from the extract of Salviae miltiorrhizae Radix in the rat. Gen Pharmacol 25: 69–73.
20. Soung DY, Rhee SH, Kim JS, Lee JY, Yang HS, et al. (2003) Peroxynitrite scavenging activity of lithospermate B from Salvia miltiorrhiza. J Pharm Pharmacol 55: 1427–32.
21. Lee BW, Chun SW, Kim SH, Lee Y, Kang ES, et al. (2011) Lithospermic acid B protects beta-cells from cytokine-induced apoptosis by alleviating apoptotic pathways and activating anti-apoptotic pathways of Nrf2-HO-1 and Sirt1. Toxicol Appl Pharmacol 252: 47–54.

22. Lee GT, Ha H, Jung M, Li H, Hong SW, et al. (2003) Delayed treatment with lithospermate B attenuates experimental diabetic renal injury. J Am Soc Nephrol 14: 709–20.
23. Hur KY, Seo HJ, Kang ES, Kim SH, Song S, et al. (2008) Therapeutic effect of magnesium lithospermate B on neointimal formation after balloon-induced vascular injury. Eur J Pharmacol 586: 226–33.
24. Hur KY, Kim SH, Choi MA, Williams DR, Lee YH, et al. (2010) Protective effects of magnesium lithospermate B against diabetic atherosclerosis via Nrf2-ARE-NQO1 transcriptional pathway. Atherosclerosis 211: 69–76.
25. Praidou A, Androudi S, Brazitikos P, Karakiulakis G, Papakonstantinou E, et al. (2010) Angiogenic growth factors and their inhibitors in diabetic retinopathy. Curr Diabetes Rev 6: 304–12.
26. Wu Y, Feng B, Chen S, Chakrabarti S (2012) ERK5 Regulates glucose-induced increased fibronectin production in the endothelial cells and in the retina in diabetes. Invest Ophthalmol Vis Sci 53: 8405–13.
27. Giacco F, Brownlee M (2010) Oxidative stress and diabetic complications. Circ Res 107: 1058–70.
28. Svoboda P, Ko SH, Cho B, Yoo SH, Choi SW, et al. (2008) Neopterin, a marker of immune response, and 8-hydroxy-2′-deoxyguanosine, a marker of oxidative stress, correlate at high age as determined by automated simultaneous high-performance liquid chromatography analysis of human urine. Anal Biochem 383: 236–42.
29. Dong QY, Cui Y, Chen L, Song J, Sun L (2008) Urinary 8-hydroxydeoxyguanosine levels in diabetic retinopathy patients. Eur J Ophthalmol 18: 94–8.
30. Park KS, Kim JH, Kim MS, Kim JM, Kim SK, et al. (2001) Effects of insulin and antioxidant on plasma 8-hydroxyguanine and tissue 8-hydroxydeoxyguanosine in streptozotocin-induced diabetic rats. Diabetes 50: 2837–41.
31. Jung M, Lee HC, Ahn CW, Park W, Choi S, et al. (2002) Effective isolation of magnesium lithospermate B and its inhibition of aldose reductase and fibronectin on mesangial cell line. Chem Pharm Bull (Tokyo) 50: 1135–6.
32. Bandello F, Lattanzio R, Zucchiatti I, Del TC (2013) Pathophysiology and treatment of diabetic retinopathy. Acta Diabetol 50: 1–20.
33. Antonetti DA, Klein R, Gardner TW (2012) Diabetic retinopathy. N Engl J Med 366: 1227–39.
34. Wang J, Xu X, Elliott MH, Zhu M, Le YZ (2010) Muller cell-derived VEGF is essential for diabetes-induced retinal inflammation and vascular leakage. Diabetes 59: 2297–305.
35. Aiello LP, Avery RL, Arrigg PG, Keyt BA, Jampel HD, et al. (1994) Vascular endothelial growth factor in ocular fluid of patients with diabetic retinopathy and other retinal disorders. N Engl J Med 331: 1480–7.
36. Miyamoto K, Khosrof S, Bursell SE, Moromizato Y, Aiello LP, et al. (2000) Vascular endothelial growth factor (VEGF)-induced retinal vascular permeability is mediated by intercellular adhesion molecule-1 (ICAM-1). Am J Pathol 156: 1733–9.
37. Leung DW, Cachianes G, Kuang WJ, Goeddel DV, Ferrara N (1989) Vascular endothelial growth factor is a secreted angiogenic mitogen. Science 246: 1306–9.
38. Xu X, Zhu Q, Xia X, Zhang S, Gu Q, et al. (2004) Blood-retinal barrier breakdown induced by activation of protein kinase C via vascular endothelial growth factor in streptozotocin-induced diabetic rats. Curr Eye Res 28: 251–6.
39. Harhaj NS, Felinski EA, Wolpert EB, Sundstrom JM, Gardner TW, et al. (2006) VEGF activation of protein kinase C stimulates occludin phosphorylation and contributes to endothelial permeability. Invest Ophthalmol Vis Sci 47: 5106–15.
40. Das EN, King GL (2007) The role of protein kinase C activation and the vascular complications of diabetes. Pharmacol Res 55: 498–510.
41. Waisbourd M, Goldstein M, Loewenstein A (2011) Treatment of diabetic retinopathy with anti-VEGF drugs. Acta Ophthalmol 89: 203–7.
42. Feit-Leichman RA, Kinouchi R, Takeda M, Fan Z, Mohr S, et al. (2005) Vascular damage in a mouse model of diabetic retinopathy: relation to neuronal and glial changes. Invest Ophthalmol Vis Sci 46: 4281–7.
43. Yang JH, Kwak HW, Kim TG, Han J, Moon SW, et al. (2013) Retinal Neurodegeneration in Type II Diabetic Otsuka Long-Evans Tokushima Fatty Rats. Invest Ophthalmol Vis Sci 54: 3844–51.
44. Geraldes P, Hiraoka-Yamamoto J, Matsumoto M, Clermont A, Leitges M, et al. (2009) Activation of PKC-delta and SHP-1 by hyperglycemia causes vascular cell apoptosis and diabetic retinopathy. Nat Med 15: 1298–306.
45. Roy S, Sato T, Paryani G, Kao R (2003) Downregulation of fibronectin overexpression reduces basement membrane thickening and vascular lesions in retinas of galactose-fed rats. Diabetes 52: 1229–34.
46. Roy S, Ha J, Trudeau K, Beglova E (2010) Vascular basement membrane thickening in diabetic retinopathy. Curr Eye Res 35: 1045–56.
47. Wu LL, Chiou CC, Chang PY, Wu JT (2004) Urinary 8-OHdG: a marker of oxidative stress to DNA and a risk factor for cancer, atherosclerosis and diabetics. Clin Chim Acta 339: 1–9.
48. Mitamura Y, Takeuchi S, Matsuda A, Tagawa Y, Mizue Y, et al. (2001) Monocyte chemotactic protein-1 in the vitreous of patients with proliferative diabetic retinopathy. Ophthalmologica 215: 415–8.
49. van Hecke MV, Dekker JM, Nijpels G, Moll AC, Heine RJ, et al. (2005) Inflammation and endothelial dysfunction are associated with retinopathy: the Hoorn Study. Diabetologia 48: 1300–6.
50. Makino N, Maeda T, Sugano M, Satoh S, Watanabe R, et al. (2005) High serum TNF-alpha level in Type 2 diabetic patients with microangiopathy is associated with eNOS down-regulation and apoptosis in endothelial cells. J Diabetes Complications 19: 347–55.
51. Limb GA, Hollifield RD, Webster L, Charteris DG, Chignell AH (2001) Soluble TNF receptors in vitreoretinal proliferative disease. Invest Ophthalmol Vis Sci 42: 1586–91.
52. Jung KI, Kim JH, Park HY, Park CK (2013) Neuroprotective effects of cilostazol on retinal ganglion cell damage in diabetic rats. J Pharmacol Exp Ther 345: 457–63.
53. Kim YH, Kim YS, Park CH, Chung IY, Yoo JM, et al. (2008) Protein kinase C-delta mediates neuronal apoptosis in the retinas of diabetic rats via the Akt signaling pathway. Diabetes 57: 2181–90.
54. Lu ZY, Bhutto IA, Amemiya T (2003) Retinal changes in Otsuka long-evans Tokushima Fatty rats (spontaneously diabetic rat) – possibility of a new experimental model for diabetic retinopathy. Jpn J Ophthalmol 47: 28–35.
55. Pescosolido N, Imperatrice B, Karavitis P (2008) Ocular disorders secondary to systemic disease and the potential role of carnitines. Drugs R D 9 Suppl 1: 15–22.
56. Nebbioso M, Federici M, Rusciano D, Evangelista M, Pescosolido N (2012) Oxidative stress in preretinopathic diabetes subjects and antioxidants. Diabetes Technol Ther 14: 257–63.

12

KDT501, a Derivative from Hops, Normalizes Glucose Metabolism and Body Weight in Rodent Models of Diabetes

Veera R. Konda*, Anuradha Desai, Gary Darland, Neile Grayson, Jeffrey S. Bland

KinDex Therapeutics, LLC, Seattle, Washington, United States of America

Abstract

Aims/Hypothesis: We developed KDT501, a novel substituted 1,3-cyclopentadione chemically derived from hop extracts, and evaluated it in various *in vitro* and *in vivo* models of diabetes and insulin sensitivity.

Methods: KDT501 was evaluated for anti-inflammatory effects in monocyte/macrophage cells; agonistic activity for peroxisome proliferator-activated receptors (PPAR); lipogenesis and gene expression profile in human subcutaneous adipocytes. Body composition, glucose, insulin sensitivity, and lipids were assessed in diet-induced obesity (DIO) mice and Zucker Diabetic Fatty (ZDF) rats after oral administration.

Results: KDT501 mediated lipogenesis in 3T3L1 and human subcutaneous adipocytes; however, the gene expression profile of KDT501 differed from that of the full PPARγ agonist rosiglitazone, suggesting that KDT501 has pleiotropic biological activities. In addition, KDT501 showed only modest, partial PPARγ agonist activity and exhibited anti-inflammatory effects in monocytes/macrophages that were not observed with rosiglitazone. In a DIO mouse model, oral administration of KDT501 significantly reduced fed blood glucose, glucose/insulin AUC following an oral glucose bolus, and body fat. In ZDF rats, oral administration of KDT501 significantly reduced fed glucose, fasting plasma glucose, and glucose AUC after an oral glucose bolus. Significant, dose-dependent reductions of plasma hemoglobin A1c, weight gain, total cholesterol, and triglycerides were also observed in animals receiving KDT501.

Conclusion: These results indicate that KDT501 produces a unique anti-diabetic profile that is distinct in its spectrum of pharmacological effects and biological mechanism from both metformin and pioglitazone. KDT501 may thus constitute a novel therapeutic agent for the treatment of Type 2 diabetes and associated conditions.

Editor: Ayyalasomayajula Vajreswari, National Institute of Nutrition, India

Funding: All authors were employees of KinDex Therapeutics and research presented was funded by KinDex Therapeutics. The funders had no role in study design, data collection and analysis, decision to publish, or preparation of the manuscript.

Competing Interests: The authors have declared that there is no duality of interest associated with this manuscript. The authors have the following interests: All authors of the manuscript work or have worked as employees of or consultants for KinDex Therapeutics, LLC, which funded this study, and this article was created during the course of that work. Phase 1 clinical development of KDT501 has been successfully completed and further clinical development studies of this compound are anticipated. There are no declarations concerning marketed products. KinDex holds the following patent relating to material pertinent to this research: US 8, 410, 178 B2. All authors also declare no conflict of interest resulting from financial or non-financial competing interests.

* E-mail: veerakonda@kindextherapeutics.com

Introduction

The molecular link between inflammation, obesity, and insulin resistance is incompletely understood; however, multiple lines of evidence suggest that inflammation plays a major role in insulin resistance. A number of groups have investigated the link between inflammation, obesity and insulin resistance [1,2]. Several studies have recently reported that obesity leads to the infiltration of macrophages and immune cells into adipose tissue, activating an inflammatory response that leads to insulin resistance [3,4]. In lean mice, adipose tissue macrophages having an alternatively activated (M2) phenotype are less inflammatory and may actually afford protection, whereas macrophages in adipose tissue of obese mice have a pro-inflammatory, classical (M1) phenotype [5,6]. These studies suggest an important link between macrophage-mediated inflammation in obesity-related insulin resistance.

PPAR-gamma (PPARγ) is the primary target of the drug class of thiazolidinediones (TZDs), which are used to treat diabetes mellitus and other diseases featuring insulin resistance. It has been shown that activation of PPARγ increases adipocyte differentiation, lipid metabolism, insulin sensitivity, and glucose homeostasis [7]. Besides their beneficial role as insulin-sensitizing agents in Type 2 diabetes mellitus (T2D), TZD drugs such as rosiglitazone and pioglitazone are known to produce adverse effects including weight gain, plasma volume expansion, edema, and cardiac hypertrophy in preclinical species [8]. The edema that can accompany the use of TZDs has been linked to congestive heart failure in humans [9].

In contrast to full PPARγ agonists, partial PPARγ agonists mitigate insulin resistance and hyperglycemia in rodent models of obesity without increasing adiposity and cardiac weight [10]. Furthermore, structurally distinct, non-TZD PPARγ modulators exhibit anti-diabetic properties with improved therapeutic indices with regard to excessive fat and cardiomegaly compared to rosiglitazone [11–14] in rodent models. Recent efforts to develop safer anti-diabetic molecules with partial PPARγ activity include the identification and validation of a partial PPARγ agonist of natural origin [15].

Several studies have reported potential anti-inflammatory effects of PPARγ ligands on monocytes/macrophages. However, it has been demonstrated that PPARγ activation is not essential for PPARγ ligands to exert anti-inflammatory effects in macrophages. For example, in a RAW264.7 cell model [16], the non-TZD PPARγ agonist L-796,449 displayed anti-inflammatory properties even though PPARγ expression was minimal or absent. As another example, abscisic acid increased PPARγ activity independent of its ligand binding mechanism [17] and reduced obesity-related inflammation and promoted glucose tolerance in db/db mice. [18]. These studies suggest that many partial or non-TZD PPARγ agonists produce anti-inflammatory activity independent of PPARγactivation or binding.

Extracts from hops (*Humulus lupulus*) have been widely used as flavoring agents in brewing. Previously, it was reported that mixtures of hop extracts show anti-inflammatory activity by inhibiting the NF-κB signaling pathway [19-21], exhibit anti-diabetic effects [22,23], and reduce systemic inflammation in high fat diet-induced obesity (DIO) mice [24]. We developed KDT501, a novel, stereochemically pure substituted 1,3-cyclopentadione, chemically derived from hop extracts and assigned the correct stereochemistry to this molecule and, for the first time, to other humulone pharmacophores [25]. In this study, we evaluated KDT501 in various *in vitro* and *in vivo* models of diabetes and insulin sensitivity.

Materials

Lipopolysaccharide (LPS), TNFα and telmisartan were purchased from Sigma (St. Louis, MO).

Milliplex MAP human cytokine/chemokine kit and adipogenesis assay kits were purchased from Millipore (Billerica, MA). 3T3-L1 cells, THP-1 cells and FBS were purchased from ATCC (Manassas, VA). RPMI-1640 medium was purchased from Hyclone (Logan, UT). Penicillin-streptomycin solution was purchased from MediaTech (Manassas, VA). PPARα, PPARγ and PPARδ assay kits, rosiglitazone, GW590735 and GW0742 were from Indigo Biosciences (State College, PA). DMEM/F12 medium was purchased from Invitrogen (Carlsbad, CA). Human subcutaneous primary adipocytes and cell culture reagents were purchased from Lonza (Walkersville, MD). All other reagents were analytical grade.

Methods

Cerep Bioprint assays

KDT501 was screened over 150 (Cerep BioPrint Panel, Poitiers, FR) biological targets, binding and enzymatic assays, as well as *in vitro* screens focused on ADME related issues. The protocols and target list are available at (http://www.cerep.fr/cerep/users/pages/catalog/profiles/DetailProfile.asp?profile = 2130).

PPARγ reporter assays

PPAR assay kits from Indigo Biosciences and supplemented protocols were used in this study. Briefly, the reporter cells were treated in triplicates with various concentrations of KDT501 (25–0.78 μM). Telmisartan (10–0.625 μM), GW590735 (10–0.03 μM), and GW0742 (1–0.01 μM) were used as positive controls for PPARγ, PPARα and PPARδ respectively. Rosiglitazone (1–0.031 μM) was used in all assays to confirm specificity to PPARγ. DMSO (0.1%) was used as a negative control. Cells were incubated for 20 hours as per the protocol and read using a luminometer (Victor2, Perkin Elmer). Average relative light unit (RLU) values from blank wells were subtracted from all the samples. The final data were compared with DMSO control and statistical analyses were performed using GraphPad Prism.

THP-1 cells

THP-1 cells were maintained in RPMI1640 in the presence of 10% serum according to manufacturer's instructions as described earlier [20]. The cells were pre-incubated with various concentrations of test compounds (KDT501, rosiglitazone, telmisartan, DHA or PGJ2) in the presence of 1% serum medium for 1 hour, then stimulated with TNF-α (10 ng/ml) or LPS (1 μg/ml) overnight (16–20 hours. Cytokines were assayed using a Milliplex MAP human cytokine/chemokine kit and Luminex 100^{TM} IS. Data were analyzed using a five-parameter logistic method and represented as Mean ±SD of four independent samples.

Lipogenesis

Murine 3T3-L1 preadipocytes were maintained in DMEM supplemented with 10% FBS as described earlier [26]. Cells were seeded at an initial density of approximately 1.5×10^6 cells in 24-well plates. After confluence, cells were treated with KDT501 (25, 12.5, 6.25, and 3.25 μM), rosiglitazone (10 μM), or DMSO on day 0. Cells were differentiated in differentiation medium consisting of 10% FBS/DMEM, 0.5 mM methylisobutylxanthine, 0.5 μM dexamethasone, and 10 μg/mL insulin. After two days, the medium was changed to progression medium consisting of 10 μg/mL insulin in 10% FBS/DMEM followed by 2 more days in maintenance medium consisting of 10% FBS/DMEM. KDT501 or rosiglitazone were included throughout the maturation phase (day 6/day 7). Human subcutaneous primary adipocytes were maintained as described for 3T3L1 adipocytes and treated with rosiglitazone (1 μM), KDT501 (10 μM), telmisartan (10 μM), DHA (10 μM) or PGJ2 (10 μM) for 10 days.

Oil O-red staining

Intracellular lipid was quantified with Oil O-Red staining using an adipogenesis assay kit from (Millipore, Billerica, MA). The medium was carefully discarded and washed twice with PBS. 300 μL Of Oil O-Red solution were added and incubated for 15 minutes at room temperature. The cells were washed, and bound dye was extracted and transferred to a 96 well plate. Absorbance was measured at 530 nm using a plate reader (Thermo Electron Corp.). Fold change relative to DMSO control was calculated from four independent wells for each condition. Data represent Mean ± SD.

Gene Expression analysis

Human subcutaneous primary adipocytes were maintained as described earlier. Cells were seeded at an initial density of approximately 2×10^6 cells in 6-well plates with PGM-2 medium (2 mL medium/well) and allowed to grow for 24 hr to confluence. Cells were treated with test compounds KDT501 (25 μM),

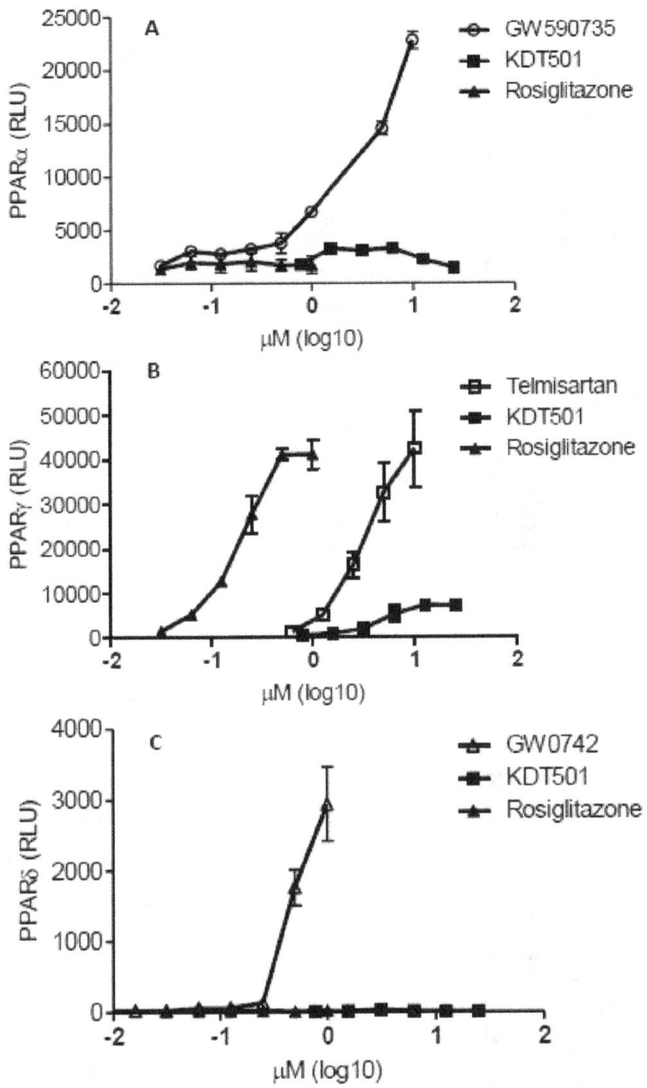

Figure 1. KDT501 agonistic effect on PPAR reporter activity. PPARα reporter cells were treated with various concentrations of GW590735 (round circles), rosiglitazone (black triangles) and KDT501 (black squares) (A). PPARγ reporter cells were treated with various concentrations of rosiglitazone, telmisartan (white squares), and KDT501 (B). PPARδ reporter cells were treated with GW0742 (white triangles), rosiglitazone and KDT501(C). Cells were treated for 20 hr and relative luminescence units (RLU) were measured as described in the methods. Agonist concentrations were transformed to log10 µM. Agonist dose- responses were plotted by non-linear regression. Data represent Mean± SD.

rosiglitazone (1 µM), telmisartan (10 µM), or DMSO in adipocyte differentiating medium. The differentiation medium consisted of indomethacin, methylisobutylxanthine, dexamethasone, and insulin from PGM-2 single aliquots. After 5 days, the cells were washed in PBS, frozen in liquid nitrogen and shipped to Expression Analysis (Durham, NC) in dry ice. Three independent plates were used for each condition.

RNA was extracted using the miRNeasy Mini Kit (Qiagen) as described by the manufacturer. RNA was isolated and expression profiling was performed using the Ambion WT Expression Kit (Life Technologies). Labeled target, which was hybridized to GeneChip Human Gene 1.0 ST Arrays (Affymetrix), was prepared essentially as described by the manufacturer. This cDNA was then used as a template for *in vitro* transcription using T7 RNA Polymerase to produce anti-sense RNA, which was then converted into single-stranded sense cDNA that was fragmented and labeled with biotin prior to hybridization to the GeneChip Arrays. Stained arrays were imaged using a Scanner 3000 (Affymetrix) and probe set analysis results were generated with Expression Console (Affymetrix) using the robust multi-array algorithm.

Gene Ontology (GO): Gene expression fold-change was calculated for test compounds ≥ absolute (log2) relative to control and with a p-value <0.05 and PADE value <15. The Bonferroni adjusted p-value (<0.05) was used for ranking and is shown as "E-Value". The GO terms for KDT501 (Probe Set 24), telmisartan (Probe Set 8) and rosiglitazone (Probe Set 74) denote direct biological pathways.

Animal Care and Use Statement

All procedures were in compliance with the U.S. Department of Agriculture's (USDA) Animal Welfare Act (9 CFR Parts 1, 2, and 3) and other appropriate agencies. All animal studies were approved by the Institutional Animal Care and Use Committee of Covance Laboratories (Greenfield, IN).

DIO Mice

C57Bl6/J male mice were 15 weeks old at the start of the experiment. In general, DIO models are initiated at an early age to evaluate effects on obesity. However, older, overweight mice were used in this study to represent middle-aged human subjects for the assessment of metabolic parameters associated with weight loss/diabetes. The mice were housed individually in cages at 72±4°F with a relative humidity of 30–70% with 12 hour light-dark cycle. High fat diet (40% Cal) TD95217 (Teklad Custom Research Diet) was used in this study. The test compounds were administered orally twice per day at 12 hour intervals (10 mL/kg) in 0.5% methylcellulose and 0.2% Tween 80 (w/v). Mice were randomly allocated on the basis of body weight to seven groups (N = 10/group), with five animals for the oral glucose tolerance test (OGTT) and 5 animals for the insulin tolerance test. KDT501 (25, 50, 100 and 200 mg/kg, calculated as the free acid), pioglitazone (30 mg/kg) and metformin (200 mg/kg) were given twice per day. Body weight and food consumption were determined weekly.

After 30 days, the mice were fasted overnight, blood was drawn through the tail vein and baseline blood glucose was measured using a glucose analyzer. One hour later, mice were given an oral gavage of glucose solution in water (4 ml/kg, 2 g/kg) and blood samples were taken at 15, 30, 60, and 120 min to determine plasma glucose and insulin levels. Five days before the start of the experiment (t = −5 days) and again at the end of the experiment (t = 28 days), body fat was determined using QNMR. With the exception of the group treated with 200 mg/kg KDT501, 10 animals/group were used in the determinations. Insulin and HbA1c glucose levels were determined on days 1, 15 and 29.

Zucker Diabetic Fatty (ZDF) Rats

Male ZDF rats were obtained from Charles River Laboratories at approximately 7 weeks of age. Rats were maintained ad lib on Purina #5008 diet, delivering approximately 17% of calories from fat. Animals with fasting glucose between 150–350 mg/dL were randomized based on glucose and body weight. Test articles were prepared in 0.5% (w/v) methylcellulose + 0.2% (w/v) Tween 80 and given by oral gavage twice daily. Rats (10/group, 6 treatment groups) were administered KDT501 (100, 150, or 200 mg/kg), metformin (200 mg/kg), pioglitazone (30 mg/kg) or vehicle

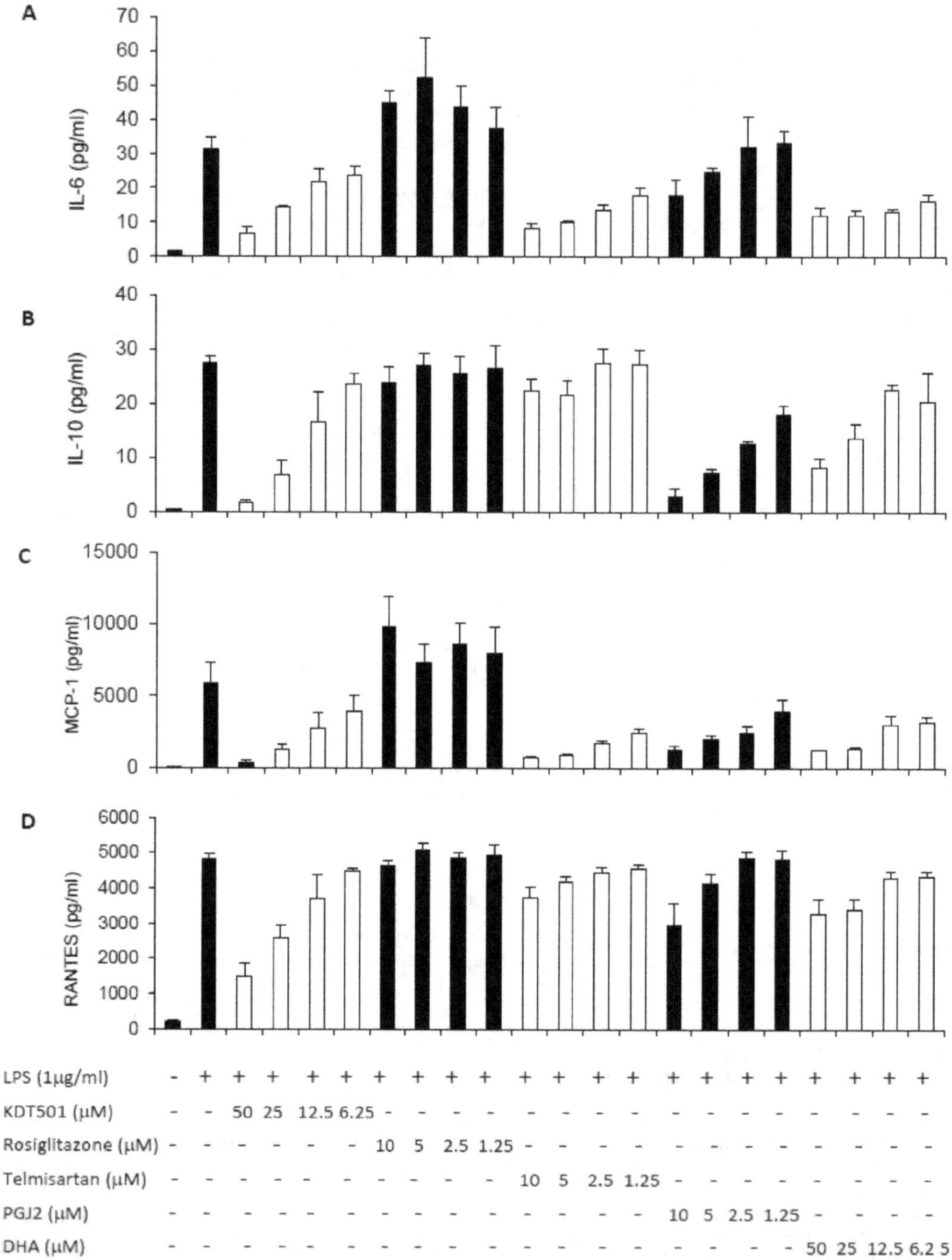

Figure 2. KDT501 reduced TNF-α and LPS-mediated inflammatory markers in THP-1 monocytes. THP-1 cells were pre-incubated in the absence or in the presence of various concentrations of KDT501, rosiglitazone, telmisartan, DHA and PGJ2 for 1 hour, and then stimulated with LPS (1 μg/mL) overnight. MCP-1, IL-6, IL-10 and RANTES levels in the medium were quantified as described in Methods. Data represent the mean ± SD from 4 independent samples. * Mean values significantly different from LPS stimulation ($p<0.05$).

control for up to 32 days. Body weights and food intake were determined weekly.

Blood was collected via tail bleed and whole blood glucose was measured on days 1, 8, 15 and 29. Blood was collected in 5 animals on days 15 and 29 for determination of glucose, insulin, lipids, hematocrit, and HbA1c. Animals were fasted overnight and OGTT was conducted on days 31 and 32 for determination of glucose and insulin levels. A second ZDF rat study was conducted and the resulting data on total cholesterol are presented.

Statistical Methods for animal studies. Statistical calculations were performed (JMP version, SAS Institute, Cary, NC). One-way ANOVA with Dunnett's test for *post hoc* determinations were used to compare vehicle treated control. Data were expressed as mean ± SEM.

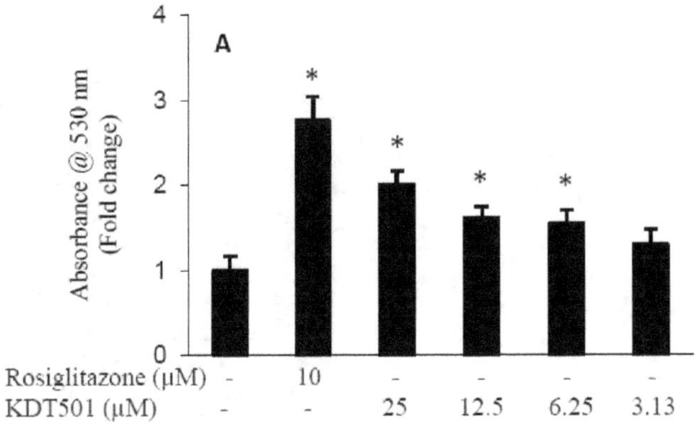

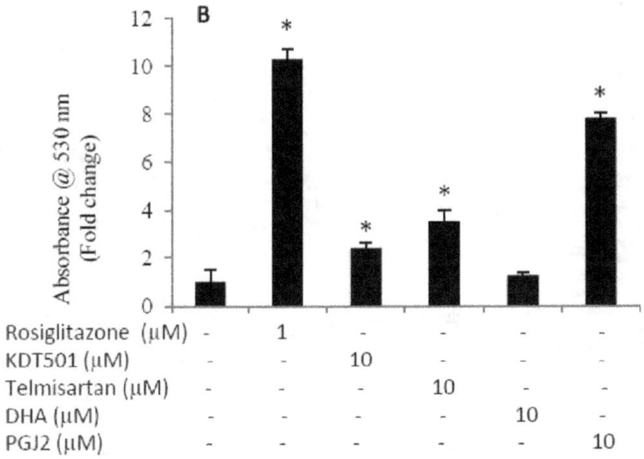

Figure 3. Effect of KDT501 on lipid accumulation in adipocytes. (A) 3T3L1 adipocytes were treated with rosiglitazone (10 uM) or various concentrations of KDT501 for 6 days. (B) Human subcutaneous adipocytes were treated with rosiglitazone (1 μM), KDT501 (10 μM), telmisartan (10 μM), DHA (10 μM) or PGJ2 (10 μM) for 10 days. Intracellular lipid was quantified with Oil Red O staining and the data represented as fold induction compared to DMSO negative control. Representative data expressed as mean ± SD from 4 independent samples. * Mean values significantly different from control ($p<0.05$).

Results

Screening for Biological targets

As a first step in our investigation, KDT501 was screened in Cerep's BioPrint Panel to identify its biological targets. Only three binding targets were identified: the ion channel, SCN2a, the type II angiotensin receptor, AGTR2, and PPARγ, with IC_{50}'s of 19, 14 and 8.4 μM, respectively. Since we were aware of the pleiotropic nature of hop components, we then embarked on a series of analyses to distinguish KDT501 at a molecular level from traditional glitazone PPARγ agonists.

Effect of KDT501 on PPAR reporter activity

High concentrations of KDT501 increased PPARγ reporter activity, but had no effect on PPARα or PPARδ reporter activity (Figure 1), suggesting that KDT501 is a specific agonist of PPARγ. Similar to rosiglitazone, telmisartan, a known PPARγ agonist, also increased PPARγ activity (Fig 1B) with lower potency (EC_{50} = 13.4 μM) compared to rosiglitazone (EC_{50} = 0.42 μM). On the other hand, KDT501 (EC_{50} = 14.0 μM) exhibited both weak and partial PPARγ activity, reaching only 29±7% (n = 3, Mean ±SEM) of rosiglitazone's maximum activation.

Anti-inflammatory properties of KDT501 in LPS-activated THP-1 cells

To further understand how KDT501 is differentiated from classical PPARγ agonists, we performed studies in monocytic THP-1 cells, an established inflammatory cell line that expresses PPARγ. Changes in cell viability were not observed for any of the compounds at the highest dose used. KDT501 (6.25 to 50 μM) dose-dependently reduced LPS stimulated inflammatory mediators MCP-1, RANTES and IL-6 (Figure 2). Telmisartan, DHA and 5-deoxy-Δ12,14- PGJ2 (PGJ2), a naturally occurring PPARγ ligand, also inhibited these cytokines in a concentration-dependent manner. On the other hand, rosiglitazone did not significantly affect any of the inflammatory markers in this study, providing an obvious distinction between KDT501 and classic TZD's, and suggesting that the anti-inflammatory properties of KDT501 are independent of PPARγ in this cell model.

Effect of KDT501 on lipogenesis in adipocytes

Since PPARγ is known to be involved in adipogenesis, we evaluated the role of KDT501 in *de novo* lipogenesis in 3T3L1 adipocytes and human subcutaneous adipocytes. Rosiglitazone (10 μM) increased lipogenesis about 2.8-fold in 3T3L1 adipocytes. KDT501 dose-dependently (3.125 to 25 μM) increased lipogenesis with maximum activation of two-fold (Figure 3A). In human subcutaneous adipocytes, rosiglitazone (1 μM), PGJ2 (10 μM), telmisartan (10 μM) and KDT501 (10 μM) increased lipogenesis by 10.3, 8.8, 3.5 and 2.4-fold respectively (Figure 3B). These data are consistent with the observed PPARγ reporter activities for the compounds and demonstrate that KDT501 is a weak, partial PPARγ agonist. No significant changes in lipogenesis were observed with DHA.

Gene expression in subcutaneous human adipocytes

Since adipocytes are one of the primary targets of classical PPARγ agonists such as rosiglitazone, we undertook a comparison of the gene expression profiles elicited by rosiglitazone and KDT501 in this cell type. The concentration necessary for maximum PPARγ activation and lipogenesis in cell-based assays was employed. For comparative purposes, we included telmisartan, which has previously been reported to exhibit weak PPARγ agonist activity [27].

In our analysis, we considered only those transcripts that were changed by at least 2-fold, regardless of test article. The data summarized in the accompanying Venn diagram reveal clear differences between KDT501 and rosiglitazone (Figure 4). Of the 62 transcripts stimulated at least 2-fold by rosiglitazone, KDT501 had stimulatory effects on only 14, 5 of which were also stimulated by telmisartan ($p<0.0001$; Fisher's exact test). Similarly, KDT501 reduced 10 transcripts, of which only 7 were common to rosiglitazone. In addition, KDT501 changed 4 transcripts (3 up and 1 down), which were not observed in either rosiglitazone or telmisartan groups. Interestingly, telmisartan changed 8 (5 up and 3 down) transcripts, which were common to both rosiglitazone and KDT501. Gene ontology data for biological processes predict that both KDT501 and telmisartan influence brown fat cell differentiation (Table 1).

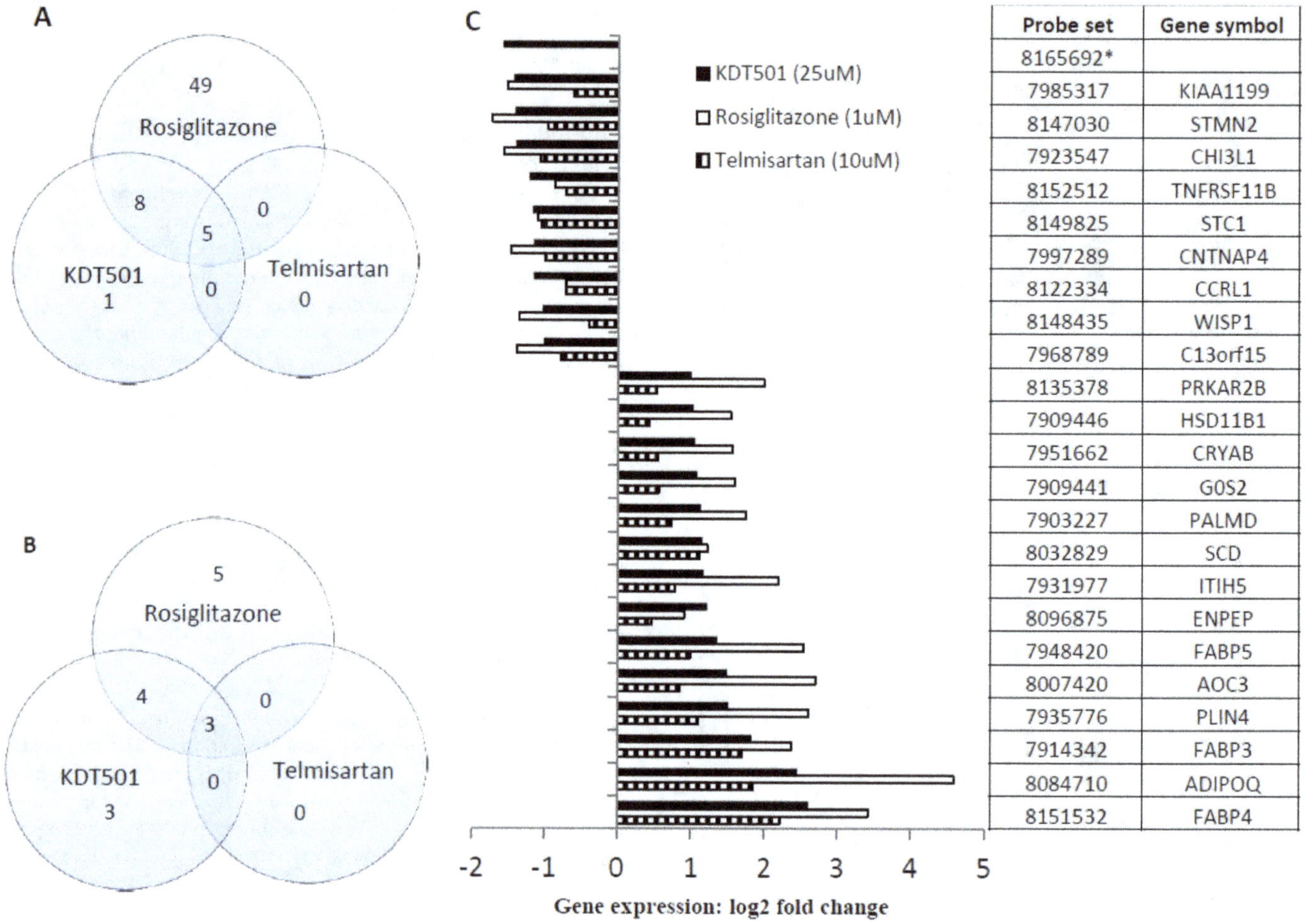

Figure 4. Human subcutaneous adipocyte gene signatures. Cells were treated with test compounds rosiglitazone (1 μM), telmisartan (10 μM) or KDT501 (25 μM) for 5 days. Gene arrays were performed and the probe sets selected were those with at least a 2-fold change as described in methods. Venn diagram represents up-regulated (A) and down regulated genes (B). KDT501-mediated (probe set 24) 3-way gene-intersection (rosiglitazone, KDT501 and telmisartan) were presented (C). * Probe set values for rosiglitazone and telmisartan are not qualified to include in the figure.

DIO mice

Body composition. Since KDT501 regulates inflammation and lipid metabolism in *in vitro* models, we evaluated KDT501 to determine its effect on glucose metabolism and weight gain in DIO mice. At the start of the experiment, the groups were well matched with regard to body weight and there were no significant differences seen in the body weight or percentage of body fat between the seven test groups. Interestingly, we also observed that the total weight loss is equivalent to fat loss (~4 g) in the high dose KDT501 (200 mg/kg bid) group (data not shown). Significant reduction in fat mass was observed by the end of the study for KDT501 (doses ≥100 mg/kg bid) and metformin (Figure 5E).

OGTT: After four weeks on a high-fat diet, animals treated with metformin and pioglitazone exhibited significantly reduced glucose and insulin AUC's (Figures 5C and 5D) compared to controls. Mice treated with KDT501 (≥100 mg/ kg) also showed significant reduction in glucose AUC. The magnitude of reduction was comparable to that seen with 30 mg/kg pioglitazone. The effect on insulin was similar, with significant reductions in the AUC for metformin and pioglitazone as well as 200 mg/ kg KDT 501, while there are indications that insulin levels were reduced at lower doses of KDT 501.

ZDF rats

Body weight gain. With the exception of groups receiving KDT501 (150 and 200 mg/kg), all animals gained weight throughout the trial (Figure 6A). Two weeks into the trial, animals receiving 200 mg/kg KDT501 began to lose weight, an effect observed one week later in the 150 mg/kg group (Figure 6A).

Effect on HbA1c. At the end of the study, 100 mg/kg of KDT501 reduced HbA1c equivalent to levels observed with metformin, while higher doses of KDT501 as well as pioglitazone reduced HbA1c levels to approximately half that of the vehicle-treated control (Figure 6B).

Non-fasting blood glucose. Administration of KDT501 (150 or 200 mg/kg) prevented the dramatic increase in blood sugar seen in vehicle-treated control animals as they progressed to frank diabetes (Figure 6C). KDT501 (200 mg/ kg) was equivalent in this regard to metformin and pioglitazone.

OGTT. The reduction seen in non-fasting blood glucose was mirrored when animals were subjected to an OGTT (Figure 6D), and all doses of KDT501 significantly reduced the AUC relative to the vehicle-treated control group (Figure 6E).

Effect on cholesterol and triglycerides. In another ZDF rat study, we evaluated the effect of KDT501 on total cholesterol and triglyceride levels in the plasma. KDT501 reduced cholester-

Table 1. Gene expression profile in human subcutaneous adipocytes.

Rank	Rosiglitazone (probe set 74)	P value	E value	Pop Hits	Enrich
1	regulation of cell-cell adhesion involved in gastrulation	4.70E-05	1.41E-04	3	167.0
2	regulation of heterotypic cell-cell adhesion	4.70E-05	1.41E-04	3	167.0
3	regulation of gastrulation	4.70E-05	1.41E-04	3	167.0
4	positive regulation of cholesterol storage	1.60E-04	8.00E-04	5	100.2
5	positive regulation of lipid storage	5.50E-04	4.95E-03	9	55.7
6	negative regulation of I-kappaB kinase/NF-kappaB cascade	5.50E-04	4.95E-03	9	55.7
7	regulation of cholesterol storage	8.40E-04	9.24E-03	11	45.5
8	regulation of embryonic development	1.20E-03	1.56E-02	13	38.5
9	positive regulation of foam cell differentiation	1.20E-03	1.56E-02	13	38.5
10	regulation of glutamate secretion	1.20E-03	1.56E-02	13	38.5
11	regulation of fatty acid biosynthetic process	1.60E-03	2.40E-02	15	33.4
12	negative regulation of endocytosis	1.60E-03	2.40E-02	15	33.4
13	response to vitamin D	1.80E-03	2.88E-02	16	31.3
14	lipid storage	2.30E-03	4.14E-02	18	27.8
15	social behavior	2.60E-03	4.94E-02	19	26.4
	KDT501 (probe set 24)				
1	response to hormone stimulus	1.50E-05	5.51E-03	367	10.5
2	response to endogenous stimulus	2.60E-05	1.05E-02	405	9.5
3	brown fat cell differentiation	6.20E-04	1.49E-02	24	53.7
4	response to steroid hormone stimulus	1.90E-04	3.65E-02	192	13.4
5	fatty acid metabolic process	2.20E-04	4.36E-02	198	13.0
	Telmisartan (probe set 8)				
1	brown fat cell differentiation	8.80E-03	1.08E-03	24	187.9
2	fat cell differentiation	1.90E-02	1.17E-02	53	85.1
3	fatty acid metabolic process	2.10E-03	1.19E-02	198	34.2
4	response to drug	2.50E-03	1.66E-02	216	31.3
5	regulation of inflammatory response	2.80E-02	3.50E-02	76	59.3
6	response to glucocorticoid stimulus	2.90E-02	3.74E-02	78	57.8
7	response to corticosteroid stimulus	3.10E-02	4.93E-02	85	53.1

Gene expression fold-change with test compounds larger than 1 log2 ratio ($\pm$1) over control with a p-value (Fisher exact) $<$0.05 and PADE value $<$15. The Bonferroni adjusted p-value ($<$0.05) was used for ranking and is shown as "E-Value". The GO terms for KDT501 (probe set 24), rosiglitazone (probe set 74) and telmisartan (probe set 8) denote direct biological pathways.

ol, but neither metformin nor pioglitazone had this effect (Figure 6F). Similar to pioglitazone, KDT501 reduced triglycerides (Figure 6G), with KDT501 (200 mg/kg) exhibiting the largest reduction by the end of the study.

Discussion

In the present study, we evaluated the effect of KDT501 on several metabolic traits associated with insulin resistance and T2D. Oral administration of KDT501 in DIO mouse and ZDF rat models of diabetes improved glucose metabolism and reduced plasma HbA1c, an important biomarker in diabetes. KDT501 dose-dependently reduced weight gain and total cholesterol in ZDF rats, while rats treated with metformin or pioglitazone gained weight. KDT501 also reduced total cholesterol, unlike metformin and pioglitazone. These results suggest that the anti-diabetic mechanism of KDT501 differs from that of both metformin and pioglitazone and that KDT501 may be a novel therapeutic for the treatment of T2D and related conditions in humans.

In recent decades, several groups have reported that inflammation plays an important role in insulin resistance. We therefore evaluated KDT501 in several inflammatory models, including monocytic cells, THP-1 cells, RAW2647 macrophages, and human synovial fibroblasts from rheumatoid arthritis subjects (data not shown). KDT501 inhibited several inflammatory mediators (MCP-1, IL-6 and RANTES) in a dose-dependent manner in LPS-activated THP-1 cells (Figure 2). Although PPARγ has been reported to be present in this human monocytic cell line [28], an observation that we have confirmed, rosiglitazone failed to affect any of these inflammatory markers. In RAW264.7 cells, the induction of LPS-activated PGE_2 and NO was reduced by KDT501, but not with rosiglitazone (results not shown). These data demonstrate that the anti-inflammatory mechanism of KDT501 differs from that of rosiglitazone and is independent of PPARγ expression, thus serving to highlight substantial differences between KDT501 and the glitazones. Several other natural compounds have been found to exhibit PPARγ-dependent (e.g., resveratrol) and independent (e.g., luteolin) anti-inflammatory properties [29] in a co-culture system of adipocytes and

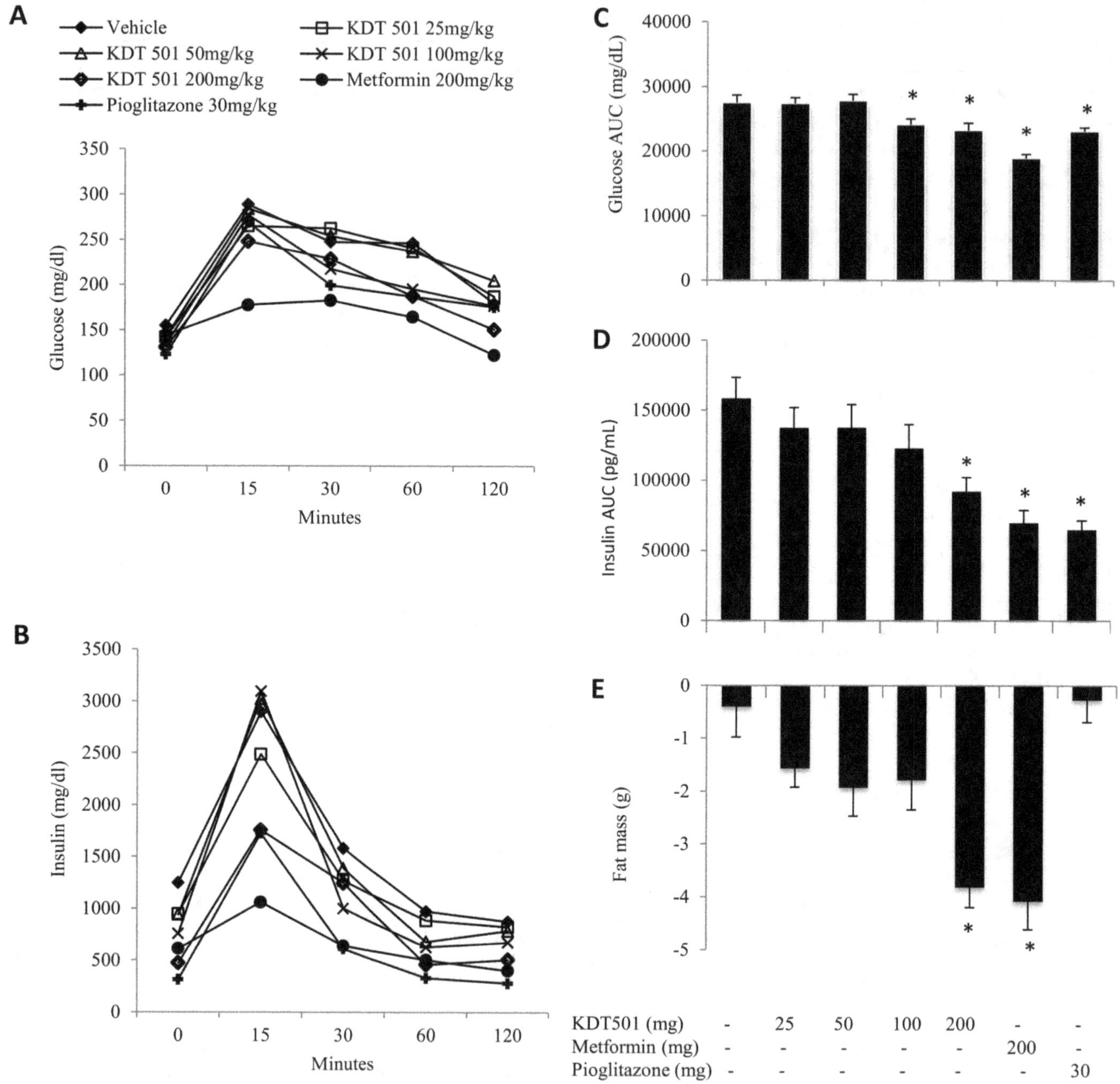

Figure 5. KDT501 reduces body fat and improves glucose metabolism. The test compounds were given orally twice daily for a month. Oral glucose tolerance test (OGTT) conducted as described in methods; glucose (A), insulin (B), glucose AUC (C) and insulin AUC (D) levels were presented. Body fat as determined by QNMR at the end of the study were presented (E). Data expressed as Mean ±SEM. * Mean values significantly different from vehicle control group ($p<0.05$).

macrophages. These studies, in combination with our findings, suggest that the anti-inflammatory activity of many partial/ non-TZD PPARγ agonists is mediated independently of PPARγ activation.

The incidence of diabetes is associated with obesity, a chronic medical condition with increasing worldwide prevalence. Many studies indicate that inflammation plays an important role in diet-induced obesity and diabetes. It has been shown that inflammatory markers such as MCP-1 are involved in the recruitment of inflammatory macrophages to adipose tissue, contributing to the development of insulin resistance and progressing, in many cases, to T2D [30,31]. MCP-1 deficiency increases M2 macrophages and ameliorates insulin sensitivity and fatty liver in diabetic mice [32]. In obese adipose tissue, 40% of all cells are infiltrating macrophages [3]. Results of the NIH-sponsored TINSAL-T2D clinical studies have demonstrated that salsalate, a non-steroidal anti-inflammatory drug, lowers HbA1c, fasting glucose and markers of inflammation in T2D patients [33].

The pleiotropic effects of many natural compounds (e.g., resveratrol, curcumin, EGCG) are well documented. KDT501 appears to be involved in the regulation of multiple insulin-sensitizing mechanisms, including the reduction of inflammation

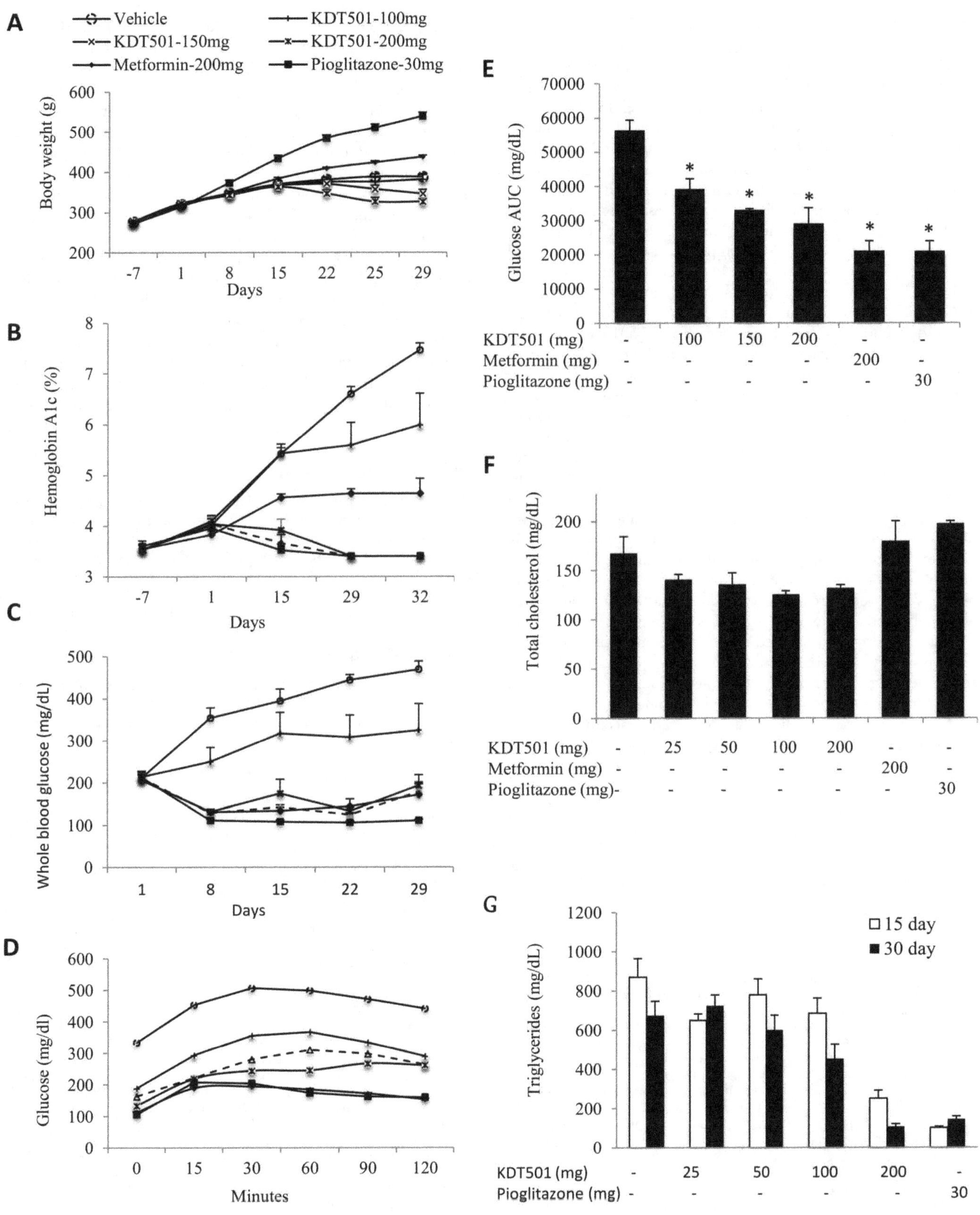

Figure 6. KDT501 reduces weight gain, improves glucose and fatty acid metabolism in ZDF rats. Vehicle control (black circles) and test compounds KDT501 (100 mg = white circles, 150 mg = white triangles, 200 mg = white squares), metformin (black diamonds) and rosiglitazone (black squares) were administered orally twice daily for up to 32 days. Weight gain (A), hemoglobin A1c (B) and whole blood glucose levels (C) were presented. At the end of the study, oral glucose tolerance tests (OGTT) were conducted as described in the methods; glucose (D) and glucose AUC levels (E) were presented. Total cholesterol levels (F) were measured in the plasma. Triglyceride levels were measured at day 15 and day 30 (G). Data expressed as Mean ±SEM. * Mean values significantly different from vehicle control group ($p<0.05$).

and activation of lipogenesis. In Cerep BioPrint assays, we identified only three biological targets, suggesting both an unusual specificity as well as a good safety profile for KDT501. KDT501 activates transcriptional activity of one of these targets, PPARγ, but not of PPARα or PPARδ, indicating ligand-binding specificity. Specificity towards PPARγ suggests reduced side effects associated with nonspecific PPAR agonists, such as PPARα-mediated hepatocarcinoma. Recent reports show that pharmacological activation of a second KDT501 target, AGTR2, in combination with PPARγ activation, ameliorates insulin resistance and reverses β-cell damage in diabetic pancreatic tissue in T2D mice [34]. AT1 receptor blockers are known to improve insulin resistance and delay the onset of diabetes [35]. AT1 receptor-mediated anti-diabetic effects are thought to be mediated through the activation of AT2 receptors by unbound angiotensin [36]. Further research is required to understand the full impact of KDT501's PPARγ and AGTR2-mediated mechanisms and their functional roles in diabetes.

Recently, it has been reported [37] that selective PPAR modulators display a selective gene regulatory profile in comparison with the full PPARγ agonist rosiglitazone. Our comparison of the gene expression profiles of human subcutaneous adipocytes treated with KDT501, rosiglitazone, and the weak PPARγ agonist telmisartan revealed that KDT501 produced not only an attenuated gene signature compared to rosiglitazone, but also regulated a different set of genes than those modulated by rosiglitazone or telmisartan. We found that saturated concentrations of telmisartan also produced an attenuated gene expression profile, compared to rosiglitazone. These data are consistent with other published gene expression profiles where partial agonists had a similar pattern of attenuated gene expression compared to full agonists [37]. Consistent with lipid accumulation data in adipocytes (Fig. 3), we observed the activation of genes involved in lipid metabolism (perilipin, fatty acid binding proteins 3, 4 & 5 etc.). We also observed the induction of adiponectin, a known PPARγ-dependent, anti-inflammatory gene in adipocytes. Interestingly, KDT501 inhibits chemokine receptor gene (CCLR1), which is known to bind MCP-1, an important inflammatory mediator that attracts macrophages to adipocytes. Gene ontology data (Table 1) suggest that rosiglitazone (probe set 77), KDT501 (probe set 24) and telmisartan (probe set 8) are involved in common (fat metabolism) as well as independent biological processes. Gene ontology data also indicate that both KDT501 and telmisartan may influence brown fat cell differentiation, which is important in thermogenesis. Additional studies are required to confirm the role of KDT501 in the regulation of brown fat physiology and thermoregulation.

Our studies show that the novel compound KDT501 improves blood glucose levels and insulin resistance in rodent models of T2D. We have also demonstrated that KDT501 moderates inflammation and adipose tissue function through a unique mechanism that is complementary and distinct from current anti-diabetic drugs. Additional research is needed to further delineate this molecule's pleiotropic mechanism and potential as a next-generation therapeutic for the treatment of human metabolic disorders.

Acknowledgments

We thank Dr. Benjamin Cravatt (The Scripps Research Institute) and Dr. John Kozarich, (ActivX) for helpful discussion and critical review and Dr. Matthew Tripp (KinDex Therapeutics) for contributing to the conception of the experiments.

Author Contributions

Conceived and designed the experiments: VK AD GD NG JB. Performed the experiments: AD. Analyzed the data: VK GD. Contributed reagents/materials/analysis tools: AD VK GD NG. Wrote the paper: AD VK GD NG JB.

References

1. Hotamisligil GS, Shargill NS, Spiegelman BM (1993) Adipose expression of tumor necrosis factor-alpha: direct role in obesity-linked insulin resistance. Science 259: 87–91.
2. Siriwardhana N, Kalupahana NS, Cekanova M, Lemieux M, Greer B, et al. (2013) Modulation of adipose tissue inflammation by bioactive food compounds. J Nutr Biochem 24: 613–623.
3. Weisberg SP, McCann D, Desai M, Rosenbaum M, Leibel RL, et al. (2003) Obesity is associated with macrophage accumulation in adipose tissue. J Clin Invest 112: 1796–1808.
4. Ferrante AW Jr (2007) Obesity-induced inflammation: a metabolic dialogue in the language of inflammation. J Intern Med 262: 408–414.
5. Lumeng CN, DelProposto JB, Westcott DJ, Saltiel AR (2008) Phenotypic switching of adipose tissue macrophages with obesity is generated by spatiotemporal differences in macrophage subtypes. Diabetes 57: 3239–3246.
6. Odegaard JI, Ricardo-Gonzalez RR, Goforth MH, Morel CR, Subramanian V, et al. (2007) Macrophage-specific PPARgamma controls alternative activation and improves insulin resistance. Nature 447: 1116–1120.
7. Brun RP, Spiegelman BM (1997) PPAR gamma and the molecular control of adipogenesis. J Endocrinol 155: 217–218.
8. Peraza MA, Burdick AD, Marin HE, Gonzalez FJ, Peters JM (2006) The toxicology of ligands for peroxisome proliferator-activated receptors (PPAR). Toxicol Sci 90: 269–295.
9. Nesto RW, Bell D, Bonow RO, Fonseca V, Grundy SM, et al. (2003) Thiazolidinedione use, fluid retention, and congestive heart failure: a consensus statement from the American Heart Association and American Diabetes Association. October 7, 2003. Circulation 108: 2941–2948.
10. Berger JP, Petro AE, Macnaul KL, Kelly LJ, Zhang BB, et al. (2003) Distinct properties and advantages of a novel peroxisome proliferator-activated protein [gamma] selective modulator. Mol Endocrinol 17: 662–676.
11. Acton JJ 3rd, Black RM, Jones AB, Moller DE, Colwell L, et al. (2005) Benzoyl 2-methyl indoles as selective PPARgamma modulators. Bioorg Med Chem Lett 15: 357–362.
12. Chang CH, McNamara LA, Wu MS, Muise ES, Tan Y, et al. (2008) A novel selective peroxisome proliferator-activator receptor-gamma modulator-SPPARgammaM5 improves insulin sensitivity with diminished adverse cardiovascular effects. Eur J Pharmacol 584: 192–201.
13. Motani A, Wang Z, Weiszmann J, McGee LR, Lee G, et al. (2009) INT131: a selective modulator of PPAR gamma. J Mol Biol 386: 1301–1311.
14. Acton JJ 3rd, Akiyama TE, Chang CH, Colwell L, Debenham S, et al. (2009) Discovery of (2R)-2-(3-{3-[(4-Methoxyphenyl)carbonyl]-2-methyl-6-(trifluoromethoxy)-1H-indol-1 -yl}phenoxy)butanoic acid (MK-0533): a novel selective peroxisome proliferator-activated receptor gamma modulator for the treatment of type 2 diabetes mellitus with a reduced potential to increase plasma and extracellular fluid volume. J Med Chem 52: 3846–3854.
15. Guasch L, Sala E, Castell-Auvi A, Cedo L, Liedl KR, et al. (2012) Identification of PPARgamma Partial Agonists of Natural Origin (I): Development of a Virtual Screening Procedure and In Vitro Validation. PLoS One 7: e50816.
16. Castrillo A, Mojena M, Hortelano S, Bosca L (2001) Peroxisome proliferator-activated receptor-gamma-independent inhibition of macrophage activation by the non-thiazolidinedione agonist L-796,449. Comparison with the effects of 15-deoxy-delta(12,14)-prostaglandin J(2). J Biol Chem 276: 34082–34088.
17. Bassaganya-Riera J, Guri AJ, Lu P, Climent M, Carbo A, et al. (2011) Abscisic acid regulates inflammation via ligand-binding domain-independent activation of peroxisome proliferator-activated receptor gamma. J Biol Chem 286: 2504–2516.
18. Guri AJ, Hontecillas R, Si H, Liu D, Bassaganya-Riera J (2007) Dietary abscisic acid ameliorates glucose tolerance and obesity-related inflammation in db/db mice fed high-fat diets. Clin Nutr 26: 107–116.
19. Desai A, Konda VR, Darland G, Austin M, Prabhu KS, et al. (2009) META060 inhibits multiple kinases in the NF-kappaB pathway and suppresses LPS-mediated inflammation in vitro and ex vivo. Inflamm Res 58: 229–234.
20. Desai A, Darland G, Bland JS, Tripp ML, Konda VR (2012) META060 attenuates TNF-alpha-activated inflammation, endothelial-monocyte interactions, and matrix metalloproteinase-9 expression, and inhibits NF-kappaB and AP-1 in THP-1 monocytes. Atherosclerosis 223: 130–136.

21. Konda VR, Desai A, Darland G, Bland JS, Tripp ML (2010) META060 inhibits osteoclastogenesis and matrix metalloproteinases in vitro and reduces bone and cartilage degradation in a mouse model of rheumatoid arthritis. Arthritis Rheum 62: 1683–1692.
22. Vroegrijk IO, van Diepen JA, van den Berg SA, Romijn JA, Havekes LM, et al. (2013) META060 protects against diet-induced obesity and insulin resistance in a high-fat-diet fed mouse. Nutrition 29: 276–283.
23. Yajima H, Ikeshima E, Shiraki M, Kanaya T, Fujiwara D, et al. (2004) Isohumulones, bitter acids derived from hops, activate both peroxisome proliferator-activated receptor alpha and gamma and reduce insulin resistance. J Biol Chem 279: 33456–33462.
24. Everard A, Geurts L, Van Roye M, Delzenne NM, Cani PD (2012) Tetrahydro iso-alpha acids from hops improve glucose homeostasis and reduce body weight gain and metabolic endotoxemia in high-fat diet-fed mice. PLoS One 7: e33858.
25. Urban J, Dahlberg CJ, Carroll BJ, Kaminsky W (2013) Absolute Configuration of Beer's Bitter Compounds. Angew Chem Int Ed Engl 52: 1553–1555.
26. Babish JG, Pacioretty LM, Bland JS, Minich DM, Hu J, et al. (2010) Antidiabetic screening of commercial botanical products in 3T3-L1 adipocytes and db/db mice. J Med Food 13: 535–547.
27. Benson SC, Pershadsingh HA, Ho CI, Chittiboyina A, Desai P, et al. (2004) Identification of telmisartan as a unique angiotensin II receptor antagonist with selective PPARgamma-modulating activity. Hypertension 43: 993–1002.
28. Pang T, Benicky J, Wang J, Orecna M, Sanchez-Lemus E, et al. (2012) Telmisartan ameliorates lipopolysaccharide-induced innate immune response through peroxisome proliferator-activated receptor-gamma activation in human monocytes. J Hypertens 30: 87–96.
29. Hirai S, Takahashi N, Goto T, Lin S, Uemura T, et al. (2010) Functional food targeting the regulation of obesity-induced inflammatory responses and pathologies. Mediators Inflamm 2010: 367838.
30. Kanda H, Tateya S, Tamori Y, Kotani K, Hiasa K, et al. (2006) MCP-1 contributes to macrophage infiltration into adipose tissue, insulin resistance, and hepatic steatosis in obesity. J Clin Invest 116: 1494–1505.
31. Weisberg SP, Hunter D, Huber R, Lemieux J, Slaymaker S, et al. (2006) CCR2 modulates inflammatory and metabolic effects of high-fat feeding. J Clin Invest 116: 115–124.
32. Nio Y, Yamauchi T, Iwabu M, Okada-Iwabu M, Funata M, et al. (2012) Monocyte chemoattractant protein-1 (MCP-1) deficiency enhances alternatively activated M2 macrophages and ameliorates insulin resistance and fatty liver in lipoatrophic diabetic A-ZIP transgenic mice. Diabetologia 55: 3350–3358.
33. Goldfine AB, Fonseca V, Jablonski KA, Pyle L, Staten MA, et al. (2010) The effects of salsalate on glycemic control in patients with type 2 diabetes: a randomized trial. Ann Intern Med 152: 346–357.
34. Ohshima K, Mogi M, Jing F, Iwanami J, Tsukuda K, et al. (2012) Direct angiotensin II type 2 receptor stimulation ameliorates insulin resistance in type 2 diabetes mice with PPARgamma activation. PLoS One 7: e48387.
35. Olivares-Reyes JA, Arellano-Plancarte A, Castillo-Hernandez JR (2009) Angiotensin II and the development of insulin resistance: implications for diabetes. Mol Cell Endocrinol 302: 128–139.
36. de Gasparo M, Catt KJ, Inagami T, Wright JW, Unger T (2000) International union of pharmacology. XXIII. The angiotensin II receptors. Pharmacol Rev 52: 415–472.
37. Tan Y, Muise ES, Dai H, Raubertas R, Wong KK, et al. (2012) Novel transcriptome profiling analyses demonstrate that selective peroxisome proliferator-activated receptor gamma (PPARgamma) modulators display attenuated and selective gene regulatory activity in comparison with PPARgamma full agonists. Mol Pharmacol 82: 68–79.

13

Apelin Ameliorates TNF-α-Induced Reduction of Glycogen Synthesis in the Hepatocytes through G Protein-Coupled Receptor APJ

Jiaojiao Chu[1,3]☯, Hangxiang Zhang[1,2]☯, Xiuqing Huang[1]☯, Yajun Lin[1], Tao Shen[1], Beidong Chen[1]☯, Yong Man[1], Shu Wang[1]*, Jian Li[1]*

1 Key Laboratory of Geriatrics, Beijing Institute of Geriatrics & Beijing Hospital, Ministry of Health, Beijing, China, **2** Department of Gerontology, Xi-Jing Hospital, Fourth Military Medical University, Xian, China, **3** Zhejiang Hospital, Hangzhou, Zhejiang Province, China

Abstract

Apelin, a novel adipokine, is the specific endogenous ligand of G protein-coupled receptor APJ. Consistent with its putative role as an adipokine, apelin has been linked to states of insulin resistance. However, the function of apelin in hepatic insulin resistance, a vital part of insulin resistance, and its underlying mechanisms still remains unclear. Here we define the impacts of apelin on TNF-α-induced reduction of glycogen synthesis in the hepatocytes. Our studies indicate that apelin reversed TNF-α-induced reduction of glycogen synthesis in HepG2 cells, mouse primary hepatocytes and liver tissues of C57BL/6J mice by improving JNK-IRS1-AKT-GSK pathway. Moreover, Western blot revealed that APJ, but not apelin, expressed in the hepatocytes and liver tissues of mice. We found that F13A, a competitive antagonist for G protein-coupled receptor APJ, suppressed the effects of apelin on TNF-α-induced reduction of glycogen synthesis in the hepatocytes, suggesting APJ is involved in the function of apelin. In conclusion, we show novel evidence suggesting that apelin ameliorates TNF-α-induced reduction of glycogen synthesis in the hepatocytes through G protein-coupled receptor APJ. Apelin appears as a beneficial adipokine with anti-insulin resistance properties, and thus as a promising therapeutic target in metabolic disorders.

Editor: Giorgio Sesti, Universita Magna-Graecia di Catanzaro, Italy

Funding: This work was supported by grants from National Basic Research Program of China (2012CB517502) and National Natural Science Foundation of China (81070634, 81270887, 81270495). The funders had no role in study design, data collection and analysis, decision to publish, or preparation of the manuscript.

Competing Interests: The authors have declared that no competing interests exist.

* E-mail: lijian@bjhmoh.cn (JL); ws3704@yahoo.com.cn (SW)

☯ These authors contributed equally to this work.

Introduction

Insulin resistance, defined as a diminished ability of cells such as adipocytes, skeletal muscle cells and hepatocytes to respond to the action of insulin, is not only the pathophysiological hallmark of type 2 diabetes and the metabolic syndrome [1], but also an independently and strongly associated factor with an increased risk of coronary disease [2,3], heart failure [4] and mortality [5].

TNF-α has been implicated in the pathogenesis of insulin resistance in vitro and in vivo [6]. Elevated plasma TNF-α levels may play an important role in insulin resistance by impairing insulin signaling [7]. Moreover, our previous study indicated that in cultured human HepG2 hepatocytes, TNF-α induced insulin-resistance, as assessed by their decreased capacity to accumulate glycogen in the presence of insulin [8].

Adipose tissue has been considered as a major endocrine organ producing several adipokines affecting insulin resistance [9]. Apelin, a novel adipokine, is the specific endogenous ligand of G protein-coupled receptor APJ [10]. The human apelin gene that is located on chromosomeXq25-26 expresses a 77-amino acid prepropeptide that is subsequently cleaved post-translationally into several active forms, including apelin-36, apelin-17, apelin-13, apelin-12, which are all agonists of apelin receptor [11,12]. Apelin has gained increasingly attention in recent years, for it appears to have numerous distinct biological activities in a variety of organs [13]. Consistent with its putative role as an adipokine, apelin has been linked to states of insulin resistance. Apelin expression was up-regulated by insulin in the adipose tissue [10], while in the pancreas, apelin could decrease insulin secretion [14]. Moreover, it has been proved that apelin is necessary for the maintenance of insulin sensitivity [15]. Interestingly, glucose utilization in the muscle and adipose tissue could be stimulated by apelin, and insulin sensitivity would be increased subsequently [16]. However, the function of apelin in hepatic insulin resistance, a vital part of insulin resistance, and its underlying mechanisms still remains unclear. Here we studied the impacts of apelin on TNF-α-induced reduction of glycogen synthesis in the hepatocytes. We show novel evidence suggesting that apelin ameliorates TNF-α-induced reduction of glycogen synthesis in the hepatocytes through G protein-coupled receptor APJ. Apelin appears as a beneficial adipokine with anti-insulin resistance properties, and thus as a promising therapeutic target in metabolic disorders.

Results

Apelin reverses TNF-α-induced reduction of glycogen synthesis in HepG2 hepatocytes and mouse primary hepatocytes

To observe effects of apelin on glycogen synthesis in the hepatocytes, human HepG2 hepatocytes were treated with 10 ng/ml TNF-α for 24 h to reduce intracellular glycogen synthesis. Then, HepG2 cells were treated with different concentrations of apelin 13 (0.1, 1, 10 nmol/L; Phoenix Pharmaceuticals, USA), followed by exposure to 10 ng/ml TNF-α for 24 h. The results indicate that glycogen content was dose-dependently increased by treatment of HepG2 cells with apelin (Fig. 1A). Next, HepG2 cells were treated with 10 nmol/L apelin for different time (2, 4, 8 h). As shown in Fig. 1B, apelin led to a time-dependently elevated glycogen content of HepG2 cells. Therefore, in the following experiments, HepG2 cells were treated with 10 nmol/L apelin for 4 h, followed by incubation 10 ng/ml TNF-α for 24 h. We also quantified cell viability in HepG2 cells treated with 10 nmol/L of apelin for 4 h and 10 ng/ml TNF-α for 24 h by a 3-(4,5-dimethylthiazol-2-yl)-2,5-diphenyltetrazoliumbromide assay to exclude the side effects associated with apelin and TNF-α, such as apoptosis. The results indicate that no cytotoxicity was seen in connection with the exposure of HepG2 cells to apelin (10 nmol/L, 4 h) and TNF-α (10 ng/ml, 24 h)(data not shown). Moreover, the glycogen content was reduced in mouse primary hepatocytes treated with 10 ng/ml TNF-α for 24 h. However, treatment of 10 nmol/L apelin impaired the effect of TNF-α on glycogen synthesis in mouse primary hepatocytes (Fig. 1C). Taken together, these results indicate that apelin could reverse TNF-α-induced reduction of glycogen synthesis.

Apelin improves insulin signaling pathway in the hepatocytes treated by TNF-α

Since insulin signaling pathway plays an important role in glycogen synthesis, we then investigated whether and how apelin improved insulin signaling pathway in the hepatocytes treated by TNF-α.As shown in Fig. 2A, JNK was activated in response to TNF-α treatment in HepG2 cells. In parallel with increased phosphorylation of JNK, phosphorylation of the residue Ser307 in IRS-1, accompanied by reduced IRS-1 levels was stimulated by TNF-α treatment. Moreover, TNF-α-induced activation of JNK led to impaired phosphorylation of AKT and GSK. However, these changes of JNK, IRS-1, AKT and GSK induced by TNF-α were reversed via apelin treatment. The effects of apelin on TNF-α-induced impaired insulin signaling pathway were further assessed in mouse primary hepatocytes (Fig. 2B). These observations suggest that apelin ameliorates TNF-α-induced reduction of glycogen synthesis in the hepatocytes by improving insulin signaling pathway.

Injection of apelin increases glycogen level and improves insulin signaling pathway in the liver tissues of TNF-α-treated C57BL/6J mice

To further assess the effects of apelin on glycogen synthesis in vivo, 12-week-old male C57BL/6J mice were injected with 7.01 μg/ml TNF-α by pumps for 7 days and the livers of mice were collected. We found a decrease of glycogen level in the liver tissues of TNF-α-treated C57BL/6J mice. However, an intraperitoneal injection of 20 nmol/kg apelin-13 led to increased glycogen level in the liver tissues of C57BL/6J mice treated by TNF-α (Fig. 3A). Moreover, as shown in Fig. 3B, insulin signaling pathway was impaired in the liver tissues treated with TNF-α. These changes of JNK, IRS-1, AKT and GSK induced by TNF-α were reversed via apelin injection.

Apelin affects TNF-α-induced reduction of glycogen synthesis in the hepatocytes through G protein-coupled receptor APJ

G protein-coupled receptor APJ has been known to be the unique receptor of apelin. In order to elucidate whether APJ is involved in the function of apelin in glycogen synthesis, we measured the expression of APJ in HepG2 cells, mouse primary hepatocytes and liver tissues of mice by Western blot. As shown in Fig. 4A, APJ receptor can be detected in HepG2 cells, mouse primary hepatocytes, as well as liver tissues of mice. F13A is an established antagonist of APJ receptor with a substitution of phenylalanine by alanine in the C-terminal of apelin-13. [17]. Therefore, to further assess the role of apelin in the maintenance of insulin sensitivity, 20 nmol/L F13A (Phoenix Pharmaceuticals, USA) was exposed to HepG2 cells and mouse primary hepatocytes

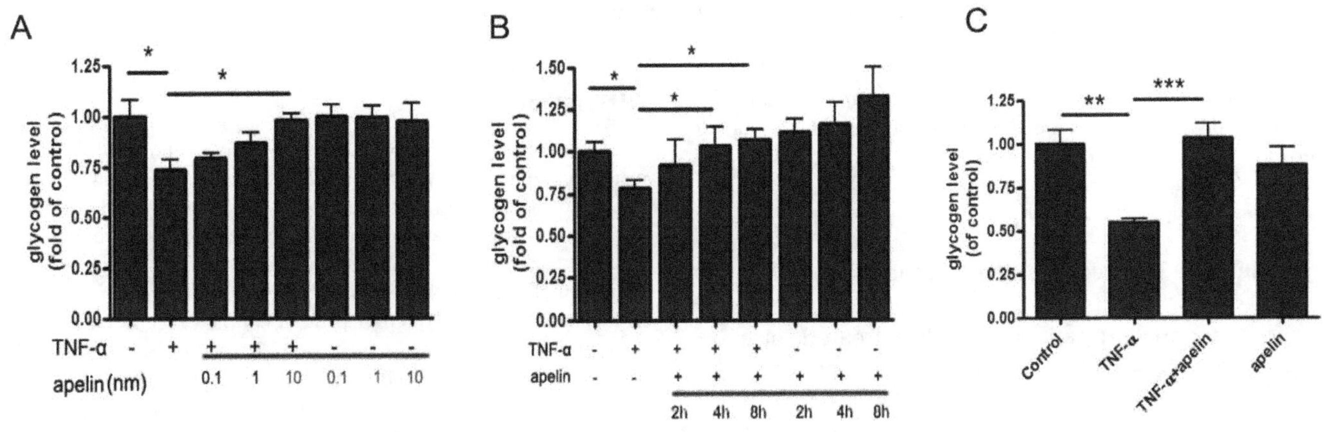

Figure 1. Apelin reverses TNF-α-induced reduction of glycogen synthesis in HepG2 hepatocytes and mouse primary hepatocytes. Exposure of HepG2 hepatocytes to apelin-13 (0.1, 1, 10 nmol/L) before treatment with 10 ng/ml TNF-α for 24 h elevated glycogen content in a dose- and time-dependent manner (A and B). The treatment of 10 nmol/L apelin-13 for 4 h reversed TNF-α-induced reduction of glycogen synthesis in mouse primary hepatocytes (C). Data represent the means ± S.E.M., n = 3 independent experiments. * $p<0.05$; ** $p<0.01$ and *** $p<0.001$ by ANOVA test (v.s. control or TNF-α).

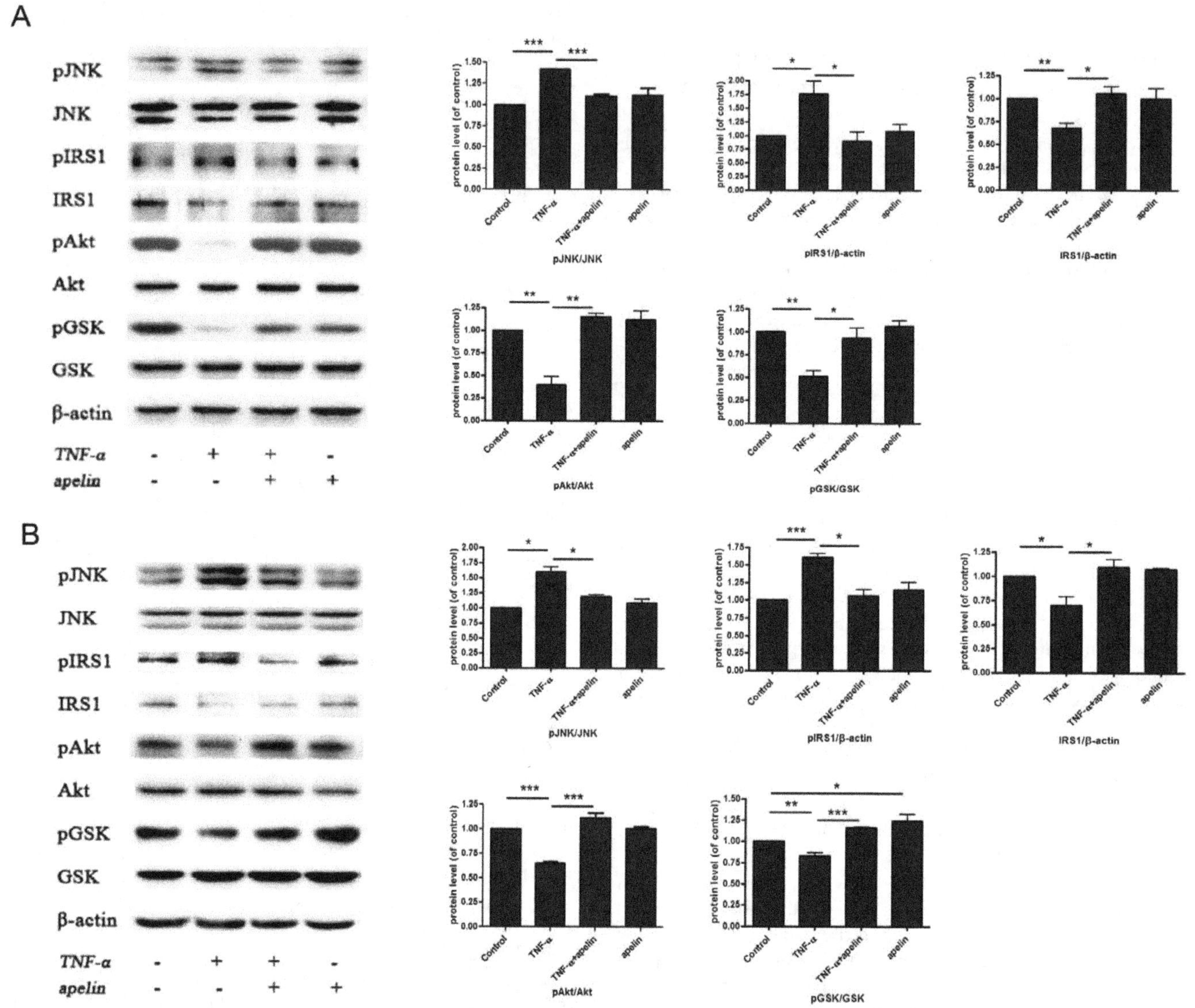

Figure 2. Apelin improves insulin signaling pathway in the hepatocytes treated by TNF-α. Apelin-13 improved insulin signaling pathway (JNK-IRS1-AKT-GSK) in HepG2 cells (A) and mouse primary hepatocytes (B) treated with 10 ng/ml TNF-α for 24 h. Data represent the means ± S.E.M., n = 3 independent experiments. * $p<0.05$; ** $p<0.01$ and *** $p<0.001$ by ANOVA test (v.s. control or TNF-α).

treated with TNF-α or/and apelin. The results reveal that regulation of apelin in glycogen synthesis and insulin signaling pathway was inhibited by treatment of F13A in HepG2 cells (Fig. 4B, C). These changes are consistent with data from mouse primary hepatocytes (Fig. 4D, E).

Injection of F13A, a competitive antagonist for APJ, suppresses the effects of apelin on glycogen synthesis and insulin signaling pathway in TNF-α-treated mice

Finally, we injected F13A (a competitive antagonist for APJ, 20 μg/mouse) or/and apelin 13 (20 nmol/kg) in TNF-α-treated C57BL/6J mice. Interestingly, injection of F13A suppressed the effects of apelin on glycogen synthesis and insulin signaling pathway in TNF-α-treated mice (Fig. 5A, B). Taken together, our results suggest that apelin ameliorates TNF-α-induced reduction of hepatic glycogen synthesis through G protein-coupled receptor APJ.

Discussion

In the present study, we found that (i) apelin can stimulate insulin signaling pathway and improve glycogen synthesis in TNF-α-treated hepatocytes and liver tissues of mice; (ii) APJ, the only known receptor for apelin, but not apelin, expressed in HepG2 cells, mouse primary hepatocytes and liver tissues of mice; and (iii) apelin ameliorates TNF-α-induced reduction of glycogen synthesis in the hepatocytes through G protein-coupled receptor APJ.

In recent years, apelin has been linked to states of insulin resistance. In clinical studies, it has been reported that the levels of plasma apelin were elevated in insulin-resistant subjects [18] and in morbidly obese individuals with type 2 diabetes [19,20], compared with normal controls. However, several recent studies have shown decreased plasma apelin concentrations in newly diagnosed and untreated patients with type 2 diabetes [21,22]. These results could be consistent with the fact that after 14 weeks of anti-diabetic treatment (rosiglitazone and metformin), plasma

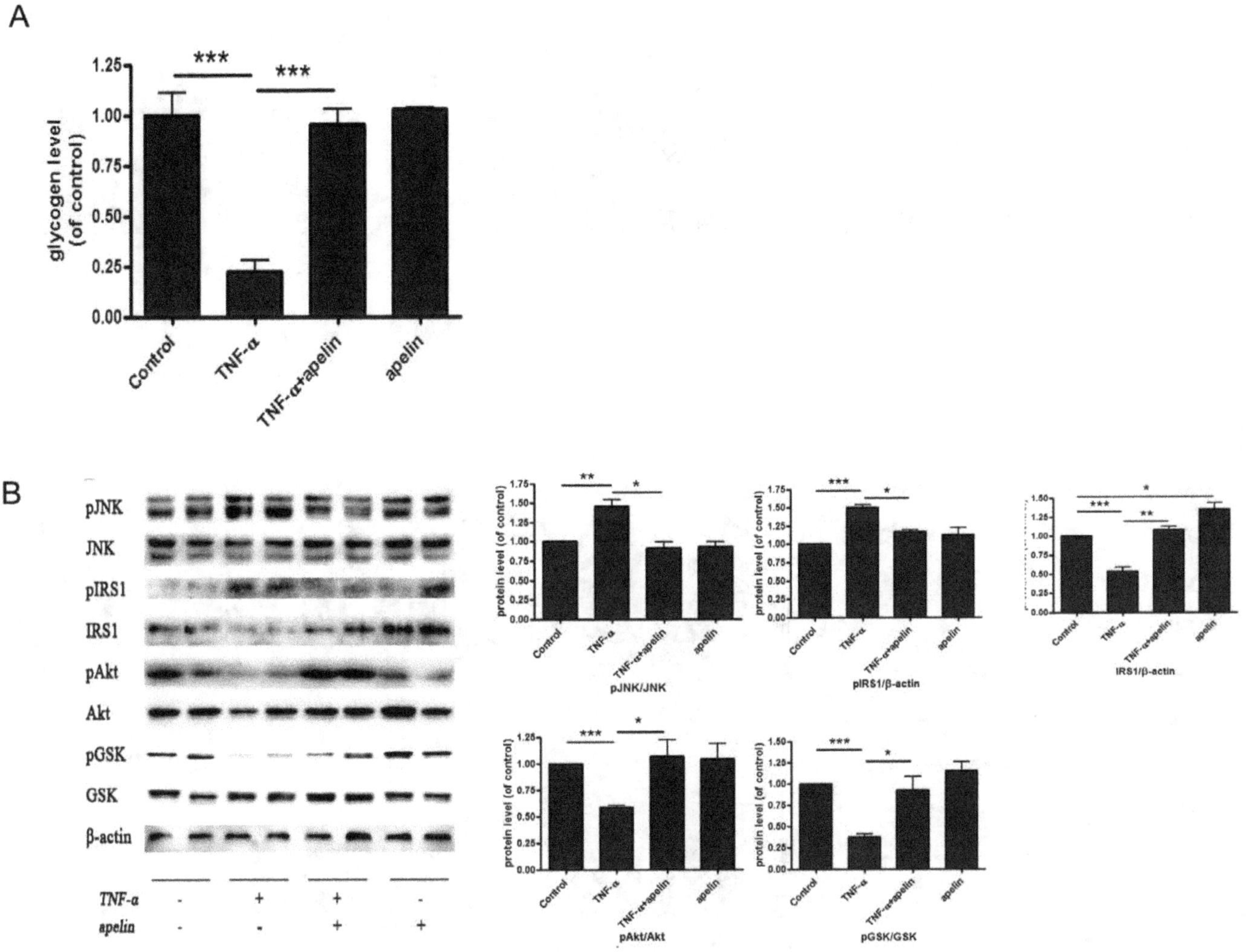

Figure 3. Injection of apelin increases glycogen level and improves insulin signaling pathway in liver tissues of TNF-α-treated C57BL/6J mice. An intraperitoneal injection of 20 nmol/kg apelin-13 led to increased glycogen level in liver tissues of C57BL/6J mice treated by TNF-α (A). Moreover, insulin signaling pathway was impaired in liver tissues treated with TNF-α. These changes of JNK, IRS-1, AKT and GSK induced by TNF-α were reversed via apelin injection (B). Data represent the means ± S.E.M., n = 5 mice per group. * $p<0.05$; ** $p<0.01$ and *** $p<0.001$ by ANOVA test (v.s. control or TNF-α).

apelin concentrations were enhanced and the glycemic profile improved [23]. Although it is difficult to reconcile these divergent findings, the data raise the possibility of alternative regulatory pathways for apelin production in the setting of insulin resistance [24]. Moreover, it has been found that changes in plasma apelin concentrations were correlated significantly with plasma triglycerides, glucose, TNF-α, HOMA-IR and HbA1c [25]. It is known that insulin resistance occurs in certain tissues, such as adipose tissue, muscle and liver. But liver becomes resistant first, followed by muscle and, last, adipose tissue. Insulin resistance in the livers led to impaired glycogen synthesis and failure to suppress glucose production [26]. Positive correlation between the levels of plasma apelin and insulin has been observed in wild type mice, heterozygous db/+ mice and homozygous db/db mice [10]. It has been reported that apelin could stimulate glucose utilization in skeletal muscle and adipose tissue in normal and insulin-resistant mice [16]. Direct administration of apelin in preclinical animal models resulted in improved insulin sensitivity [16,27]. Moreover, the mice with a generalized deficiency of apelin have abnormal insulin tolerance and insulin sensitivity, however, administration of exogenous apelin to these mice reversed these abnormalities [15]. These observations indicate that apelin directly increases insulin sensitivity and suggest that the elevations in circulating apelin concentrations observed in states of insulin resistance are compensatory [24]. In our study, human HepG2 hepatocytes were treated with 10 ng/ml TNF-α for 24 h to decrease intracellular glycogen synthesis. The results indicate that glycogen content was dose-dependently increased by treatment of HepG2 cells with apelin. Moreover, treatment of 10 nmol/L apelin impaired the effect of TNF-α on glycogen synthesis in mouse primary hepatocytes. Similarly, an intraperitoneal injection of 20 nmol/kg apelin 13 led to increased glycogen levels in the liver tissues of TNF-α-treated C57BL/6J mice. Taken together, these results suggest that apelin can reverse TNF-α-induced reduction of glycogen synthesis.

It has been reported that apelin is secreted predominantly from endothelial cells [28]. More recently, apelin has been found to be present in adipocytes [10,29]. To date, evidence suggests that apelin is expressed in CNS and a range of peripheral rat tissues, including heart, liver, kidney, testis, ovary, and adipose tissue, with

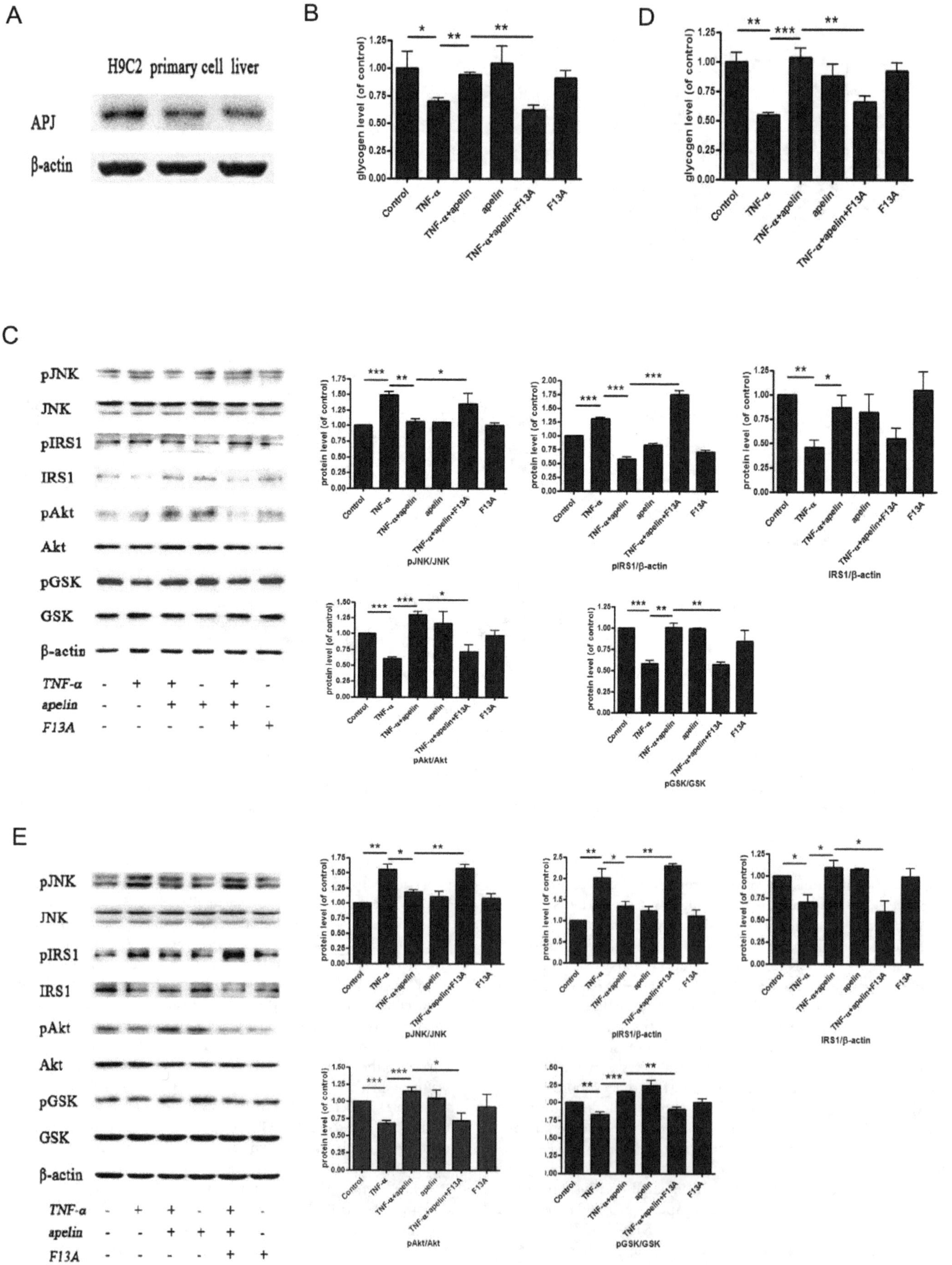
A
H9C2 primary cell liver
APJ
β-actin
B
D
glycogen level (of control)
Control
TNF-α
TNF-α+apelin
apelin
TNF-α+apelin+F13A
F13A
C
pJNK
JNK
pIRS1
IRS1
pAkt
Akt
pGSK
GSK
β-actin
TNF-α
apelin
F13A
protein level (of control)
pJNK/JNK
pIRS1/β-actin
IRS1/β-actin
pAkt/Akt
pGSK/GSK
E

Figure 4. Apelin affects TNF-α-induced reduction of glycogen synthesis in the hepatocytes through G protein-coupled receptor APJ. APJ expressed in HepG2 cells, primary mouse hepatocytes and liver tissues of mice (A). 20 nmol/L F13A, a competitive antagonist for APJ, was exposed to HepG2 cells and mouse primary hepatocytes treated with TNF-α or/and apelin. The regulation of apelin in glycogen synthesis and insulin signaling pathway was inhibited by treatment of F13A in HepG2 cells (B and C) and mouse primary hepatocytes (D and E). Data represent the means ± S.E.M., n = 3 independent experiments. * $p<0.05$; ** $p<0.01$ and *** $p<0.001$ by ANOVA test.

highest levels in the lung and the mammary gland [30]. However, we found that no apelin is expressed in HepG2 cells and mouse primary hepatocytes (data not shown). This corroborates previous report [30]. Therefore, in our experiments, exogenous apelin 13 was used to treat HepG2 and mouse primary hepatocytes, and administrate C57BL/6J mice.

Insulin signaling pathway plays a critical role in regulation of glycogen synthesis. There is strong evidence for oxidative stress-dependent changes in intracellular signaling, resulting in insulin resistance in vivo [31]. From a mechanistic perspective, increased reactive oxygen species (ROS) can trigger activation of stress-sensitive serine/threonine kinase signaling pathways, such as JNK, that, in turn, phosphorylate multiple targets, including the insulin receptor and IRS proteins [32]. Increased serine phosphorylation of IRS-1 reduces its ability to undergo tyrosine phosphorylation and may accelerate the degradation of IRS-1, followed by reduced AKT phosphorylation. It is demonstrated that AKT phosphorylated and inhibited GSK-3, followed by suppressed glycogen synthase activity, resulting in decreased glycogen synthesis. We found that ROS levels were increased in HepG2 cells by exposure to TNF-α. However, apelin significantly inhibited the generation of ROS in response to TNF-α (data not shown). It has been reported that through increased apelin production, RAS blockers could prevent the generation of ROS in differentiating adipocytes [33]. Inhibition of ROS production by apelin has also been shown in other cell types [34,35]. Our results also show that in parallel with increased phosphorylation of JNK, phosphorylation of the residue Ser307 in IRS-1, accompanied by reduced IRS-1 levels was stimulated by TNF-α treatment in HepG2 cells. Moreover, TNF-α-induced activation of JNK led to impaired phosphorylation of AKT and GSK. However, these changes of JNK, IRS-1, AKT and GSK induced by TNF-α were reversed via apelin treatment. The effects of apelin on TNF-α-induced impaired insulin signaling pathway were further assessed in mouse primary hepatocytes and liver tissues of C57BL/6J mice.

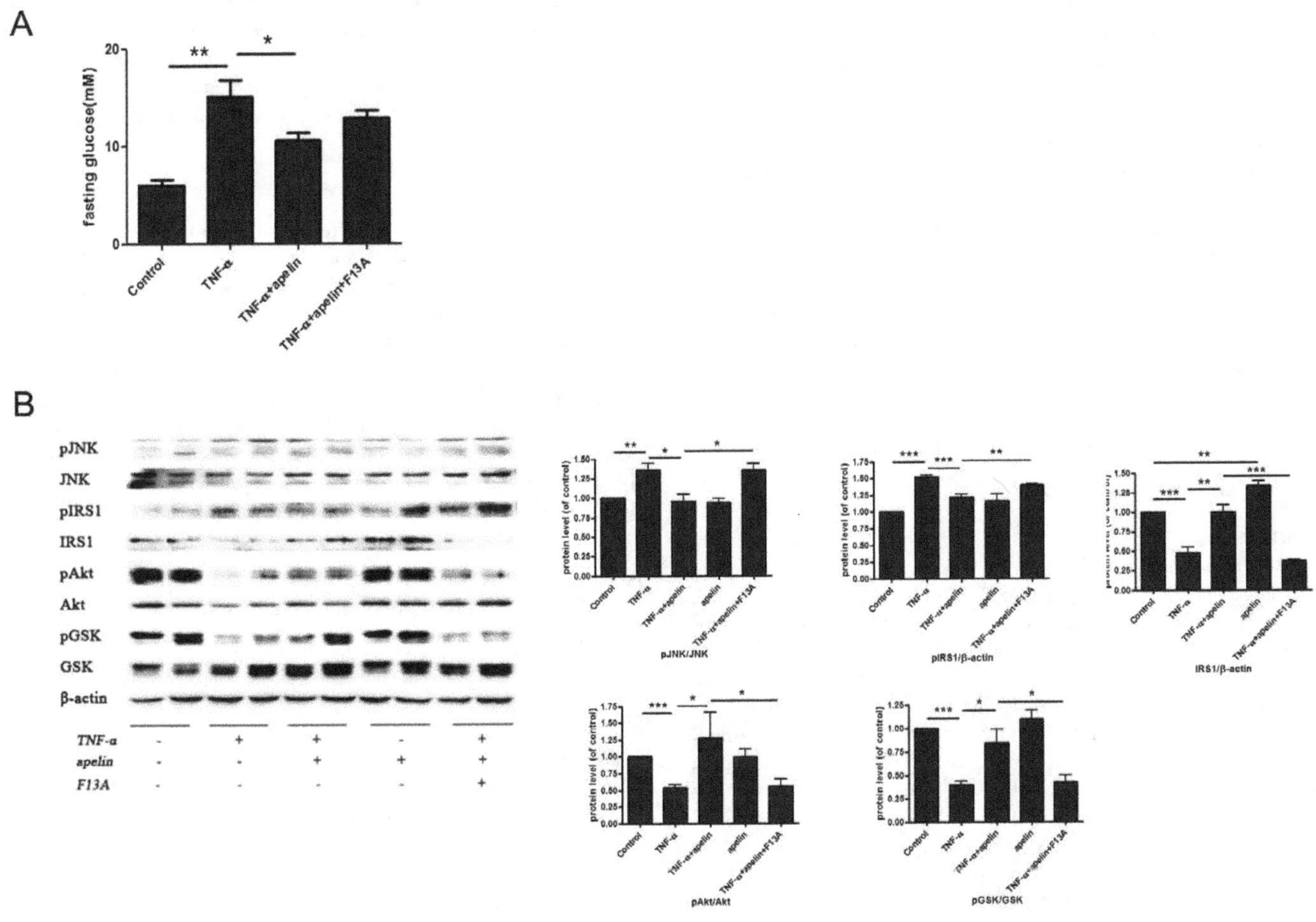

Figure 5. Injection of F13A suppresses the effects of apelin on glycogen synthesis and insulin signaling pathway in TNF-α-treated mice. F13A (20 μg/mouse) or/and apelin 13 (20 nmol/kg) was injected in TNF-α-treated C57BL/6J mice. Injection of F13A suppressed the effects of apelin on glycogen synthesis (A) and insulin signaling pathway (B) in TNF-α-treated mice. Data represent the means ± S.E.M., n = 5 mice per group. * $p<0.05$; ** $p<0.01$ and *** $p<0.001$ by ANOVA test.

It is consider that apelin is the specific ligand of G protein-coupled receptor APJ. Up to date, there is no evidence for multiple receptor subtypes of APJ [36,37]. No apelin expression can be detected in liver cells despite of the general distribution in other tissues [30,38]. As for APJ, opinions vary about whether APJ is expressed in hepatocytes [16,30,38]. In the present study, we measured the expression of APJ in HepG2 cells, mouse primary hepatocytes and liver tissues of mice by Western blot. The results indicate that APJ expressed in HepG2 cells, mouse primary hepatocytes and liver tissues of mice. As apelin exists in blood, we consider that apelin could enter the liver with blood-steam, activate receptor APJ in the cellular membrane of hepatocytes, and then stimulate down-stream signal molecule. Notably, F13A could competitively bind to APJ which blocking the activation the receptor by apelin. [39] Therefore, F13A is used as a competitive antagonist for APJ.In this study, 20 nmol/L F13A was exposed to HepG2 cells and mouse primary hepatocytes treated with TNF-α or/and apelin. The results reveal that regulation of apelin in glycogen synthesis and insulin signaling pathway was inhibited by treatment of F13A in HepG2 cells and mouse primary hepatocytes. These changes are consistent with data from in TNF-α-treated C57BL/6J mice.

In previous study, 10 C57BL/6J mice matched for age, body weight and glucose level were enrolled in plasma insulin level measurement by an ELISA kit (Linco) according to the manufacturer's protocol. These mice were separated into 2 groups randomly. The plasma insulin levels of mice in these 2 groups were 2.82±0.90 ng/ml and 3.00±1.71 ng/ml respectively ($p = 0.85$), suggesting that insulin levels were comparable among the different groups. Therefore, the plasma insulin concentration was not measured at the beginning of the treatment in the present study. It is a limitation in the present study.

In summary, this study provides novel evidence suggesting that apelin ameliorates TNF-α-induced reduction of glycogen synthesis in the hepatocytes through G protein-coupled receptor APJ. Apelin appears as a beneficial adipokine with anti-insulin resistance properties, and thus as a promising therapeutic target in metabolic disorders. However, further studies are needed to determine what the downstream signaling pathway of AJP is and how AJP signaling pathway is connected to insulin signaling pathway.

Materials and Methods

Animals

12-week-old male C57BL/6J mice were provided from Peking University Health Science Center. The mice matched for age, body weight and glucose level were separated for 5 groups (control, TNF-α, apelin, TNF-α+ apelin, TNF-α+apelin+F13A) with 5 mice per group and fed a standard laboratory diet in a temperature-controlled (20–24°C) and humidity-controlled (45–55%) environment. A 12 h/12 h light/dark cycle was maintained. For all experiments examining chronic TNF-α exposure, Alzet osmotic pumps (Durect, Cupertino, CA) with a 7-day pumping capacity and infusion rate of 1 µl/h were used. Pumps were filled to capacity with 7.01 µg/ml TNF-α diluted in carrier (0.9% NaCl and 0.1% BSA). For apelin treatment, an intraperitoneal injection of 20 nmol/kg apelin-13 were performed for 10 min before the mice were sacrificed. For F13A treatment, 20 ug/mouse F13A were intraperitoneal injected for 30 min before the mice were sacrificed. Following induction of halothane general anesthesia, pumps were implanted into the intrascapular subcutaneous space. Incisions were closed with interrupted absorbable sutures. Liver tissues were removed surgically and frozen immediately in liquid nitrogen for further analysis.

All animal procedures were performed in accordance with the National Institutes of Health Animal Care and Use Guidelines. All animal protocols were approved by the Animal Ethics Committee at the Beijing Institute of Geriatrics.

Cell culture

HepG2 cells (American Type Culture Collection) were cultured in minimum Eagle's medium (low glucose; Invitrogen) supplemented with 10% fetal bovine serum (Hyclone), 100units/ml penicillin (Invitrogen), and 0.1 mg/ml streptomycin (Invitrogen). Cells were maintained at 37°C with humidified air and CO2 (5%). Experiments on hepatocytes were performed in the presence of 10 ng/ml TNF-α for 24 h.

Isolation of mouse primary hepatocytes

Male C57BL/6J mice (8-week-old) were provided from Peking University Health Science Center. Primary hepatocytes were isolated by a two-step collagenase perfusion (0.2 mg/ml type IV collagenase (Sigma) in Hanks balanced salt solution), as described previously [40,41].The hepatocytes were collected by centrifugation at 800 rpm for 8 min. Immediately after harvesting, the cells were suspended in pre-warmed William's E medium (Sigma) supplemented with 10% fetal bovine serum, 20 ng/ml dexamethasone (Sigma), ITS (5 mg/l insulin, 5 mg/l trasferrin, 5 µg/l sodium selenate) (Sigma) and 10 µg/ml gentamicin (Invitrogen). Hepatocytes were plated in collagen-coated 25 cm2flask at 1×106 cells.

Western blot analysis

Cell lysates (15–30 µg of protein) were separated by 10% SDS-PAGE, transferred to PVDF membrane (Millipore), blocked with 5% nonfat dry milk, and probed with antibodies at 4°C overnight. The blots were incubated with HRP-conjugated anti-IgG, followed by detection with ECL (Millipore). Antibodies against IRS1, phospho-IRS1, JNK, phospho-JNK, AKT, phospho-AKT, GSK and phospho-GSK were all purchased from Cell Signal Technology, USA. Antibody against apelin receptor APJ was obtained from Phoenix Pharmaceuticals, USA. To check insulin signaling molecules, cells were treated with 10 nmol/L insulin (Usbio) for 10 min before the protein was collected.

Analysis of glycogen contents

Glycogen levels were measured in cells or liver tissues incubated for 3 h in the presence of 10 nmol/L insulin (Usbio), using a glycogen assay kit (Biovision).

Statistical analysis

All values are represented as means ±SEM. of the indicated number of measurements. A one-way ANOVA test was used to determine significance, requiring $p<0.05$ for statistical significance.

Author Contributions

Conceived and designed the experiments: JC SW JL. Performed the experiments: JC HZ XH BC. Analyzed the data: JC HZ XH SW JL. Contributed reagents/materials/analysis tools: YL TS YM. Wrote the paper: JC JL.

References

1. Goldstein BJ (2002) Insulin resistance as the core defect in type 2 diabetes mellitus. Am J Cardiol 90: 3G–10G.
2. Lempiainen P, Mykkanen L, Pyorala K, Laakso M, Kuusisto J (1999) Insulin resistance syndrome predicts coronary heart disease events in elderly nondiabetic men. Circulation 100: 123–128.
3. Mlinar B, Marc J, Janez A, Pfeifer M (2007) Molecular mechanisms of insulin resistance and associated diseases. Clin Chim Acta 375: 20–35.
4. Ingelsson E, Arnlov J, Lind L, Sundstrom J (2006) Metabolic syndrome and risk for heart failure in middle-aged men. Heart 92: 1409–1413.
5. Lakka HM, Laaksonen DE, Lakka TA, Niskanen LK, Kumpusalo E, et al. (2002) The metabolic syndrome and total and cardiovascular disease mortality in middle-aged men. JAMA 288: 2709–2716.
6. Hotamisligil GS, Shargill NS, Spiegelman BM (1993) Adipose expression of tumor necrosis factor-alpha: direct role in obesity-linked insulin resistance. Science 259: 87–91.
7. Liang H, Yin B, Zhang H, Zhang S, Zeng Q, et al. (2008) Blockade of tumor necrosis factor (TNF) receptor type 1-mediated TNF-alpha signaling protected Wistar rats from diet-induced obesity and insulin resistance. Endocrinology 149: 2943–2951.
8. Li L, He Q, Huang X, Man Y, Zhou Y, et al. (2010) NOX3-derived reactive oxygen species promote TNF-alpha-induced reductions in hepatocyte glycogen levels via a JNK pathway. FEBS Lett 584: 995–1000.
9. Rosen ED, Spiegelman BM (2006) Adipocytes as regulators of energy balance and glucose homeostasis. Nature 444: 847–853.
10. Boucher J, Masri B, Daviaud D, Gesta S, Guigne C, et al. (2005) Apelin, a newly identified adipokine up-regulated by insulin and obesity. Endocrinology 146: 1764–1771.
11. Tatemoto K, Hosoya M, Habata Y, Fujii R, Kakegawa T, et al. (1998) Isolation and characterization of a novel endogenous peptide ligand for the human APJ receptor. Biochem Biophys Res Commun 251: 471–476.
12. Medhurst AD, Jennings CA, Robbins MJ, Davis RP, Ellis C, et al. (2003) Pharmacological and immunohistochemical characterization of the APJ receptor and its endogenous ligand apelin. J Neurochem 84: 1162–1172.
13. Falcao-Pires I, Ladeiras-Lopes R, Leite-Moreira AF (2010) The apelinergic system: a promising therapeutic target. Expert Opin Ther Targets 14: 633–645.
14. Sorhede Winzell M, Magnusson C, Ahren B (2005) The apj receptor is expressed in pancreatic islets and its ligand, apelin, inhibits insulin secretion in mice. Regul Pept 131: 12–17.
15. Yue P, Jin H, Aillaud M, Deng AC, Azuma J, et al. (2010) Apelin is necessary for the maintenance of insulin sensitivity. Am J Physiol Endocrinol Metab 298: E59–67.
16. Dray C, Knauf C, Daviaud D, Waget A, Boucher J, et al. (2008) Apelin stimulates glucose utilization in normal and obese insulin-resistant mice. Cell Metab 8: 437–445.
17. Devic E, Rizzoti K, Bodin S, Knibiehler B, Audigier Y (1999) Amino acid sequence and embryonic expression of msr/apj, the mouse homolog of Xenopus X-msr and human APJ. Mech Dev 84: 199–203.
18. Li L, Yang G, Li Q, Tang Y, Yang M, et al. (2006) Changes and relations of circulating visfatin, apelin, and resistin levels in normal, impaired glucose tolerance, and type 2 diabetic subjects. Exp Clin Endocrinol Diabetes 114: 544–548.
19. Soriguer F, Garrido-Sanchez L, Garcia-Serrano S, Garcia-Almeida JM, Garcia-Arnes J, et al. (2009) Apelin levels are increased in morbidly obese subjects with type 2 diabetes mellitus. Obes Surg 19: 1574–1580.
20. Daviaud D, Boucher J, Gesta S, Dray C, Guigne C, et al. (2006) TNFalpha up-regulates apelin expression in human and mouse adipose tissue. FASEB J 20: 1528–1530.
21. Erdem G, Dogru T, Tasci I, Sonmez A, Tapan S (2008) Low plasma apelin levels in newly diagnosed type 2 diabetes mellitus. Exp Clin Endocrinol Diabetes 116: 289–292.
22. Zhang Y, Shen C, Li X, Ren G, Fan X, et al. (2009) Low plasma apelin in newly diagnosed type 2 diabetes in Chinese people. Diabetes Care 32: e150.
23. Kadoglou NP, Tsanikidis H, Kapelouzou A, Vrabas I, Vitta I, et al. (2010) Effects of rosiglitazone and metformin treatment on apelin, visfatin, and ghrelin levels in patients with type 2 diabetes mellitus. Metabolism 59: 373–379.
24. Xu S, Tsao PS, Yue P (2011) Apelin and insulin resistance: another arrow for the quiver? J Diabetes 3: 225–231.
25. Castan-Laurell I, Dray C, Attane C, Duparc T, Knauf C, et al. (2011) Apelin, diabetes, and obesity. Endocrine 40: 1–9.
26. Gao D, Nong S, Huang X, Lu Y, Zhao H, et al. (2010) The effects of palmitate on hepatic insulin resistance are mediated by NADPH Oxidase 3-derived reactive oxygen species through JNK and p38MAPK pathways. J Biol Chem 285: 29965–29973.
27. Higuchi K, Masaki T, Gotoh K, Chiba S, Katsuragi I, et al. (2007) Apelin, an APJ receptor ligand, regulates body adiposity and favors the messenger ribonucleic acid expression of uncoupling proteins in mice. Endocrinology 148: 2690–2697.
28. Kleinz MJ, Davenport AP (2004) Immunocytochemical localization of the endogenous vasoactive peptide apelin to human vascular and endocardial endothelial cells. Regul Pept 118: 119–125.
29. Glassford AJ, Yue P, Sheikh AY, Chun HJ, Zarafshar S, et al. (2007) HIF-1 regulates hypoxia- and insulin-induced expression of apelin in adipocytes. Am J Physiol Endocrinol Metab 293: E1590–1596.
30. Kleinz MJ, Davenport AP (2005) Emerging roles of apelin in biology and medicine. Pharmacol Ther 107: 198–211.
31. Katakam AK, Chipitsyna G, Gong Q, Vancha AR, Gabbeta J, et al. (2005) Streptozotocin (STZ) mediates acute upregulation of serum and pancreatic osteopontin (OPN): a novel islet-protective effect of OPN through inhibition of STZ-induced nitric oxide production. J Endocrinol 187: 237–247.
32. Bloch-Damti A, Bashan N (2005) Proposed mechanisms for the induction of insulin resistance by oxidative stress. Antioxid Redox Signal 7: 1553–1567.
33. Hung WW, Hsieh TJ, Lin T, Chou PC, Hsiao PJ, et al. (2011) Blockade of the renin-angiotensin system ameliorates apelin production in 3T3-L1 adipocytes. Cardiovasc Drugs Ther 25: 3–12.
34. Foussal C, Lairez O, Calise D, Pathak A, Guilbeau-Frugier C, et al. (2010) Activation of catalase by apelin prevents oxidative stress-linked cardiac hypertrophy. FEBS Lett 584: 2363–2370.
35. Zeng XJ, Yu SP, Zhang L, Wei L (2010) Neuroprotective effect of the endogenous neural peptide apelin in cultured mouse cortical neurons. Exp Cell Res 316: 1773–1783.
36. O'Dowd BF, Heiber M, Chan A, Heng HH, Tsui LC, et al. (1993) A human gene that shows identity with the gene encoding the angiotensin receptor is located on chromosome 11. Gene 136: 355–360.
37. Katugampola SD, Maguire JJ, Matthewson SR, Davenport AP (2001) [(125)I]-(Pyr(1))Apelin-13 is a novel radioligand for localizing the APJ orphan receptor in human and rat tissues with evidence for a vasoconstrictor role in man. Br J Pharmacol 132: 1255–1260.
38. Kawamata Y, Habata Y, Fukusumi S, Hosoya M, Fujii R, et al. (2001) Molecular properties of apelin: tissue distribution and receptor binding. Biochim Biophys Acta 1538: 162–171.
39. Lee DK, Saldivia VR, Nguyen T, Cheng R, George SR, et al. (2005) Modification of the terminal residue of apelin-13 antagonizes its hypotensive action. Endocrinology 146: 231–236.
40. Seglen PO (1976) Preparation of isolated rat liver cells. Methods Cell Biol 13: 29–83.
41. Casciano DA (2000) Development and utilization of primary hepatocyte culture systems to evaluate metabolism, DNA binding, and DNA repair of xenobiotics. Drug Metab Rev 32: 1–13.

14

Phytol/Phytanic Acid and Insulin Resistance: Potential Role of Phytanic Acid Proven by Docking Simulation and Modulation of Biochemical Alterations

Mohamed M. Elmazar[1], Hanan S. El-Abhar[2]*, Mona F. Schaalan[3], Nahla A. Farag[4]

1 British Universityin Cairo (BUE), Cairo, Egypt, **2** Department of Pharmacology & Toxicology, Faculty of Pharmacy, Cairo University, Cairo, Egypt, **3** Department of Biochemistry, Faculty of Pharmacy, Misr International University (MIU), Cairo, Egypt, **4** Department of Pharmaceutical Medicinal Chemistry, Faculty of Pharmacy, Misr International University (MIU), Cairo, Egypt

Abstract

Since activation of PPARγ is the main target for the antidiabetic effect of TZDs, especially when it heterodimerizes with RXR, we aimed to test the potential antidiabetic effect of phytol (250 mg/kg), the natural precursor of phytanic acid, a RXR ligand and/or pioglitazone (5 mg/kg) to diabetic insulin-resistant rats. Regarding the molecular docking simulation on PPARγ, phytanic acid, rather than phytol, showed a binding mode that mimics the crystal orientation of rosiglitazone and pioglitazone, forming H bonds with the same amino acids (S289, H 323, H 449 and Y 473), and the least energy level, which emphasizes their importance for PPARγ molecular recognition, activation, hence antidiabetic activity. In addition, docking on the RXRα/PPARγ heterodimer, revealed that phytanic acid has higher binding affinity and lesser energy score on RXRα, compared to the original ligand, retinoic acid. Phytanic acid binds by 3H bonds and shares retinoic acid in arginine (R 316). These results were further supported biochemically, where oral phytol and/or pioglitazone (5 mg/kg) improved significantly glucose homeostasis, lipid panel, raised serum adiponectin level and lowered TNF-α, reaching in most cases the effect of the 10 mg/kg pioglitazone. The study concluded that the insulin sensitizing/anti-diabetic effect of phytol is mediated by partly from activation of nuclear receptors and heterodimerization of RXR with PPARγ by phytanic acid.

Editor: Franco Folli, University of Texas Health Science Center at San Antonio, United States of America

Funding: The authors have no support or funding to report.

Competing Interests: The authors have declared that no competing interests exist.

* E-mail: Hanabhar@yahoo.com

Introduction

Type-2 diabetes and obesity are rampant metabolic disorders in modern society [1], originating from the slothful lifestyle along with the high consumption of westernized diet which is rich in dietary fat content and fructose in soft drinks [2]. Furthermore, excessive accumulation of triglycerides (TGs) and certain fatty acid derivatives in skeletal muscles and other tissues mediate many of the adverse effects of insulin resistance syndrome [3], which is associated with a constellation of pathological metabolic disorders [1].

Current antidiabetics, including insulin secretagogues, insulin sensitizers or their combination, provide a sensible therapeutic approach [4]. Thiazolidinediones (TZDs), the insulin sensitizers, act by activating the nuclear receptors peroxisome proliferator–activated receptors (PPARs) [5] and selectively PPARγ subtype. The latter heterodimerizes with retinoid X receptor (RXR), to trigger transcription factors in adipocytes and skeletal muscles [6]. Albeit the positive effect of oral hypoglycemics, several side effects can develop, and over time, some patients lose response towards them; factors that could hinder their efficacy and safety. Accordingly, attention has been driven towards finding RXR agonists that can safely and effectively potentiate or replace TZDs. Synthetic ligands for RXR-dubbed as 'rexinoids'- function as TZDs where they ameliorate insulin resistance [7], lower hyperglycemia in type-2 diabetes and obesity [8] and enhance pre-adipocytes differentiation [9]. Moreover, the combined effect of rexinoids with TZDs was greater than either agent alone [7].

Phytol, a branched-chain fatty alcohol present as part of the chlorophyll pigment, is released only in the ruminants' digestive system, presumably by bacteria present in their gut [10], hence, it is present in the animals' adipose tissues and dairy products at a relatively high amounts [11]. Gloerich et al. [12] reported increased levels of phytol and its metabolites, viz., phytenic, phytanic and prystanic acids, in plasma and liver of mice fed phytol enriched diet, and suggested that once phytol is taken up by the body, it is transported to the liver to be metabolized into phytanic acid through three enzymatic steps [13], which are believed to be under the control of PPARα [12]. In humans and mammals phytanic acid appears as an oxidized product of phytol following ingestion of fat-containing foods of animal origin or vegetables and their absorption in small intestine. Phytol, therefore, is a precursor of the natural rexinoid phytanic acid that, besides triggering RXR, it activates the full spectrum of PPARs [14]. It also boosts the transcriptional activity of the PPAR/RXR heterodimers [3] and other nuclear receptors, viz., retinoic acid receptor (RAR) [15] where phytol and its metabolite, potentiate the teratogenic effects induced by a synthetic RARα agonist in mice.

Previous *in vitro* studies reported that phytanic acid activates several PPARs subtypes [14–16], and PPARγ agonists are widely used in the treatment of type 2 diabetes. Therefore, the present work pointed toward verifying the potential antidiabetic effect of phytol by comparing it, and its metabolite, with the TZDs using molecular docking techniques (Molsoft ICM 3.4-8C program) in an unprecedented attempt to visualize the orientation, binding modes and affinities of these compounds to the active sites of their receptor(s). The goal extended also to validate the *in vivo* effect of phytol alone and its modulatory action on pioglitazone using an insulin-resistant diabetic rat model [17].

Materials and Methods

1. Method of the drug modeling studies

All docking studies were performed using "Internal Coordinate Mechanics (Molsoft ICM 3.4-8C)". Molsoft, a flexible docking program, enables the prediction of favorable protein-ligand complex structures with reasonable accuracy and speed [18]. ICM docking is currently the most accurate predictive tool of the binding geometry of biologically active compounds [18,19,20].

Phytol, phytanic acid, and pioglitazone were first docked on the crystal structures of PPARγ (2PRG), which is originally complexed with its ligand rosiglitazone, as found in RCSB Protein Data Bank (PDB entry 2PRG) [21]. In addition, we performed another docking study of phytanic acid and/or pioglitazone into the crystal structures of the RXRα/PPARγ (1FM6) heterodimer, that was available through the RCSB Protein Data Bank (PDB entry 1FM6) [22], and contains two binding sites for two ligands. One active site is in complex with the 9-cis retinoic acid (9cRAR) which is a selective agonist to RXRα, and the other is complexed with rosigitazone which is the binding ligand of PPARγ receptor.

1.A. Preparation of small molecules. ChemDraw 3D structures were constructed using Chem 3D ultra 8.0 software [Molecular Modeling and Analysis; Cambridge Soft Corporation, USA (2004)], and then they were energetically minimized using MOPAC (semi-empirical quantum mechanics), Jop Type with 100 iterations and minimum RMS gradient of 0.01, and saved as MDL MolFile (*.mol).

1.B. Generation of ligand and protein structures. The crystal structures of target protein PPARγ (2PRG) and RXRα/ PPARγ heterodimer (1FM6) active sites were retrieved from the Protein Data Bank (http://www.rcsb.org/pdb/welcome.do). All bound waters, ligands and cofactors were removed from the protein. The amino acids of the binding site where defined using data in pdbsum (http://www.ebi.ac.uk/thoronton-srv/databases/pdbsum).

1.C. Docking using Molsoft ICM 3.4-8C program. The docking procedure was accomplished in the following sequence:

I. Conversion of PDB file into an ICM object: This conversion involves addition of hydrogen bonds, assignment of atoms' types, and charges from the residue templates.

II. Docking of ICM small molecule in the following sequence:

Setup Docking Project: Set project name, setup the receptor, review and adjust binding site, and make **receptor maps**

Start docking simulation

Display of the result

ICM stochastic global optimization algorithm attempts to find the global minimum of the energy function that includes five grid potentials describing interaction of the flexible ligand with the receptor and internal conformational energy of the ligand, during this process a stack of alternative low energy conformations is saved. The mode of interaction of rosiglitazone within 2PRG, and 1FM6 was used as a standard docked model. All agonists were compared according to the best binding free energy (minimum) obtained among all the run.

2. Materials and method of the experimental model

2.A. Drugs and chemicals. Streptozotocin (STZ) and phytol were purchased from Sigma Aldrich Co. (St Louis, MO, USA), pioglitazone from Medical Union Pharmaceutical Co. (Ismailia, Egypt), and long acting insulin (Monotard) from Eli Lilly (USA). Cholesterol and lard were obtained from commercial sources, and fructose from El-Nasr Chemical-Co. (AbouZaabal, Cairo, Egypt). Phytol was diluted with cottonseed oil and pioglitazone was suspended in 1% Na-CMC.

2.B. Animals. Adult male Wistar albino rats (80–120 g; National Research Center Laboratory, Cairo, Egypt) were oused (three rats/cage), in polypropylene cages, kept on a 12 hr light/ dark cycle, and constant environmental conditions. Animals were fed commercially available normal pellet and water *ad libitum*, prior to the dietary manipulation. Experimental design and animal handling were performed according to the guidelines of the Animal Care and Use and after approval of the Ethics Committee of Faculty of Pharmacy, Cairo, Egypt.

2.C. Development of diabetic insulin-resistant rats. Rats were divided into two dietary regimen-groups, normal fat diet (NFD; n = 20), and high fat diet (HFD; n = 80) with fructose (20%) in drinking water, until the rats' body weights reached 220±40 g. The composition of NPD [3.15 kcal/g; fat (5%), protein as casein (21%), carbohydrate as starch (60%), fibers (3%), vitamins and minerals (4.5%)] and this group served as normal control. While the HFD was[4.1 kcal/g; fructose (60%), lard (10%), Casein (20.7%), Cellulose (4.2%), Mineral Mix (3.5%), Vitamin Mix (1%), Calcium Carbonate (0.3%) and DL-Methionine (0.3%)]. During the 6th week, animals received a daily single dose of Monotard (0.5 IU/kg, i.p). By the end of this week, and after an overnight food deprivation, HFD fed rats received freshly prepared STZ in citrate buffer (35 mg/kg, i.p, single dose) [17]. NFD group received either vehicle or same dose of STZ and the results recorded in table 1. As no significant difference was reported between both groups, the NFD receiving vehicle was considered as the normal reference group.

Periodic estimation of body weight (BW) and levels of fasting serum glucose, triglycerides (TGs), total cholesterol (TC) and insulin were determined. Only animals with persistent blood glucose levels between 200–350 mg/dl, hyperinsulinemia, and hypercholesterolemia, for 7 days after STZ, were considered diabetic insulin resistant and were used in the study and permitted HFD and fructose during the treatment period.

Table 1. Effect of STZ (35 mg/kg, i.p.) on NPD -fed rats.

Parameters	NPD	NPD+STZ
Glucose(mg/dl)	93±10	110±15
Insulin(μIU/ml)	11±2	9.5±1
TG(mg/dl)	50+6	57±7
TC(mg/dl)	100±12	80±9.5
HDL-C(mg/dl)	40±3.5	38±4
LDL-C(mg/dl)	47±5.5	50±5

Values are means±SD; NPD: Normal pellet diet.

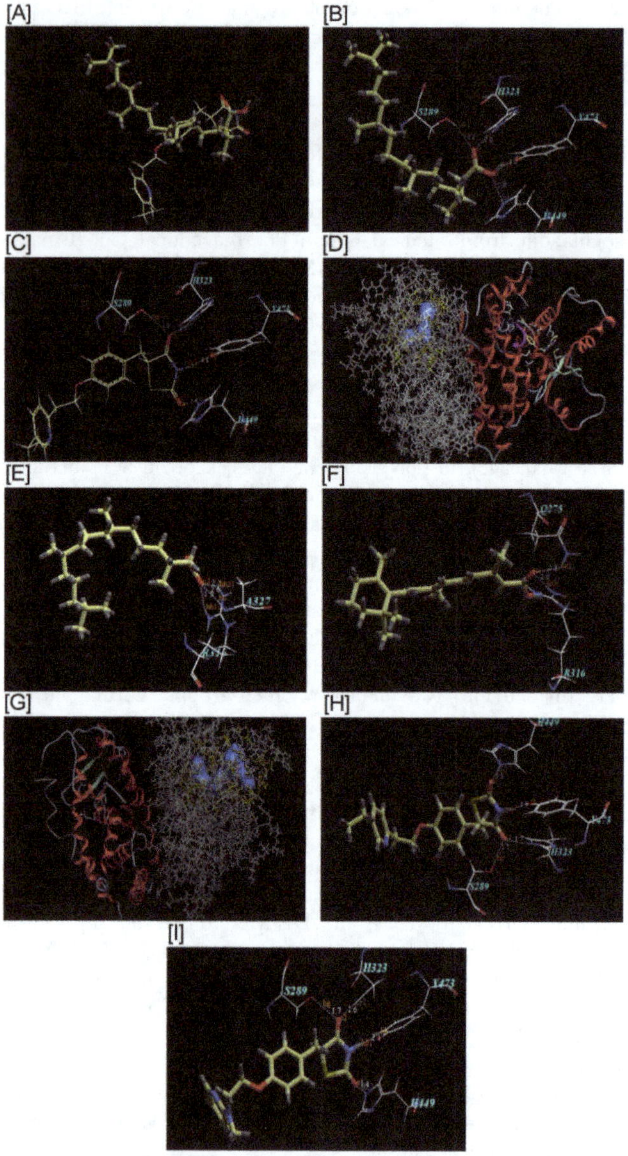

Figure 1. The docking modes of phytanic acid in the crystal structures of PPARγ binding protein and RXR receptor in terms of orientation, fitting and binding affinity as compared with phytol rosiglitazone, pioglitazone and retinoic acid. A: The superimposition of phytanic acid (wire and stick) and pioglitazone (wire) into the binding site of PPAR γ, (for interpretation of the references to color in the text, the reader is referred to the web version of this article). **B**: The binding mode of phytanic acid into the binding site of PPAR γ. It exhibits an ICM score of (−111.09) and forms 4 hydrogen bonds shown as white dotted lines (Table 2). These encompass one hydrogen bond between O of carbonyl moiety with S-289 of distance 2.17 A; another bond between O of CO with H323 of distance 2.03 and another two H bonds between O of OH with H- 449 of distance 1.89 A and between H of OH with Y 473 of distances 1.22A. (For interpretation of the references to color in the text, the reader is referred to the web version of this article). **C**: The binding mode of pioglitazone into the binding site of PPAR γ. It exhibits an ICM score of (−105.43) and forms 4 hydrogen bonds shown as white dotted lines (Table 2). These encompass two hydrogen bonds between O of CO with S 289 and H323 of distance 1.20 A and 0.70 A, respectively and another two between H of NH with Y-473 and O of CO with H-449 of distance 1.80 A and 2.76 A, respectively. (For interpretation of the references to color in the text, the reader is referred to the web version of this article). **D**: The binding mode of phytanic acid docked in RXR α binding site (left), while PPAR γ is bound with its ligand rosiglitazone (right). **E**: The binding mode of phytanic acid into the binding site of RXRα. It exhibits an ICM score of −114.75 and forms 3 hydrogen bonds shown as white dotted lines (Table 3). These include two hydrogen bonds between O of 2-oxo of carboxylic acid moiety with R-316 of distance 1.92 A and 2.15 A, and another bond with A-327of distance 2.63 A. (For interpretation of the references to color in the text, the reader is referred to the web version of this article). **F**: The binding mode of retinoic acid into the binding site of RXR α revealed an ICM score of (−86.79) and the existence of 2 hydrogen bonds shown as white dotted lines (Table 3) between O of 2-oxo moiety with R-316, and Q-275 of distance 1.96 A and 2.32 A, respectively. (For interpretation of the references to color in the text, the reader is referred to the web version of this article). **G**: The binding mode of pioglitazone docked in PPARγ binding site, while RXR α with its ligand 9-cis retinoic acid. **H**: The binding mode of pioglitazone into the binding site of PPARγ revealed having an ICM score of −106.37 and the existence of 4 hydrogen bonds shown as white dotted lines (Table 3). Two hydrogen bonds are shown between O of 2-oxo moiety with S-289, and H-323 of distance 1.66 A and 1.66 A, respectively. One H bond between another O of 4-oxo moiety with H-449 of distance 1.47 A and another H bond between H of NH of TZD with Y-473 of distances 1.89 A. (For interpretation of the references to color in the text, the reader is referred to the web version of this article). **I**: The binding mode of rosiglitazone into the binding site of PPAR γ revealed having an ICM score of −104.37 and the existence of 4 hydrogen bonds shown as white dotted lines (Table 3). Two hydrogen bonds exist between O of 2-oxo moiety with S-289, and H-323 of distance 1.66 A and 1.64 A, respectively. One H bond exists between another O of 4-oxo moiety with H-449 of distance 1.43 A and another H bond between H of NH of TZD with Y-473 of distances 1.79 A. (For interpretation of the references to color in the text, the reader is referred to the web version of this article).

2.D. Intra-peritoneal glucose (GTT) and insulin glucose (IGTT) tolerance tests. One week after STZ administration, two groups (n = 6) of 6 hr-food deprived diabetic rats, were given glucose (2 g/kg, ip) [17] without (GTT) and with (IGTT) insulin injection (0.4 I.U/kg; i.p), with a slight modification of Levy et al. [23] to suit animals' sensitivity. Droplets of blood from the tail vein were withdrawn (under brief ether anesthesia) every 30 min., and up to 120 min. to evaluate the resulting glucose concentrations. Two groups of non-diabetic rats (n = 6) were similarly tested.

2.E. Effect of phytol and pioglitazone on diabetic insulin-resistant rats. One week after STZ administration, five groups of diabetic rats (n = 7) were given daily oral doses of cottonseed oil (0.5 ml/kg, group DV), phytol (250 mg/kg, group DP_h), pioglitazone (5 and 10 mg/kg, groups DP_5 and DP_{10}) or a combination of phytol with pioglitazone (5 mg/kg) (group DP_hP_5). All drug regimens continued for 2 weeks, and the last dose of any treatment was given 24 hours before rats were euthanized. Animals were fasted 18 hours before the time of carnage, to minimize feeding induced variations in lipid and glucose pattern.

2.F. Collection of samples for analysis. Before killing, rats were weighed, then euthanized and serum was separated from the collected blood to assess levels of glucose, fructosamine, insulin, TGs, TC, LDL-C, HDL-C, TNF-α and adiponectin, as well as, the activity of ALT. Rats were then euthanized and liver, visceral fat (VF) and epididymal fat (EF) were carefully dissected out, weighed and their weights were expressed as a ratio of body weight (BW) multiplied by a factor of 100. Glucose and lipid profiles were assessed colorimetrically using commercially available kits, while HOMA-index was calculated according to Matthews et al. [24]. RIA techniques were adopted to determine concentrations of insulin and adiponectin, whereas TNF-α was measured by an ELISA kit (R&D Systems, Minneapolis, USA). Liver specimens were used to determine TGs and TC after lipid extraction [25].

2.G. Measurement of Phytanic Acid. Extraction and derivitization of serum samples for analysis of phytanic acid was

Table 2. ICM scores of phytol, phytanic acid, pioglitazone, and rosiglitazone docked in PPARγ of the 2 PRG crystal structure binding sites and hydrogen bonds formed with amino acid residues.

Compounds	ICM scores	No. of hydrogen bonds	Involved group of amino acid	Atom of ligand involved	Length of hydrogen bond
Phytol	−102.57	2	S289 ..... hg	O of OH	1.85 A
			H323 .....he2	O of OH	1.86 A
Phytanic acid	−111.09	4	S289 .... hg	O of CO	2.17 A
			H323 .....he2	O of CO	2.03 A
			H449 .... he2	O of OH	1.89 A
			Y473 ... oh	H of OH	1.22 A
Pioglitazone	−105.43	4	S289 .... hg	O of CO (TZD)	1.20 A
			H323.... he2	O of CO (TZD)	0.70 A
			H449 ..... he2	O of CO (TZD)	2.76 A
			Y473.... oh	H of NH (TZD)	1.80 A
Rosiglitazone	−103.26	4	S289..... hg	O of CO (TZD)	1.79 A
			H323..... he2	O of CO (TZD)	1.59A
			H449.... he2	O of OH (TZD)	1.39 A
			Y473..... oh	H of NH (TZD)	1.81 A

performed using gas liquid chromatography/mass spectroscopy analysis. Serum was subjected to saponification using ethanolic KOH with triheneicosanoic acid as internal standard. The free fatty acid moieties were extracted into hexane and converted to the more volatile fatty acid methyl esters (FAME), which were extracted and injected onto a GLC column. The separation of FAME and the analysis of phytanic acid was performed on a Trace 2000 GC from ThermoQuest with an AS 2000 autosampler and a Finnigan trace mass spec. Phytanic acid methyl ester as a reference standard was purchased from Sigma-Aldrich [26].

The analysis results reveal that the administration of 250 mg phytol to the experimental rats released 18 μg/ml±2.5 phytanic acid in the serum.

2.H. Statistical analysis. Results are expressed as means ± SD and differences between groups were tested for significance using analysis of variance (ANOVA), followed by Tukey post hoc test, $P<0.05$. To test for an interaction between individual treatments when given in combination, a factorial design test is used. Correlation coefficient (r) between serum glucose, insulin and HOMA-index with serum TNF-α, adiponectin, ALT and VFW/BW ratio was carried out in untreated and treated hyperglycemic animals using linear regression analysis.

Results

Table 2, Figure 1A–C depict the docking results of phytanic acid in the crystal structures of PPARγ binding protein (2PRG) in

Table 3. ICM scores of phytanic acid, retinoic acid, pioglitazone, and rosiglitazone docked in 1FM6 crystal structure binding site and hydrogen bonds formed with amino acid residues.

Compounds	ICM scores	No. of hydrogen bonds	Involved group of amino acid	Atom of ligand involved	Length of hydrogen bond
Phytanic acid	−114.75	3	R316 ... hh12	O of CO	1.92 A
			R316..... hh21	O of CO	2.15 A
			A327......hn	O of CO	2.63 A
Retinoic acid	−86.79	2	R316..hh21	O of CO	1.96 A
			Q275.....hh21	O of CO	2.32 A
Pioglitazone	−106.37	4	S289....hg	O of CO (TZD)	1.66 A
			H323...he2	O of CO (TZD)	1.66 A
			H449....he2	O of CO (TZD)	1.47 A
			Y473...oh	H of NH (TZD)	1.89 A
Rosiglitazone	−104.37	4	S289....hg	O of CO (TZD)	1.66 A
			H323...he2	O of CO (TZD)	1.64 A
			H449....he2	O of CO (TZD)	1.43 A
			Y473...oh	H of NH (TZD)	1.79 A

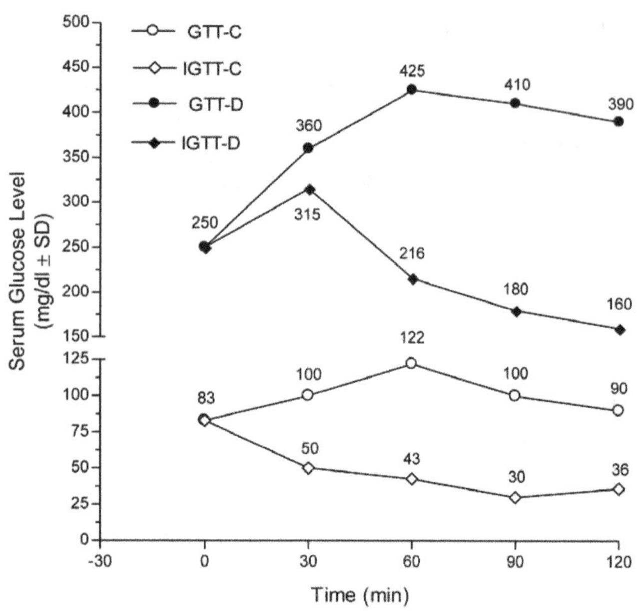

Figure 2. The glucose tolerance curve of the experimental groups. The glucose tolerance curve depicts the effect of 2 g/kg, ip, glucose without (GTT, ○), and with concurrent insulin injection (0.4 IU/kg, ip) (IGTT, ◇) in serum of normal control (hollow-C) and insulin-resistant rats (solid-D), after 0, 30, 60, 90, and 120 min. Values are means (± S.D.) of six animals. As compared with the normal control group, P≤0.05 (unpaired Student's t test).

terms of orientation, fitting and binding affinity as compared with rosiglitazone, pioglitazone and phytol. Docking simulations showed a binding mode of phytanic acid very similar to the crystal orientation of the TZD head group of rosiglitazone, and pioglitazone as well. Phytanic acid fitted with the PPARγ ligand binding domain interacting via hydrogen bonding with Ser- 289, His-323, His-449, and Tyr-473. Interestingly, the ICM score values of phytanic acid on PPARγ proved that it has the least energy levels with the highest binding affinity compared to those of pioglitazone and rosiglitazone (ICM score: −111.09, −105.43 and −103.26, respectively). On the other hand, phytol complexed only to two amino acids, viz., Ser-289 and His-323 by two hydrogen bonds, and it showed the highest energy level with the least binding affinity (ICM score: −102.57). Table 3 and figures 1D–F and G–I show the second docking results, which revealed that phytanic acid on RXRα, has a higher binding affinity and lesser energy score as compared to retinoic acid, the natural ligand (ICM scores: −114.75 for phytanic acid vs −86.79 for retinoic acid). While phytanic acid was complexed to RXR receptor via 3 H bonds (2R and 1A), it shared retinoic acid in arginine R 316. The pioglitazone binding affinities and complexing properties of the heterodimer mimicked those of rosiglitazone and the binding to the PPARγ single receptor, having an ICM score of −106.37 vs −104.37for rosiglitazone. Pioglitazone again bound to the receptor by complexing to the same four amino acids (S, H, H and Y) via 4 H bonds.

Regarding the biochemical results, comparisons were related to the DV group since no significant difference between DV and D groups was reported. GTT and IGTT in diabetic and non-diabetic rats were shown in figure 2. Glucose injection caused a marked steady rise of serum glucose level in diabetic rats over that of non-diabetic ones along the tested period. Nevertheless, the co-administration of insulin with glucose increased serum glucose level only at the 30 minutes point followed by a steady decrease in diabetic rats. However, in non-diabetic rats, the same pattern was observed, but without initial rise at the 30 minutes point. Compared to normal group, the levels of glucose, fructosamine, and insulin, along with HOMA index and TNF-α were elevated by 3.0, 2.3, 3.2, 9.5 and 13 folds, respectively in diabetic rats; however, adiponectin level was significantly lower than the control group only when using Student's t test (data not shown) (Fig. 3). Serum TG, TC, LDL-C and ALT were elevated markedly in diabetic animals (Fig. 4), while HDL-C was 30% lower as compared to non-diabetic group, with a consequent increase in TC/HDL ratio (76%). Diabetic rats gained more BW (27%), LW (30%) and LW/BW ratio (15%) (Fig. 5). In addition, VFW/BW and EFW/BW ratios were elevated by 3.3 and 2.2 folds, respectively, as well as the liver content of TGs (2.5 folds) and TC (6.4 folds).

Phytol repressed insulin and fructosamine levels back to normal, decreased those of glucose, HOMA-index and TNF-α, as compared to control group and increased adiponectin level by 4 folds (Fig. 3). Phytol also reduced serum levels of TGs (34%), TC (10%), ALT (33%), and TC/HDL-C ratio (18%) as presented in figure 4. It also leveled off LW (22%), VFW/BW (18%) and EFW/BW ratios (21%), along with liver contents of TGs (24%) and TC (26%), as compared to diabetic non-treated rats (Fig. 5). Groups DP_5 and DP_{10} showed a reduced glucose (50%; 63%), insulin (55%; 70%), fructosamine (54%; 55%) and TNF-α (76%; 48%) levels, as well as HOMA-index (77%; 89%), whilst adiponectin was raised by 4 and 4.8 folds, respectively (Fig. 3). Pioglitazone (5 mg/kg) improved serum lipid homeostasis and ALT activity, effects that reached to normal levels in DP_{10}group (Fig. 4). Both doses of pioglitazone reduced hepatic TGs (17%; 41%) and TC (22%; 44%), as well as, LW (17%; 23%), VFW/BW ratio (16%; 45%), and EFW/BW ratio (28%; 52%), while BW was lowered only in DP_{10} group (Fig. 5).

DP_hP_5 group showed recovered glucose and lipid homeostasis, insulin, HOMA-index, TNF-α and ALT to reach values virtually close to those of the control non-diabetic rats (Fig. 3 and 4). In addition, this combination raised serum levels of adiponectin (4.3 folds) (Fig. 3) and HDL-C (24%), (Fig. 4), while reduced VFW/BW and EFW/BW ratios, along with BW, LW and liver contents of TGs and TC (Fig. 5).

To detect the possible interactions between phytol and pioglitazone, the results of DV, DP_h, DP_5 and DP_hP_5 groups were statistically analyzed using factorial design. There was an additive effect of the combination compared with individual treatments only on BW and VFW/BW ratio. Although in all other parameters measured, there was a significant interaction, where the combined effect was higher than that of either individual treatment, yet this interaction did not reach an additive effect statistically. Using linear regression analysis, glucose, insulin and HOMA-index correlate positively with TNF-α, ALT and VFW/BW ratio and negatively with adiponectin, $P<0.001$(Table 4).

Discussion

To the best of the author's knowledge, the present work is the first in vivo study to verify the antidiabetic/insulin sensitizing action of phytol. The docking study proved that phytanic acid has high affinity to interact with PPARγ in a pattern similar to that of the TZD agonists, via 4 hydrogen bonding with the same amino acids, viz., Ser- 289, His-323, His-449, and, Tyr-473. Hence, these 4 amino acids are considered indispensable for the PPARγ molecular recognition, activation and antidiabetic biological activity. Moreover, the current finding emphasized that phytanic

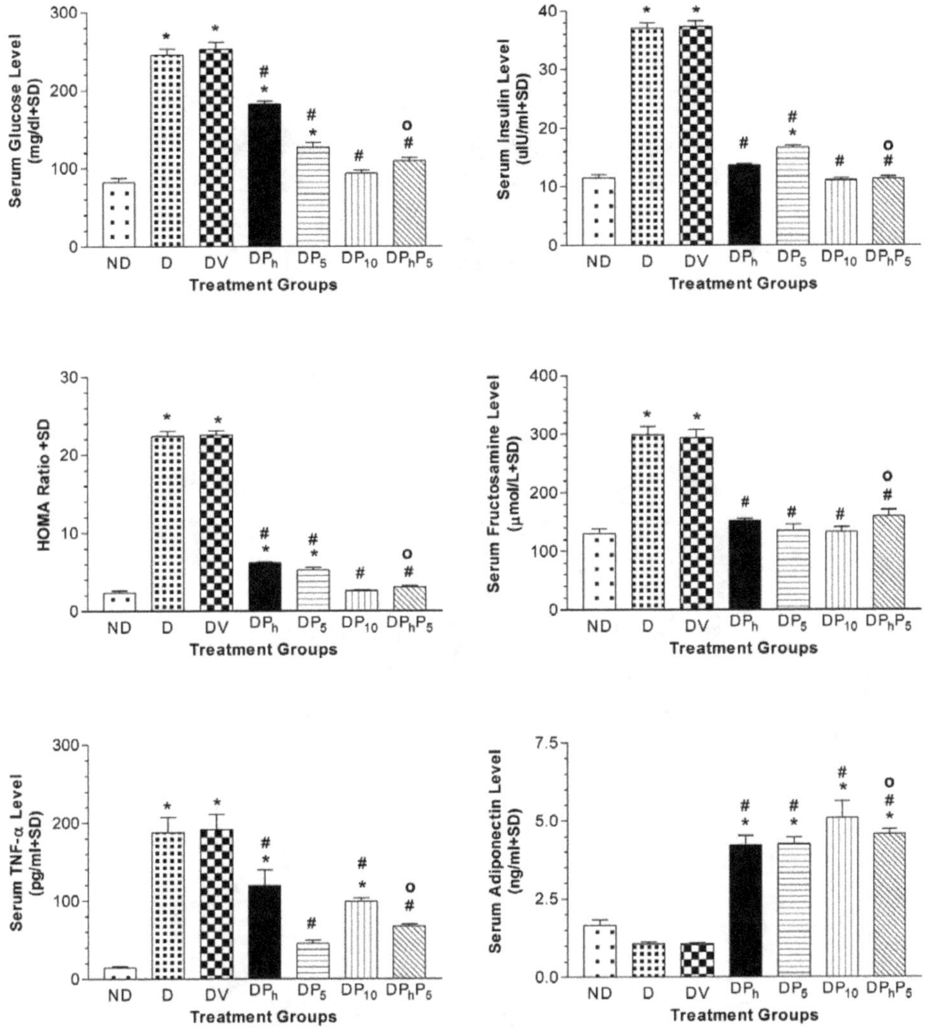

Figure 3. Effect of diabetes (DV) and different oral drug regimens on glucose homeostasis indicators. Effect of diabetes (DV) and different oral drug regimens, viz., phytol (DP_h, 250 mg/kg); pioglitazone (DP_5, 5 mg/kg); pioglitazone (DP_{10}, 10 mg/kg); phytol and pioglitazone (DP_hP_5); on serum levels of glucose, insulin, fructosamine, TNF-α, adiponectin and insulin resistance (HOMA-ratio) (mean of 7 animals ± S.D). As compared with non-diabetic [ND] (*) and diabetic [DV] (#) groups using one way ANOVA followed by Tukey post hoc test, $P<0.05$. (^{O}) Significant interaction when P_h and P_5 were combined using Factorial Design.

acid complexes to RXR with lesser energy than retinoic acid, the natural ligand, and shared retinoic acid in arginine R 316 which highlights the vital role of arginine R 316 for the dimer activity.

Therefore, the phytol-induced glucose homeostasis salvage is partly attributed to the ability of phytanic acid to boost the expression of transcriptional activity of PPARs/RXR heterodimers that regulates several genes' expression [3], via the binding to PPAR-responsive element (PPRE). This insinuates that either partner, RXR or PPARγ, can regulate the transcriptional activity by interacting with its own ligand. In this essence, phytol mimics its synthetic candidates, which through activating RXR could have a marked impact on whole body metabolism, including insulin-sensitization and improved glycemic control, in a comparable action to TZDs.

Phytanic acid by activating RXR and/or PPARγ can activate GLUT2 gene, and glucokinase mRNA, effects that facilitate hepatic glucose influx [14,27]. In addition, agonists of this nuclear receptor increase the expression and translocation of GLUT4 in adipocytes, and the catabolism of glucose along with the decrease in hepatic glucose output [28].

Furthermore, the dyslipidemic effect of phytol, which coincides relatively with a previous study [29] may be attributed again to the phytanic acid-induced activation of PPARs/RXR heterodimerization, a dimer that induces various genes involved in lipid homeostasis [30]. In the presence of decreased glucose level [28], stimulation of PPARα, enhances lipid metabolism through up-regulating enzymes involved in β-oxidative degradation of fatty acids [14,28], a critical fate in regulation of VLDL synthesis [31]. PPARα-dependent and -independent β-oxidation enzymes are induced by phytol feeding, as reported previously [12]. The ability of phytol to lower FFAs [12] could improve glucose profile by enhancing hepatic glucose uptake, decreasing gluconeogenesis, suppressing hepatic glucose production, and mobilizing lipids from muscle, leading to enhanced muscle sensitivity to insulin, and suppressing delivery of TG's substrates to the liver [31].

Besides its action on redressing altered glucose panel and improving dyslipidemic state observed in this model, phytol also elevated adiponectin and decreased that of TNF-α and ALT; results that play a role in its antidiabetic effect. Moreover, visceral and epidydimal fat contents correlate positively with insulin

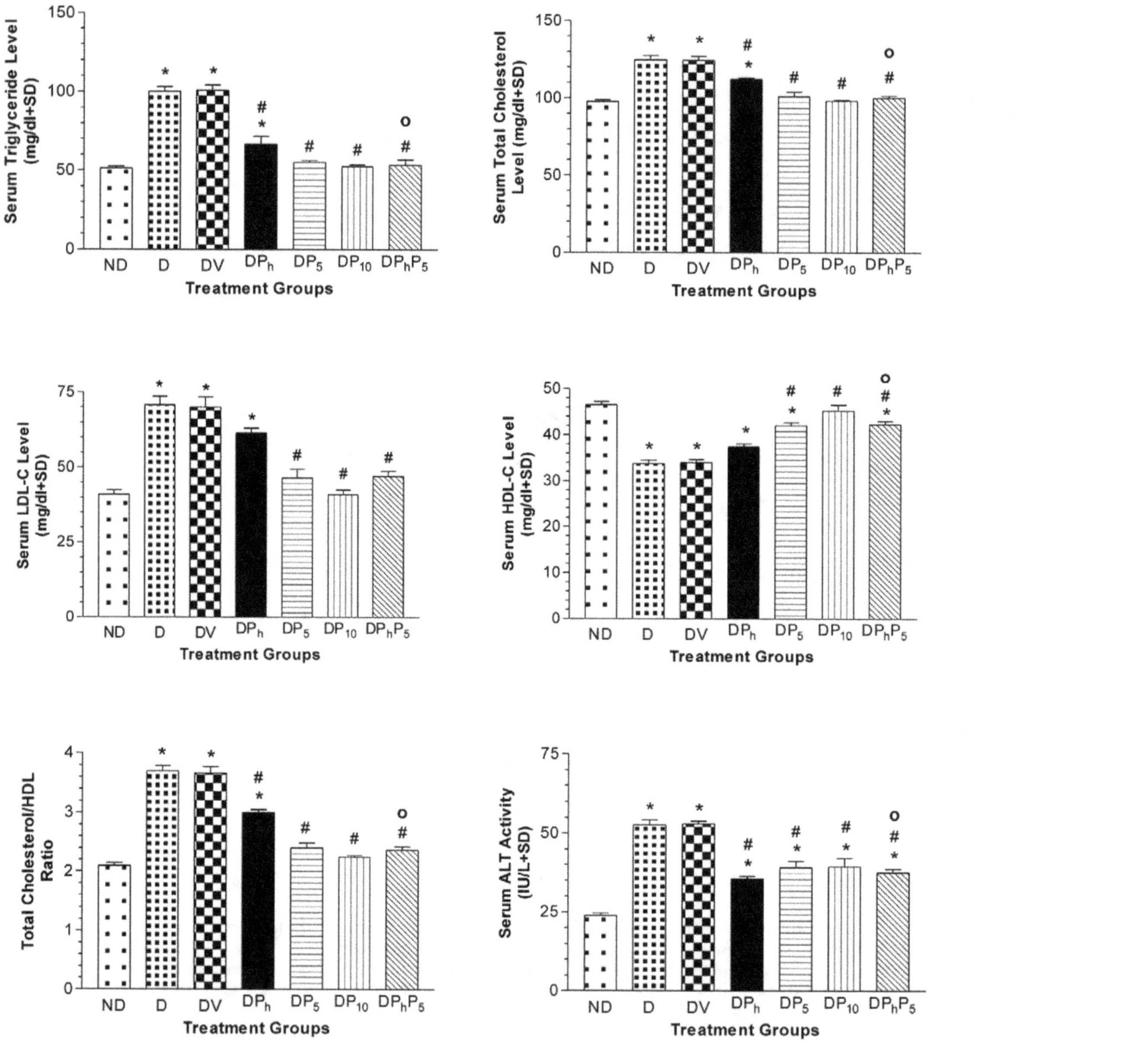

Figure 4. Effect of diabetes (DV) and different oral drug regimens on the serum lipid profile. Effect of diabetes (DV) and different oral drug regimens, viz., phytol (DP_h, 250 mg/kg); pioglitazone (DP_5, 5 mg/kg); pioglitazone (DP_{10}, 10 mg/kg); phytol and pioglitazone (DP_hP_5); on serum levels of triglycerides, total cholesterol, LDL-C, HDL-C, ALT and TC/HDL ratio (mean of 7 animals ± S.D). As compared with non-diabetic [ND] (*) and diabetic [DV] (#) groups using one way ANOVA followed by Tukey post hoc test, $P<0.05$. (^{O}) Significant interaction when P_h and P_5 were combined using Factorial Design.

resistance [32], hence, phytol-mediated decrease in VFW/and EFW/BW ratios, offers another mechanism for improved insulin sensitivity.

White adipose tissue (WAT), represented herein by epidydimal fat content, participates in the induction of whole-body insulin resistance, partly by the macrophage infiltration-induced chronic inflammation of WAT and/or the release of TNF-α, which is highly expressed in WAT [33]. TNF-α is a critical mediator in insulin resistance induction [34,35], inhibition of which by phytol could convey the improvement of insulin sensitivity along with glucose disposal.

In the current study, phytol boosted the adiponectin level, another adipocytokine that is closely associated with improved insulin sensitivity [36]. The adiponectin promoter contains a functional PPRE to which PPARγ/RXR heterodimer binds directly and increases its activity in adipocytes [37]. Our docking results confirmed the binding of phytanic acid with the RXR in the heterodimer; a finding that can verify the phytol-induced increase in adiponectin. Adiponectin antidiabetic properties result from enhancement of insulin-induced tyrosine phosphorylation of the IR [36], activation of IRS-1-mediated phosphatidylinositol-3 kinase (PI-3K) and glucose uptake in hepatic and skeletal muscle cells [37]. Besides, it enhances muscle β-oxidation, stimulates glucose utilization, suppresses hepatic glucose production [38], and decreases TNF-α level [39].

Another possible mechanism for the insulin sensitizing/anti-diabetic effect of phytol is its ability to lower ALT activity; an enzyme found primarily in the liver and is considered an indicator

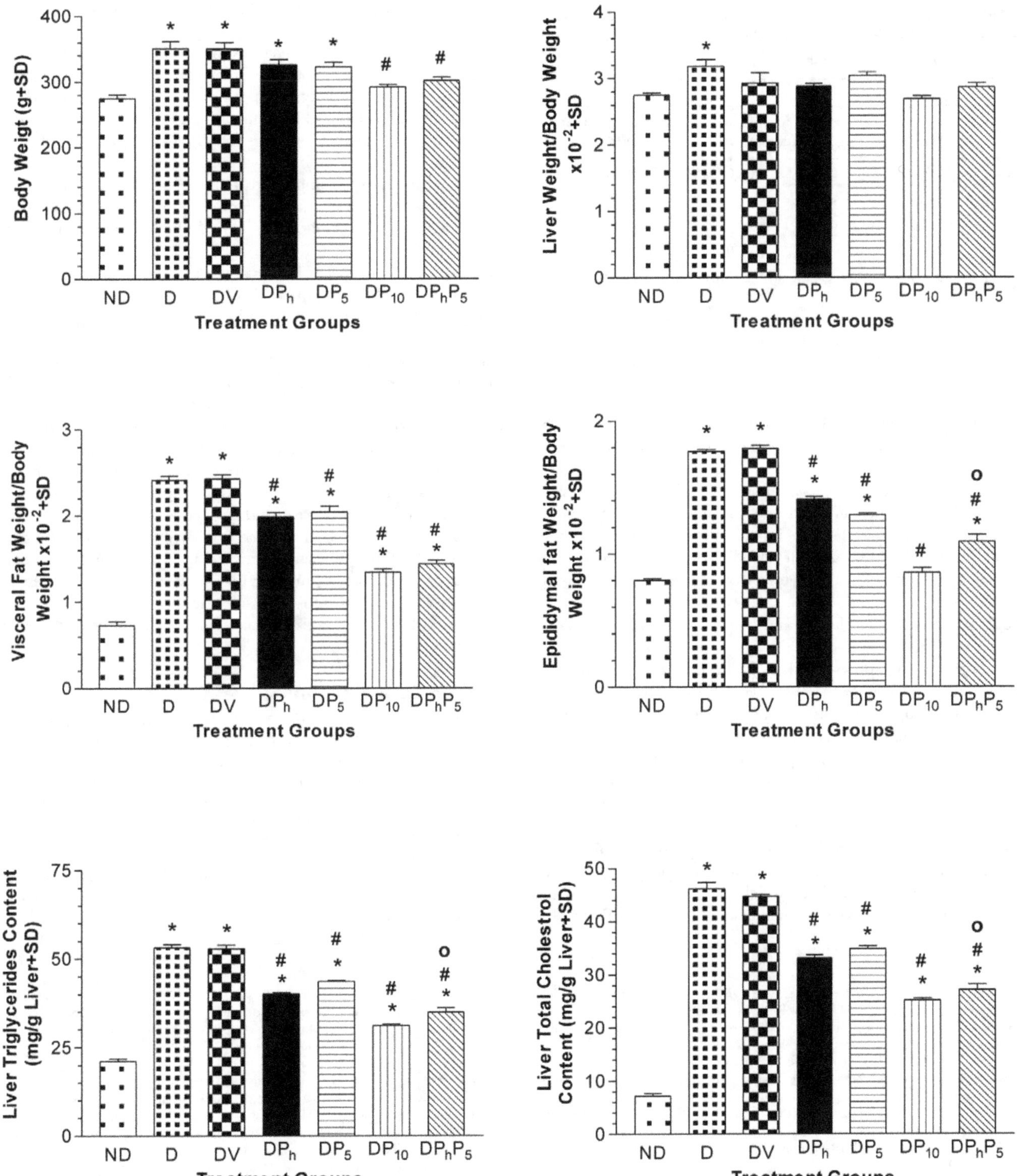

Figure 5. Effect of diabetes (DV) and different oral drug regimens on liver weight:, visceral fat:, and epidydimal fat:body weight ratios and on hepatic triglycerides and total cholesterol contents. Effect of diabetes (DV) and different oral drug regimens, viz., phytol (DP_h, 250 mg/kg); pioglitazone (DP_5, 5 mg/kg); pioglitazone (DP_{10}, 10 mg/kg); phytol and pioglitazone (DP_hP_5); on body weight, ratios of liver weight/body weight, visceral fat weight/body weight, and epidydimal weight/body weight, and contents of liver triglycerides and total cholesterol(mean of 7 animals ± S.D). As compared with non-diabetic [ND] (*) and diabetic [DV] (#) groups using one way ANOVA followed by Tukey post hoc test, $P<0.05$. (O) Significant interaction when P_h and P_5 were combined using Factorial Design.

Table 4. Correlation coefficient (*r*) between serum glucose, insulin and HOMA-R with TNF-α, adiponectin, ALT and visceral fat weight/body weight ratio.

	TNF-α	Adiponectin	ALT	Visceral fat/ BWT
Glucose	0.7089	−0.8567	0.6915	0.8664
	P<0.001	P<0.001	P<0.001	P<0.001
Insulin	0.7299	−0.9163	0.8255	0.8345
	P<0.001	P<0.001	P<0.001	P<0.001
HOMA-R	0.7590	−0.9196	0.8264	0.8319
	P<0.001	P<0.001	P<0.001	P<0.001

Correlation was carried out in untreated and treated hyperglycemic animals only.

of hepatocellular health. ALT level is influenced by disorders such as obesity, insulin resistance, and type-2 diabetes, ailments that wane normal hepatocellular function. Elevated ALT level may result from impaired insulin signaling, since insulin suppresses genes encoding gluconeogenic enzymes, including ALT [40], and/or increased level of TNF-α via inducing hepatic fatty changes [40] characterized by high ALT level. All these disturbances were corrected by treatment with phytol, as presented in the present work

Pioglitazone effect on glucose and lipid homeostasis, acquiesce with previous studies, [40–42], as well as its ability to increase adiponectin and to suppress TNF-α, and ALT [43–45]. Most of these actions are attributed to the effect of TZDs on PPARγ, as they activate multiple gene cassettes by their robust binding to this nuclear receptor; findings that support our docking results.

As a member of the TZDs, pioglitazone was reported to increase body weight via the activation of PPARγ that causes pre-adipocytes differentiation into mature fat cells and upregulates a number of genes responsible for lipogenesis [32]. However, the present results showed no weight gain in pioglitazone-treated rats; a finding that coincides with earlier studies reporting negative influence of pioglitazone on body weight of high-fat fed rats, with [46], or without [42] STZ. Pioglitazone, unlike rosiglitazone, possesses partial PPARα effect [47] which may clarify its negative influence on body weight.

As PPARs exert their effects by heterodimerizing with RXR, therefore, interaction of either partner with its ligand can regulate the transcriptional activity; this points again to the docking results of both phytanic acid and pioglitazone. In a previous *in vitro* study, co-treatment of cells with ligands for PPAR and RXR resulted in an additive effect [14]. This may explain the results of the current study, where phytol improved almost all altered parameters induced by the current animal model, and its co-administration with pioglitazone (5 mg/kg) exerted better effect, reaching approximately that of the higher pioglitazone dose (10 mg/kg). However, the combined effect was not statistically additive except on decreased body weight, and VFW/BW ratio, both of which have good impact on insulin sensitivity.

In conclusion, phytol has a potential role in the management of insulin resistance and metabolic disorders that accompany diabetes and/or obesity, through activating RXR via its metabolite, and modulating other factors that imply in metabolic disorders. Moreover, molecular docking studies of phytanic acid on the two crystal structures of PPARγ binding protein, and RXRα/PPARγ heterodimer showed good alignment with the experimental findings and verified/confirmed the antidiabetic biological activity of phytol and its active metabolite, phytanic acid. Phytol can be administered with lower doses of TZDs to maintain the full therapeutic action, but with lesser side effects. Therefore, addition of nutraceuticals, at meaningful doses, to antidiabetic agents would have substantial efficacy, and presumably could be used as aids to good glucose tolerance and insulin sensitivity.

Author Contributions

Conceived and designed the experiments: MME HSE MFS NAF. Performed the experiments: MME HSE MFS NAF. Analyzed the data: MME HSE MFS NAF. Wrote the paper: HSE. Responsible for the experimentation of the research: MFS. Assessed the Biochemicals: MFS. Collected data: MFS. Performed the statistical analysis: MME. Interpreted data: MME. Illustrated figures: MME. Contributed to the interpretation of data: HSE. Drafted the article: HSE. Revised the article critically for important intellectual content: HSE. Gave final approval of the article version to be published: HSE. Responsible for the molecular docking studies using Molsoft, flexible docking program "Internal Coordinate Mechanics (Molsoft ICM 3.4-8C)": NAF.

References

1. Astrup A, Finer N (2000) Redefining type-2 diabetes: 'Diabesity' or 'obesity dependent diabetes mellitus'? Obesity Reviews 1: 57–9
2. Basciano H, Federico L, Adeli K (2005) Fructose, insulin resistance, and metabolic dyslipidemia. Nutrition and Metabolism 2: 1–5
3. McCarty MF (2005) Up-regulation of PPARgamma coactivator-1alpha as a strategy for preventing and reversing insulin resistance and obesity. Medical Hypotheses 64: 399–407
4. DeFronzo RA (1999) Pharmacologic therapy for type-2 diabetes mellitus. Ann Intern Med 131: 281–303
5. Spiegelman BM (1998) PPAR-γ: adipogenic regulator and thiazolidinedione receptor. Diabetes 47: 507–14.
6. McCarty MF (2001) The chlorophyll metabolite phytanic acid is a natural rexinoid–potential for treatment and prevention of diabetes. Medical Hypotheses 56: 217–19
7. Mukherjee R, Davies PJ, Crombie DL, Bischoff ED, Cesario RM, et al. (1997) Sensitization of diabetic and obese mice to insulin by retinoid X receptor agonists. Nature 386: 407–10
8. Villarroya F, Iglesias R, Giralt M (2004) Retinoids and retinoid receptors in the control of energy balance: novel pharmacological strategies in obesity and diabetes. Curr Med Chem 11: 795–805
9. Canan Koch SS, Dardashti LJ, Cesario RM, Croston GE, Boehm MF, et al. (1999) Synthesis of retinoid X receptor-specific ligands that are potent inducers of adipogenesis in 3T3-L1 cells. J Med Chem 42: 742–50
10. Hansen RP (1966) Occurence of phytanic acid in rumen bacteria. Nature 210: 841
11. Brown PJ, Mei G, Gibberd FB, Burston D, Mayne PD, et al. (1993) Diet and Refsum's disease. The determination of phytanic acid and phytol in certain foods and the application of this knowledge to the choice of suitable convenience foods for patients with Refsum's disease. J Hum Nutr Diet 6: 295–305
12. Gloerich J, van Vlies N, Jansen GA, Denis S, Ruiter JP, et al. (2005) A phytol-enriched diet induces changes in fatty acid metabolism in mice both via PPAR alpha dependent and - independent pathways. J Lipid Res 46: 716–26
13. van den Brink DM, van Miert JN, Dacremont G, Rontani JF, Wanders RJ (2005) Characterization of the final step in the conversion of phytol into phytanic acid. J BiolChem 280: 26838–44
14. Heim M, Johnson J, Boess F, Bendik I, Weber P, et al. (2002) Phytanic acid, a natural peroxisome proliferator-activated receptor (PPAR) agonist, regulates glucose metabolism in rat primary hepatocytes. FASEB J 16: 718–20
15. Elmazar MMA, Nau H (2004) Potentiation of the teratogenic effects induced by coadministration of retinoic acid or phytanic acid/phytol with synthetic retinoid receptor ligands. Arch Toxicol 78: 660–8.
16. Gloerich J, van den Brink DM, Ruiter JPN, van Vlies N, Vaz FM, et al. (2007) Metabolism of phytol to phytanic acid in the mouse, and the role of PPARα in its regulation. J Lipid Res 48:77–85.
17. Schaalan M, El-Abhar HS, Barakat M, El-Denshary ES (2009) Westernized-like-diet-fed rats: effect on glucose homeostasis, lipid profile, and adipocyte hormones and their modulation by rosiglitazone and glimepiride. J Diabetes Complications 23: 199–208.
18. Murcko MA, Stouten PFW (1997) In:Charifson PS (ed) Practical Application of Computer-Aided Drug Design, Marcel Dekker, New York, pp 355.

19. Anderson A, Weng ZJ (1999) Molecular Graphics & Modeling 17,180.
20. Halperin I, Ma B, Wolfson H, Nussinov R (2002) Proteins: Structure, Function, and Genetics, 47, 409.
21. Nolte RT, Wisely GB, Westin S, Cobb JE, Lambert MH, et al. (1998) Ligand binding and co-activator assembly of the peroxisome proliferator-activated receptor-gamma. Nature 395: 137–143
22. Gampe RT Jr, Montana VG, Lambert MH, Miller AB, Bledsoe RK, et al. (2000) Asymmetry in the PPARgamma/RXRalpha crystal structure reveals the molecular basis of heterodimerization among nuclear receptors. Mol Cell 5: 545–555
23. Levy J, Gavin JR 3rd, Fausto A, Gingerich RL, Avioli LV (1984) Impaired insulin action in rats with non-insulin-dependent diabetes. Diabetes 33:901–6
24. Matthews DR, Hosker JP, Rudenski AS, Naylor BA, Treacher DF, et al. (1985) Homeostasis model assessment: Insulin resistance and b-cell function from fasting plasma glucose and insulin concentrations in man. Diabetologia 28: 412–19.
25. Bligh EG, Dyer WJ (1959) A rapid method of total lipid extraction and purification. Can J BiochemPhysiol 37: 911–17.
26. Allen NE, Grace PB, Ginn A, Travis RC, Roddam AW, et al. (2008) Phytanic acid: measurement of plasma concentrations by gas-liquid chromatography-mass spectrometry analysis and associations with diet and other plasma fatty acids. Br J Nutr. ;99(3):653–9.
27. Kim HI, Kim JW, Kim SH, Cha JY, Kim KS, et al. (2000) Identification and functional characterization of the peroxisomal proliferator response element in rat GLUT2 promoter. Diabetes 49: 1517–24
28. Jay MA, Ren J (2007) Peroxisome proliferator-activated receptor (PPAR) in metabolic syndrome and type-2 diabetes mellitus. Curr Diabetes Rev 3: 33–9
29. Van den Branden C, Vamecq J, Wybo I, Roels F (1986) Phytol and peroxisome proliferation. Pediatr Res 20: 411–5
30. Hashimoto T, Shimizu N, Kimura T, Takahashi Y, Ide T (2006) Polyunsaturated fats attenuate the dietary phytol–induced increase in hepatic fatty acid oxidation in mice. J Nutr 136: 882–6
31. Miyazaki Y, Mahankali A, Matsuda M, Glass L, Mahankali S, et al (2001) Improved glycemic control and enhanced insulin sensitivity in type 2 diabetic subjects treated with pioglitazone. Diabetes Care 24: 710–9
32. Miyazaki Y, Mahankali A, Matsuda M (2002) Effect of pioglitazone on abdominal fat distribution and insulin sensitivity in type-2 diabetic patients. J ClinEndocrinolMetab 87: 2784–91
33. Tsuchida A, Yamauchi T, Takekawa S (2005) Peroxisome proliferator–activated receptor (PPAR)-α activation increases adiponectin receptors and reduces obesity-related inflammation in adipose tissue comparison of activation of PPARα, PPARγ, and their combination. Diabetes 54: 3358–70
34. Yamauchi T, Kamon J, Waki H (2001) The fat-derived hormone adiponectin reverses insulin resistance associated with both lipoatrophy and obesity. Nat Med 7: 941–6.
35. Hotamisligil GS, Murray DL, Choy LN, Spiegelman BM (1994)Tumor necrosis factor α inhibits signaling from the insulin receptor. Proc Nat AcadSci USA 91: 4854–8.
36. Stefan N, Vozarova B, Funahashi T (2002) Plasma adiponectin concentration is associated with skeletal muscle insulin receptor tyrosine phosphorylation, and low plasma concentration precedes a decrease in whole-body insulin sensitivity in humans. Diabetes 50:1884–8.
37. Iwaki M, Matsuda M, Maeda N (2003) Induction of adiponectin, a fat-derived antidiabetic and antiatherogenic factor, by nuclear receptors. Diabetes 52: 1655–63.
38. Yamauchi T, Kamon J, Minokoshi Y (2002) Adiponectin stimulates glucose utilization and fatty-acid oxidation by activating AMP activated protein kinase. Nat Med 8: 1288–95.
39. Maeda N, Takahashi M, Funahashi T (2001) PPARγ ligands increase expression and plasma concentrations of adiponectin, an adipose-derived protein. Diabetes 50: 2094–99.
40. Vozarova B, Stefan N, Lindsay RS (2002) High alanine aminotransferase is associated with decreased hepatic insulin sensitivity and predicts the development of type-2 diabetes. Diabetes 51: 1889–95.
41. Hofmann C, Lorenz K, Colca JR (1991) Glucose transport deficiency in diabetic animals is corrected by treatment with the oral antihyperglycemic agent pioglitazone. Endocrinology 129: 1915–25.
42. Srinivasan K, Patole PS, Kaul CL, Ramarao P (2004) Reversal of glucose intolerance by pioglitazone in high fat diet-fed rats. Methods Find Exp Clin Pharmacol 26: 327–33.
43. Vijay SK, Mishra M, Kumar H, Tripathi K (2009) Effect of pioglitazone and rosiglitazone on mediators of endothelial dysfunction, markers of angiogenesis and inflammatory cytokines in type-2 diabetes. Acta Diabetol 46: 27–33.
44. Iwata M, Haruta T, Usui I, Takata Y, Takano A, et al. (2001) Pioglitazone ameliorates tumor necrosis factor-α–induced insulin resistance by a mechanism independent of adipogenic activity of peroxisome proliferator–activated receptor-γ. Diabetes 50: 1083–92.
45. Miyazaki Y, Mahankali A, Wajcberg E, Bajaj M, Mandarino LJ, et al. (2004) Effect of pioglitazone on circulating adipocytokine levels and insulin sensitivity in type 2 diabetic patients. J Clin Endocrinol Metab 89: 4312–19.
46. Ding S, Shen Z, Chen Y, Sun S, Liu Q, et al. (2005) Pioglitazone can ameliorate insulin resistance in low-dose streptozotocin and high sucrose-fat diet induced obese rats. Acta Pharmacologica Sinica 26: 575–80.
47. Sakamoto J, Kimura H, Moriyama S, Odaka H, Momose Y, et al. (2000) Activation of human peroxisome proliferators-activated receptor (PPAR) types by pioglitazone. Biochem Biophys Res Commun 278: 704–11.

15

Is Serum Zinc Associated with Pancreatic Beta Cell Function and Insulin Sensitivity in Pre-Diabetic and Normal Individuals?

Khanrin P. Vashum[1]*, Mark McEvoy[1], Abul Hasnat Milton[1], Md. Rafiqul Islam[1,2], Stephen Hancock[1], John Attia[1]

1 Centre for Clinical Epidemiology and Biostatistics (CCEB), School of Medicine and Public Health, The University of Newcastle, and Hunter Medical Research Institute, Newcastle, New South Wales, Australia, **2** Ministry of Health and Family Welfare, Government of Bangladesh, Dhaka, Bangladesh

Abstract

Aim: To determine if there is a difference in serum zinc concentration between normoglycaemic, pre-diabetic and type-2 diabetic groups and if this is associated with pancreatic beta cell function and insulin sensitivity in the former 2 groups.

Method: Cross sectional study of a random sample of older community-dwelling men and women in Newcastle, New South Wales, Australia. Beta cell function, insulin sensitivity and insulin resistance were calculated for normoglycaemic and prediabetes participants using the Homeostasis Model Assessment (HOMA-2) calculator.

Result: A total of 452 participants were recruited for this study. Approximately 33% (N = 149) had diabetes, 33% (N = 151) had prediabetes and 34% (N = 152) were normoglycaemic. Homeostasis Model Assessment (HOMA) parameters were found to be significantly different between normoglycaemic and prediabetes groups ($p<0.001$). In adjusted linear regression, higher serum zinc concentration was associated with increased insulin sensitivity ($p = 0.01$) in the prediabetic group. There was also a significant association between smoking and worse insulin sensitivity.

Conclusion: Higher serum zinc concentration is associated with increased insulin sensitivity. Longitudinal studies are required to determine if low serum zinc concentration plays a role in progression from pre-diabetes to diabetes.

Editor: Yiqing Song, Brigham & Women's Hospital, and Harvard Medical School, United States of America

Funding: The University of Newcastle and Vincent Fairfax Family Foundation funded the Hunter Community study and this study was funded by Lions District Diabetes foundation, Australia. The funders had no role in study design, data collection and analysis, decision to publish, or preparation of the manuscript.

Competing Interests: The authors have declared that no competing interests exist.

* E-mail: Khanrin.vashum@newcastle.edu.au

Introduction

Diabetes, a disorder of metabolism with defects in either insulin secretion, insulin action or both, is increasing globally due to population growth, aging, urbanization, unhealthy eating habits, and increasing prevalence of obesity and physical inactivity [1]. Diabetes is a leading cause of morbidity and mortality with an estimated 346 million adults being affected worldwide in 2011 [1]. The prevalence is continuing to rise and is expected to double between 2005–2030. [1,2].

Type 2 diabetes is often asymptomatic and may remain undiagnosed for several years [3]. It is characterized by insulin resistance, hyperinsulinaemia, beta cell dysfunction and subsequent beta cell failure [4]. Numerous influences on the onset of diabetes have been proposed, one of which may be the abnormal homeostasis of trace elements such as zinc [5]. [6]. Zinc is involved in the synthesis, storage, and secretion of monomeric insulin, as well as conversion to a dimeric form for storage and secretion as crystalline insulin [7,8]. Zinc is essential in insulin action and carbohydrate metabolism [9]. Oxidative stress also plays an important role in the pathogenesis of diabetes and its complications, and zinc is a structural component of key antioxidant enzymes such as superoxide dismutase, which is vital for intra- and extracellular antioxidant defence [10].

Animal models have shown that peripheral insulin resistance contributes to impaired glucose tolerance in non-diabetic, zinc deficient rats [11]. Oral administration of zinc complex in KKA(y) mice daily also caused significant improvements in hyperglycaemia, glucose intolerance and insulin resistance [12]. Conversely, a zinc deficient diet led to increased fasting blood glucose levels and reduced circulating insulin in db/db mice [13]. Human studies on the other hand have had conflicting results regarding zinc supplementation in type 2 diabetes. A lower incidence of type 2 diabetes has been reported in women who had a higher intake of dietary zinc [14]. A Cochrane review found that there was insufficient evidence to suggest the use of zinc supplementation in the prevention of type 2 diabetes [15]. By contrast, a systematic review and meta-analysis of 25 articles, which included 22 studies on type 2 diabetes, concluded that zinc supplementation has beneficial effects on glycaemic control [16]. The review however had several limitations including differences in zinc doses, sample size, study duration, limited availability of data on zinc intake and variation in baseline parameters.

Pre-diabetes is a condition that increases the risk of developing type 2 diabetes and often precedes diabetes. In Australia the prevalence of pre-diabetes is estimated at 16.4%, more than double the prevalence of type-2 diabetes [17]. Pre-diabetic individuals have a six fold increased risk of developing type 2 diabetes compared with those with normal glucose values [17]. People with Pre-diabetes have impaired fasting glucose (IFG), impaired glucose tolerance (IGT), or both; blood glucose is higher than normal but not high enough to be classified as diabetes and this state is reversible [17]. Reversion to normal glucose tolerance occurs in about 25% over 3–5 years of observation, while the rest remain stable or progress to overt diabetes. However, with longer observation, the majority of individuals with IFG or IGT appear to develop diabetes [18]. People in the pre-diabetic stage are not only at an increased risk of developing diabetes but also have an increased risk of developing cardiovascular and other macro-vascular disease [17].

This study therefore set out to determine if there is a difference in serum zinc concentration between normal, pre-diabetic and type-2 diabetic groups of community-dwelling men and women aged 55–85 years. A further aim was to determine if serum zinc concentration is associated with pancreatic beta cell function and insulin sensitivity in pre-diabetic and normal individuals. The use of a pre-diabetic group who has not yet developed nephropathy is an important improvement in establishing that low zinc is not simply an epiphenomenon due to loss of zinc secondary to diabetic nephropathy.

Methods

A random sample of participants aged between 55 and 85 years was selected from the Hunter Community Study (HCS), a cohort of community-dwelling men and women in Newcastle, New South Wales (NSW), Australia. Approval to conduct the research was granted by the University of Newcastle Human Research Ethics Committees and Hunter New England Research Ethics. This study has been described in detail elsewhere [19]. In brief, participants were randomly selected from the NSW State Electoral roll and contacted between mid December 2004 and May 2007. A modified Dillman recruiting strategy [20] was used whereby two letters of introduction and an invitation to participate were posted to the selected persons. An HCS research assistant telephoned persons who did not respond to initial postal contacts. If contact was not established after five attempts, the individual was classified as a non-responder. Persons who could not speak English and those living in a residential aged care facility were deemed ineligible. Once written consent to participate was obtained from eligible study subjects, they were asked to complete a series of self-reported postal questionnaires.

In addition to completing the postal questionnaires, participants were invited to attend the HCS data collection centre (clinic) to enable a series of clinical measures to be ascertained. The clinic measures included blood pressure, height, weight, waist-circumference and blood collection for routine biochemical analysis (including fasting blood glucose). The clinic measures assessed also included consent to link study information with data from Medicare Australia (Medicare and Pharmaceutical Benefit Scheme) and local health databases.

Classification of diabetic status

As part of the clinical assessment in the HCS, fasting blood glucose was measured and participants were categorized into three groups according to American Diabetic Association (ADA) guidelines:

- Normal (normoglycemic): fasting blood glucose concentration <5.6 mmol/l,
- Prediabetic: fasting blood glucose concentration 5.6–6.9 mmol/l, and
- Diabetic: fasting blood glucose concentration ≥ 7 mmol/l or previously diagnosed as diabetic or currently taking diabetic medications (oral hypoglycaemic agents, insulin etc).

Measurement of serum zinc and serum insulin

Blood was collected in EDTA tubes and centrifuged at 4°C and 3000 g for 10 min. to separate serum, which was stored for three years at -80°C before analysis. Serum zinc concentration was measured using Inductively Coupled Plasma Mass Spectrometry (ICP-MS, Perkin Elmer Sciex) as ICP-MS has greater precision and sensitivity compared to the older classic atomic absorption spectroscopy (AAS) technique often used to measure zinc. Analysis of serum insulin was performed using a BECKMAN-COULTER 'DXI 800'.

Calculation of HOMA parameters

Measured serum insulin and fasting blood glucose concentration was used to calculate steady state beta cell function (%B), insulin sensitivity (%S) and insulin resistance (IR) for normal and prediabetic participants by using the Homeostasis Model Assessment (HOMA2) calculator (University of Oxford, website; http://www.dtu.ox.ac.uk/homacalculator/index.php). The HOMA2 calculator is an updated version (computer model) of the original HOMA model (HOMA1). HOMA2 also accounts for variations in hepatic and peripheral glucose resistance and the reduction of peripheral glucose-stimulated glucose uptake. However, the HOMA2 calculator is not appropriate for use in frank diabetes as it needs further validation in this group [21].

Measurement of other exposure variables

Participant's age, gender, education, income, smoking, alcohol intake, self-reported medical history (clinician diagnosis), self reported medications and use of zinc supplements or multivitamins with zinc, Body Mass Index (BMI) and Glomerular filtration rate (GFR) were collected. Education was categorized as primary school only, secondary school not completed, secondary school completed, trade or technical college qualification, and University or other tertiary qualification. Smoking was categorized as current, never, or former smoker. Alcohol intake was quantified and classified according to Australian National Health & Medical Research (NHMRC) guidelines [22] as number of drinks per month. BMI was calculated from participants' height and weight, which was measured during their clinic visit and grouped according to the guidelines for BMI classification by the World Health Organization (WHO).

Statistical analysis

To detect a mean difference as low as 1.7 mmol/L ($\pm$5 mmol/L) in serum zinc concentration among three groups (normal, pre-diabetic and diabetic) with 95% confidence interval and 80% power, a sample size of 375 was calculated. Assuming a 15% refusal and dropout rate, recruiting a total of 450 eligible participants was estimated to be sufficient to observe the differences for this study, i.e. 150 in each group. The statistical analysis was performed using STATA software version 11.0 supplied by STATA Corporation, Texas, USA. Initially, baseline characteristics of the study participants compared by the participants' fasting blood glucose status and presented as mean, standard deviation and proportion were analysed using a chi-square test for categorical variables and analysis of variance (ANOVA) for continuous variables. For markers that did not follow a normal distribution, non-parametric tests were performed.

Homeostasis Model Assessment (HOMA2) calculator was used to calculate the HOMA parameters i.e. beta cell function (%B), insulin sensitivity (%S) and insulin resistance (IR) for normal and prediabetic participants. Multiple linear regression analyses were then performed for all three HOMA parameters for normoglycaemic and prediabetic group separately to determine factors associated with each outcome. Number of medications used was considered in the multivariate analyses, but dropped out of final models (except for insulin resistance in the pre-diabetic group).

Results

A total of 452 participants with measurement of fasting blood glucose concentration were randomly recruited for this study. The baseline characteristics of the participants according to their fasting blood glucose concentration are shown in Table 1. Of the participants, roughly a third (N = 149) were diabetic, a third prediabetic (N = 151) and a third (N = 152) were normoglycaemic. Participants were roughly evenly split between males and females. Age was found to be significantly different with an overall average age of 66.6 years (±7.5), however the normoglycaemic group (65.6±7.3 years) was slightly younger compared to the diabetic group (67.9±7.7 years). Significant differences among the groups were also seen in household income, BMI, hypertension status, use of antihypertensive medication and the number of medications that the participants were taking. Overall, more than 80% of the participants across all the groups were on some form of medication. Only 6% (N = 27) of the total participants were taking zinc supplements or multivitamins with zinc but this was not significantly different between the groups. More than 50% in the normal group had never smoked but the rate of current smokers was similar across all the groups. Alcohol intake (number of drinks/month) was similar across the three groups with roughly 50% being classified as safe drinkers. The mean glomerular filtration rate (GFR) was also found to be similar across the three groups.

Table 2 shows the median of the blood/serum laboratory findings and HOMA parameters, as these biochemical and HOMA parameters were not normally distributed. Median fasting serum glucose concentration was 4.8 mmol/L, 5.8 mmol/L and 6.8 mmol/L in normalglycaemic, pre-diabetic and diabetic participants respectively. The median serum zinc concentration was found to be similar across all three groups (13 umol/L) however; median serum insulin concentration was different between normalglycaemic and prediabetic groups with this being higher in the prediabetic group (76 Vs 54 mIU/L). Furthermore, to examine whether serum zinc concentration was associated with the HOMA parameters, steady state beta cell function (%B), insulin sensitivity (%S) and insulin resistance (IR) for normoglycaemic and pre-diabetic groups were calculated. The pre-diabetic group had a lower median of beta cell function and median insulin sensitivity than the normoglycaemic group and higher median insulin resistance compared to the normoglycemic group.

The non-parametric Kruskal-Wallis test was used to test differences by glycaemic status (Table 2). As median serum zinc concentration was similar across all groups no statistical significant difference was found. However, median insulin concentration was significantly different between normoglycaemic and prediabetic groups ($p<0.001$). Moreover, all the HOMA parameters i.e, beta cell function (%B), insulin sensitivity (%S) and insulin resistance (IR) were found to be statistically significantly different between groups [$p<0.001$ (table 2)].

Multiple linear regression analyses for HOMA parameters was carried out separately by the participants' glycaemic status i.e normoglycaemic and prediabetics groups (Table 3 & 4). After adjusting for multiple possible confounders, the prediabetic group showed significant association between serum zinc concentration and insulin sensitivity ($p = 0.01$) indicating that insulin sensitivity increases with an increase in serum zinc concentration. Significant positive association of household income with beta cell function ($p = 0.03$) and insulin resistance ($p = 0.04$) was also observed in the prediabetic group. The same analysis also showed that insulin resistance increases with increasing number of medications ($p = 0.02$). However, similar stratified analysis for the normoglycaemic group did not show any significant association of HOMA parameters with serum zinc or household income.

We also found that beta cell function was higher in those with higher BMI in both the nomoglycaemic ($p = 0.001$) and prediabetic ($p = 0.009$) group. In the normoglycaemic group, insulin resistance ($p<0.001$) was also higher in those with higher BMI. Moreover, an association was found between smoking status and insulin sensitivity in the normoglycaemic group indicating that current smokers had lower insulin sensitivity ($P = 0.004$) and that insulin resistance increases with an increase in the number of medications ($p = 0.02$).

Discussion

This study has demonstrated that higher serum zinc concentration is associated with increased insulin sensitivity even after adjusting for a number of potential confounders. Furthermore, we also found that the higher the BMI, the higher the beta cell function in both groups and the higher the insulin resistance in the normoglycaemic group. Current smoking status in the normoglycaemic group was associated with lower insulin sensitivity and higher insulin resistance compared to those who had never smoked or were previous smokers. In the prediabetic group, increase in household income led to increase in beta cell function and insulin resistance.

Previous studies have reported reduced concentrations of serum zinc in prediabetics and diabetes mellitus [23,24] however, like other studies in both developed and developing countries [25,26], our study did not find any difference in serum zinc concentration amongst the diabetic, pre-diabetic and normoglycaemic groups. Zargar et al found that serum zinc concentration was not altered in diabetes mellitus whereas Ekmekcioglu et al found a higher zinc concentration in whole blood and plasma, although the levels between healthy and diabetic individuals did not differ statistically in these blood fractions. Serum zinc concentration varies under the influence of lifestyle factors such as smoking and alcohol consumption [27], as well as metabolic and hormonal influences [25].

Another method that is broadly used to assess zinc status is the determination of zinc concentration in urine. Hyperzincuria has been described to be a regular finding in type 2 diabetes and has been associated with hyperglycemia [5,9]. Increased urinary loss can imply a decrease in total body zinc. The serum zinc

Table 1. Baseline characteristics by participants fasting blood glucose status.

Characteristic	Overall (n = 452)	Normal (n = 152)	Pre-diabetic (n = 151)	Diabetic (n = 159)	p-value
Age (mean±SD)	66.6 (7.4)	65.6 (7.3)	66.3 (7.0)	67.9 (7.7)	0.03
Sex (n, %)					>0.05
Male	238 (53.72)	69 (46.62)	89(60.54)	80 (54.05)	
Female	205 (46.28)	79(53.38)	58(39.46)	68(45.95)	
Education (n, %)					>0.05
Primary schooling only	14 (3.17)	7 (4.73)	1 (0.68)	6 (4.08)	
Secondary schooling completed	108 (24.43)	41 (27.70)	36 (24.49)	31 (21.09)	
Secondary schooling not completed	98 (22.17)	29 (19.59)	28 (19.05)	41(27.89)	
Trade qualification or TAFE	103 (23.30), 89 (20.14)	39 (6.35), 24 (16.22)	34 (23.13), 38 (25.85)	30(20.41), 27(18.37)	
University or other tertiary study	24 (5.43)	5 (3.38)	9 (6.12)	10 (6.80)	
Others	6 (1.36)	3 (2.03)	1 (0.68)	2 (1.36)	
Household income/year (n,%)					0.003
Less than 5000	8 (1.81)	1 (0.68)	2(1.36)	5 (3.40)	
$5000–$9,999 per year	22 (4.98)	7 (4.73)	8 (5.44)	7 (4.76)	
$10,000–$19,999 per year	98 (22.17)	25 (16.89)	31 (21.09)	42 (28.57)	
$20,000–$29,999 per year	92 (20.81)	31 (20.95)	26 (17.69)	35 (23.810	
$30,000–$39,999 per year	47 (10.63)	27 (18.240	11 (7.48)	9 (6.12)	
$40,000–$49,999 per year	38 (8.60)	13 (8.78)	15 (10.20)	10 (6.80)	
$50,000–$69,999 per year	51 (11.54)	22 (14.86)	17 (11.56)	12 (8.16)	
$70 000 or more per year	61 (13.80)	18 (12.160	30 (20.41)	13 (8.84)	
Missing	25(5.66)	4 (2.70)	7 (4.76)	14 (9.52)	
Smoking status (n, %)					>0.05
Smoked never	209 (47.18)	77 (52.03)	63 (42.86)	69 (46.62)	
Previous smoker	192 (43.34)	59 (39.86)	70 (47.62)	63 (42.57	
Current smoker	35 (7.90)	11 (7.43)	13 (8.84)	11 (7.43)	
Missing	7 (1.58)	1 (0.68)	1 (0.68)	5 (3.38)	
Alcohol use (n, %)					>0.05
No	91 (20.54)	33 (22.30)	19 (12.93)	39 (26.35)	
Safe drinker	236 (53.27)	83 (56.08)	81 (55.78)	71 (49.97)	
Moderate drinker	28 (6.32)	9 (6.08)	11 (7.48)	8 (5.41)	
Hazardous drinker-binge	27 (6.09)	8 (5.41)	11 (7.48)	8 (5.41)	
Hazardous drinker-chronic	18 (4.06)	5 (3.38)	9 (6.12)	4 (2.70)	
Missing	43 (9.71)	10 (6.76)	15 (10.20)	18 (12.16)	
Hypertension (n, %)					<0.001
Yes	237 (47.57)	61 (40.13)	80 (52.98)	96 (64.43)	
No	215 (52.34)	91 (59.87)	71 (47.02)	53 (35.57)	
BMI (n, %)					<0.001
<25	49 (10.89)	28 (18.54)	10 (6.67)	11 (7.38)	
25.00–29.99	185 (41.11)	75 (49.67)	63 (42)	47 (31.54)	
≥30	216 (48)	48 (31.79)	77 (51.33)	91 (61.07)	
Taking any medicines (n, %)					<0.001
Yes	387 (85.62)	122 (80.26)	126 (83.44)	139 (93.29)	
No	64 (14.38)	30 (19.74)	25 (16.56)	10 (6.71)	
Taking antihypertensive (n, %)					<0.001
Yes	243 (53.76)	60 (39.47)	80 (52.98)	103 (69.13)	
No	209 (46.24)	92 (60.53)	71 (47.02)	46 (30.87)	
Taking anti diabetic (n, %)					
Yes	78 (17.26)			78 (52.35)	

Table 1. Cont.

Characteristic	Overall (n = 452)	Normal (n = 152)	Pre-diabetic (n = 151)	Diabetic (n = 159)	p-value
No	374 (82.74)	152 (100)	151 (100)	71 (47.65)	
Taking zinc supplements or multivitamins with zinc (n, %)					>0.05
Yes	27 (5.97)	9 (5.92)	6 (3.97)	12 (8.05)	
No	425 (94.03)	143 (94.08)	145 (96.03)	137 (91.95)	
GFR (ml/mt) (mean± SD)	75.3 (17)	77.4 (17.3)	73.9 (14.4)	74.5 (18.6)	>0.05

concentrations in our participants were within normal limits (10–18 umol/L); however as we did not measure zinc excretion, altered levels of zinc in the tissues cannot be ruled out. However, mean GFR was above 70 mls/min in all three groups and the absence of a significant difference in GFR between the groups suggests that there is no impairment in renal function and hence there is unlikely to be a difference in urinary zinc excretion secondary to diabetic nephropathy.

Another explanation for these findings could be the dietary habits of the Australian study population; those involved in this study may all consume food with relatively high levels of zinc. Although zinc deficiency is widespread and 33% of the world's population is affected [28], a recent study on the global prevalence of zinc deficiency showed that in Australia, the estimated prevalence of inadequate zinc intake was <15% [29] whereas in developing countries it was >25%. In developing countries, pulses and cereals represent the major source of zinc. However, in the United States and other developed countries, meat provides 40–60%, pulses about 20–40% and dairy products about 10–30% of the dietary zinc [30]. Although the sample of people in this study was randomly selected, they may have been relatively healthy and hence zinc replete.

We also examined total serum iron concentration amongst the groups, as zinc is known to interact with iron and decrease zinc absorption [31]. The mean total serum iron was 17.47 (±5.38) μmol/L and there was minimal difference in the mean total serum iron concentration between the groups and no statistical difference was seen ($p = 0.13$, results not presented).

The HOMA parameters findings however indicate that zinc may play a role in progression of diabetes with results showing that serum zinc concentration is associated with insulin sensitivity in the pre-diabetic group. There are many probable mechanisms for this; zinc is important with regard to metabolic diseases such as insulin resistance, metabolic syndrome (MS) and diabetes mainly because it is required for insulin storage in the pancreas and stabilization of insulin hexamers. The anti-oxidative properties of zinc may also delay progression of insulin resistance and diabetes [32]. Furthermore, some studies have suggested that zinc supplementation may improve insulin sensitivity [33,34] and that zinc status affects some risk factors related to insulin resistance [35].

This study found that increasing BMI was associated with increasing beta cell function in both groups and also an increase in insulin resistance in the normoglycaemic group. Previous studies showed that higher BMI was associated with insulin resistance with or without other associated conditions [36–38]. Release of chemokines and inflammatory cytokines from adipose tissue in obesity may result in chronic systemic low grade inflammation that leads to the development of insulin resistance [36]. On the other hand there are still areas of significant uncertainty and gaps of knowledge that limit a full understanding of beta cell function in obesity. It has been found that obesity is associated with a modest expansion of beta cell mass, however any effect of various factors (e.g. duration of obesity or recent changes in body weight) on beta cell mass in humans is unknown [39].

The result of this study also showed that there was an association between current smoking status and insulin sensitivity and insulin resistance. This finding is similar to a recent study which showed that smokers were less insulin sensitive compared with nonsmokers;the mechanisms responsible for this are unclear

Table 2. Laboratory findings and Homeostasis Model Assessment (HOMA) using for beta cell efficiency in normal and pre-diabetic groups.

	Laboratory findings			Beta cell efficiency using HOMA-2 calculator		
Patient status	Mean fasting blood glucose mmol/l ± SD (Median)	Mean serum zinc, umol/L ±SD (Median)	Mean serum insulin, mIU/L ±SD (Median)	Mean % of beta cell function ±SD (Median)	Mean % of insulin sensitivity ±SD (Median)	Mean insulin resistance ±SD (Median)
Normal (n = 152)	4.8±0.4 (4.8)	13.11±1.72 (13)	63.86±39.33 (54)	115.67±46.46 (110.7)	146.33±217.80 (98.5)	1.17±0.71 (1.01)
Prediabetic (n = 151)	5.9±0.3 (5.8)	13.15±1.67 (13)	89.95±61.86 (76)	93.55±46.16 (88.8)	141.08±310.30 (68.5)	1.72±1.14 (1.46)
Diabetic (n = 149)	7.1±2.1 (6.8)	13.46±3.61 (13)	-	-	-	-
Non-parametric Kruskal-Wallis P value	†<0.001	†>0.05	<0.001	<0.001	<0.001	<0.001

†Across all groups.

Table 3. Adjusted linear regression analysis for HOMA parameters in participants with normal fasting glucose.

Exposure indicators	HOMA2 Parameters								
	Beta Cell function			Insulin Sensitivity			Insulin Resistance		
	Coefficient	P value	95% CI[†]	Coefficient	P value	95% CI[†]	Coefficient	P value	95% CI[†]
Serum Zinc	1.43	0.55	−3.30 to 6.17	9.05	0.35	−9.94 to 28.03	−0.007	0.93	−0.064 to 0.059
Age	0.27	0.66	−0.93 to 1.47	−1.82	0.46	−6.62 to 3.00	0.003	0.65	−0.012 to 0.019
Gender	4.77	0.59	−12.51 to 22.04	−31.16	0.37	−100.41 to 38.08	−0.056	0.62	−0.28 to 0.17
BMI	2.91	0.001	1.27 to 4.56	−2.64	0.43	−9.22 to 3.95	0.050	<0.001	0.028 to 0.071
Education	−0.01	0.80	−0.07 to 0.05	0.03	0.84	−0.23 to 0.28	−0.0003	0.40	−0.001 to 0.0005
House hold income	−0.83	0.74	−5.72 to 4.05	3.73	0.71	−15.84 to 23.31	−0.007	0.82	−0.070 to 0.056
Smoking class	8.55	0.22	−5.12 to 22.22	−80.79	0.004	−135.60 to −25.98	0.22	0.02	0.04 to 0.39
Alcohol use	−5.61	0.22	−14.62 to 3.41	29.02	0.11	−7.13 to 65.17	−0.079	0.18	−0.19 to 0.037
Constant	−6.98	0.91	−128.90 to 114.92	256.87	0.30	−231.74 to 745.48	−0.398	0.62	−1.975 to 1.178

[†]CI: Confidence Interval.

Table 4. Adjusted linear regression analysis for HOMA parameters in pre-diabetic participants.

Exposure indicators	HOMA2 Parameters								
	Beta Cell function			Insulin Sensitivity			Insulin Resistance		
	Coefficient	P value	95% CI[†]	Coefficient	P value	95% CI[†]	Coefficient	P value	95% CI[†]
Serum Zinc	0.45	0.85	−4.34 to 5.25	48.63	0.01	10.59 to 86.67	0.135	0.06	−0.007 to 0.28
Age	0.83	0.20	−0.445 to 2.10	−4.50	0.36	−14.59 to 5.58	0.011	0.51	−0.022 to 0.043
Gender	12.45	0.16	−5.15 to 30.05	−103.95	0.12	−243.50 to 35.60	0.092	0.71	−0.40 to 0.58
BMI	2.18	0.009	0.560 to 3.80	−3.39	0.66	−16.27 to 9.48	0.030	0.17	−0.013 to 0.074
Education	−3.25	0.34	−9.92 to 3.41	12.23	0.53	−40.63 to 65.09	−0.128	0.18	−0.31 to 0.06
House hold income	4.81	0.03	0.50 to 9.12	−12.28	0.46	−46.45 to 21.88	0.126	0.04	0.003 to 0.248
Smoking class	3.64	0.57	−9.11 to 16.40	−96.90	0.06	−198.04 to 4.24	−0.017	0.92	−0.357 to 0.322
Alcohol use	0.42	0.92	−7.49 to 8.32	−17.34	0.59	−80.04 to 45.36	0.022	0.84	−0.201 to 0.246
No. of medicatons	–	–	–	–	–	–	0.114	0.02	0.018 to 0.210
Constant	−71.47	0.34	−218.43 to 75.50	168.84	0.77	−996.58 to 1334.25	−2.44	0.23	−6.474 to1.583

[†]CI: Confidence Interval.

[40]. Bergman et al. also reported that smoking cessation is associated with an improvement in insulin sensitivity in the absence of changes in adiposity or body weight. Since the association between the number of medications consumed and increased insulin resistance was only observed in the prediabetic group, this is likely an indication of metabolic disorders and associated risks, e.g. obesity, hypertension, lipid abnormalities, and atherosclerotic cardiovascular disease [41].

A strength of this study is the large sample size with a similar number of participants in all groups compared to previous studies. Zinc measurement was done using ICP-MS rather than atomic absorption spectroscopy (AAS) as studies have showed that ICP-MS provides much lower detection limits, high precision, high accuracy and reliable isotopic analysis compared to other methods for measuring trace elements [42,43]. Also, the coefficients of variation (CV%) for ICP-MS for serum zinc analysis was 13% which indicates low laboratory error. A potential limitation of our study is the absence of information on family history of diabetes and we did not consider other important trace elements such as copper, which may influence serum zinc concentration.

In conclusion, though no significant difference was found in the serum zinc concentration between normoglycaemic, prediabetes, and diabetes groups, this study suggests that zinc may still plays a vital role in diabetes as higher serum zinc concentration is associated with increased insulin sensitivity. The associations of BMI with beta cell function, and insulin sensitivity with smoking status should be explored further as these are important risk factors that may be modified as a means of preventing the progression to full diabetes. Further studies are needed to confirm these findings and the results need to be replicated in longitudinal studies.

Acknowledgments

The authors would like to thank the men and women participating in the HCS as well as all the staff, investigators and collaborators who have supported or been involved in the project to date.

Author Contributions

Conceived and designed the experiments: KPV MM MRI AHM SH JA. Performed the experiments: KPV MM JA AHM. Analyzed the data: KPV MM MRI JA SH. Contributed reagents/materials/analysis tools: KPV MM AHM MRI JA SH. Wrote the paper: KPV MM JA MRI AHM SH.

References

1. Wild S, Roglic G, Green A, Sicree R, King H (2004) Global prevalence of diabetes estimates for the year 2000 and projections for 2030. Diabetes Care 27: 1047–1053.
2. WHO (2012) Diabetes fact sheet No. 312. World Health Organization.
3. Engelgau MM, Narayan K, Herman WH (2000) Screening for type 2 diabetes. Diabetes Care 23: 1563–1580.
4. Stumvoll M, Goldstein BJ, van Haeften TW (2005) Type 2 diabetes: principles of pathogenesis and therapy. The Lancet 365: 1333–1346.
5. Kazi TG, Afridi HI, Kazi N, Jamali MK, Arain MB, et al. (2008) Copper, chromium, manganese, iron, nickel, and zinc levels in biological samples of diabetes mellitus patients. Biological Trace Element Research 122: 1–18.
6. Chen H, Tan C (2012) Prediction of type-2 diabetes based on several element levels in blood and chemometrics. Biological Trace Element Research 147: 67–74.
7. Meyer JA, Spence DM (2009) A perspective on the role of metals in diabetes: past findings and possible future directions. Metallomics 1: 32–41.
8. Noormagi A, Gavrilova J, Smirnova J, Tõugu V, Palumaa P (2010) Zn (II) ions co-secreted with insulin suppress inherent amyloidogenic properties of monomeric insulin. Biochem J 430: 511–518.
9. Chausmer AB (1998) Zinc, insulin and diabetes. Journal of the American College of Nutrition 17: 109–115.
10. Zheng Y, Li XK, Wang Y, Cai L (2008) The Role of Zinc, Copper and Iron in the Pathogenesis of Diabetes and Diabetic Complications: Therapeutic Effects by Chelators*. Hemoglobin 32: 135–145.
11. Tallman DL, Taylor CG (1999) Potential interactions of zinc in the neuroendocrine-endocrine disturbances of diabetes mellitus type 2. Canadian journal of physiology and pharmacology 77: 919–933.
12. Adachi Y, Yoshida J, Kodera Y, Kiss T, Jakusch T, et al. (2006) Oral administration of a zinc complex improves type 2 diabetes and metabolic syndromes. Biochemical & Biophysical Research Communications 351: 165–170.
13. Simon SF, Taylor CG (2001) Dietary zinc supplementation attenuates hyperglycemia in db/db mice. Experimental Biology & Medicine 226: 43–51.
14. Sun Q, van Dam RM, Willett WC, Hu FB (2009) Prospective study of zinc intake and risk of type 2 diabetes in women. Diabetes Care 32: 629–634.
15. Beletate V, El Dib RP, Atallah AN (2007) Zinc supplementation for the prevention of type 2 diabetes mellitus. Cochrane Database of Systematic Reviews: CD005525.
16. Jayawardena R, Ranasinghe P, Galappatthy P, Malkanthi R, Constantine G, et al. (2012) Effects of zinc supplementation on diabetes mellitus: a systematic review and meta-analysis. Diabetology & Metabolic Syndrome 4: 13.
17. Twigg SM, Kamp MC, Davis TM, Neylon EK, Flack JR (2007) Prediabetes: a position statement from the Australian Diabetes Society and Australian Diabetes Educators Association. Medical journal of Australia 186: 461.
18. Nathan DM, Davidson MB, DeFronzo RA, Heine RJ, Henry RR, et al. (2007) Impaired fasting glucose and impaired glucose tolerance implications for care. Diabetes Care 30: 753–759.
19. McEvoy M, Smith W, D'Este C, Duke J, Peel R, et al. (2010) Cohort profile: The Hunter Community Study. International journal of epidemiology 39: 1452–1463.
20. Dillman DA (1978) Mail and telephone surveys: Wiley New York.
21. Wallace TM, Levy JC, Matthews DR (2004) Use and abuse of HOMA modeling. Diabetes Care 27: 1487–1495.
22. Health N, Council MR (2009) Australian guidelines to reduce health risks from drinking alcohol. NHMRC Canberra.
23. Islam MR, Arslan I, Attia J, McEvoy M, McElduff P, et al. (2013) Is Serum Zinc Level Associated with Prediabetes and Diabetes?: A Cross-Sectional Study from Bangladesh. PLoS One 8: e61776.
24. Rahim A, Iqbal K (2011) To assess the levels of zinc in serum and changes in the lens of diabetic and senile cataract patients. JPMA - Journal of the Pakistan Medical Association 61: 853–855.
25. Ekmekcioglu C, Prohaska C, Pomazal K, Steffan I, Schernthaner G, et al. (2001) Concentrations of seven trace elements in different hematological matrices in patients with type 2 diabetes as compared to healthy controls. Biological Trace Element Research 79: 205–219.
26. Zargar AH, Shah NA, Masoodi SR, Laway BA, Dar FA, et al. (1998) Copper, zinc, and magnesium levels in non-insulin dependent diabetes mellitus. Postgraduate Medical Journal 74: 665–668.
27. Schuhmacher M, Domingo J, Corbella J (1994) Zinc and copper levels in serum and urine: relationship to biological, habitual and environmental factors. Science of the total environment 148: 67–72.
28. Usha D, Girish H, Venugopal PM, Pratibha D, Archana S, et al. (2009) Zinc Deficiency: Descriptive Epidemiology and Morbidity among Preschool Children in Peri-urban Population in Delhi, India. Journal of Health Population and Nutrition 27: 632–639.
29. Wessells KR, Brown KH (2012) Estimating the Global Prevalence of Zinc Deficiency: Results Based on Zinc Availability in National Food Supplies and the Prevalence of Stunting. PLoS One 7: e50568.
30. Nriagu J (2010) Zinc deficiency in human health. Encyclopedia of Environmental Health: 789–800.
31. Olivares M, Pizarro F, Ruz M (2007) New insights about iron bioavailability inhibition by zinc. Nutrition 23: 292–295.
32. Wiernsperger N, Rapin J (2010) Trace elements in glucometabolic disorders: an update. Wiernsperger and Rapin Diabetology & Metabolic Syndrome 2.
33. Hashemipour M, Kelishadi R, Shapouri J, Sarrafzadegan N, Amini M, et al. (2009) Effect of zinc supplementation on insulin resistance and components of the metabolic syndrome in prepubertal obese children. Hormones (Athens) 8: 279–285.
34. Marreiro DN, Geloneze B, Tambascia MA, Lerário AC, Halpern A, et al. (2004) Participation of zinc in insulin resistance. Arquivos Brasileiros de Endocrinologia & Metabologia 48: 234–239.
35. Singh RB, Niaz MA, Rastogi SS, Bajaj S, Gaoli Z, et al. (1998) Current zinc intake and risk of diabetes and coronary artery disease and factors associated with insulin resistance in rural and urban populations of North India. Journal of the American College of Nutrition 17: 564–570.
36. Ognjanovic S, Jacobs DR, Steinberger J, Moran A, Sinaiko AR (2012) Relation of chemokines to BMI and insulin resistance at ages 18–21. Int J Obes (Lond).
37. Ferrannini E, Natali A, Bell P, Cavallo-Perin P, Lalic N, et al. (1997) Insulin resistance and hypersecretion in obesity. European Group for the Study of Insulin Resistance (EGIR). J Clin Invest 100: 1166–1173.
38. Trirogoff ML, Shintani A, Himmelfarb J, Ikizler TA (2007) Body mass index and fat mass are the primary correlates of insulin resistance in nondiabetic stage 3–4 chronic kidney disease patients. Am J Clin Nutr 86: 1642–1648.
39. Ferrannini E, Camastra S, Gastaldelli A, Sironi AM, Natali A, et al. (2004) Beta-Cell Function in Obesity Effects of Weight Loss. Diabetes 53: S26–S33.
40. Bergman BC, Perreault L, Hunerdosse D, Kerege A, Playdon M, et al. (2012) Novel and reversible mechanisms of smoking-induced insulin resistance in humans. Diabetes 61: 3156–3166.
41. DeFronzo RA, Ferrannini E (1991) Insulin resistance: a multifaceted syndrome responsible for NIDDM, obesity, hypertension, dyslipidemia, and atherosclerotic cardiovascular disease. Diabetes Care 14: 173–194.
42. Forrer R, Gautschi K, Lutz H (2001) Simultaneous measurement of the trace elements Al, As, B, Be, Cd, Co, Cu, Fe, Li, Mn, Mo, Ni, Rb, Se, Sr, and Zn in human serum and their reference ranges by ICP-MS. Biological Trace Element Research 80: 77–93.
43. Lee J-H, Kim JH (2012) Comparison of serum zinc levels measured by inductively coupled plasma mass spectrometry in preschool children with febrile and afebrile seizures. Annals of laboratory medicine 32: 190–193.

16

Metabolic Side-Effects of the Novel Second-Generation Antipsychotic Drugs Asenapine and Iloperidone

Heidi N. Boyda[1], Ric M. Procyshyn[2,3], Catherine C. Y. Pang[1], Erin Hawkes[1], Daniel Wong[1], Chen Helen Jin[1], William G. Honer[2,3], Alasdair M. Barr[1,3]*

1 Department of Anesthesiology, Pharmacology and Therapeutics, University of British Columbia, Vancouver, British Columbia, Canada, **2** Department of Psychiatry, University of British Columbia, Vancouver, British Columbia, Canada, **3** British Columbia Mental Health and Addictions Services, British Columbia Mental Health and Addictions Research Institute, Vancouver, British Columbia, Canada

Abstract

Background: The second generation antipsychotic (SGA) drugs are widely used in psychiatry due to their clinical efficacy and low incidence of neurological side-effects. However, many drugs in this class cause deleterious metabolic side-effects. Animal models accurately predict metabolic side-effects for SGAs with known clinical metabolic liability. We therefore used preclinical models to evaluate the metabolic side-effects of glucose intolerance and insulin resistance with the novel SGAs asenapine and iloperidone for the first time. Olanzapine was used as a comparator.

Methods: Adults female rats were treated with asenapine (0.01, 0.05, 0.1, 0.5, 1.0 mg/kg), iloperidone (0.03, 0.5, 1.0, 5.0, 10.0 mg/kg) or olanzapine (0.1, 0.5, 1.5, 5.0, 10.0 mg/kg) and subjected to the glucose tolerance test (GTT). Separate groups of rats were treated with asenapine (0.1 and 1.0 mg/kg), iloperidone (1.0 and 10 mg/kg) or olanzapine (1.5 and 15 mg/kg) and tested for insulin resistance with the hyperinsulinemic-euglycemic clamp (HIEC).

Results: Asenapine showed no metabolic effects at any dose in either test. Iloperidone caused large and significant glucose intolerance with the three highest doses in the GTT, and insulin resistance with both doses in the HIEC. Olanzapine caused significant glucose intolerance with the three highest doses in the GTT, and insulin resistance with the higher dose in the HIEC.

Conclusions: In preclinical models, asenapine shows negligible metabolic liability. By contrast, iloperidone exhibits substantial metabolic liability, comparable to olanzapine. These results emphasize the need for appropriate metabolic testing in patients treated with novel SGAs where current clinical data do not exist.

Editor: Frederick G. Hamel, Omaha Veterans Affairs Medical Center, United States of America

Funding: The current research was supported by grants from the British Columbia Provincial Health Services Authority and NSERC grant 356069-09 to AMB, and NSERC grant 355912-11 to CCYP. AMB is a CIHR New Investigator and HNB is a CIHR Banting scholar. The funders had no role in study design, data collection and analysis, decision to publish, or preparation of the manuscript.

Competing Interests: Dr. Procyshyn has received consulting and lectures fees from AstraZeneca, Bristol-Myers Squibb, Janssen, Sunovion, Pfizer, Otsuka. Dr. Honer has received consulting fees or sat on paid advisory boards for Novartis, Roche Canada and the Canadian Agency for Drugs and Technology in Health; and has received royalties for the licenses of antibody manufacturers from the University of British Columbia. Dr. Barr is on the advisory board or received consulting fees from Roche Canada and Eli Lilly Canada; and received educational grant support from BMS Canada. All other authors reported no biomedical financial interests or potential conflicts of interest.

* E-mail: albarr@interchange.ubc.ca

Introduction

The second generation antipsychotic (SGA) drugs represent the preferred choice of pharmacological treatment for schizophrenia. Many SGAs are also approved for additional indications, and are widely used off-label for other psychiatric disorders [1]. Despite the lower incidence of extrapyramidal side-effects with SGAs compared to their predecessors, over the last decade it has become clear that the majority of SGAs are associated with substantial unwanted side-effects. These side-effects are predominantly metabolic disturbances which include the components of metabolic syndrome [2–5]: weight-gain, adiposity, hyperlipidemia, glucose intolerance and insulin resistance. Pharmacological interventions, such as anti-diabetic drugs, may be only partly successful in reversing metabolic changes [6,7], leaving those with SGA drug-induced metabolic side-effects at substantially increased risk of developing cardiovascular disease and Type 2 Diabetes Mellitus (DM) [8,9], resulting in increased morbidity and mortality.

However, within the SGA class, there is considerable variation with regards to metabolic liability [10–12]. This has been most commonly assessed by weight-gain. Numerous studies have confirmed a continuum of metabolic liability, with the drugs clozapine and olanzapine causing greatest weight-gain, through intermediate effects with drugs including risperidone and quetiapine, to least weight-gain with ziprasidone and aripiprazole. Importantly, even the latter drugs are not body-weight-neutral, as weight-gain is greater than with placebo [13], particularly in patients taking antipsychotic drugs for the first time [14]. Fewer studies have examined the effects of SGAs on glucose control and insulin resistance, likely due to the greater difficulty of such measurements. Nevertheless, the pattern resembles that for weight-gain, with greatest insulin resistance caused by clozapine and olanzapine, and least by ziprasidone and aripiprazole [15]. Considerable evidence indicates that the effects of SGAs on insulin resistance and other metabolic indices, such as dyslipidemia [16], are not simply due to drug-induced weight-gain. Studies have reported new-onset diabetes in the absence of obesity or substantial weight-gain in SGA-treated patients [17], while acute effects of SGAs in non-psychiatric subjects included rapid-onset glucose intolerance in the absence of major weight-gain [18–20].

The metabolic side-effects of SGAs have been modeled in preclinical rodent paradigms [21], using sophisticated techniques such as the glucose tolerance test and hyperinsulinemic-euglycemic clamp [22]. Acute and chronic studies of SGA-induced insulin resistance and glucose intolerance have largely replicated clinical findings. Furthermore, the animal models are strongly homologous with clinical data, as drugs with greater metabolic liability in humans exert stronger metabolic effects in the preclinical paradigms [16,23–31]. These models are therefore useful not only in helping to understand the biological basis of metabolic side-effects, but also in predicting such effects in novel antipsychotic drugs.

The two novel SGA drugs asenapine and iloperidone were both approved by the US Food and Drug Administration in 2009 for the treatment of schizophrenia [32]. While the clinical efficacy of these new drugs compared to placebo has been confirmed in registration trials, little is known about the metabolic side-effects of these compounds [12]. Some data are published regarding weight-gain, but to our knowledge, there has been no reported documentation of glucose intolerance and insulin resistance with these drugs, which are the core symptoms of Type 2 DM. Given the utility of preclinical models in predicting metabolic dysregulation caused by SGAs, we conducted a study of both glucose tolerance and insulin resistance with asenapine and iloperidone, using established procedures, across a wide range of doses. For reference, we concurrently measured metabolic dysregulation in animals treated with olanzapine, as this drug is known to reliably cause metabolic dysregulation.

Materials and Methods

Animals

Adult female Sprague-Dawley rats (250–275 g) from Charles River (Montreal, Canada) were habituated to the UBC colony for one week. Females are the preferred sex for rodent models of antipsychotic drug-induced metabolic dysregulation because they exhibit more consistent metabolic abnormalities than males [21,33,34]. Rats were pair-housed and maintained on a 12-hour light-dark cycle (lights on at 07:00hours) under ambient temperature (22±1°C), with food and water available *ad libitum*. Approval by the UBC Animal Care and Use Committee was established for all procedures; animals were treated in accordance with the NIH Guidelines for the Care and Use of Laboratory Animals [35].

Pharmacological Agents and Solutions

Antipsychotic drugs included asenapine [Sigma-Aldrich Inc., St. Louis, MO,], iloperidone and olanzapine [Toronto Research Chemicals Inc., Toronto, ON]. All dosing solutions were prepared daily. Asenapine was formulated in a vehicle composed of 0.9% saline with the addition of 10 μL 1 M hydrochloric acid; iloperidone and olanzapine were formulated in 50% polyethylene glycol 400, 40% distilled water and 10% ethanol (PEG solution) [36]. Antipsychotics were dissolved in a volume of 1 ml/kg. For clamp experiments, recombinant human insulin (Humulin R) [Eli Lily, Indianapolis, IN) and dextrose (50%) were formulated in 0.9% w/v saline. All other chemicals were of reagent grade.

Intraperitoneal Glucose Tolerance Test (IGTT) (see Fig. 1A for Sequence of Events)

All rats were given a baseline IGTT prior to drug administration, as described previously [26]. Briefly, animals were fasted overnight for 16±2 hours; the following morning animals were wrapped in a towel to minimize stress, and a drop of saphenous venous blood was procured with a 25-gauge needle for baseline blood glucose measurement. Subsequently, animals received a glucose challenge (1 g/kg/ml, i.p.) followed by repeated sampling of blood glucose readings every 15 min for two hours. Glucose measurements were determined by handheld glucometer (One Touch Ultra). Based on total glucose levels, rats were rank ordered and randomly matched to one of six treatment groups (vehicle or five different doses of asenapine [n = 8–9 per group]) the following week. There was always one week minimum duration between subsequent IGTTs.

For the asenapine IGTT, rats were fasted as above. Baseline blood glucose levels were measured, and then a single dose of asenapine (0.01, 0.05, 0.1, 0.5 or 1.0 mg/kg) or vehicle was administered by s.c. injection; each rat received only one dose. A second measurement of blood glucose was taken 30 minutes later, to assess drug treatment on fasting glucose levels. Subsequently, a saphenous blood draw using heparinized collecting tubes was performed to obtain plasma samples for analysis of insulin levels; extracted blood samples were centrifuged (10,000 RPM, 10 Min, 4°C) and samples stored at −80°C. Immediately afterwards, the IGTT commenced, whereby animals received a challenge injection of 1 g/ml/kg of glucose. Glucose levels were monitored and recorded every 15 minutes for two hours duration. Animal handlers were blinded to drug treatment. One week after the asenapine IGTT, rats received another baseline IGTT, for re-randomization for treatment with iloperidone the following week. Rats received either vehicle or iloperidone (0.03, 0.5, 1.0, 5.0 or 10.0 mg/kg). Following another baseline IGTT and re-randomization, rats received the final antipsychotic treatment with vehicle or olanzapine (0.1, 0.5, 1.5, 5.0 or 10.0 mg/kg).

Surgical Preparations for Hyperinsulinemic-Euglycemic Clamp (HIEC)

Rats were prepared for surgery under isoflurane anesthesia and pre-operative ketoprofen (5 mg/kg, s.c). Heparinized saline-filled polyethylene cannulae (PE50) were inserted into the right common carotid artery and both exterior jugular veins. The arterial cannula was used to sample blood for measurement of glucose levels and venous cannulae were used for the infusion of insulin and dextrose. All cannulae were tunneled subcutaneously to the nape of neck and exteriorized. Animals recovered for 24 hours prior to the HIEC: two animals did not make a full recovery and were excluded.

HIEC Procedures (see Fig. 1B for Sequence of Events)

Overnight fasted rats (16±2 hours) were habituated to the cage prior. The two venous cannulae were connected to auxiliary

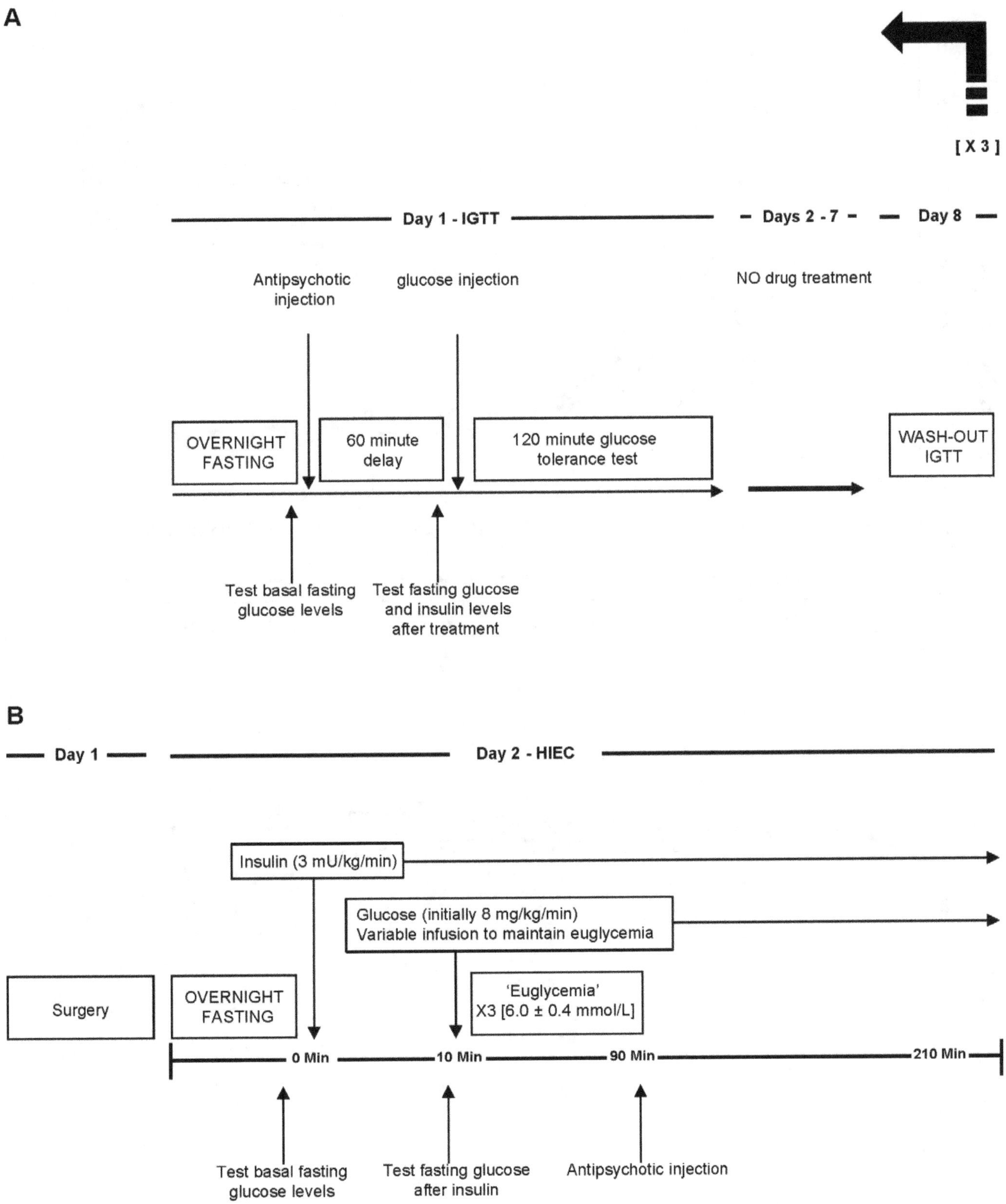

Figure 1. Experimental protocol. Describing (**A**) the intraperitoneal glucose tolerance test and (**B**) the hyperinsulinemic-euglycemic clamp with acute antipsychotic drug treatment.

heparinized saline-filled PE50 tubing, directly attached to infusion-only pumps (Harvard Apparatus, Holliston, MA). After a baseline blood glucose reading from the arterial cannula, insulin infusion (3 mU/kg/min) was initiated (t = 0 min) and kept running at

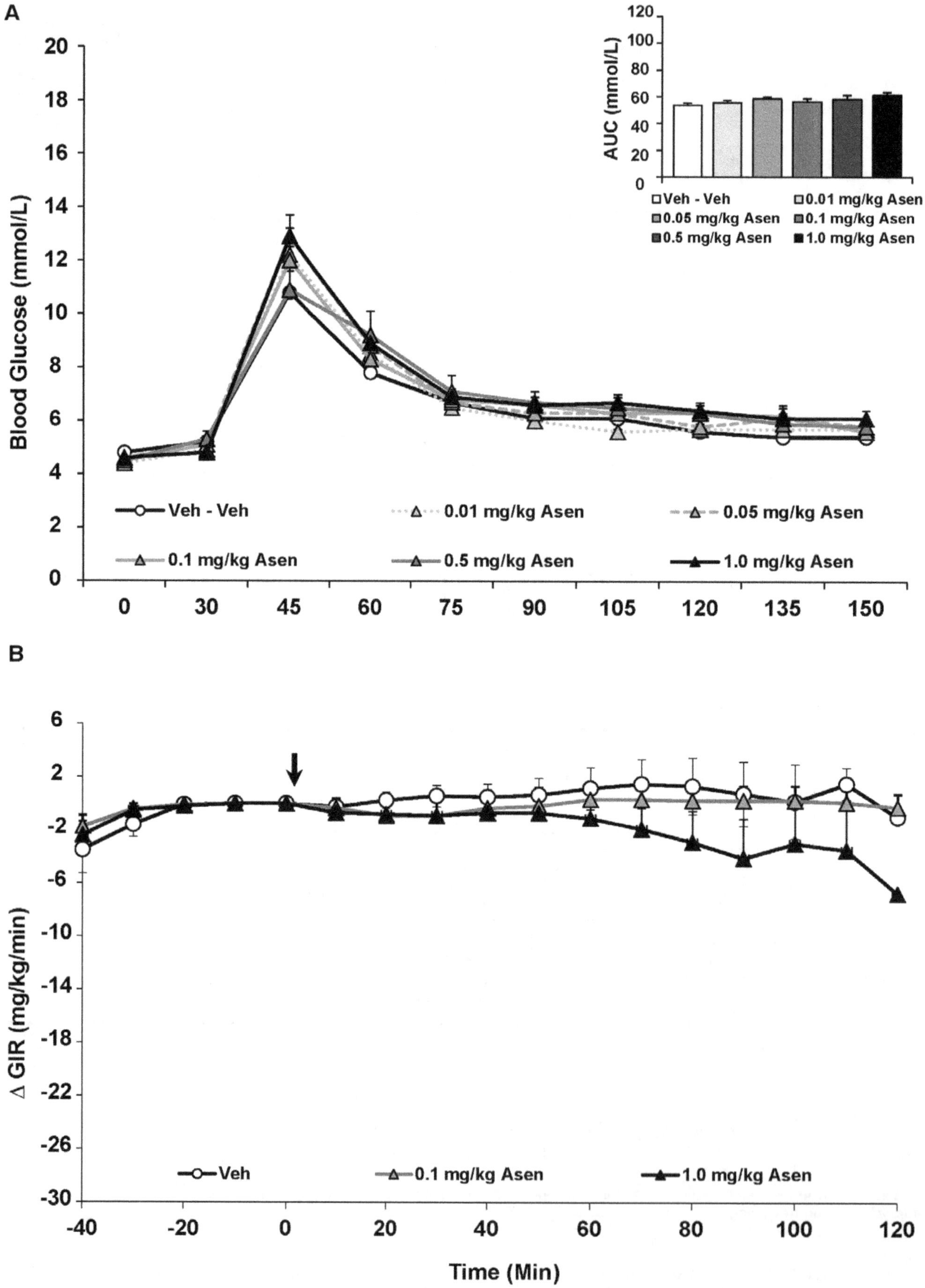
A
Blood Glucose (mmol/L)
AUC (mmol/L)
Veh - Veh
0.01 mg/kg Asen
0.05 mg/kg Asen
0.1 mg/kg Asen
0.5 mg/kg Asen
1.0 mg/kg Asen
B
Δ GIR (mg/kg/min)
Veh
0.1 mg/kg Asen
1.0 mg/kg Asen
Time (Min)

Figure 2. Acute effects of the antipsychotic drug asenapine on glucose levels in adult female rats. (**A**) Animals (n = 8–10 per group) received a single injection of vehicle or asenapine (0.01, 0.05, 0.1, 0.5, 1 mg/kg, s.c). Glucose levels were recorded prior to drug treatment in overnight-fasted rats at Time 0, and then 30 minutes following drug administration (*x-axis*). Immediately following this glucose measurement, all rats were subjected to a glucose tolerance test by receiving an intraperitoneal challenge injection of 1 mg/ml/kg of glucose, and blood glucose levels were measured every 15 minutes for the next two hours. Total cumulative glucose levels for each treatment group are summed as the "area under the curve" during the glucose tolerance test by graph inset (*top right*). Values represent group means ± SEM. (**B**) A separate cohort of animals (n = 6–8 per group) were fasted overnight and subjected to the hyperinsulinemic-euglycemic clamp. After animals reached euglycemia (three consecutive blood glucose readings of 6.0±0.4 mmol/L), rats were treated with vehicle, low (0.1 mg/kg) or high dose (1.0 mg/kg) asenapine (arrow at t = 0 min). Glucose levels were recorded every 10 minutes and the glucose infusion rate was adjusted as needed. Glucose infusion rates for each treatment group are presented as change in glucose infusion rate from euglycemia. Values represent group means ± SEM.

a constant rate for the entire experiment. Dextrose (50% w/v) infusion commenced at 8 mg/kg/min (0.96 ml/kg/hr) at t = 10 min and the glucose infusion rate (GIR) was adjusted as needed, every 10 minutes, to maintain glucose concentrations at 6.0 mmol/L. Euglycemia was determined when three consecutive blood glucose measurements presented 6.0±0.4 mmol/L at the same GIR. Animals then randomly received a single s.c injection of either vehicle or asenapine (0.1, 1.0 mg/kg), iloperidone (1.0, 10.0 mg/kg) or olanzapine (1.5, 15.0 mg/kg) [n = 5–7 per group], and the clamp was continued for 120 minute duration. The sample size of n = 5–7 animals per group is consistent with previously published studies [27,28]. Handlers were blinded to drug treatment.

Plasma Insulin Measurement by ELISA

Insulin levels were measured using the ultra-sensitive rat insulin ELISA kit (Crystal Chem Inc., IL, USA). Plasma samples (5 µl) were added and analyzed, in duplicate, on 96 well plates. Samples were incubated, followed by repeated washes. Substrate was added and absorbance measured at 450 nm –630 nm, as previously [37,38]. Calibrators were prepared and used to generate a calibration curve. A reference (non-fasted) animal's plasma added to all plates served as reference standard; confirming a high intra-plate reliability, with mean run-to-run correlations of 0.996 (range 0.994–0.999).

Insulin Resistance

Determination of insulin resistance in rats was accomplished using the homeostatic model assessment of insulin resistance (HOMA-IR) equation (1) [39]. The product of both the fasting levels of glucose (expressed as mmol/L) and insulin (µU/ml) 30 minutes post-drug administration is divided by a constant of 22.5. Greater insulin resistance is represented via a larger calculated HOMA-IR score.

$$(I_0 \times G_0) \div 22.5 \qquad (1)$$

where I_0 and G_0 are fasting insulinemia and glycaemia.

Statistical Analysis

Metabolic indices during the IGTT were analyzed by one-way analysis of variance (ANOVA), with drug dose as the between group factor. For the IGTT, glucose data were summed as the area-under-the-curve throughout the 120 minute procedure [36]. For the HIEC data, all drugs were included in the overall ANOVA, as the same vehicle group was use for all between-drug comparisons. Alpha value was set at $p<0.05$. LSD post-hoc tests were conducted when a main effect or interaction between main effects was significant. Data were analyzed with SPSS software, Chicago, IL, version 20.

Results

IGTT

Analysis of the IGTT with asenapine revealed no significant effect of drug treatment on fasting glucose levels or glucose intolerance following glucose challenge (Figure 2A). Interestingly, asenapine affected fasting insulin levels [$F_{(5,43)} = 3.03$, $p<0.05$], whereby the three lower doses of the drug *decreased* insulin levels compared to controls, although this was only significant for the lowest asenapine dose ($p<0.05$) (Table 1). Similarly, asenapine significantly affected insulin resistance [$F_{(5,43)} = 2.59$, $p<0.05$], measured by HOMA-IR, as insulin resistance was significantly reduced with the lowest asenapine dose (0.01 mg/kg) and a strong trend with the next two doses (0.05 and 0.1 mg/kg) (Table 1).

By contrast, while iloperidone had no effect on fasting glucose levels, it exhibited a strongly significant effect on glucose tolerance during the IGTT [$F_{(5,43)} = 13.06$, $p<0.0001$] (Figure 3A). Post-hoc analysis revealed a dose-dependent effect whereby the three highest doses of iloperidone (1.0, 5.0 and 10.0 mg/kg) increasingly elevated glucose intolerance compared to controls ($p<0.05$), with the two highest doses causing increased glucose intolerance compared to both controls and the three lower doses of the drug ($p<0.001$). There was manifest as a striking increase of 88% and 91% in glucose levels with the two highest doses of iloperidone compared to vehicle-treated rats. Regarding insulin, the ANOVA indicated a main effect of drug on fasting insulin levels [$F_{(5,43)} = 8.47$, $p<0.0001$] (Table 1), reflecting a dose-dependent elevation of insulin levels. Insulin was significantly higher than controls with the three highest doses of iloperidone ($p<0.05$). Similarly, HOMA-IR values also significantly increased by drug treatment [$F_{(5,43)} = 7.90$, $p<0.0001$] (Table 1), as the three highest doses of iloperidone induced greater insulin resistance compared to controls ($p<0.01$).

The effects of olanzapine on glucose metabolism were consistent with our previous findings [26,36]. There was no effect of olanzapine treatment on fasting glucose levels, but a strong effect on glucose tolerance in the IGTT [$F_{(5,43)} = 8.47$, $p<0.0001$] (Figure 4A). There was a dose-dependent effect of olanzapine, whereby the three higher doses increased glucose levels versus controls. This was highly significant for the 5 and 15 mg/kg doses ($p<0.001$), which increased glucose levels by 24% and 69% compared to controls. Olanzapine also significantly increased insulin levels [$F_{(5,43)} = 2.90$, $p<0.05$] (Table 1). All doses increased insulin levels: this was a trend for the 0.5 and 1.5 mg/kg doses ($p = 0.06$), while the two highest doses (5 and 10 mg/kg) caused larger increases ($p<0.01$). The effect of olanzapine on HOMA-IR values was a non-significant trend [$F_{(5,43)} = 2.05$, $p = 0.09$] to increase values. Importantly, values on the washout IGTT given the week after olanzapine treatment did not differ from the baseline IGTT values prior to SGA treatment, indicating that glucose tolerance did not change during the course of the study.

Table 1. Mean concentration of fasting glucose, insulin and HOMA-IR scores in antipsychotic drug treated rats.

Antipsychotic Drug	Measure	Treatment Dose (mg/kg)					
Asenapine		**0**	**0.01**	**0.05**	**0.1**	**0.5**	**1.0**
	G_0	5.1±0.3	4.9±0.3	5.1±0.2	5.0±0.1	5.4±0.4	4.8±0.2
	I_0	24.6±5.7	16.3±2.2*	21.7±3.0	20.4±3.1	29.7±4.4	33.3±3.5
	HOMA-IR	5.7±1.5	3.4±0.4*	4.9±0.7	4.5±0.7	7.2±1.3	7.2±1.0
Iloperidone		**0**	**0.03**	**0.5**	**1.0**	**5.0**	**10.0**
	G_0	4.6±0.2	4.9±0.2	4.6±0.2	4.9±0.2	5.1±0.2	5.2±0.3
	I_0	21.6±3.6	21.6±2.6	28.2±5.0	40.1±4.9*	44.9±3.6*	58.8±7.7*
	HOMA-IR	4.6±0.8	4.7±0.5	5.9±1.2	8.8±1.2*	10.2±0.8*	13.8±2.2*
Olanzapine		**0**	**0.1**	**0.5**	**1.5**	**5.0**	**15.0**
	G_0	5.0±0.2	5.3±0.2	5.3±0.3	5.7±0.3	5.2±0.2	5.0±0.2
	I_0	19.7±1.7	32.5±6.0	35.9±5.7	36.3±2.7	41.4±6.6*	47.8±5.8*
	HOMA-IR	4.5±0.5	7.8±1.5	8.7±1.6	9.2±1.1	9.6±1.5	10.8±1.5

I_0 = fasting insulin levels (µU/ml); G_0 = fasting glucose levels (mmol/L); HOMA-IR = homeostasis model assessment of insulin resistance (µU·mmol)/(ml·L).
Rats were treated with five separate doses of asenapine, iloperidone, olanzapine or vehicle. Values represented as means ± SEM at t = 30 min during the IGTT.
*indicates different from vehicle-treated animals, $p<0.05$.

HIEC

Average basal glucose levels were similar for all groups prior to euglycemia and administration of antipsychotic drugs. Insulin resistance during the HIEC is indicated by a reduction in the GIR, and therefore the primary analysis compared the effects of antipsychotics on GIR.

For the overall ANOVA, specific antipsychotic drug (asenapine, iloperidone, olanzapine or vehicle) and dose (vehicle, lower or higher dose) were represented by between-subjects factors. The results indicated significant main effects of both drug [$F_{(2,34)} = 12.76$, $p<0.0001$], dose [$F_{(2,34)} = 20.78$, $p<0.0001$] and a drug × dose interaction [$F_{(2,34)} = 2.93$, $p<0.05$]. Drug effects were evident as asenapine treatment, regardless of dose, had no effect on the GIR compared to vehicle-treated rats (Figure 2B). By contrast, both iloperidone and olanzapine, regardless of dose, significantly decreased the GIR compared to vehicle-treated rats ($p<0.01$) (Figure 3B & 4B). Furthermore, both iloperidone ($p<0.01$) and olanzapine ($p<0.05$) decreased GIR significantly more than asenapine. For iloperidone, both doses (1.0 and 10.0 mg/kg) caused significant decreases in the GIR. In both iloperidone dose groups this was evident by 30 mins post treatment, and by 40 mins the higher-dose group had a significantly lower GIR than the lower-dose group. In the olanzapine group, only the higher dose of the drug (15 mg/kg) significantly decreased infusion rate throughout the duration of the HIEC ($p<0.01$). The higher dose olanzapine group showed significantly decreased GIR compared to both controls and lower-dose animals within 30 mins of treatment. While the magnitude of the decrease in GIR was greater with iloperidone than olanzapine, this effect did not quite achieve statistical significance.

Discussion

In the present study, we assessed the metabolic side-effects of the novel SGA drugs asenapine and iloperidone for the first time, as well as olanzapine for reference. Two separate techniques were used to measure metabolic dysregulation, including both the glucose tolerance test and the hyperinsulinemic-euglycemic clamp. Consistent with previous preclinical studies, olanzapine caused dose-dependent glucose intolerance in the IGTT and insulin resistance in the clamp [26,27,40–47]. By contrast, the novel SGA drug asenapine was largely devoid of metabolic effects at the doses tested, causing only a slight reduction in insulin levels and HOMA-IR values with the lowest dose. In comparison, the novel SGA drug iloperidone showed potent dose-dependent effects on metabolic function. The three highest doses in the IGTT substantially increased glucose intolerance, to a greater degree than that observed with olanzapine. Similarly, both low- and high-dose iloperidone increased insulin resistance in the euglycemic clamp.

These overall findings reconfirm the powerful effect of the SGA olanzapine in animal models of glucose control and uptake, and demonstrate for the first time that similar-to-greater magnitude effects were observed with iloperidone, while asenapine shows minimal metabolic liability. The glucose tolerance test assesses glucose "intolerance" by measuring the capacity of the fasted subject to restore glucose levels to the normal range over time after a glucose challenge; this procedure is widely used in both clinical and preclinical studies of prediabetes and Type 2 DM [48]. The glucose tolerance test has been viewed positively for its physiological relevance and practicality in measuring metabolic side-effects in animals or humans, as it reflects how glucose will be controlled after a meal [49]. However, as both glucose and insulin levels are free to vary in this test, it is necessary to use "clamp" procedures, such as the hyperinsulinemic-euglycemic clamp, to confirm the presence of whole-body insulin resistance, which provides a specific measure of cell-mediated glucose uptake via the action of insulin. These procedures should be considered as complementary, and the high degree of correlation between them with the current results provides converging evidence for drug-specific metabolic liability. The only exception to this was in rats treated with the 1.5 mg/kg dose of olanzapine, where animals in the IGTT displayed significant glucose intolerance, but the same dose did not cause significant insulin resistance in the clamp. It is therefore possible that the IGTT is more sensitive at detecting SGA-induced metabolic dysregulation.

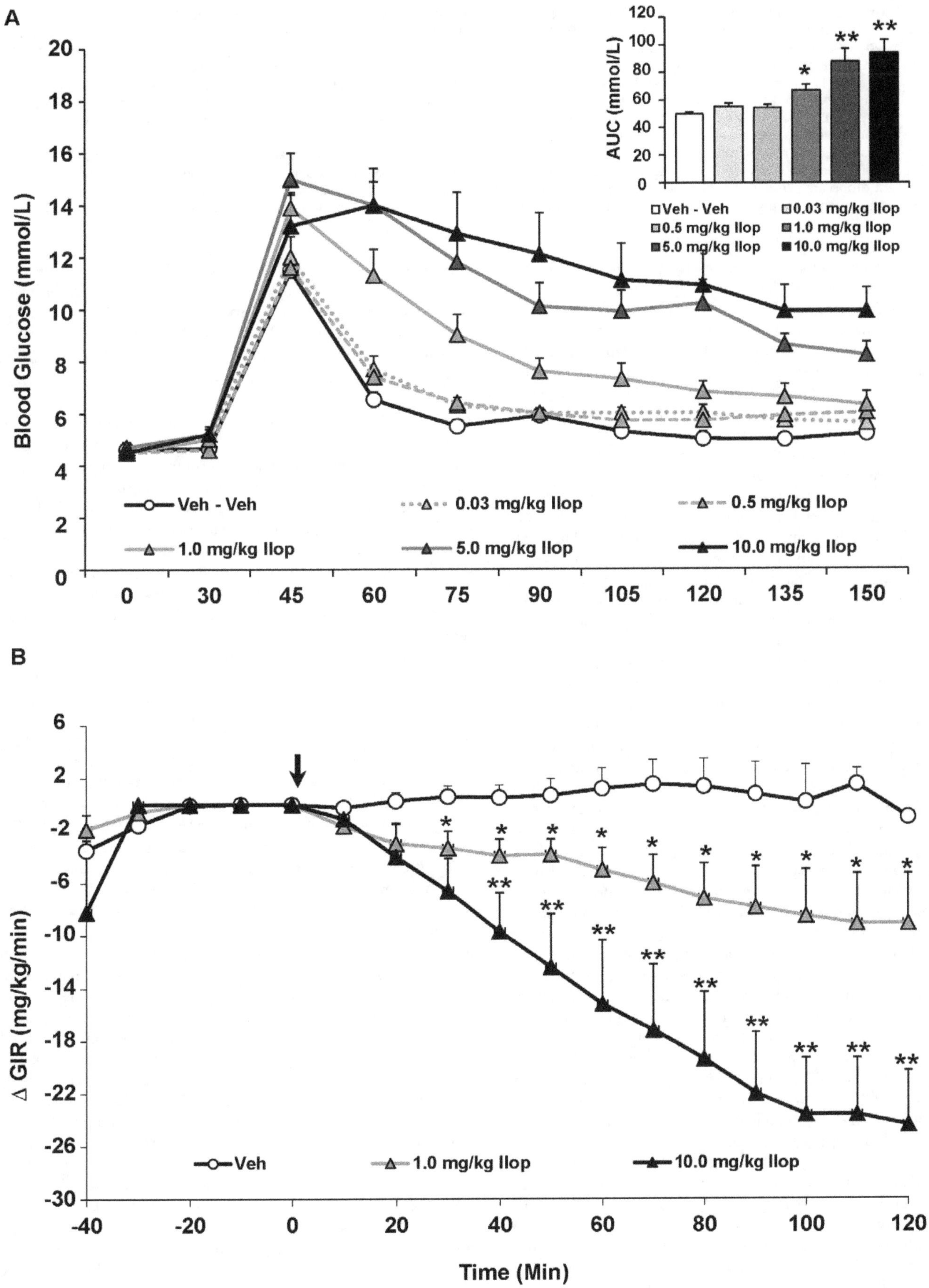
A
Blood Glucose (mmol/L)
AUC (mmol/L)
Veh - Veh
0.03 mg/kg Ilop
0.5 mg/kg Ilop
1.0 mg/kg Ilop
5.0 mg/kg Ilop
10.0 mg/kg Ilop
B
Δ GIR (mg/kg/min)
Veh
1.0 mg/kg Ilop
10.0 mg/kg Ilop
Time (Min)

Figure 3. Acute effects of the atypical antipsychotic drug iloperidone on glucose levels in adult female rats. (**A**) Animals (n = 8–10 per group) received a single injection of vehicle or iloperidone (0.03, 0.5, 1.0, 5.0, 10.0 mg/kg, s.c). Glucose levels were recorded prior to drug treatment in overnight-fasted rats at Time 0, and then 30 minutes following drug administration (*x-axis*). Immediately following this glucose measurement, all rats were subjected to a glucose tolerance test by receiving an intraperitoneal challenge injection of 1 mg/ml/kg of glucose, and blood glucose levels were measured every 15 minutes for the next two hours. Total cumulative glucose levels for each treatment group are summed as the "area under the curve" during the glucose tolerance test by graph inset (*top right*). Values represent group means ± SEM. * indicates different from vehicle-treated animals, $p<0.05$; ** indicates different from vehicle and 0.03–1.0 mg/kg iloperidone-treated animals, $p<0.01$ (**B**). A separate cohort of animals (n = 6–8 per group) were fasted overnight and subjected to the hyperinsulinemic-euglycemic clamp. After animals reached euglycemia (three consecutive blood glucose readings of 6.0±0.4 mmol/L), rats were treated with vehicle, low (1.0 mg/kg) or high dose (10.0 mg/kg) iloperidone (arrow at t = 0 min). Glucose levels were recorded every 10 minutes and the glucose infusion rate was adjusted as needed. Glucose infusion rates for each treatment group are presented as change in glucose infusion rate from euglycemia Values represent group means ± SEM. * indicates different from vehicle-treated animals, $p<0.05$; ** indicates different from vehicle and 1.0 mg/kg iloperidone-treated animals, $p<0.05$.

As noted above, numerous studies have previously reported metabolic dysregulation following both acute and chronic treatment with olanzapine. We recently reported that rats treated daily with olanzapine for ten weeks showed no change in the magnitude of glucose intolerance in the IGTT compared to their first challenge with the drug [36], indicating that acute treatment with SGAs can model chronic drug-treatment effects. However, to our knowledge, there are no studies of glucose intolerance or insulin resistance with the SGAs asenapine and iloperidone, in either animals or humans. Clinically, in three short-term phase 3 trials of iloperidone for schizophrenia, non-fasting glucose levels in all three dose ranges were significantly increased compared to placebo-treated subjects, whereas the risperidone comparator group did not differ from placebo [50]. Both risperidone- and iloperidone-treated subjects exhibited significant weight-gain versus placebo. A separate 28 day clinical trial of iloperidone in head-to-head comparison with ziprasidone noted greater weight-gain in the iloperidone arm [51], with 21% of iloperidone subjects (versus 7% of ziprasidone and 3% of placebo) displaying clinically significant weight-gain. Changes in glucose levels, which were not specified with regards to fasting status, were 7.9 mg/dL for iloperidone versus 4.7 mg/dL for ziprasidone. An analysis of three long-term safety trials of iloperidone, with haloperidol as comparator, noted both greater weight-gain and increases in glucose levels at six weeks and 52 weeks following treatment in the iloperidone group [52]. Thus, clinical data suggest that both fasting and non-fasting glucose levels are increased by iloperidone, compared to other antipsychotic drugs including risperidone, ziprasidone and haloperidol, none of which may be considered high metabolic risk. However, data from preclinical studies with SGAs indicate that fasting levels of glucose in the absence of a glucose challenge may underestimate loss of glycemic control. For example, in the present study, fasting glucose levels were not increased by any of the SGAs, yet for two drugs severe glucose intolerance was observed when the glucose challenge was applied.

There are a larger number of studies that have reported the effects of asenapine on weight-gain and fasting glucose levels, in both schizophrenia and bipolar disorder, although a full summary of these findings is beyond the scope of the present discussion. Asenapine causes less weight-gain and glucose elevation than olanzapine [53–55]. When compared head-to-head against haloperidol, neither drug caused significant weight-gain versus placebo, and fasting glucose abnormalities were actually marginally lower in the two doses of asenapine than in the haloperidol-treated group [56]. A short term study of asenapine only, with no comparator, for psychosis in the elderly reported a non-significant decrease in the number of subjects meeting criteria for metabolic syndrome compared to baseline [57]. Clinical data therefore indicate minimal effects of asenapine on weight-gain and fasting glucose. Similarly, preclinical evidence indicates that the antipsychotic drug sulpiride may also have negligible effects on glycemic control and may even improve glucose clearance in female rats. Compared to both control and risperidone-treated animals, sulpiride administration was associated with a 13% reduction in the area under the curve for the GTT, despite increased body weight gain [33].

A potential issue regarding the current findings is the choice of SGA doses, as metabolic effects can be dose-dependent [58]. Clinical studies can compare metabolic side-effects between antipsychotic drugs at doses of equivalent clinical efficacy, using standardized measures such as chlorpromazine equivalency [59–61]. This is not possible in animal models, and so "head-to-head" comparison between drugs represents a theoretical challenge, despite its common practice. It has been suggested that dosing based on dopamine D_2 receptor occupancy may represent one strategy, but issues remain regarding route of administration and inconsistent effects for all SGAs [62]. We chose our current dosing based on the behavioral effects of drugs in preclinical screens and models of schizophrenia. Behavioral effects in the latter share some homology with clinical symptomatology in humans [63]. Previous behavioral paradigms with asenapine in rats have shown potent antipsychotic-like effects below a dose of 0.2 mg/kg. Franberg and colleagues reported improvement in the conditioned avoidance response task with doses from 0.05–0.2 mg/kg [64] while doses from 0.01–0.075 mg/kg reversed phencyclidine (PCP)-induced deficits in a novel object recognition task [65]. Marston and colleagues demonstrated that 0.03 mg/kg asenapine reversed low-dose amphetamine hyperactivity, while 0.1 mg/kg reversed high-dose amphetamine hyperactivity [66]. In the same study, 0.03–0.1 mg/kg asenapine reversed apomorphine-induced deficits in prepulse inhibition (PPI) of the acoustic startle reflex. Thus, the 100-fold dose range in the current study more than encompasses the dosing required to produce behavioral effects, and the total absence of metabolic effects at doses as high as 0.5 and 1.0 mg/kg strongly indicates the metabolic liability of asenapine is low at behaviorally relevant doses. Regarding iloperidone, an initial report observed behavioral effects at doses between 0.7–5.2 mg/kg [67] while Barr and colleagues reported that both 1.0 and 3.0 mg/kg iloperidone reversed apomorphine-induced PPI deficits [68]. However, 3.0 mg/kg of iloperidone did not reverse the effects on PPI of 1.5 mg/kg of PCP, which is a dose commonly used to screen for antipsychotics, indicating that higher doses of iloperidone would have been needed to demonstrate antipsychotic efficacy. By comparison, 10 mg/kg olanzapine robustly reversed PPI deficits caused by 1.5 mg/kg PCP [69], implying that both iloperidone and olanzapine may be reasonably well-matched dose-wise in the current study. The clinically approved daily dose of iloperidone for psychosis is 12–24 mg [32], while olanzapine is 10–20 mg [70] and therefore very similar. Thus, the greater glucose intolerance and insulin resistance caused by iloperidone versus olanzapine at similar doses

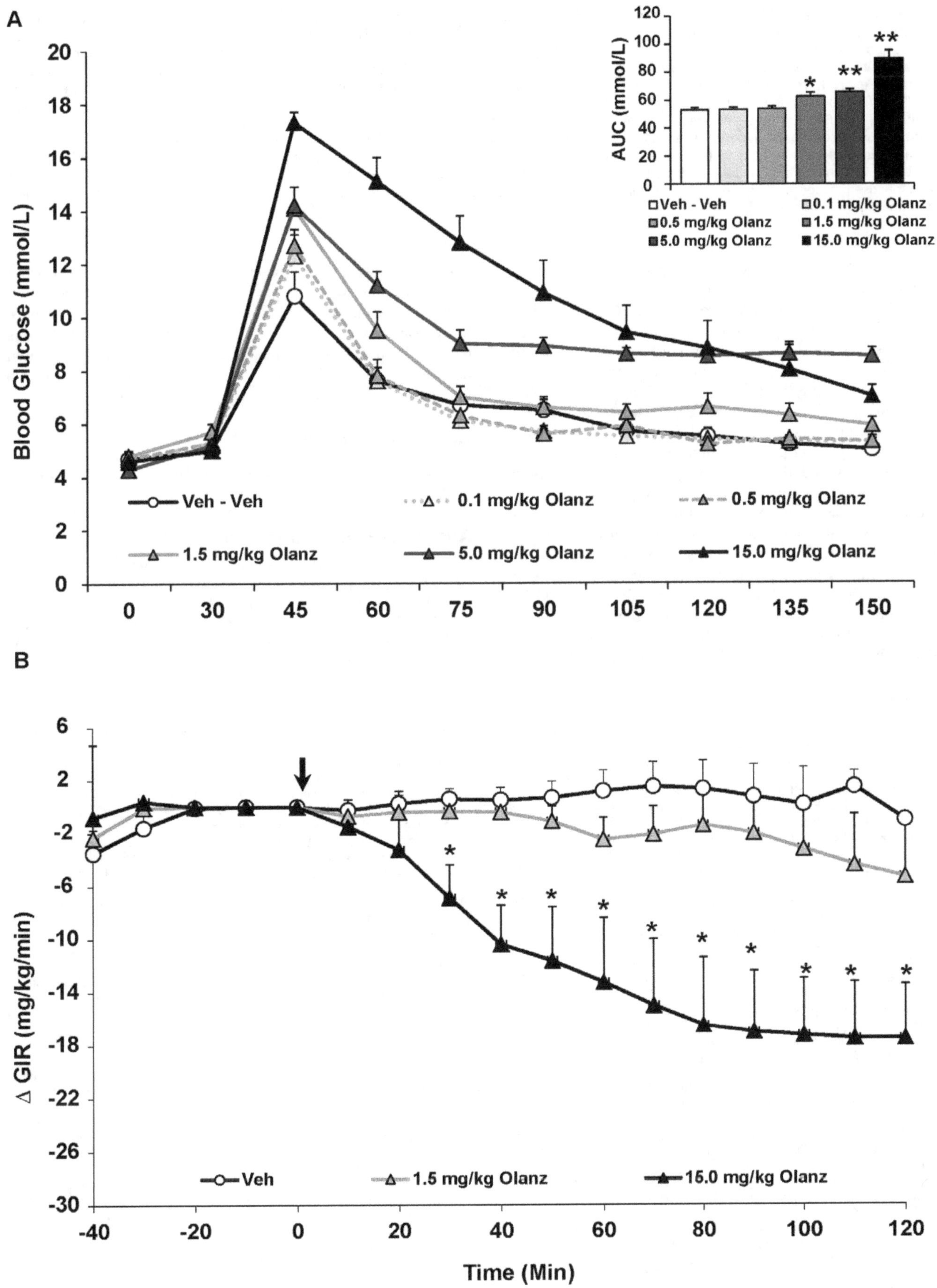
A
Blood Glucose (mmol/L)
AUC (mmol/L)
*
**
**
Veh - Veh
0.1 mg/kg Olanz
0.5 mg/kg Olanz
1.5 mg/kg Olanz
5.0 mg/kg Olanz
15.0 mg/kg Olanz
B
Δ GIR (mg/kg/min)
Veh
1.5 mg/kg Olanz
15.0 mg/kg Olanz
Time (Min)

Figure 4. Acute effects of the atypical antipsychotic drug olanzapine on glucose levels in adult female rats. (**A**) Animals (n = 8–10 per group) received a single injection of vehicle or olanzapine (0.1, 0.5, 1.5, 5.0, 15.0 mg/kg, s.c). Glucose levels were recorded prior to drug treatment in overnight-fasted rats at Time 0, and then 30 minutes following drug administration (*x-axis*). Immediately following this glucose measurement, all rats were subjected to a glucose tolerance test by receiving an intraperitoneal challenge injection of 1 mg/ml/kg of glucose, and blood glucose levels were measured every 15 minutes for the next two hours. Total cumulative glucose levels for each treatment group are summed as the "area under the curve" during the glucose tolerance test by graph insets (*top right*). Values represent group means ± SEM. * indicates different from vehicle-treated animals, $p<0.05$; ** indicates different from vehicle-treated animals, $p<0.01$ (**B**). A separate cohort of animals (n = 6–8 per group) were fasted over-night and subjected to the hyperinsulinemic-euglycemic clamp. After animals reached euglycemia (three consecutive blood glucose readings of 6.0±0.4 mmol/L), rats were treated with vehicle, low (1.5 mg/kg) or high dose (15.0 mg/kg) olanzapine (arrow at t = 0 min). Glucose levels were recorded every 10 minutes and the glucose infusion rate was adjusted as needed. Glucose infusion rates for each treatment group are presented as change in glucose infusion rate from euglycemia. Values represent group means ± SEM. * indicates different from vehicle and low-dose olanzapine-treated animals, $p<0.05$.

(e.g. 5 mg/kg) indicates that iloperidone may have acute metabolic effects at least as strong as olanzapine.

The results of the current study strongly suggest that metabolic testing of patients treated with novel SGAs is warranted. Although, like numerous preclinical studies, the current results were based on acute treatment without weight-gain, there is an increasing body of evidence demonstrating weight-independent and drug-specific effects on glucose intolerance and insulin resistance. Results from the Clinical Antipsychotic Trial of Intervention Effectiveness (CATIE) study observed that 42.7% of patients treated with SGAs had metabolic dysregulation [71]. When controlling for Body Mass Index, CATIE men were 85% and CATIE women 137% more likely to have metabolic syndrome than the normal population. Newcomer and colleagues used the glucose tolerance test in adiposity-matched patients to show that those treated with SGAs had greater glucose elevations than patients treated with first generation drugs [72]. Importantly, in the first double-blind, placebo-controlled crossover trial, it was recently demonstrated that acute 3-day treatment of normals with 10 mg of olanzapine caused significant impairments in the glucose tolerance test [18]. The glucose area-under-the-curve increased by 42%, which is highly consistent with our present findings in rats. Future clinical evaluation of glucose intolerance and insulin resistance in novel SGA-treated patients should therefore remain a priority, using techniques specifically designed to challenge metabolic regulation, despite the greater difficulty of using such protocols, given the long-term health implications for loss of glycemic control.

Acknowledgments

We acknowledge the technical assistance of Su-Lin Lim in the euglycemic clamp experiments.

Author Contributions

Conceived and designed the experiments: HNB RMP CCYP EH DW CHJ WGH AMB. Performed the experiments: HNB RMP CCYP EH DW CHJ WGH AMB. Analyzed the data: HNB RMP CCYP EH DW CHJ WGH AMB. Contributed reagents/materials/analysis tools: HNB RMP CCYP EH DW CHJ WGH AMB. Wrote the paper: HNB RMP CCYP EH DW CHJ WGH AMB.

References

1. Procyshyn RM, Honer WG, Wu TK, Ko RW, McIsaac SA, et al. (2010) Persistent antipsychotic polypharmacy and excessive dosing in the community psychiatric treatment setting: a review of medication profiles in 435 Canadian outpatients. J Clin Psychiatry 71: 566–573.
2. Gohlke JM, Dhurandhar EJ, Correll CU, Morrato EH, Newcomer JW, et al. (2012) Recent advances in understanding and mitigating adipogenic and metabolic effects of antipsychotic drugs. Front Psychiatry 3: 62.
3. Procyshyn RM, Wasan KM, Thornton AE, Barr AM, Chen EY, et al. (2007) Changes in serum lipids, independent of weight, are associated with changes in symptoms during long-term clozapine treatment. J Psychiatry Neurosci 32: 331–338.
4. Newcomer JW (2007) Antipsychotic medications: metabolic and cardiovascular risk. J Clin Psychiatry 68 Suppl 4: 8–13.
5. Henderson DC (2008) Managing weight gain and metabolic issues in patients treated with atypical antipsychotics. J Clin Psychiatry 69: e04.
6. Baptista T, Rangel N, El Fakih Y, Uzcategui E, Galeazzi T, et al. (2009) Rosiglitazone in the assistance of metabolic control during olanzapine administration in schizophrenia: a pilot double-blind, placebo-controlled, 12-week trial. Pharmacopsychiatry 42: 14–19.
7. Carrizo E, Fernandez V, Connell L, Sandia I, Prieto D, et al. (2009) Extended release metformin for metabolic control assistance during prolonged clozapine administration: a 14 week, double-blind, parallel group, placebo-controlled study. Schizophr Res 113: 19–26.
8. Leung JY, Barr AM, Procyshyn RM, Honer WG, Pang CC (2012) Cardiovascular side-effects of antipsychotic drugs: the role of the autonomic nervous system. Pharmacol Ther 135: 113–122.
9. Liao CH, Chang CS, Wei WC, Chang SN, Liao CC, et al. (2011) Schizophrenia patients at higher risk of diabetes, hypertension and hyperlipidemia: a population-based study. Schizophr Res 126: 110–116.
10. Baptista T, ElFakih Y, Uzcategui E, Sandia I, Talamo E, et al. (2008) Pharmacological management of atypical antipsychotic-induced weight gain. CNS Drugs 22: 477–495.
11. Rummel-Kluge C, Komossa K, Schwarz S, Hunger H, Schmid F, et al. (2010) Head-to-head comparisons of metabolic side effects of second generation antipsychotics in the treatment of schizophrenia: A systematic review and meta-analysis. Schizophr Res.
12. Gallego JA, Nielsen J, De Hert M, Kane JM, Correll CU (2012) Safety and tolerability of antipsychotic polypharmacy. Expert Opin Drug Saf 11: 527–542.
13. Citrome L (2007) Risk-benefit analysis of available treatments for schizophrenia. Psychiatric Times 1: 27–30.
14. Kahn RS, Fleischhacker WW, Boter H, Davidson M, Vergouwe Y, et al. (2008) Effectiveness of antipsychotic drugs in first-episode schizophrenia and schizophreniform disorder: an open randomised clinical trial. Lancet 371: 1085–1097.
15. Chaggar PS, Shaw SM, Williams SG (2011) Effect of antipsychotic medications on glucose and lipid levels. J Clin Pharmacol 51: 631–638.
16. Skrede S, Ferno J, Vazquez MJ, Fjaer S, Pavlin T, et al. (2012) Olanzapine, but not aripiprazole, weight-independently elevates serum triglycerides and activates lipogenic gene expression in female rats. Int J Neuropsychopharmacol 15: 163–179.
17. Newcomer JW (2005) Second-generation (atypical) antipsychotics and metabolic effects: a comprehensive literature review. CNS Drugs 19 Suppl 1: 1–93.
18. Albaugh VL, Singareddy R, Mauger D, Lynch CJ (2011) A double blind, placebo-controlled, randomized crossover study of the acute metabolic effects of olanzapine in healthy volunteers. PLoS One 6: e22662.
19. Vidarsdottir S, de Leeuw van Weenen JE, Frolich M, Roelfsema F, Romijn JA, et al. (2010) Effects of olanzapine and haloperidol on the metabolic status of healthy men. J Clin Endocrinol Metab 95: 118–125.
20. Sacher J, Mossaheb N, Spindelegger C, Klein N, Geiss-Granadia T, et al. (2008) Effects of olanzapine and ziprasidone on glucose tolerance in healthy volunteers. Neuropsychopharmacology 33: 1633–1641.
21. Boyda HN, Tse L, Procyshyn RM, Honer WG, Barr AM (2010) Preclinical models of antipsychotic drug-induced metabolic side effects. Trends Pharmacol Sci 31: 484–497.
22. Hahn M, Chintoh A, Giacca A, Xu L, Lam L, et al. (2011) Atypical antipsychotics and effects of muscarinic, serotonergic, dopaminergic and histaminergic receptor binding on insulin secretion in vivo: an animal model. Schizophr Res 131: 90–95.
23. Davey KJ, O'Mahony SM, Schellekens H, O'Sullivan O, Bienenstock J, et al. (2012) Gender-dependent consequences of chronic olanzapine in the rat: effects on body weight, inflammatory, metabolic and microbiota parameters. Psychopharmacology (Berl) 221: 155–169.
24. Weston-Green K, Huang XF, Deng C (2012) Alterations to melanocortinergic, GABAergic and cannabinoid neurotransmission associated with olanzapine-induced weight gain. PLoS One 7: e33548.
25. Smith GC, Chaussade C, Vickers M, Jensen J, Shepherd PR (2008) Atypical antipsychotic drugs induce derangements in glucose homeostasis by acutely

increasing glucagon secretion and hepatic glucose output in the rat. Diabetologia 51: 2309–2317.
26. Boyda HN, Tse L, Procyshyn RM, Wong D, Wu TK, et al. (2010) A parametric study of the acute effects of antipsychotic drugs on glucose sensitivity in an animal model. Prog Neuropsychopharmacol Biol Psychiatry 34: 945–954.
27. Houseknecht KL, Robertson AS, Zavadoski W, Gibbs EM, Johnson DE, et al. (2007) Acute effects of atypical antipsychotics on whole-body insulin resistance in rats: implications for adverse metabolic effects. Neuropsychopharmacology 32: 289–297.
28. Chintoh AF, Mann SW, Lam L, Giacca A, Fletcher P, et al. (2009) Insulin resistance and secretion in vivo: Effects of different antipsychotics in an animal model. Schizophr Res 108: 127–133.
29. Jassim G, Skrede S, Vazquez MJ, Wergedal H, Vik-Mo AO, et al. (2011) Acute effects of orexigenic antipsychotic drugs on lipid and carbohydrate metabolism in rat. Psychopharmacology (Berl).
30. Ferno J, Vik-Mo AO, Jassim G, Havik B, Berge K, et al. (2009) Acute clozapine exposure in vivo induces lipid accumulation and marked sequential changes in the expression of SREBP, PPAR, and LXR target genes in rat liver. Psychopharmacology (Berl) 203: 73–84.
31. Weston-Green K, Huang XF, Deng C (2011) Olanzapine treatment and metabolic dysfunction: a dose response study in female Sprague Dawley rats. Behav Brain Res 217: 337–346.
32. Citrome L (2011) Iloperidone, asenapine, and lurasidone: a brief overview of 3 new second-generation antipsychotics. Postgrad Med 123: 153–162.
33. Baptista T, Araujo de Baptista E, Ying Kin NM, Beaulieu S, Walker D, et al. (2002) Comparative effects of the antipsychotics sulpiride or risperidone in rats. I: bodyweight, food intake, body composition, hormones and glucose tolerance. Brain Res 957: 144–151.
34. Weston-Green K, Huang XF, Deng C (2010) Sensitivity of the female rat to olanzapine-induced weight gain–far from the clinic? Schizophr Res 116: 299–300.
35. National Research Council (US) (2011) Committee for the Guide for the Care and Use of Laboratory Animals. Washington (DC): National Academies Press. 8th Edition.
36. Boyda HN, Procyshyn RM, Tse L, Wong D, Pang CC, et al. (2012) Intermittent treatment with olanzapine causes sensitization of the metabolic side-effects in rats. Neuropharmacology 62: 1391–1400.
37. Barr AM, Fish KN, Markou A, Honer WG (2008) Heterozygous reeler mice exhibit alterations in sensorimotor gating but not presynaptic proteins. Eur J Neurosci 27: 2568–2574.
38. Barr AM, Young CE, Sawada K, Trimble WS, Phillips AG, et al. (2004) Abnormalities of presynaptic protein CDCrel-1 in striatum of rats reared in social isolation: relevance to neural connectivity in schizophrenia. Eur J Neurosci 20: 303–307.
39. Mather K (2009) Surrogate measures of insulin resistance: of rats, mice, and men. Am J Physiol Endocrinol Metab 296: E398–399.
40. Boyda HN, Procyshyn RM, Tse L, Hawkes E, Jin CH, et al. (In Press) Differential effects of 3 classes of antidiabetic drugs on olanzapine-induced glucose dysregulation and insulin resistance in female rats. J Psychiatry Neurosci 37: 110140.
41. Albaugh VL, Henry CR, Bello NT, Hajnal A, Lynch SL, et al. (2006) Hormonal and metabolic effects of olanzapine and clozapine related to body weight in rodents. Obesity (Silver Spring) 14: 36–51.
42. Chintoh AF, Mann SW, Lam L, Lam C, Cohn TA, et al. (2008) Insulin resistance and decreased glucose-stimulated insulin secretion after acute olanzapine administration. J Clin Psychopharmacol 28: 494–499.
43. Martins PJ, Haas M, Obici S (2011) Central nervous system delivery of the antipsychotic olanzapine induces hepatic insulin resistance. Diabetes 59: 2418–2425.
44. Smith GC, Vickers MH, Shepherd PR (2011) Olanzapine effects on body composition, food preference, glucose metabolism and insulin sensitivity in the rat. Arch Physiol Biochem.
45. Victoriano M, Hermier D, Even PC, Fromentin G, Huneau JF, et al. (2009) Early perturbation in feeding behaviour and energy homeostasy in olanzapine-treated rats. Psychopharmacology (Berl) 206: 167–176.
46. Cooper GD, Pickavance LC, Wilding JP, Halford JC, Goudie AJ (2005) A parametric analysis of olanzapine-induced weight gain in female rats. Psychopharmacology (Berl) 181: 80–89.
47. Patil BM, Kulkarni NM, Unger BS (2006) Elevation of systolic blood pressure in an animal model of olanzapine induced weight gain. Eur J Pharmacol 551: 112–115.
48. Monzillo LU, Hamdy O (2003) Evaluation of insulin sensitivity in clinical practice and in research settings. Nutr Rev 61: 397–412.
49. Muniyappa R, Lee S, Chen H, Quon MJ (2008) Current approaches for assessing insulin sensitivity and resistance in vivo: advantages, limitations, and appropriate usage. Am J Physiol Endocrinol Metab 294: E15–26.
50. Weiden PJ, Cutler AJ, Polymeropoulos MH, Wolfgang CD (2008) Safety profile of iloperidone: a pooled analysis of 6-week acute-phase pivotal trials. J Clin Psychopharmacol 28: S12–19.
51. Cutler AJ, Kalali AH, Weiden PJ, Hamilton J, Wolfgang CD (2008) Four-week, double-blind, placebo- and ziprasidone-controlled trial of iloperidone in patients with acute exacerbations of schizophrenia. J Clin Psychopharmacol 28: S20–28.
52. Kane JM, Lauriello J, Laska E, Di Marino M, Wolfgang CD (2008) Long-term efficacy and safety of iloperidone: results from 3 clinical trials for the treatment of schizophrenia. J Clin Psychopharmacol 28: S29–35.
53. McIntyre RS, Cohen M, Zhao J, Alphs L, Macek TA, et al. (2010) Asenapine for long-term treatment of bipolar disorder: a double-blind 40-week extension study. J Affect Disord 126: 358–365.
54. Buchanan RW, Panagides J, Zhao J, Phiri P, den Hollander W, et al. (2012) Asenapine versus olanzapine in people with persistent negative symptoms of schizophrenia. J Clin Psychopharmacol 32: 36–45.
55. McIntyre RS, Cohen M, Zhao J, Alphs L, Macek TA, et al. (2009) A 3-week, randomized, placebo-controlled trial of asenapine in the treatment of acute mania in bipolar mania and mixed states. Bipolar Disord 11: 673–686.
56. Kane JM, Cohen M, Zhao J, Alphs L, Panagides J (2011) Efficacy and safety of asenapine in a placebo- and haloperidol-controlled trial in patients with acute exacerbation of schizophrenia. J Clin Psychopharmacol 30: 106–115.
57. Dubovsky SL, Frobose C, Phiri P, Greef R, Panagides J (2011) Short-term safety and pharmacokinetic profile of asenapine in older patients with psychosis. Int J Geriatr Psychiatry.
58. Simon V, van Winkel R, De Hert M (2009) Are weight gain and metabolic side effects of atypical antipsychotics dose dependent? A literature review. J Clin Psychiatry 70: 1041–1050.
59. Barr AM, Honer WG, Johnson JL, Wu TK, Procyshyn RM (2010) A comparison of antipsychotic drug-defined daily doses versus chlorpromazine equivalent doses in patients with or without extrapyramidal motor symptoms. J Clin Psychopharmacol 30: 741–743.
60. Barr AM, Procyshyn RM, Hui P, Johnson JL, Honer WG (2008) Self-reported motivation to smoke in schizophrenia is related to antipsychotic drug treatment. Schizophr Res 100: 252–260.
61. Barr AM, Panenka WJ, Honer WG, Khara S, Procyshyn RM (2011) Excessive antipsychotic dosing in a Canadian outpatient population. Psychiatr Serv 62: 682–683.
62. Kapur S, VanderSpek SC, Brownlee BA, Nobrega JN (2003) Antipsychotic dosing in preclinical models is often unrepresentative of the clinical condition: a suggested solution based on in vivo occupancy. J Pharmacol Exp Ther 305: 625–631.
63. Braff DL, Geyer MA, Swerdlow NR (2001) Human studies of prepulse inhibition of startle: normal subjects, patient groups, and pharmacological studies. Psychopharmacology (Berl) 156: 234–258.
64. Franberg O, Wiker C, Marcus MM, Konradsson A, Jardemark K, et al. (2008) Asenapine, a novel psychopharmacologic agent: preclinical evidence for clinical effects in schizophrenia. Psychopharmacology (Berl) 196: 417–429.
65. Snigdha S, Idris N, Grayson B, Shahid M, Neill JC (2011) Asenapine improves phencyclidine-induced object recognition deficits in the rat: evidence for engagement of a dopamine D1 receptor mechanism. Psychopharmacology (Berl) 214: 843–853.
66. Marston HM, Young JW, Martin FD, Serpa KA, Moore CL, et al. (2009) Asenapine effects in animal models of psychosis and cognitive function. Psychopharmacology (Berl) 206: 699–714.
67. Strupczewski JT, Bordeau KJ, Chiang Y, Glamkowski EJ, Conway PG, et al. (1995) 3-[[(Aryloxy)alkyl]piperidinyl]-1,2-benzisoxazoles as D2/5-HT2 antagonists with potential atypical antipsychotic activity: antipsychotic profile of iloperidone (HP 873). J Med Chem 38: 1119–1131.
68. Barr AM, Powell SB, Markou A, Geyer MA (2006) Iloperidone reduces sensorimotor gating deficits in pharmacological models, but not a developmental model, of disrupted prepulse inhibition in rats. Neuropharmacology 51: 457–465.
69. Bakshi VP, Geyer MA (1995) Antagonism of phencyclidine-induced deficits in prepulse inhibition by the putative atypical antipsychotic olanzapine. Psychopharmacology (Berl) 122: 198–201.
70. Mitchell M, Riesenberg R, Bari MA, Marquez E, Kurtz D, et al. (2006) A double-blind, randomized trial to evaluate the pharmacokinetics and tolerability of 30 or 40 mg/d oral olanzapine relative to 20 mg/d oral olanzapine in stable psychiatric subjects. Clin Ther 28: 881–892.
71. McEvoy JP, Meyer JM, Goff DC, Nasrallah HA, Davis SM, et al. (2005) Prevalence of the metabolic syndrome in patients with schizophrenia: baseline results from the Clinical Antipsychotic Trials of Intervention Effectiveness (CATIE) schizophrenia trial and comparison with national estimates from NHANES III. Schizophr Res 80: 19–32.
72. Newcomer JW, Haupt DW, Fucetola R, Melson AK, Schweiger JA, et al. (2002) Abnormalities in glucose regulation during antipsychotic treatment of schizophrenia. Arch Gen Psychiatry 59: 337–345.

Direct Inhibitory Effects of Pioglitazone on Hepatic Fetuin-A Expression

Akinobu Ochi[1], Katsuhito Mori[1]*, Masanori Emoto[1], Shinya Nakatani[1], Tomoaki Morioka[1], Koka Motoyama[1], Shinya Fukumoto[1], Yasuo Imanishi[1], Hidenori Koyama[2], Eiji Ishimura[1], Masaaki Inaba[1]

1 Department of Metabolism, Endocrinology and Molecular Medicine, Osaka City University Graduate School of Medicine, Osaka, Japan, **2** Department of Internal Medicine, Division of Endocrinology and Metabolism, Hyogo College of Medicine, Nishinomiya, Japan

Abstract

Fetuin-A, a circulating glycoprotein synthesized in the liver, is involved in insulin resistance and type 2 diabetes. However, regulation of fetuin-A synthesis has remained obscure. We previously reported that pioglitazone treatment significantly reduced serum fetuin-A levels in patients with type 2 diabetes. To clarify whether pioglitazone can directory inhibit hepatic fetuin-A synthesis, we investigated the effects of pioglitazone on fetuin-A expression both in vitro and in vivo. Pioglitazone treatment suppressed mRNA and protein expression of fetuin-A in Fao hepatoma cells. Interestingly, rosiglitazone but not metformin, also inhibited fetuin-A expression. In addition, GW 9662, an inhibitor of peroxisome proliferator-activated receptor (PPAR) γ, reversed pioglitazone-induced suppression of fetuin-A, suggesting that thiazolidinedione derivatives may have common characteristics with regard to fetuin-A suppression, possibly through PPARγactivation. Finally, oral administration of pioglitazone to mice for 8 weeks resulted in suppression of hepatic fetuin-A mRNA. These findings suggest that pioglitazone may partially ameliorate insulin resistance through its direct inhibitory effects on fetuin-A expression in the liver.

Editor: Jean-Marc A. Lobaccaro, Clermont Université, France

Funding: This study was supported, in part, by a Grant-in-Aid for Scientific Research (C) (No.25461250) from the Japan Society for the Promotion of Science (to Mori). No additional funding was received for this study. The funders had no role in study design, data colletion and analysis, decision to publish, or preparation of the manuscript.

Competing Interests: The authors declare no conflict of interest associated with this manuscript.

* E-mail: ktmori@med.osaka-cu.ac.jp

Introduction

Fetuin-A (alpha-2-HS-glycoprotein; AHSG) is mainly synthesized in the liver and has multiple functions in human physiology and pathology [1,2]. Among them, fetuin-A known as one of most important hepatokines [3] is involved in insulin resistance and type 2 diabetes, although its precise role is poorly understood. Cross-sectional studies have demonstrated a positive correlation between fetuin-A levels and insulin resistance [4]. Prospective studies also have shown that high fetuin-A levels predict the incidence of type 2 diabetes [5] [6]. As one of its mechanisms, both in vitro and in vivo studies have suggested a direct inhibitory effect of fetuin-A on insulin receptor autophosphorylation, which alters downstream signaling [7]. In addition, a recent report has made a breakthrough in this area. It is well known that free fatty acids (FFAs) stimulate secretion of proinflammatory cytokines from adipocytes through Toll-like receptor 4 (TLR4), resulting in insulin resistance [8]. However, it remained obscure how FFAs can induce adipose tissue inflammation, since FFAs appear to not bind to TLR4 directly [9]. Facing such criticism, Pal and Dasgupta et al. clearly demonstrated that fetuin-A acts as an adaptor protein between FFAs and TLR4 [10]. These findings suggest that fetuin-A may amplify insulin resistance through this pathway. In response, Stefan et al. reported the probability that an interaction between FFAs and fetuin-A could induce insulin resistance in humans [11]. Therefore, although the regulation of fetuin-A synthesis is incompletely understood, fetuin-A is an attractive target for the development of novel diabetes treatments.

Pioglitazone, one of thiazolidinedione derivatives, is an established insulin-sensitizing agent used by patients with type 2 diabetes. Its unique action is predominantly exerted through peroxisome proliferator-activated receptor (PPAR) γin adipocytes [12]. We previously reported that treatment with pioglitazone significantly reduced serum fetuin-A levels in patients with type 2 diabetes [13]. Intriguingly, other representative insulin-sensitizing therapies, such as metformin (500 mg/day or 750 mg/day) and aerobic exercise, did not affect fetuin-A levels [13], although it has been reported that high dose of metformin (2500 mg/day or 3000 mg/day) decreased plasma fetuin-A levels [14]. Therefore, fetuin-A-mediated improvement of insulin resistance is likely to be a particular property of pioglitazone. However, in the previous clinical study we could not conclude whether pioglitazone directly inhibited fetuin-A synthesis in the liver because the pleiotropic effects of pioglitazone on glucose and lipid metabolism [12] may have indirectly modulated fetuin-A levels.

To clarify the direct inhibitory effect of pioglitazone on fetuin-A synthesis, we examined the effects of pioglitazone on fetuin-A expression in cultured hepatocytes. We also investigated whether administration of pioglitazone to mice could suppress fetuin-A expression in the liver, resulting in decreased circulating fetuin-A levels.

Materials and Methods

Reagents

All cell culture plasticware was purchased from Becton, Dickinson and Company (NJ, USA). Pioglitazone hydrochloride, rosiglitazone, glimepiride, GW9662, and dimethyl sulfoxide (DMSO) were obtained from Wako Pure Chemical Industries Ltd. (Osaka, Japan). Metformin (1,1-dimethyl biguanide hydrochloride) was purchased from Sigma Aldrich (MO, USA).

Cell Culture

Rat hepatoma cells (Fao cells) were provided courtesy by Dr. Rohit N. Kulkarni (Joslin Diabetes Center, Boston, MA) [15]. Cells were cultured and maintained in RPMI-1640 medium (Invitrogen, CA, USA) supplemented with 10% heat-inactivated FBS (Invitrogen), 100 U/mL penicillin, and 100 µg/mL streptomycin (Invitrogen) in humidified air with 5% CO2 at 37°C [15]. The culture medium was replaced every 2 days. After cultures reached confluence, cells were serum-starved overnight and subsequently incubated for different periods (0, 6, 12, 18, and 24 h) and at different doses (0, 2, 5, and 10 mM) of pioglitazone. Similarly, cells were treated with or without rosiglitazone (10 µM), metformin (1 or 2 mM), or glimepiride (1, 5, or 10 µM) for 24 h. Cells were preincubated with GW9662 for 1 h before addition of pioglitazone.

RNA Isolation and Real-time Quantitative RT-PCR

RNA [2 µg, isolated from cells by using TRIzol Reagent (Invitrogen)] was used to synthesize cDNA by reverse transcription with the High Capacity cDNA Reverse Transcription Kit (Applied Biosystems, CA, USA) according to manufacturer's instructions. Expression of rat or mouse *Ahsg* mRNA, and 18S ribosomal RNA were measured quantitatively using the Taqman Real-Time PCR technique (Applied Biosystems). Ready-to-use primers for rat or mouse fetuin-A mRNA and 18S ribosomal RNA were purchased from Applied Biosystems (Taqman Gene Expression Assays) and used according to manufacturer's instructions. A cycle threshold (Ct) value was measured for each sample, and mRNA expression levels were determined by a comparative Ct method using 18S ribosomal RNA as endogenous control (Applied Biosystems) [16].

Western Blotting

After each treatment, the cells were washed twice with ice-cold buffer (137 mM NaCl, 1 mM $MgCl_2$, 1 mM $CaCl_2$, 0.1 mM Na_2VO_4, 20 mM Tris-HCl at pH 7.6) and lysed in the same buffer supplemented with 1% Nonidet P-40, 10% glycerol, 2 mM EDTA, 10 mM sodium pyrophosphate, 10 mM NaF, 2 mM Na_2VO_4, 2 mM phenylmethylsulfonyl fluoride, and 8 µg/mL leupeptin. After removal of insoluble materials, the protein concentration was determined using the BCA protein assay (Thermo Scientific, MI, USA). Cell lysates or culture supernatant medium (40 µg protein per lane) were mixed with a sample-loading buffer and separated on a 10% SDS-PAGE gel. Proteins were transferred to nitrocellulose membranes (GE Healthcare, Buckinghamshire, UK) and immunoblotted with rat fetuin-A antibody (Santa Cruz Biotechnology Inc, CA, USA) and α-tubulin antibody (Cell Signaling Technology, MA, USA) [17]. Protein bands were identified by ECL (GE Healthcare, NJ, USA) and quantified using a densitometer (Lumino Shot^{TM} 400Jr) (TAKARA Bio Inc, Shiga, Japan).

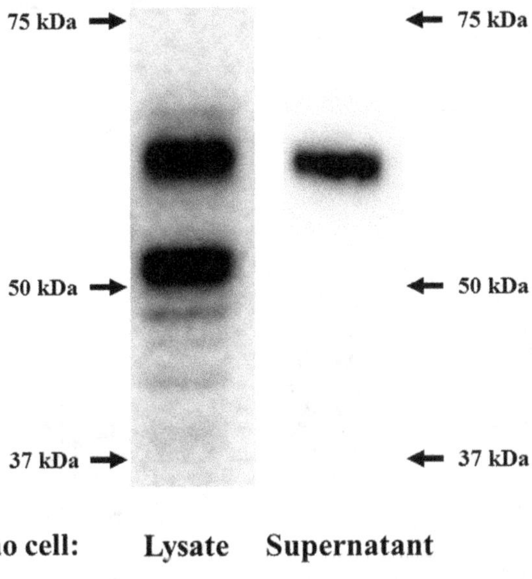

Figure 1. Fetuin-A expression in hepatocytes and its post-translational modifications. Lysates from Fao cells (left panel) and the supernatant from cultured Fao cells (right panel) were run on a 10% SDS-PAGE gel, transferred to a membrane, and probed using an anti-fetuin-A antibody.

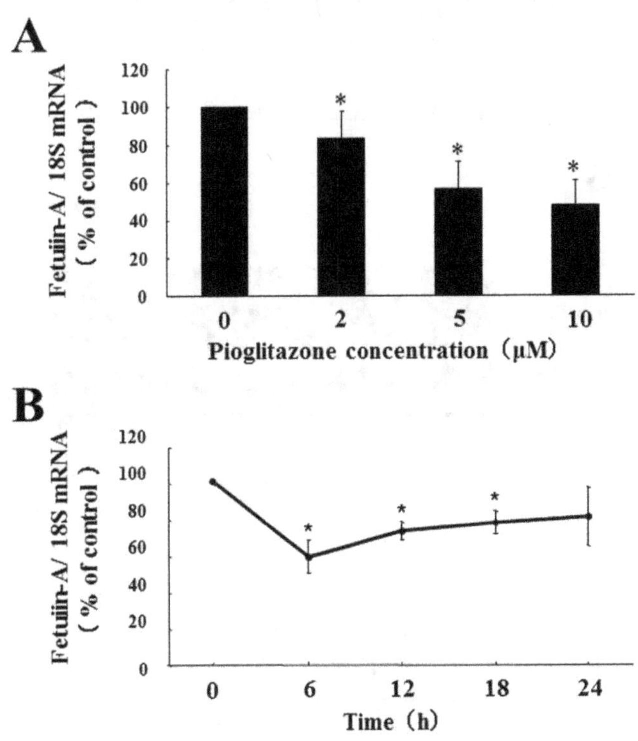

Figure 2. Effects of pioglitazone on expression of fetuin-A mRNA in Fao cells. Fao cells were treated with pioglitazone at different doses (0, 2, 5, and 10 µM for 24 h) (A) or for different periods (0, 6, 12, 18, and 24 h with 10 µM) (B). Total RNA was isolated from Fao cells treated with or without pioglitazone, and the levels of fetuin-A mRNA expression were determined using quantitative real-time RT-PCR. Levels of fetuin-A mRNA were determined using a comparative cycle threshold method, using 18S ribosomal RNA as endogenous reference, and fetuin-A mRNA levels without pioglitazone (A) or at 0 h (B) were defined as 100% (CTL). Mean ± SD were calculated from at least three independent experiments. *$P<0.05$ vs. CTL.

Animal Experiments

All procedures in this study were approved by the Animal Care and Use committee at the Osaka City University Graduate School of Medicine, Osaka, Japan [16]. Male C57BL/6J mice were maintained in a temperature-controlled (24°C) facility with a 12-h light/12-h dark cycle and fed a standard chow *ad libitum*. At 7 weeks, the mice were divided into a group bred with pioglitazone, delivered as a food admixture at 10 mg/kg/day, (Pio group: $n=6$) and a group bred without pioglitazone (CTL group: $n=6$). Mice were fed with the appropriate diet from 7 to 20 weeks of age. Body weight was monitored weekly. Blood glucose levels were also measured weekly using a portable glucose meter (Glu-test Sensor, Sanwa, Japan). At 20 weeks of age, mice were fasted overnight, and then sacrificed under the anesthesia with pentobarbital; liver tissues and blood samples were collected. Hepatic mRNA expression in CTL or Pio group was examined as mentioned above. Serum fetuin-A levels in CTL or Pio group were measured by enzyme-linked immunosorbent assay kit (Mouse fetuin-A/ AHSG ELISA kit, Adipo Bioscience, CA, USA).

Statistical Analysis

Each experiment was repeated at least thrice to confirm the results. All data are expressed as mean ± standard deviation (SD). Student's t-test was used for comparisons between two groups. Statistically significant differences among more than three groups were analyzed using ANOVA with post hoc analysis (Dunnet or Scheffe test). All analyses were performed using StatView 5 (SAS Institute Inc., Cary, NC, USA) designed for Windows. The level of statistical significance was set at $P<0.05$.

Results

Fetuin-A Expression in Hepatocytes and its Posttranslational Modification

Fetuin-A is known to be posttranslationally modified, including serine and threonine phosphorylations and glycosylations [7]. Therefore, the apparent molecular weight of fetuin-A on an immunoblot is approximately 60 kDa, which is much higher than deduced molecular weight based on the amino acid sequence. We

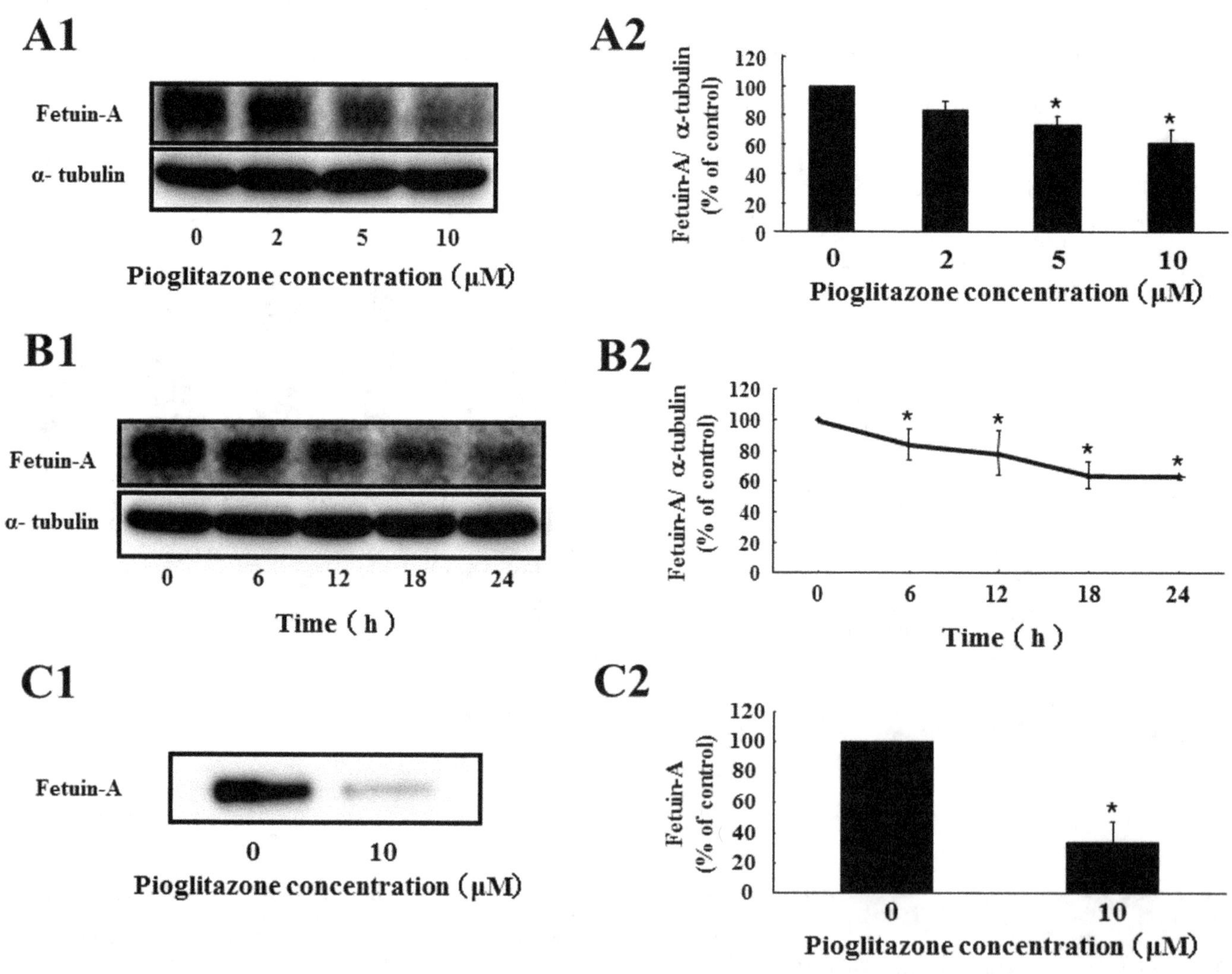

Figure 3. Effects of pioglitazone on fetuin-A protein expression in Fao cells. Fao cells were treated with pioglitazone at different doses (0, 2, 5, and 10 μM for 24 h) (A) or for different periods of time (0, 6, 12, 18, and 24 h with 10 μM) (B). Western blots of cell lysates from Fao cells treated with or without pioglitazone were probed with anti-fetuin-A antibody (A1) (B1). Fetuin-A protein levels were determined using α-tubulin as an endogenous reference, and fetuin-A levels without pioglitazone (A2) or at 0 h (B2) were defined as 100% (CTL). Western blots of Fao cell supernatants with or without 10 μM pioglitazone for 24 h were probed with anti-fetuin-A antibody (C1). Fetuin-A protein levels from experiments without pioglitazone were defined as 100% (CTL). Mean ± SD were calculated from at least three independent experiments. *$P<0.05$ vs. CTL.

detected two primary bands using a cell lysate from Fao cells (Fig. 1, left panel). The lower band may correspond to the endogenous fetuin-A protein before apparent modification. To confirm this, we transfected HEK 293 cells, which are believed not to have the ability to perform liver-specific posttranslational modification, with mouse fetuin-A (*Ahsg*) cDNA, provided courtesy by Dr. Jiang (Thomas Jefferson University, PA, USA) [18]. As expected, we observed only one band, which migrated at approximately 50 kDa in the immunoblot (data not shown). Next, culture medium from Fao cells was subjected to immunoblotting for fetuin-A. Only the upper band (60 kDa) was detected, suggesting that only fully modified fetuin-A is secreted from hepatocytes (Fig. 1, right panel).

Inhibitory Effects of Pioglitazone on both mRNA Expression and Protein Expression of Fetuin-A

To investigate whether pioglitazone can directly suppress fetuin-A expression in hepatocytes, we cultured Fao cells with or without pioglitazone. Pioglitazone downregulated fetuin-A mRNA expression (51.8% decrease by 10 μM pioglitazone for 24 h) in a dose-dependent manner (Fig. 2A). Pioglitazone (10 μM) significantly suppressed fetuin-A mRNA levels at 6 h (38.5% decrease) and maintained this suppression at 24 h (Fig. 2B). Next, we examined the effects of pioglitazone on fetuin-A protein expression in Fao cells and found that pioglitazone inhibited fetuin-A protein expression in dose- (Fig. 3 A1 and A2) and time- (Fig. 3 B1 and B2) dependent manner (38.8% decrease by 10 μM pioglitazone for 24 h). We also investigated whether pioglitazone decreased the levels of fetuin-A secreted into the cultured medium. As expected, pioglitazone strikingly suppressed fetuin-A secretion (66.3% decrease by 10 μM pioglitazone for 24 h) (Fig. 3 C1 and C2). These findings suggest that pioglitazone directly suppresses fetuin-A expression in heoatocytes and subsequently reduces secretion of posttranslationally modified fetuin-A.

Specificity of Pioglitazone-induced Fetuin-A Suppression

To examine the specificity of pioglitazone-induced fetuin-A suppression, we used rosiglitazone, another thiazolidinedione derivative. Rosiglitazone significantly suppressed fetuin-A protein expression (31.8% decrease by 10 μM rosiglitazone for 24 h) (Fig. 4A1 and 4A2). On the other hand, metformin, another insulin-sensitizing drug, did not affect fetuin-A expression (Fig. 4B1 and 4B2). In addition, the sulfonylurea glimepiride, a representative antidiabetic drug, had no effect on fetuin-A expression (data not shown). These findings suggest that pioglitazone-induced

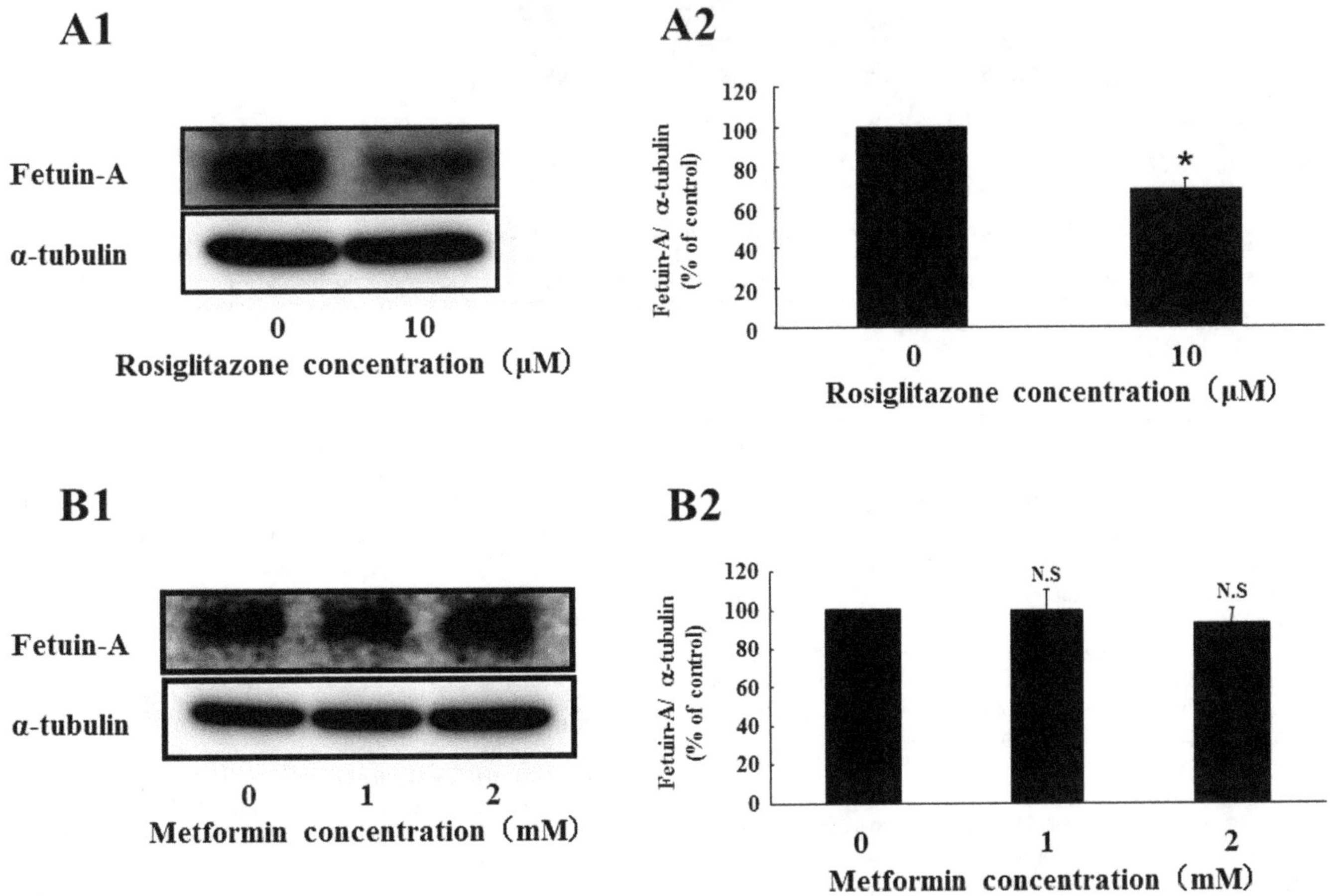

Figure 4. Effects of rosiglitazone or metformin on expression of fetuin-A protein in Fao cells. Fao cells were treated with rosiglitazone (0 and 10 μM) or metformin (0, 1, and 2 mM) for 24 h. Western blots of cell lysates from Fao cells treated without or with rosiglitazone or metformin were probed with anti-fetuin-A antibody (A1) (B1). Fetuin-A protein levels were determined using α-tubulin as an endogenous reference, and fetuin-A protein levels without rosiglitazne (A2) or metformin (B2) was defined as 100% (CTL). Mean ± SD were calculated from at least three independent experiments. $^{*}P<0.05$ vs. CTL.

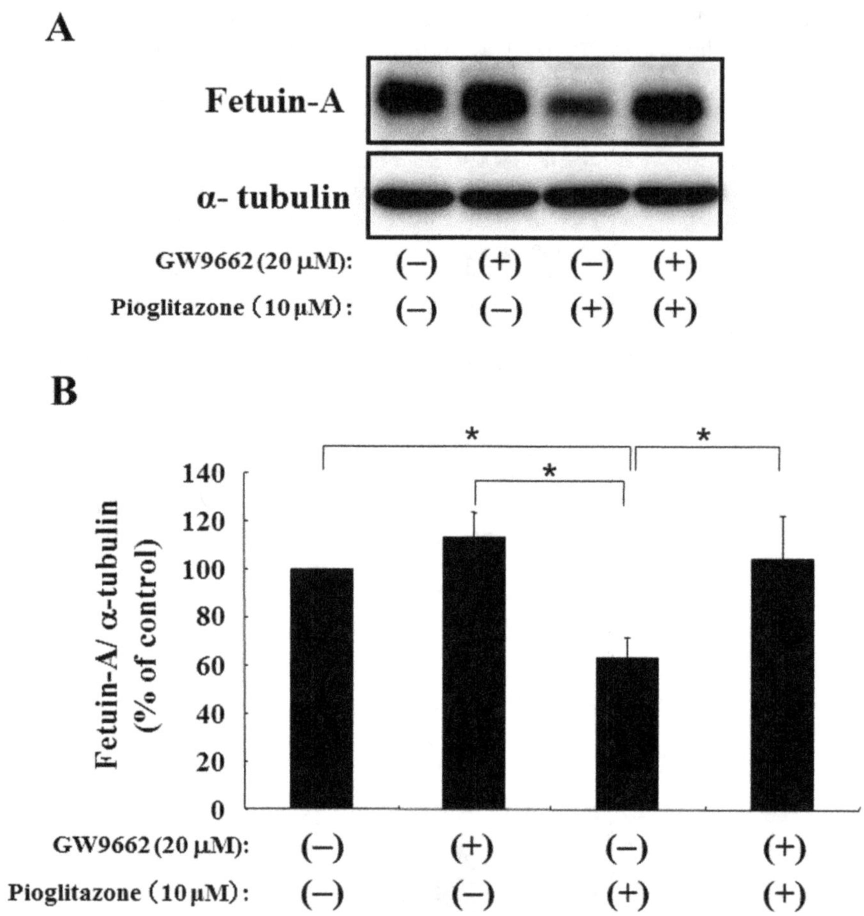

Figure 5. Effects of a PPARγ inhibitor (GW9662) on pioglitazone-induced suppression of fetuin-A in Fao cells. Fao cells were treated in the absence or presence of 10 μM pioglitazone for 24 h with or without 1-h preincubation with 20 μM GW9662, an inhibitor of PPARγ. Western blots of cell lysates from Fao cells were probed with anti-fetuin-A antibody (A). Fetuin-A protein levels were determined using α-tubulin as an endogenous reference, and the fetuin-A protein level without both pioglitazone and GW9662 was defined as 100% (CTL). Mean ± SD was calculated from at least three independent experiments. *$P<0.05$ between each group.

fetuin-A suppression may be a class effect of thiazolidinedione derivatives. However, it is not common in insulin-sensitizing drugs.

Involvement of PPARγ in Pioglitazone-induced Suppression of fetuin-A

To have better insight into the mechanism, we investigated whether pioglitazone-induced suppression operated through PPARγ, a receptor for thiazolidinedione derivatives. GW9662, an inhibitor of PPARγ, did not change fetuin-A expression significantly (Fig. 5A). Interestingly, treatment with GW9662 reversed pioglitazone-induced suppression of fetuin-A to non-treatment levels (Fig. 5B). These findings suggest that pioglitazone suppresses fetuin-A expression though PPARγ.

Effects of Pioglitazone on Hepatic Fetuin-A Expression and Serum Fetuin-A Level in Mice

To minimize the impact of metabolic disorders, such as diabetes, dyslipidemia, and hepatic steatosis, on fetuin-A levels, we administered pioglitazone to healthy mice and investigated its effects on hepatic fetuin-A expression and circulating fetuin-A levels in vivo. Pioglitazone treatment induced significant body weight gain from week 13 onward (Fig. 6 A1), but did not affect casual plasma glucose levels (Fig. 6 A2). Importantly, hepatic expression of fetuin-A mRNA in the Pio group was significantly suppressed compared with that in the CTL group (27.1% inhibition, $P<0.05$). On the other hand, although serum levels of fetuin-A in the Pio group tended to be lower than those in CTL group, the difference did not reach statistical significance (29.7 vs. 35.3 μg/mL, $P=0.253$).

Discussion

Because of the critical role of fetuin-A in insulin resistance and type 2 diabetes, it is imperative to clarify how fetuin-A synthesis is regulated. We previously reported that pioglitazone, but not metformin, reduced serum fetuin-A levels in patients with type 2 diabetes [13]. However, its regulatory mechanisms have been unclear. In this study, we first demonstrated the direct inhibitory effect of piogliazone on fetuin-A expression, through PPARγ activation, in cultured hepatocytes. We also found that piogliazone treatment significantly inhibited hepatic fetuin-A expression in mice.

Considering the pleiotropic effects of pioglitazone, several possibilities remain with regard to pioglitazone-induced suppression of fetuin-A. First, the involvement of hepatic steatosis should be considered because circulating fetuin-A levels were positively associated with liver fat content evaluated by proton magnetic

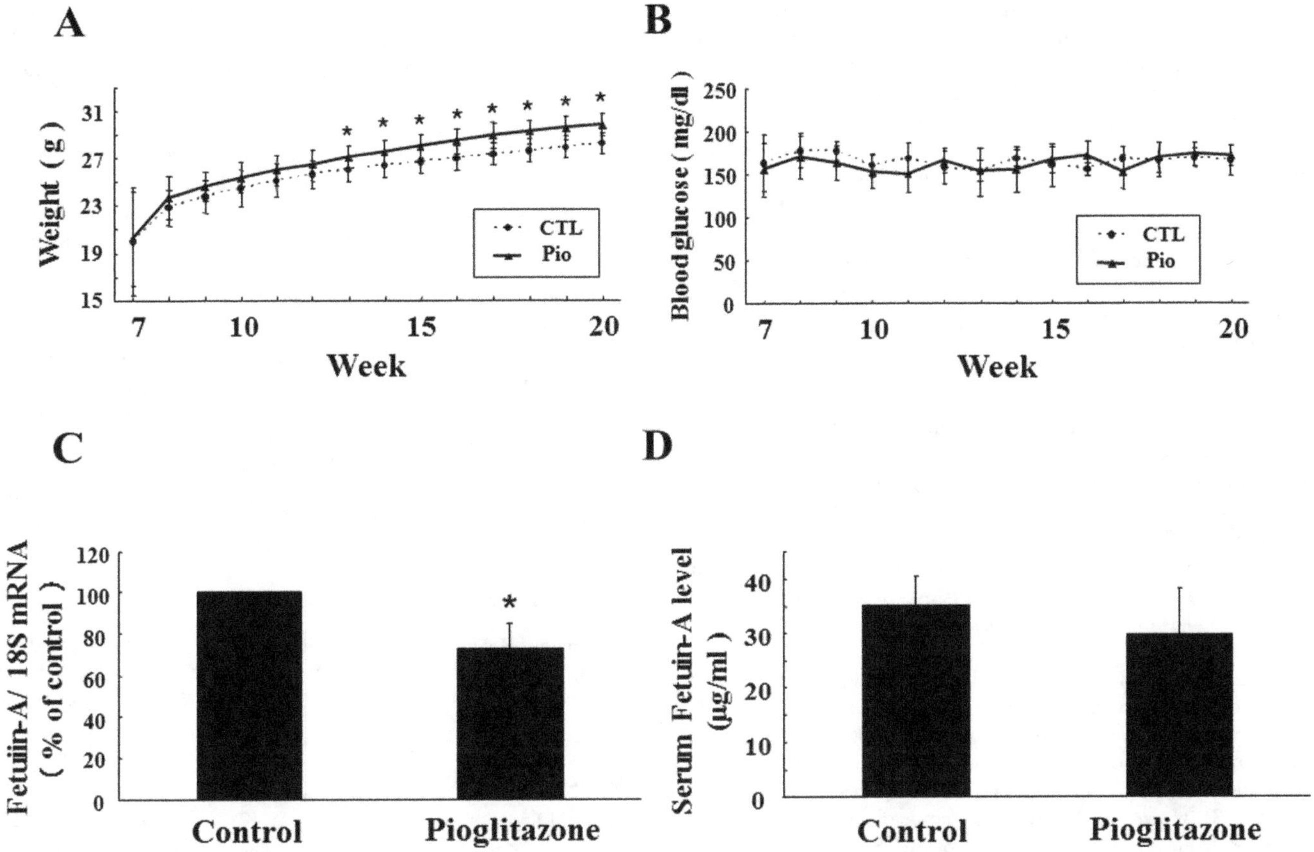

Figure 6. Effects of pioglitazone on hepatic fetuin-A expression and circulating fetuin-A levels in mice. Male C57BL/6J mice at 7 weeks of age were divided into a group bred with pioglitazone delivered as a food mixture at 10 mg/kg/day (Pio group: $n=6$) and a group without pioglitazone (CTL group: $n=6$). Body weight (A) and casual blood glucose levels (B) were monitored weekly in mice in each group from 7 weeks of age until 20 weeks of age. At 20 weeks of age, mice were sacrificed and liver tissues and blood samples were collected. Total RNA was isolated from mice in each group. Fetuin-A mRNA expression was determined using quantitative real-time RT-PCR. Fetuin-A mRNA expression levels were determined using a comparative cycle threshold method, with 18S ribosomal RNA as anendogenous reference. The fetuin-A mRNA level in the CTL group was defined as 100% (C). Circulating fetuin-A levels in the CTL- or Pio group were measured using an ELISA kit (D). Columns represented mean ± SD. $^{*}P<0.05$ vs. CTL.

resonance spectroscopy in humans [19]. In addition, lifestyle intervention decreased both circulating fetuin-A levels and fat accumulation in the liver [19]. Interestingly, pioglitazone, but not metformin, could improve hepatic lipid content [20]. When taken together, pioglitazone can ameliorate hepatic steatosis, resulting in decreased circulating fetuin-A levels. Second, it has been reported that FFAs enhance fetuin-A expression in hepatocytes [21]. Pioglitazone is known to improve dyslipidemia, including high levels of FFAs [12]. Therefore, pioglitazone may decrease serum fetuin-A levels through reduction of FFAs. Finally, alteration of the adipokine profile caused by pioglitazone treatment could change fetuin-A levels. In this case, pioglitazone would act mainly on adipocytes through PPARγ, leading to upregulation of adiponectin, a representative adipokine [22]. Because adiponectin has been reported to alleviate fatty liver disease [23], pioglitazone may suppress fetuin-A levels by increasing adiponectin levels. All the speculations mentioned above describe indirect effects of pioglitazone on fetuin-A suppression. However, our findings suggest that pioglitazone can exert direct suppression of hepatic fetuin-A expression, though pioglitazone-induced indirect effects also could modify fetuin-A levels in vivo.

In one of its many roles, fetuin-A is well known to be a powerful calcification inhibitor [1,2]. Its physiological role in the mortality of hemodialysis patients, its significance as an inhibitor of vascular calcification [24], and the techniques required to protect patients from ectopic calcification [25] have been established in detail. On the other hand, many clinical studies suggest that fetuin-A is involved in metabolic disorders, including diabetes and metabolic syndrome. Although fetuin-A can directly inhibit insulin receptor signaling in vitro [7], it has been unclear how fetuin-A acts on glucose and lipid metabolism with major force in vivo. Though we previously observed that pioglitazone treatment for 6 months reduced fetuin-A levels by approximately 13% [13], it has been a large open question whether such a slight alteration in fetuin-A, which is a very abundant serum protein, has a critical impact on systemic metabolism. Recently, Pal and Dasgupta et al. shed light on this deep question [10]. They proved that fetuin-A is necessary for lipid-induced chronic inflammation in adipose tissue, which is profoundly involved in metabolic disorders, including insulin resistance. FFAs activate intracellular NF-κB-associated genes, which encode inflammatory cytokines such as IL-6 and TNF-α through TLR4. In this process, fetuin-A functions as an adaptor between FFAs and TLR4 [10]. Therefore, small alterations in fetuin-A levels may lead to a substantial impact on metabolism through amplification mechanisms mediated by inflammatory cytokines. To confirm that these findings are relevant to the pathogenesis of insulin resistance in humans, Stefan et al. investigated the relationships between insulin resistance and circulating levels of fetuin-A and FFAs. They found a significant association between fetuin-A and insulin resistance in subjects with high FFAs but not in subjects with low FFAs. The positive association between FFAs and insulin resistance in subjects with high fetuin-A but not with low fetuin-A was also observed, suggesting that an interaction of FFAs with fetuin-A induces insulin resistance in humans [11].

PPARγ is predominantly expressed in adipocytes; its expression in liver is low. However, hepatic PPARγ plays a critical role in hepatic steatosis and in whole-body lipid and glucose homeostasis [26]. In this study, we found significant suppression of hepatic fetuin-A expression. Nevertheless, circulating fetuin-A levels were not significantly decreased in the pioglitazone-treated group compared with the control group. One possibility may be a relative small sample size ($n = 6$ in each group). Another explanation could be the condition of mice. To exclude the influence of metabolic disorders on fetuin-A expression, we chose healthy mice. Therefore, we may find an apparent reduction in circulating fetuin-A levels if we perform similar experiments in diabetic model mice because hepatic PPARγ expression is elevated in rodent models of diabetes or obesity [27].

With regard to the effect of metformin on fetuin-A expression, there seems to be inconsistent findings. Haukeland et al. found that metformin treatment for 6 months decreased plasma fetuin-A levels in patients with non-alcoholic fatty liver disease [14]. On the other hand, we found no changes in serum fetuin-A levels after intervention by metformin for 6 months in patients with type 2 diabetes [13]. However, the seemingly contradictory findings may be derived from the different dosages of metformin (500 mg/day or 750 mg/day [13] vs. 2500 mg/day or 3000 mg/day [14]). Similarly, Haukeland et al. reported that fetuin-A secretion from HepG2 cells decreased in the presence of metformin in a dose-dependent manner [14]. Again, the different amounts of metformin might lead to inconsistent results in in vitro studies. In fact, we detected the decrease of fetuin-A expression by treatment with high dose of 5 mM metformin in Fao cells (data not shown). Apart from this, it has been reported that high glucose enhanced fetuin-A promoter activity in HepG2 cells through activation of the ERK 1/2 signaling pathway, resulting in an increase of fetuin-A protein expression [28]. Therefore, to evaluate fetuin-A levels in patients with diabetes, glycemic levels should be also considered in addition to drug intervention.

In conclusion, pioglitazone can directly suppress hepatic fetuin-A expression both in vitro and in vivo. This appears to be a unique characteristic of thiazolidinedione derivatives compared with other antidiabetic drugs. Because emerging evidence suggests that fetuin-A may serve as a therapeutic target for metabolic disorders, including insulin resistance and type 2 diabetes, discovery of a liver-specific PPARγ agonist will provide the potential for an entirely new approach to treating metabolic disorders through fetuin-A regulation.

Acknowledgments

We thank Dr. Rohit N. Kulkarni (Joslin Diabetes Center, Boston, MA) for providing Fao cells, and Dr. Jiang (Thomas Jefferson University, PA, USA) for mouse fetuin-A (*Ahsg*) cDNA. We also thank Masayo Monden for her technical assistance.

Author Contributions

Conceived and designed the experiments: K. Mori AO. Performed the experiments: AO SN TM K. Motoyama. Analyzed the data: AO. Contributed reagents/materials/analysis tools: AO. Wrote the paper: K. Mori AO. Contributed to the discussion and reviewed and edited the manuscript: ME SF YI HK EI MI.

References

1. Mori K, Emoto M, Inaba M (2011) Fetuin-A: a multifunctional protein. Recent Pat Endocr Metab Immune Drug Discov 5: 124–146.
2. Mori K, Emoto M, Inaba M (2012) Fetuin-A and the cardiovascular system. Adv Clin Chem 56: 175–195.
3. Stefan N, Haring HU (2013) The role of hepatokines in metabolism. Nat Rev Endcrinol 9: 144–152.
4. Mori K, Emoto M, Yokoyama H, Araki T, Teramura M, et al. (2006) Association of serum fetuin-A with insulin resistance in type 2 diabetic and nondiabetic subjects. Diabetes Care 29: 468.
5. Ix JH, Wassel CL, Kanaya AM, Vittinghoff E, Johnson KC, et al. (2008) Fetuin-A and incident diabetes mellitus in older persons. JAMA 300: 182–188.
6. Stefan N, Fritsche A, Weikert C, Boeing H, Joost HG, et al. (2008) Plasma fetuin-A levels and the risk of type 2 diabetes. Diabetes 57: 2762–2767.
7. Auberger P, Falquerho L, Contreres JO, Pages G, Le Cam G, et al. (1989) Characterization of a natural inhibitor of the insulin receptor tyrosine kinase: cDNA cloning, purification, and anti-mitogenic activity. Cell 58: 631–640.
8. Shi H, Kokoeva MV, Inouye K, Tzameli I, Yin H, et al. (2006) TLR4 links innate immunity and fatty acid-induced insulin resistance. J Clin Invest 116: 3015–3025.
9. Erridge C, Samani NJ (2009) Saturated fatty acids do not directly stimulate Toll-like receptor signaling. Arterioscler Thromb Vasc Biol 29: 1944–1949.
10. Pal D, Dasgupta S, Kundu R, Maitra S, Das G, et al. (2012) Fetuin-A acts as an endogenous ligand of TLR4 to promote lipid-induced insulin resistance. Nat Med 18: 1279–1285.
11. Stefan N, Haring HU (2013) Circulating fetuin-A and free fatty acids interact to predict insulin resistance in humans. Nat Med 19: 394–395.
12. Derosa G (2010) Efficacy and tolerability of pioglitazone in patients with type 2 diabetes mellitus: comparison with other oral antihyperglycaemic agents. Drugs 70: 1945–1961.
13. Mori K, Emoto M, Araki T, Yokoyama H, Lee E, et al. (2008) Effects of pioglitazone on serum fetuin-A levels in patients with type 2 diabetes mellitus. Metabolism 57: 1248–1252.
14. Haukeland JW, Dahl TB, Yndestad A, Gladhaug IP, Loberg EM, et al. (2012) Fetuin-A in nonalcoholic fatty liver disease: in vivo and in vitro studies. Eur J Endorinol 166: 503–510.
15. Backer JM, Kahn CR, White MF. (1989) Tyrosine phosphorylayion of the insulin receptor during insulin-stimulated internalization in rat hepatoma cells. J Biol Chem 264: 1694–1701.
16. Monden M, Koyama H, Otsuka Y, Morioka T, Mori K, et al. (2013) Receptor for advanced glycation end products regulates adipocyte hypertrophy and insulin sensitivity in mice: involvement of Toll-like receptor 2. Diabetes 62: 478–489.
17. Mori K, Giovannone B, Smith RJ (2005) Distinct Grb10 domain requirements for effects on glucose uptake and insulin signaling. Mol Cell Endocrinol 230: 39–50.
18. Jiang Q, Dibra F, Lee MD, Oldenburg R, Uitto J (2010) Overexpression of fetuin-a counteracts ectopic mineralization in a mouse model of pseudoxanthoma elasticum (abcc6(−/−)). J Invest Dermatol 130: 1288–1296.
19. Stefan N, Hennige AM, Staiger H, Machann J, Schick F, et al. (2006) Alpha2-Heremans-Schmid glycoprotein/fetuin-A is associated with insulin resistance and fat accumulation in the liver in humans. Diabetes Care 29: 853–857.
20. Roden M (2006) Mechanisms of Disease: hepatic steatosis in type 2 diabetes–pathogenesis and clinical relevance. Nat Clin Pract Endocrinol Metab 2: 335–348.
21. Dasgupta S, Bhattacharya S, Biswas A, Majumdar SS, Mukhopadhyay S, et al. (2010) NF-kappaB mediates lipid-induced fetuin-A expression in hepatocytes that impairs adipocyte function effecting insulin resistance. Biochem J 429: 451–462.
22. Kadowaki T, Yamauchi T, Kubota N, Hara K, Ueki K, et al. (2006) Adiponectin and adiponectin receptors in insulin resistance, diabetes, and the metabolic syndrome. J Clin Invest 116: 1784–1792.
23. Xu A, Wang Y, Keshaw H, Xu LY, Lam KS, et al. (2003) The fat-derived hormone adiponectin alleviates alcoholic and nonalcoholic fatty liver diseases in mice. J Clin Invest 112: 91–100.
24. Hermans MM, Brandenburg V, Ketteler M, Kooman JP, van der Sande FM, et al. (2007) Association of serum fetuin-A levels with mortality in dialysis patients. Kidney Int 72: 202–207.
25. Heiss A, DuChesne A, Denecke B, Grotzinger J, Yamamoto K, et al. (2003) Structural basis of calcification inhibition by alpha 2-HS glycoprotein/fetuin-A. Formation of colloidal calciprotein particles. J Biol Chem 278: 13333–13341.

20-Hydroxyeicosatetraenoic Acid Impairs Endothelial Insulin Signaling by Inducing Phosphorylation of the Insulin Receptor Substrate-1 at Ser^{616}

Xuguang Li[1]*, Gang Zhao[2], Ben Ma[2], Rui Li[2], Jiang Hong[1], Shaowen Liu[1], Dao Wen Wang[2]

1 Department of Cardiology, Shanghai First People's Hospital, School of Medicine, Shanghai Jiao Tong University, Shanghai, People's Republic of China, **2** Department of Internal Medicine, Tongji Hospital, Tongji Medical College, Huazhong University of Science and Technology, Wuhan, People's Republic of China

Abstract

20-hydroxyeicosatetraenoic acid (20-HETE) induces endothelial dysfunction and is correlated with diabetes. This study was designed to investigate the effects of 20-HETE on endothelial insulin signaling.Human umbilical vein endothelial cells (HUVECs) or C57BL/6J mice were treated with 20-HETE in the presence or absence of insulin, and p-ERK1/2, p-JNK, IRS-1/PI3K/AKT/eNOS pathway, were examined in endothelial cells and aortas by immunoblotting. eNOS activity and nitric oxide production were measured. 20-HETE increased ERK1/2 phosphorylation and IRS-1 phosphorylation at Ser^{616}; these effects were reversed by ERK1/2 inhibition. We further observed that 20-HETE treatment resulted in impaired insulin-stimulated IRS-1 phosphorylation at Tyr^{632} and subsequent PI3-kinase/Akt activation. Furthermore, 20-HETE treatment blocked insulin-stimulated phosphorylation of eNOS at the stimulatory Ser^{1177} site, eNOS activation and NO production; these effects were reversed by inhibiting ERK1/2. Treatment of C57BL/6J mice with 20-HETE resulted in ERK1/2 activation and impaired insulin-dependent activation of the IRS-1/PI3K/Akt/eNOS pathway in the aorta. Our data suggest that the 20-HETE activation of IRS-1 phosphorylation at Ser^{616} is dependent on ERK1/2 and leads to impaired insulin-stimulated vasodilator effects that are mediated by the IRS-1/PI3K/AKT/eNOS pathway.

Editor: Jin Q. Cheng, H.Lee Moffitt Cancer Center & Research Institute, United States of America

Funding: This work was supported by the National Natural Science Foundation of China (No. 81300090 and No. 30930039,http://www.nsfc.gov.cn/) and the Young Physician Training Project of Shanghai. The funders had no role in study design, data collection and analysis, decision to publish, or preparation of the manuscript.

Competing Interests: The authors have declared that no competing interests exist.

* E-mail: li.xg@163.com

Introduction

Insulin promotes vasorelaxation and capillary recruitment in peripheral tissues and is a potent pro-angiogenic molecule that regulates neovascularization and EC migration [1]. These functions are mediated by a signaling cascade involving insulin receptor substrate-1 (IRS-1), PI3-kinase (PI3K), Akt, endothelial NO synthase (eNOS), and the generation of NO [2]. Accumulating experimental evidence suggests that both endothelial NO synthase (eNOS) and nitric oxide (NO) are involved in the pathogenesis of diabetes and insulin resistance [3]. Associated micro- and macro-vascular complications of metabolic disorders (e.g., retinopathy, nephropathy, hypertension, atherosclerosis, and coronary artery disease) are preceded by a state of endothelial dysfunction that is characterized by impaired NO bioavailability and vasorelaxation. Altered eNOS expression, NO production, and endothelial dysfunction, are important features of insulin-resistant conditions and diabetes [4].

The synthesis of 20-hydroxyeicosatetraenoic acid (20-HETE), the ω-hydroxylation product of arachidonic acid, is catalyzed by enzymes of the cytochrome P450 (P450) 4 gene family (CYP4A, -4B, and -4F) [5]. Increased 20-HETE levels have been observed in pathological conditions including ischemic cerebrovascular diseases, cardiac ischemia-reperfusion injury, kidney diseases, hypertension, and diabetes mellitus [6–8]. Evidence has accumulated that suggests a role for 20-HETE in vascular disorders such as atherosclerosis and hypertension [9–13], which are associated with endothelial dysfunction and insulin resistance. Moreover, the 20-HETE inhibitor HET0016 attenuated the development of diabetes-induced vascular dysfunction [14–16]. These findings indicate that the effects of 20-HETE on the development of hypertension and vascular dysfunction constitute the mechanisms by which 20-HETE contributes to endothelial dysfunction in diabetes and other insulin-resistant conditions.

Furthermore, evidence suggests that 20-HETE activates the mitogen-activated protein kinase (MAPK) pathway by stimulating ERK1/2 phosphorylation in endothelial cells [17]. Several serine residues in IRS-1 have been identified as negative regulatory sites, including Ser^{616} (orthologous to Ser^{612} in rat IRS-1), which is activated by mitogen-activated protein kinase (MAPK) [18]. It remains unclear, however, whether activation of this kinase by 20-HETE would affect the phosphorylation of IRS-1 at Ser^{616}, thus impairing activation of the insulin vasodilatory signaling pathway involving PI 3-kinase/Akt/eNOS.

The present study investigated whether 20-HETE affects insulin signaling that involves the production of NO in endothelial cells.

Materials and Methods

Materials

L-[^{14}C]arginine and L-[^{14}C]citrulline were obtained from PerkinElmer Inc. (Santa Clara, CA, USA). Antibodies for phospho-ERK1/2, ERK1/2, phospho-JNK, JNK, IRS-1, phospho-IRS-1 (Ser^{312}), phospho-IRS-1 (Ser^{616}), phospho-IRS-1 (Ser^{612}), phospho-IRS-1 (Tyr^{632}), phospho-IRS-1 (Tyr^{628}), the p85 subunit of PI3K, phospho-protein kinase B (AKT; Ser^{473}), AKT, eNOS, phospho-eNOS(Ser^{1177}), and β-actin were obtained from Santa Cruz Biotechnology (Santa Cruz, CA, USA). PD98059 (a reversible MEK1 inhibitor), SP600125 (inhibitor of JNK), N^G-nitro-L-arginine (L-NNA, inhibitor of NOS), cGMP ELISA kit and 20-Hydroxyeicosatetraenoic acid (20-HETE) were obtained from the Cayman Chemical Company (Ann Arbor, MI, USA). Other reagents were obtained from Sigma (St. Louis, MO, USA).

Endothelial Cell Culture

Human umbilical vein endothelial cells(HUVECs) were obtained from Lonza, and were cultured according to the manufacturer's instruction. The ECM was consisted of 10% fetal bovine serum, 1% endothelial cell growth supplement.

Animals

C57BL/6J mice(6 weeks old) were obtained from Shanghai Experimental Animal Center, Chinese academy of science. All animals were maintained in a pathogen-free environment and given radiation-sterilized food pellets and distilled water. Experiments were carried out according to the National Institutes of Health Guide for Care and Use of Laboratory Animals and were approved by the Bioethics Committee of Shanghai Jiao Tong University. All surgery was performed under sodium pentobarbital anesthesia, and all efforts were made to minimize suffering.

The Effects of 20-HETE on the Phosphorylation of ERK1/2 and JNK, and on the Serine Phosphorylation of IRS-1

First of all, human umbilical vein endothelial cells (HUVECs) were cultured for 18 hours in serum-deprived medium and incubated for various concentrations of 20-HETE (1 nm, 2 nm, 5 nm, 10 nm). Human umbilical vein endothelial cells (HUVECs) were cultured for 18 hours in serum-deprived medium and incubated for various times in the presence or absence of 5 nmol/L 20-HETE. The MEK1 inhibitor PD98059 (50 nmol/L) or JNK inhibitor SP600125 (30 nm) was added to the cells 30 minutes before the addition of 20-HETE. Equal amounts of cell lysates were incubated with p-Ser^{312}-IRS-1, p-Ser^{616}-IRS-1, phospho-ERK1/2, or phospho-JNK antibodies. To normalize the blots for protein levels, immunoblotting was performed with anti-phosphospecific antibodies; the blots were then stripped and reprobed with anti-IRS-1, anti-ERK1/2, or anti-JNK antibody.

The Effects of 20-HETE on the Tyrosine Phosphorylation of IRS-1, the Association of IRS-1 with the p85 Subunit of PI3-Kinase, and Akt and eNOS Phosphorylation

Human umbilical vein endothelial cells (HUVECs) were cultured for 18 hours in serum-deprived medium containing 10 mmol/L glucose and incubated for 30 minutes in the presence or absence of 5 nmol/L 20-HETE; the cells were then stimulated with 100 nmol/L insulin. PD98059 (50 nmol/L) was added to the cells 30 minutes before the addition of 20-HETE. Equal amounts of cell lysates were separately incubated with anti-Tyrosine-IRS-1, anti-PI3K(P85 subunit), p-Ser^{473}-AKT, and p-Ser^{1177}-eNOS. To normalize the blots for protein levels, immunoblotting was performed with anti-phosphospecific antibodies; the blots were then stripped and reprobed with IRS-1, AKT, eNOS, and β-actin antibodies.

NOS activity and cGMP production

NOS activity was determined in whole-cell lysates of HUVECs using a NOS detection system (Sigma, Saint Louis, Mo, USA) according to the manufacturer's instructions; this system measures the ability of NOS to convert L-[^{14}C] arginine to L-[^{14}C] citrulline. The data were normalized based on the amount of protein used and the reaction time. The amount of cyclic GMP production in the medium by the HUVECs was assessed by a cGMP assay kit (Cayman, Ann Arbor, MI) according to the manufacturer's instructions.

In vivo insulin stimulation

Based on results from a previous study and preliminary studies [19], the mice were injected with 20-HETE (10 mg/kg body weight) via the tail vein 1 h before insulin injection. In experiments using MEK inhibitor PD98059, the substance was injected i.p. at 10 mg/kg of body weight 2 h before 20-HETE injection. The animals were then stimulated with insulin (i.p., 0.75 mU/g of body weight) and euthanized with sodium pentobarbital (40 mg/kg of body weight). Aortas were immediately collected and snap-frozen in liquid nitrogen. Insulin signaling studies were then performed on aortic lysates as described above.

Assessment of Insulin-induced Vasorelaxation

The insulin-induced aortic rings relaxation experiments were performed according to a previously described method [20,21]. Briefly, insulin (10^{-8}–10^{-5} M) was added in a cumulative manner. Arteries were incubated in the presence and absence of N^G-nitro-L-arginine (L-NNA; 10^{-4} M), 20-HETE (1 μM) and PD98059 (10 μM). For insulin curves, relaxation at each concentration was measured and expressed as percent maximum relaxation, where 100% is equivalent to loss of all tension developed in response to phenylephrine.

Immunoblotting

The protein contents of extracts were determined using the Bradford method. Extracts were resolved using SDS-PAGE and transferred to polyvinylidene difluoride (PVDF) filter membranes. Proteins were detected by immunoblotting and visualized using enhanced chemiluminescence. Procedures were performed as described previously [22].

Statistical analysis

The data are presented as the means ± SEM. Comparisons among groups were performed using one-way ANOVA, followed by a Scheffe F-test. $P<0.05$ was accepted as statistically significant.

Results

20-HETE-induced Phosphorylation of ERK1/2 and Site-Specific Serine Phosphorylation of IRS-1

Increased serine phosphorylation of IRS-1 has been shown to inhibit the ability of IRS-1 to be tyrosine phosphorylated by the insulin receptor and to bind and activate PI3-kinase. Specifically, it has been shown that this function is performed by ERK1/2 at Ser^{616} of IRS-1. As shown in the present study, 20-HETE treatment caused a dose-dependent increase in the phosphorylation of ERK1/2 but not JNK in HUVECs (Fig. 1A and B), with the maximal effects occurring at 5 nm. These stimulatory effects of

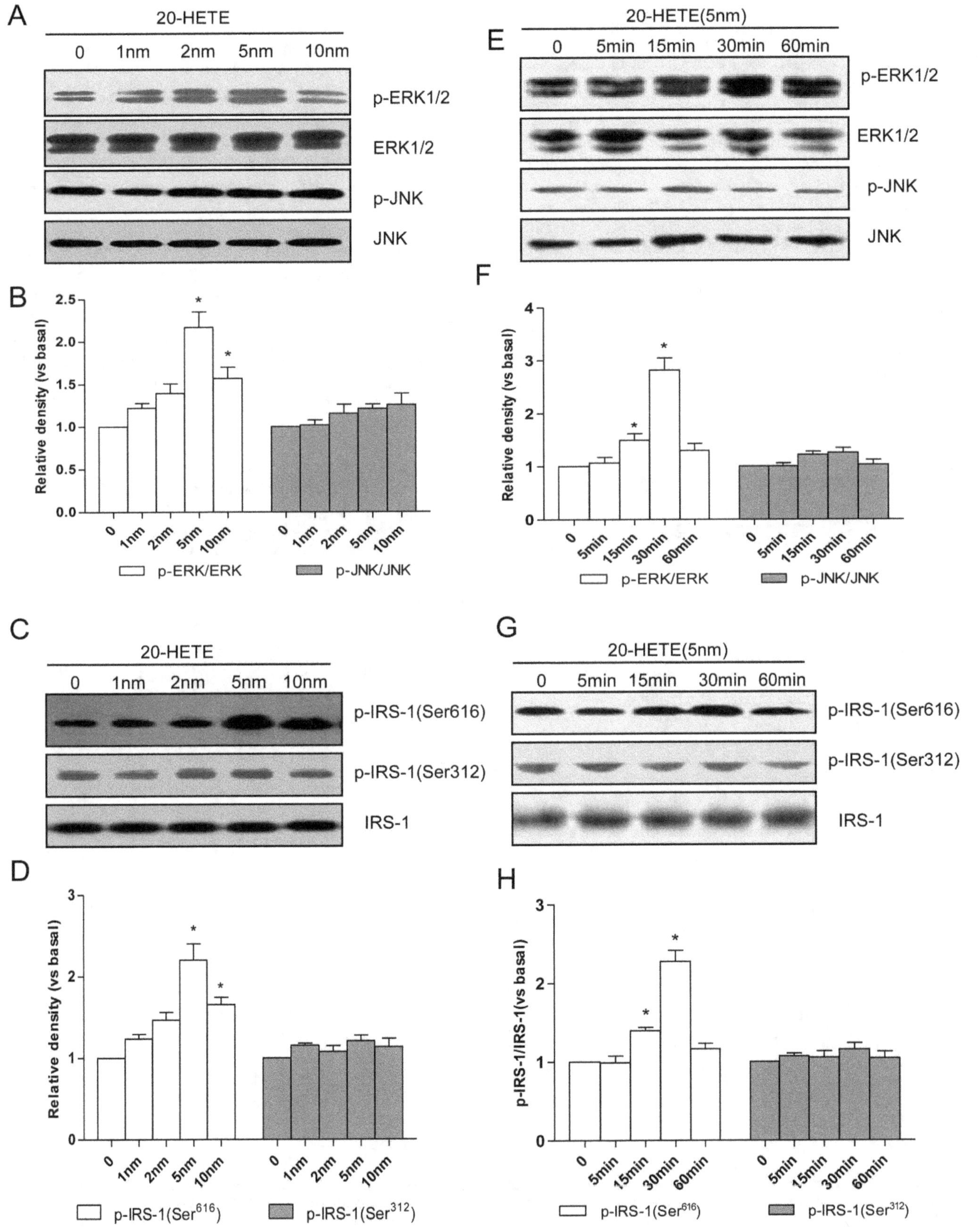

Figure 1. Concentration and time course of the effects of 20-HETE on JNK phosphorylation, ERK1/2 phosphorylation, and IRS-1 Serine phosphorylation in HUVECs. (A) A representative immunoblot of ERK1/2 phosphorylation and JNK phosphorylation induced by different concentration of 20-HETE; (B) Statistical analysis of the phosphorylation of ERK1/2 and JNK in Figure 1A; (C) A representative immunoblot of the Ser^{616} and Ser^{312} phosphorylation of IRS-1 induced by different concentration of 20-HETE; (D) Statistical analysis of the phosphorylation of IRS-1 at Ser^{616}

and Ser^{312} in Figure 1C; (E) A representative immunoblot of ERK1/2 phosphorylation and JNK phosphorylation induced by 20-HETE at different time; (F) Statistical analysis of the phosphorylation of ERK1/2 and JNK in Figure 1E; (G) A representative immunoblot of the Ser^{616} and Ser^{312} phosphorylation of IRS-1 induced by 20-HETE at different time; (H) Statistical analysis of the phosphorylation of IRS-1 at Ser^{616} and Ser^{312} in Figure 1G;Each bar represents the mean ± SD of three independent experiments; *: $P<0.05$. measurements in 20-HETE-treated cells versus measurements in non-20-HETE-treated cells.

20-HETE were accompanied by time-dependent increases in IRS-1 phosphorylation at Ser^{616} but not at Ser^{312} (Fig. 1C and D). Additionally, 20-HETE treatment also induced a time-dependent increase in the phosphorylation of ERK1/2 but not JNK in HUVECs (Fig. 1E and F), with the maximal effects occurring after 30 min of incubation. These stimulatory effects of 20-HETE were accompanied by time-dependent increases in IRS-1 phosphorylation at Ser^{616} but not at Ser^{312} (Fig. 1G and H). The ERK1/2 inhibitor PD98059 or JNK inhibitor SP600125 (30 nm) was added to the cells 30 minutes before 20-HETE addition. The results showed that PD98059 blocked 20-HETE-induced phosphorylation of ERK1/2 (Fig. 2A and C; $P<0.05$). Consequently, the 20-HETE-induced phosphorylation of IRS-1 at Ser^{616} was also reversed by treatment with PD98059 (Fig. 2B and C; $P<0.05$). However, 20-HETE or SP600125 does not affect the phosphorylation of JNK and IRS-1 phosphorylation at Ser^{312} (Fig. 2D, E and F).

20-HETE impaired Insulin-Stimulated Tyrosine Phosphorylation of IRS-1 and PI3K/Akt activation

Because the serine phosphorylation of IRS-1 converts IRS-1 into an inhibitor of the intrinsic IR tyrosine kinase, we tested the possibility that the increased Ser616 phosphorylation of IRS-1 induced by 20-HETE would be associated with impaired insulin-stimulated tyrosine phosphorylation of IRS-1. As shown in Figure 3A, exposure of HUVECs to 20-HETE resulted in an

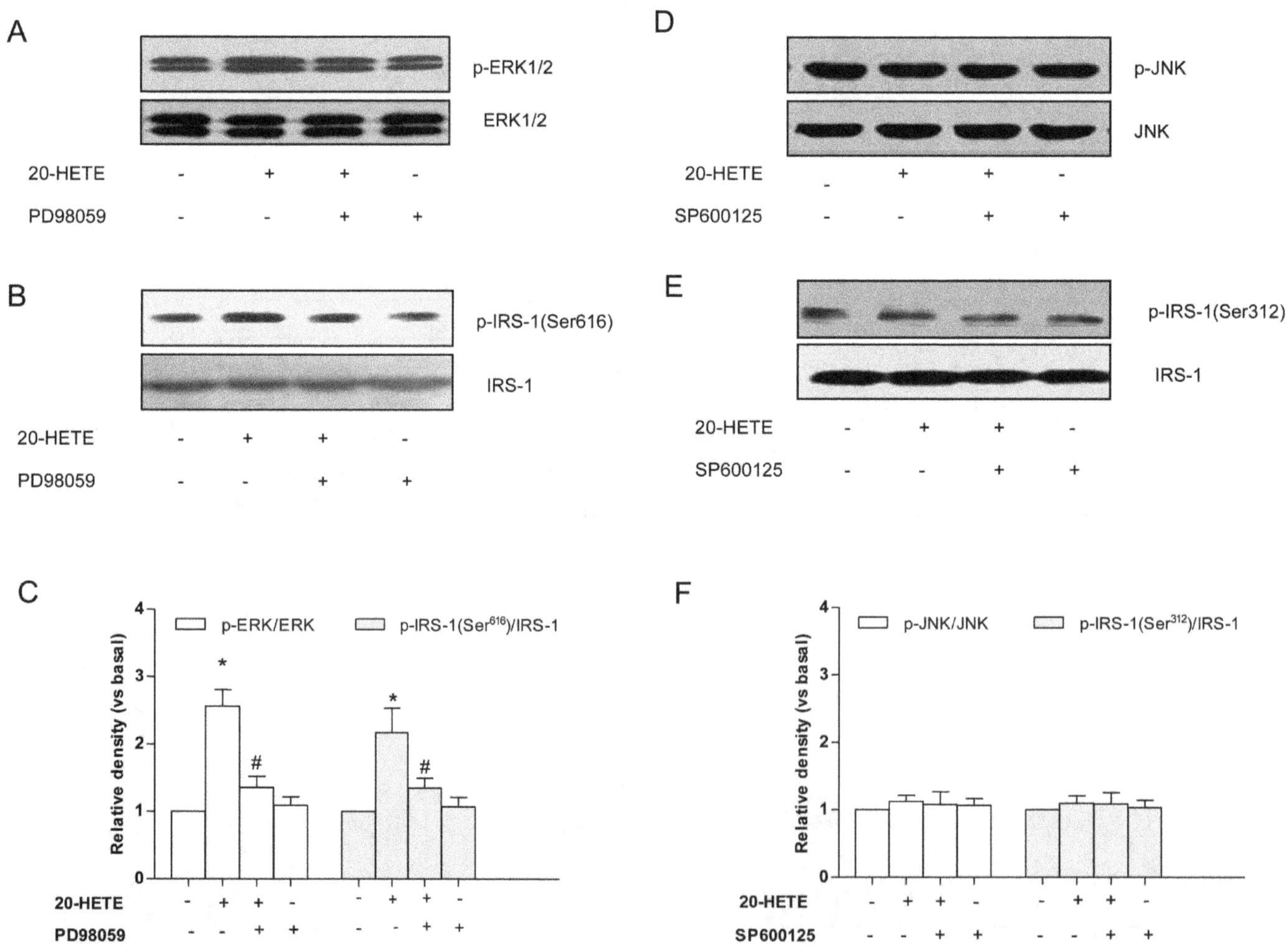

Figure 2. The effects of the ERK1/2 inhibitor on 20-HETE-stimulated IRS-1 Serine phosphorylation and ERK1/2 phosphorylation in HUVECs. PD98059 (50 nmol) or SP600125 (20 nm) was added to the cells 30 min before the addition of 20-HETE. (A) A representative immunoblot of ERK1/2 phosphorylation; (B) A representative immunoblot of the Ser^{616} phosphorylation of IRS-1; (C) Statistical analysis of the phosphorylation of ERK1/2 and the phosphorylation of IRS-1 at Ser^{616}; (D) A representative immunoblot of JNK phosphorylation; (E) A representative immunoblot of the Ser^{312} phosphorylation of IRS-1; (F) Statistical analysis of the phosphorylation of JNK and the phosphorylation of IRS-1 at Ser^{312}. Each bar represents the mean ± SD of three independent experiments; *: $P<0.05$. measurements in 20-HETE-treated cells versus measurements in non-20-HETE-treated cells. #: $P<0.05$. measurements in PD98059-treated cells versus measurements in 20-HETE-treated cells.

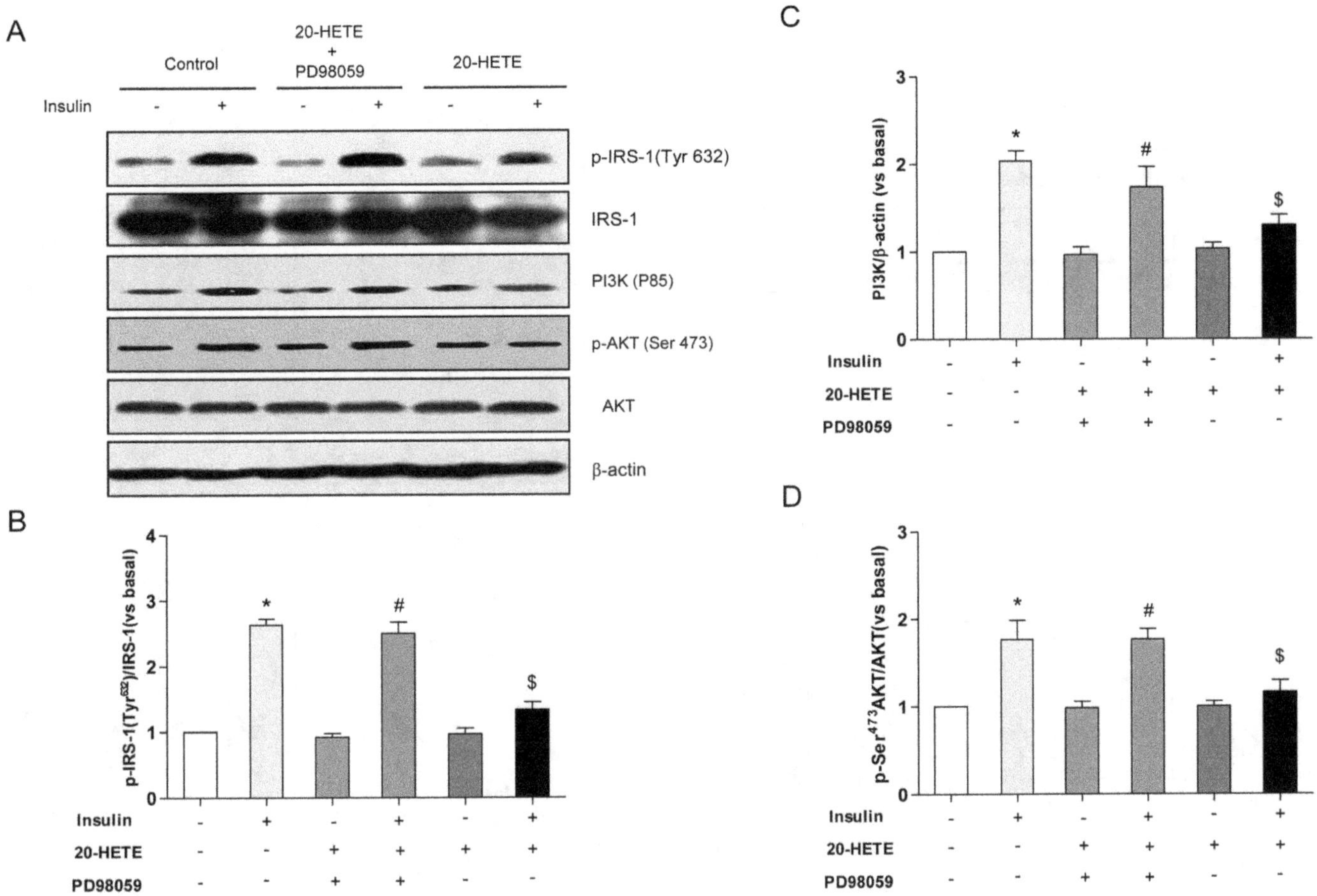

Figure 3. The effects of 20-HETE on the insulin-stimulated tyrosine phosphorylation of IRS-1 and on PI3K/Akt activation. HUVECs were treated with 20-HETE in the presence or absence of PD98059, and 100 nmol insulin was then added for 10 min. (A) A representative immunoblot of the Tyr^{632} phosphorylation of IRS-1; PI3K and the Ser^{473} phosphorylation of Akt (B) Statistical analysis of the tyrosine phosphorylation of IRS-1; (C) Statistical analysis of P13K(p85) expression; (D) Statistical analysis of the Ser^{473} phosphorylation of Akt. Each bar represents the mean ± SD of three independent experiments; *: $P<0.05$, versus control; #: $P<0.05$, versus 20-HETE + PD98059; $: $P<0.05$, versus insulin.

approximately 30% inhibition of insulin-stimulated Tyr632 phosphorylation of IRS-1. The inhibitory effect of 20-HETE was reversed by treatment with PD98059. Because the association of PI3K/Akt with tyrosine-phosphorylated IRS-1 is essential for downstream insulin signaling, the effect of 20-HETE on IRS-1/p85/Akt docking was examined by immunoblotting with anti-p85 and anti-Ser473 Akt antibodies. As shown in Figure 3C and D, respectively, insulin increased the binding of IRS-1 to the p85 subunit 1.8-fold and increased Ser473 Akt phosphorylation 1.6-fold. Treatment with 20-HETE decreased the insulin-stimulated binding of IRS-1 to the p85 subunit by 30% and decreased Ser473 Akt activation by 40%. These inhibitory effects of 20-HETE were reversed by PD98059. Besides that, both ERK1/2 and JNK were phosphorylated by insulin treatment, which were accompanied by IRS-1 phosphorylation at Ser616 and Ser 312(Figure S1 and S2). However, 20-HETE treatment did not reinforce these stimulatory effects of insulin (Figure S1 and S2).

20-HETE Impaired the Insulin-stimulated Activation of eNOS and eNOS Activity

Insulin increased the phosphorylation of eNOS on Ser^{1177} 1.6-fold (Figure 4A and B). Treatment with 20-HETE decreased insulin-stimulated Ser^{1177} eNOS phosphorylation by 30% (based on the levels in 20-HETE-treated, insulin-stimulated cells versus the levels in non-20-HETE-treated, insulin-stimulated cells; $P<0.05$). Treatment of HUVECs with PD98059 reversed the inhibitory effect of 20-HETE (Figure 4A and B, $P<0.05$). We next determined whether 20-HETE would affect the eNOS activation and cGMP production induced by insulin. Insulin stimulated eNOS activity 1.7-fold whereas 20-HETE treatment decreased insulin-stimulated eNOS activity by 30% (Figure 4C; $P<0.05$). Treatment of HUVECs with PD98059 partially reversed the inhibitory effects of 20-HETE on insulin-stimulated eNOS activity (Figure 4C; $P<0.05$). NO production was reflected by measuring cGMP levels, insulin stimulated cGMP production 3.5-fold, whereas 20-HETE treatment decreased of insulin-stimulated cGMP production by 75% (Figure 4D; $P<0.05$). Treatment of HUVECs with PD98059 partially reversed the inhibitory effects of 20-HETE on insulin-stimulated cGMP production (Figure 4D).

20-HETE Induced Serine Phosphorylation of IRS-1 in C57BL/6J Mouse Aortas

In mice treated for 1 h with 20-HETE, the phosphorylation of IRS-1 at Ser^{612} (orthologous to Ser^{616} in human IRS-1) in the aortas was increased 3.2-fold (Figure 5A and B; $P<0.05$). These stimulatory effects of 20-HETE were accompanied by increased phosphorylation of ERK1/2 (Figure 5A and C; $P<0.05$). These

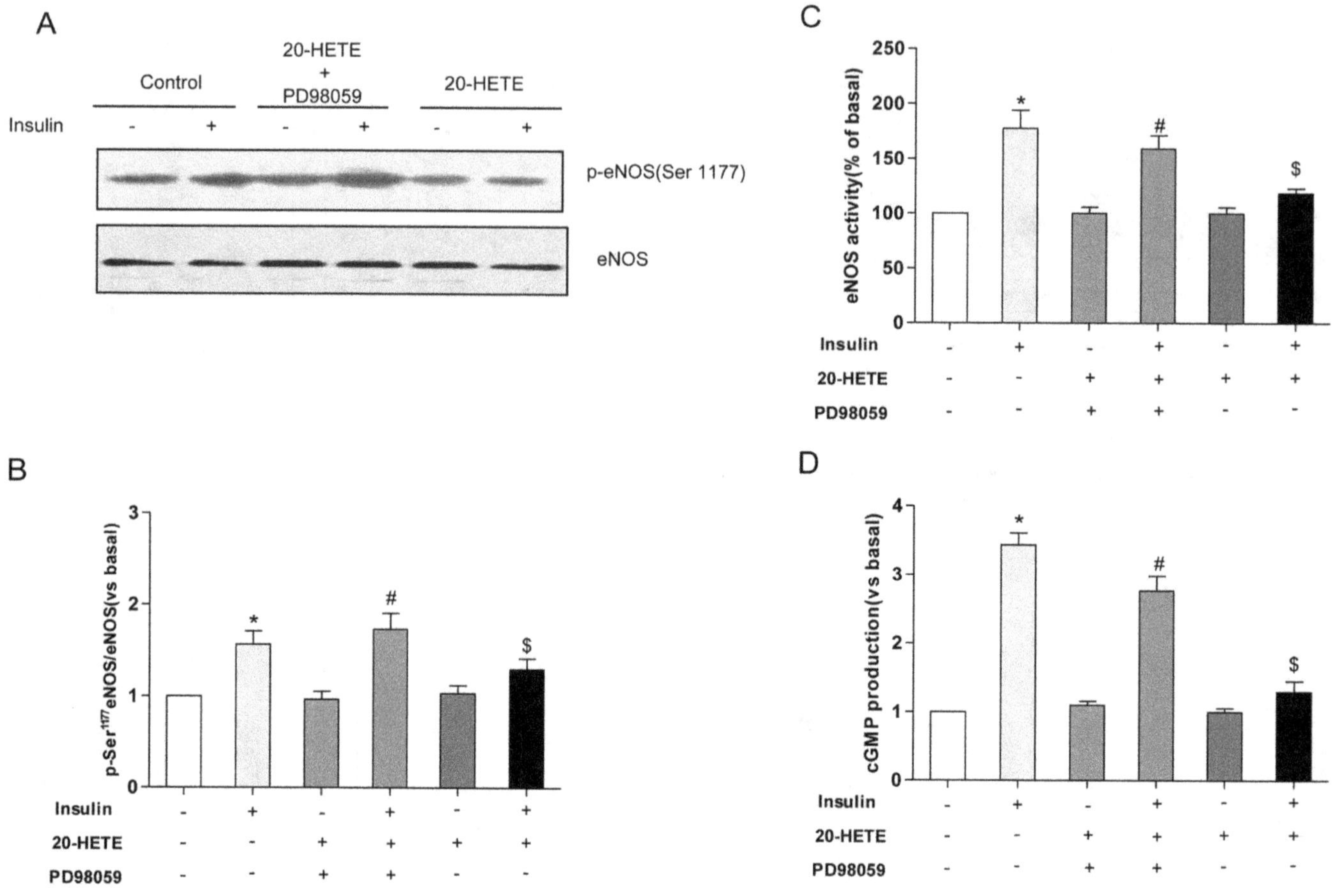

Figure 4. The effects of 20-HETE on the insulin-stimulated activation of eNOS and eNOS activity. HUVECs were treated as indicated in Figure 3. (A) A representative immunoblot of the phosphorylation of eNOS at Ser^{1177}; (B) Statistical analysis of the phosphorylation of eNOS at Ser^{1177}; (C) NOS activity was determined in cell lysates of HUVECs using a NOS detection system according to the manufacturer's instructions; (D) The release of NO into the medium by HUVECs was assessed by measuring cGMP level. Each bar represents the mean ± SD of three independent experiments; *: $P<0.05$, versus control; #: $P<0.05$, versus 20-HETE + PD98059; $: $P<0.05$, versus insulin.

effects of 20-HETE were reversed by treatment with PD98059 (Figure 5A, B, and C; $P<0.05$).

20-HETE Impaired Insulin-stimulated Activation of the Tyrosine Phosphorylation of IRS-1, PI3-kinase, Akt, and eNOS C57BL/6J Mouse Aortas

We tested whether 20-HETE would also affect the activation of the insulin-stimulated IRS-1/PI3KAkt/eNOS pathway in vivo in mice treated for 1 h with 20-HETE. Insulin increased the Tyr^{628} phosphorylation of IRS-1 (corresponding to Tyr^{632} in human IRS-1) and PI3K activation (Figure 6A, B and C; $P<0.05$). Insulin stimulated Akt phosphorylation on Ser^{473} 1.6-fold and the phosphorylation of eNOS on Ser^{1177} 2-fold in the mouse aortas (comparing the levels in the aortas of insulin-stimulated mice versus basal levels; Figure 6A, D, and E; $P<0.05$). Treatment with 20-HETE resulted in 40 and 50% decreases of insulin-stimulated Akt and eNOS phosphorylation, respectively (Figure 6A, D, and E; $P<0.05$). Treatment of mice with PD98059 reversed the inhibitory effect of 20-HETE (Figure 6A, D, and E; $P<0.05$).

20-HETE Inhibited Insulin-induced Vasodilation

To evaluate endothelial function, the vasorelaxation responses to insulin were examined in mouse aortas. Insulin-induced concentration-dependent relaxations of aortic rings were obtained from the C57BL/6 mice, and the relaxations were significantly inhibited in the presence of either L-NNA (inhibitor of NOS) or 20-HETE, but PD98059 (inhibitor of ERK1/2) blocked the inhibitory effect of 20-HETE significantly (Figure S3).

Discussion

In this study, we inquired whether 20-HETE-induced alterations in insulin signaling contribute to an impairment of endothelial insulin action. The current study is the first to provide strong direct evidence that exposure of HUVECs to 20-HETE inhibited insulin-stimulated NOS activity and NO production. This event was associated with an increased ERK1/2 activity that was paralleled by increased IRS-1 phosphorylation at Ser^{616} and decreased insulin-stimulated IRS-1 tyrosine phosphorylation. This study is potentially of great significance, because it brings into being a new face to a prominent eicosanoid and suggests a feed-forward amplification of endothelial dysfunction and insulin resistance induced by 20-HETE.

It is well accepted that the serine phosphorylation of IRS-1 is a negative regulator of insulin signaling [23]. ERK1/2 regulates stress responses, inflammation, and apoptosis, and has been implicated in the pathogenesis of endothelial dysfunction and insulin resistance [24]. ERK1/2 activation has been shown to result in an increased phosphorylation at Ser^{612} of IRS-1

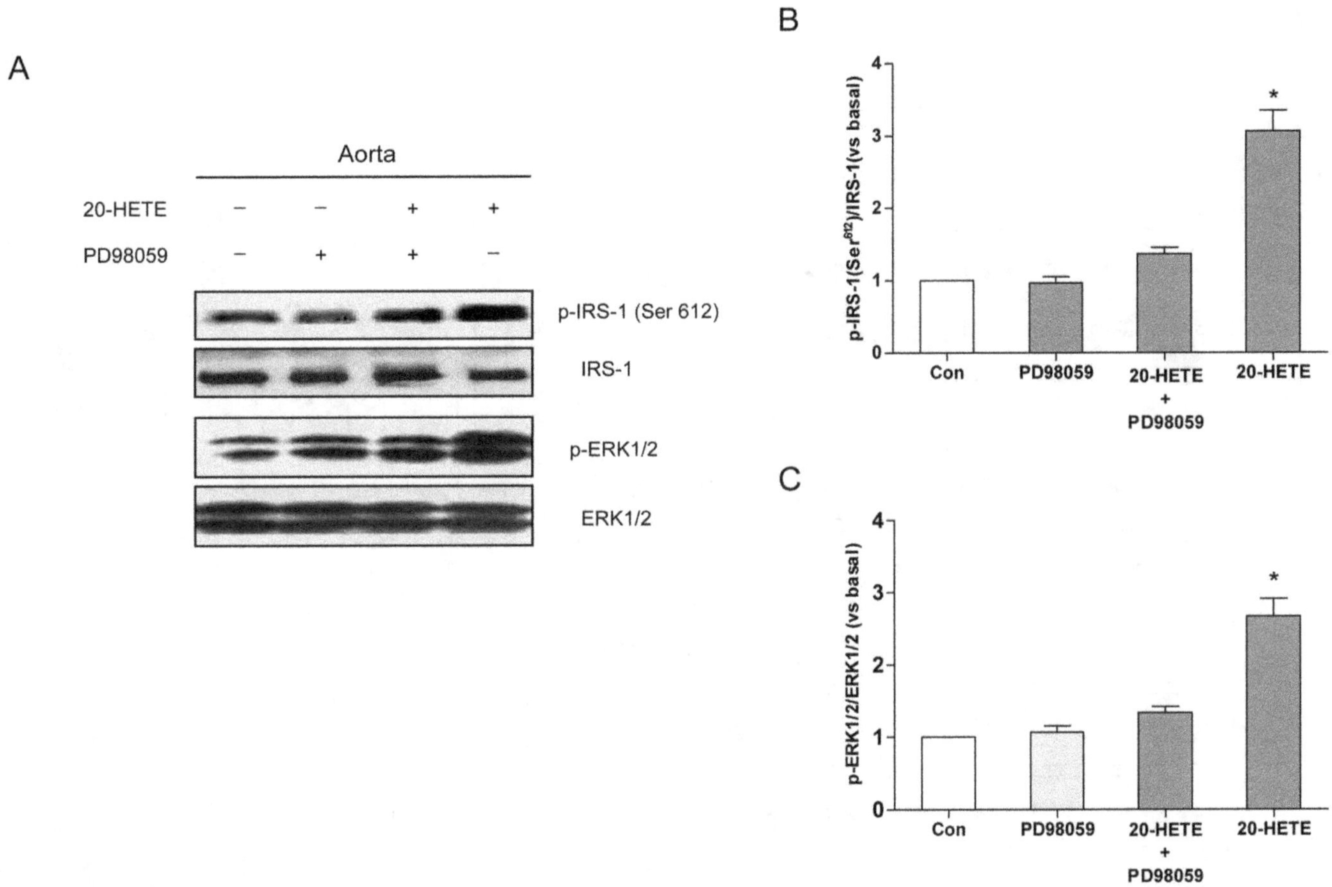

Figure 5. The effects of 20-HETE on the serine phosphorylation of IRS-1 in C57BL/6J mouse aortas. (A) A representative immunoblot of the Ser^{616} phosphorylation of IRS-1 and of ERK1/2 phosphorylation; (B) Statistical analysis of the phosphorylation of IRS-1 at Ser^{616}; (C) Statistical analysis of ERK1/2 phosphorylation. Each bar represents the mean ± SD of three independent experiments; *: $P<0.05$, measurements in 20-HETE-treated aorta versus measurements in non-20-HETE-treated aorta.

(orthologous to Ser^{616} in human IRS-1), thereby inhibiting the insulin-stimulated tyrosine phosphorylation of IRS-1 and subsequent activation of PI3K [25]. Because 20-HETE activates ERK1/2 in cultured vascular endothelial cells [17,26], we examined the possibility that the 20-HETE-induced phosphorylation at Ser^{616} of IRS-1, which is mediated by ERK1/2, may account for the inhibitory effects of 20-HETE on the insulin signaling pathway that is involved in NO production. Similar to previous researchers [17], we found that HUVECs exhibited increased ERK1/2 activity in a time-dependent manner when exposed to 20-HETE. Interestingly, IRS-1 phosphorylation at Ser^{616} was increased with a concomitant increase in ERK1/2 activity. The specific inhibitor of ERK1/2, PD98059, completely abolished 20-HETE-induced IRS-1 serine phosphorylation and ERK1/2 phosphorylation. These data suggest that 20-HETE may induce ERK1/2-dependent endothelial insulin resistance and dysfunction. The vasodilatory effects of insulin are mediated by the IRS-1/PI-3 kinase/Akt/eNOS signaling pathway that leads to increased endothelial NO production. A growing body of evidence indicates that the serine phosphorylation of IRS-1, which is induced by a variety of factors, interferes with the ability of IRS-1 to be tyrosine-phosphorylated upon insulin stimulation and reduces its ability to engage the p85 subunit of PI 3-kinase [27,28]. Our findings demonstrate that the exposure of HUVECs to 20-HETE results in decreased NO production upon insulin stimulation and is associated with impairment of tyrosine phosphorylation of IRS-1 and its corresponding association with the p85 subunit of PI 3-kinase, leading to the defective activation of Akt and eNOS.

The phosphorylation of eNOS (at Ser1177 in humans) and its association with 90-kDa heat shock protein (HSP90) are both required for eNOS activation [29]. In primary human endothelial cells, previous studies show that impairment of the insulin signaling involving IRS-1/PI3-kinase/Akt induced by either Ang II or IL-6 in IRS-1 resulted in a decrease in the ability of insulin to phosphorylate eNOS at the positive regulatory site Ser1177 and to dephosphorylate the inhibitory site Thr495 [18,30]. Accordingly, the present study demonstrated that the impaired activation of the insulin-dependent IRS-1/PI3-kinase/Akt pathway in HUVECs exposed to 20-HETE was associated with a decrease in Ser1177phosphorylation, resulting in a reduction in NOS activity. These findings are in contrast to those reported in bovine aortic endothelial cells (BAECs), in which the addition of 5 nM 20-HETE (the same concentration that used in the current study) had no effect on the basal and ionophore-stimulated levels of eNOS phosphorylation at either Ser1179 or Thr497 but inhibited the association of eNOS with HSP90 [10]. This disparity might have arisen because the cells are different in that they originate from different vascular beds that respond to 20-HETE with opposing outcomes.

Additionally, as demonstrated in this study, the inhibition of ERK1/2 activity with its specific inhibitor PD98059 completely

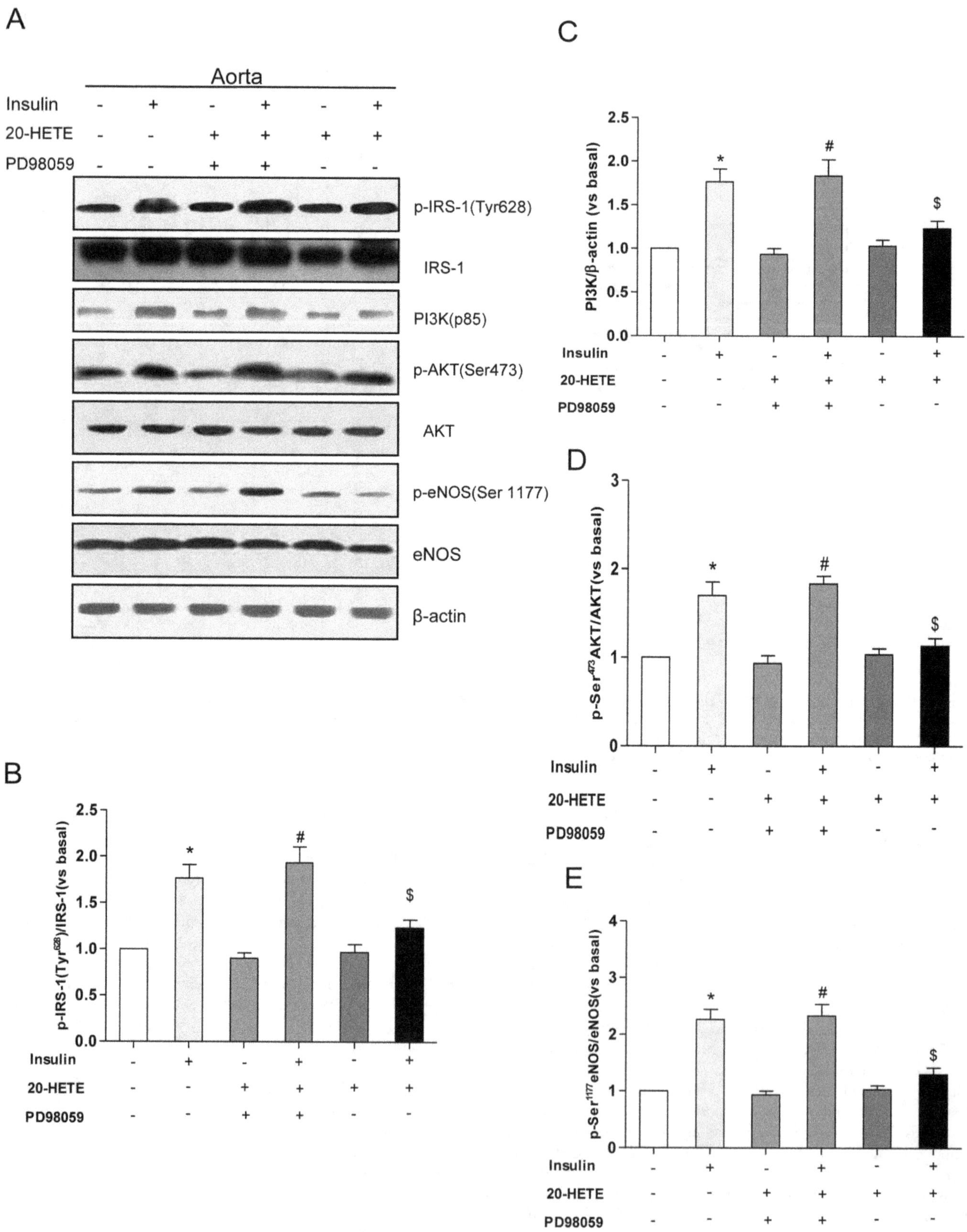

Figure 6. The effects of 20-HETE on the insulin-stimulated activation of the tyrosine phosphorylation of IRS-1, PI3K, Akt, and eNOS in C57BL/6J mouse aortas. (A) A representative immunoblot of the Tyr^{628} phosphorylation of IRS-1, p85, Ser^{473}-AKT, and Ser^{1177}-eNOS; (B) Statistical analysis of the tyrosine phosphorylation of IRS-1; (C) Statistical analysis of P13K(p85) expression; (D) Statistical analysis of the Ser^{473} phosphorylation of Akt; (E) Statistical analysis of the Ser^{1177} phosphorylation of eNOS. Each bar represents the mean ± SD of three independent experiments; *: $P<0.05$, versus control; #: $P<0.05$, versus 20-HETE + PD98059; $: $P<0.05$, versus insulin.

abolished 20-HETE-induced IRS-1 serine phosphorylation and restored the insulin sensitivity of IRS-1 tyrosine phosphorylation, Akt phosphorylation, and eNOS activity in the presence of 20-HETE. This strongly suggests that 20-HETE induces endothelial cell insulin resistance via an ERK1/2-dependent pathway.

The results obtained in aortas isolated from C57BL/6J mice support the likelihood that our findings in cultured endothelial cells may have physiological relevance. These in vivo findings demonstrate that 20-HETE induces phosphorylation at Ser^{612} of IRS-1 mediated by ERK1/2 and impairs the ability of insulin to stimulate eNOS Ser^{1177} phosphorylation via blunting the IRS-1/PI3-kinase/Akt pathway. Insulin-stimulated vasodilation were also attenuated by 20-HETE significantly, suggesting that 20-HETE impaired the endothelial function by terminating insulin signaling.

A close relationship between chronic inflammation and insulin resistance has been well established, and the IKKβ pathway is a target for insulin resistance [31]; in addition, IκB was activated by 20-HETE (data not shown), which is consistent with pervious observations that 20-HETE stimulates NFκB activation and promotes proinflammatory cytokine production via an ERK1/2-dependent pathway [17]. Additionally, 20-HETE increases superoxide production, activates NAPDH oxidase in endothelial cells and promotes the development of vascular dysfunction [32,33]. Oxidative stress plays a pivotal role in the development of diabetes complications, both microvascular and cardiovascular in origin. The metabolic abnormalities of diabetes cause mitochondrial superoxide overproduction in the endothelial cells of both large and small vessels, as well as in the myocardium [34]. Therefore, the proinflammatory and pro-oxide stress effects of 20-HETE on endothelial cells may exacerbate endothelial insulin resistance and dysfunction.

20-HETE is believed to be a prohypertensive eicosanoid, and inhibition of 20-HETE in experimental models of hypertension reduces blood pressure [35]. Clinic evidence has indicated a significant positive association between 20-HETE excretion and BMI [36], and obesity has been linked with insulin resistance [37], which may be a rational explanation for the inhibitory effect of 20-HETE on insulin vascular action. Based on the results, 20-HETE production and/or action might be a therapeutic target to treat hypertension associated with insulin resistance states. Taken together, these data support the concept that 20-HETE impairs the ability of insulin to stimulate NOS activity by regulating the reciprocal phosphorylation of eNOS at Ser^{1177} via mechanisms involving the activation of PI3-kinase/Akt. The inhibitory effects of 20-HETE are likely to be mediated by the activation of ERK1/2, which induces the phosphorylation of IRS-1 at Ser^{616}, leading to the dysfunction of IRS-1 as a docking protein. This provides support for the hypothesis that 20-HETE may play an important role in the pathophysiology of cardiovascular disease associated with hypertension and insulin resistance.

Supporting Information

Figure S1 The effects of 20-HETE on the insulin-stimulated JNK phosphorylation, ERK1/2 phosphorylation, and IRS-1 Serine phosphorylation in HUVECs. HUVECs were treated with 20-HETE in the presence or absence of PD98059, and 100 nmol insulin was then added for 10 min. Insulin stimulates phosphorylation of ERK1/2 and JNK. (A) A representative immunoblot of ERK1/2 phosphorylation and JNK phosphorylation induced by different concentration of 20-HETE; (B) Statistical analysis of the phosphorylation of ERK1/2 in Figure S1-A; (C) Statistical analysis of the phosphorylation of JNK in Figure S1-A. Each bar represents the mean ± SD of three independent experiments; *: $P<0.05$, versus control.

Figure S2 The effects of 20-HETE on the insulin-stimulated IRS-1 Serine phosphorylation in HUVECs. HUVECs were treated with 20-HETE in the presence or absence of PD98059, and 100 nmol insulin was then added for 10 min. Insulin induced IRS-1 phosphorylation at Ser^{616} and at Ser^{312}. (A) A representative immunoblot of the phosphorylation of IRS-1 at Ser^{312} and Ser^{616}; (B) Statistical analysis of the phosphorylation of JNK and the phosphorylation of IRS-1 at Ser^{616} in Figure S2-A; (C) Statistical analysis of the phosphorylation of IRS-1 at Ser^{312} in Figure S2-A. Each bar represents the mean ± SD of three independent experiments; *: $P<0.05$, versus control.

Figure S3 The effects of 20-HETE on the insulin-induced vasorelaxation. Insulin-induced concentration-dependent relaxations of aortic rings, but the relaxations were significantly inhibited in the presence of either L-NNA (inhibitor of NOS) or 20-HETE, but PD98059 (inhibitor of ERK1/2) reversed the inhibitory effect of 20-HETE. *: $P<0.05$, measurements in insulin + L-NNA versus control (insulin); #: $P<0.05$, measurements in insulin +20-HETE versus control (insulin); &: $P<0.05$, measurements in insulin +20-HETE +PD98059 versus insulin +20-HETE.

Acknowledgments

We wish to thank Hongwei Hou for excellent technical assistance.

Author Contributions

Conceived and designed the experiments: XL DWW. Performed the experiments: XL GZ BM RL. Analyzed the data: XL JH SL. Contributed reagents/materials/analysis tools: XL GZ BM RL. Wrote the paper: XL SL.

References

1. Muniyappa R, Montagnani M, Koh KK, Quon MJ (2007) Cardiovascular actions of insulin. Endocr Rev 28: 463–491.
2. Zeng G, Nystrom FH, Ravichandran LV, Cong LN, Kirby M, et al. (2000) Roles for insulin receptor, PI3-kinase, and Akt in insulin-signaling pathways related to production of nitric oxide in human vascular endothelial cells. Circulation 101: 1539–1545.
3. Huang PL (2009) eNOS, metabolic syndrome and cardiovascular disease. Trends Endocrinol Metab 20: 295–302.
4. Mather KJ, Steinberg HO, Baron AD (2013) Insulin resistance in the vasculature. J Clin Invest 123: 1003–1004.
5. Hardwick JP (2008) Cytochrome P450 omega hydroxylase (CYP4) function in fatty acid metabolism and metabolic diseases. Biochem Pharmacol 75: 2263–2275.
6. Miyata N, Roman RJ (2005) Role of 20-hydroxyeicosatetraenoic acid (20-HETE) in vascular system. J Smooth Muscle Res 41: 175–193.
7. Lai G, Wu J, Liu X, Zhao Y (2012) 20-HETE induces hyperglycemia through the cAMP/PKA-PhK-GP pathway. Mol Endocrinol 26: 1907–1916.
8. Chen YJ, Li J, Quilley J (2008) Deficient renal 20-HETE release in the diabetic rat is not the result of oxidative stress. Am J Physiol Heart Circ Physiol 294: H2305–2312.
9. Cheng J, Garcia V, Ding Y, Wu CC, Thakar K, et al. (2012) Induction of angiotensin-converting enzyme and activation of the renin-angiotensin system contribute to 20-hydroxyeicosatetraenoic acid-mediated endothelial dysfunction. Arterioscler Thromb Vasc Biol 32: 1917–1924.
10. Cheng J, Ou JS, Singh H, Falck JR, Narsimhaswamy D, et al. (2008) 20-hydroxyeicosatetraenoic acid causes endothelial dysfunction via eNOS uncoupling. Am J Physiol Heart Circ Physiol 294: H1018–1026.
11. Cheng J, Wu CC, Gotlinger KH, Zhang F, Falck JR, et al. (2010) 20-hydroxy-5,8,11,14-eicosatetraenoic acid mediates endothelial dysfunction via IkappaB

kinase-dependent endothelial nitric-oxide synthase uncoupling. J Pharmacol Exp Ther 332: 57–65.
12. Singh H, Cheng J, Deng H, Kemp R, Ishizuka T, et al. (2007) Vascular cytochrome P450 4A expression and 20-hydroxyeicosatetraenoic acid synthesis contribute to endothelial dysfunction in androgen-induced hypertension. Hypertension 50: 123–129.
13. Orozco LD, Liu H, Perkins E, Johnson DA, Chen BB, et al. (2013) 20-HETE inhibition attenuates balloon injury-induced neointima formation and vascular remodeling in rat carotid arteries. J Pharmacol Exp Ther.
14. Benter IF, Yousif MH, Canatan H, Akhtar S (2005) Inhibition of Ca2+/calmodulin-dependent protein kinase II, RAS-GTPase and 20-hydroxyeicosatetraenoic acid attenuates the development of diabetes-induced vascular dysfunction in the rat carotid artery. Pharmacol Res 52: 252–257.
15. Wang Z, Yadav AS, Leskova W, Harris NR (2011) Inhibition of 20-HETE attenuates diabetes-induced decreases in retinal hemodynamics. Exp Eye Res 93: 108–113.
16. Yousif MH, Benter IF, Dunn KM, Dahly-Vernon AJ, Akhtar S, et al. (2009) Role of 20-hydroxyeicosatetraenoic acid in altering vascular reactivity in diabetes. Auton Autacoid Pharmacol 29: 1–12.
17. Ishizuka T, Cheng J, Singh H, Vitto MD, Manthati VL, et al. (2008) 20-Hydroxyeicosatetraenoic acid stimulates nuclear factor-kappaB activation and the production of inflammatory cytokines in human endothelial cells. J Pharmacol Exp Ther 324: 103–110.
18. Andreozzi F, Laratta E, Sciacqua A, Perticone F, Sesti G (2004) Angiotensin II impairs the insulin signaling pathway promoting production of nitric oxide by inducing phosphorylation of insulin receptor substrate-1 on Ser312 and Ser616 in human umbilical vein endothelial cells. Circ Res 94: 1211–1218.
19. Miyata N, Seki T, Tanaka Y, Omura T, Taniguchi K, et al. (2005) Beneficial effects of a new 20-hydroxyeicosatetraenoic acid synthesis inhibitor, TS-011 [N-(3-chloro-4-morpholin-4-yl) phenyl-N'-hydroxyimido formamide], on hemorrhagic and ischemic stroke. J Pharmacol Exp Ther 314: 77–85.
20. Padilla J, Jenkins NT (2013) Induction of endoplasmic reticulum stress impairs insulin-stimulated vasomotor relaxation in rat aortic rings: role of endothelin-1. J Physiol Pharmacol 64: 557–564.
21. Taguchi K, Kobayashi T, Matsumoto T, Kamata K (2011) Dysfunction of endothelium-dependent relaxation to insulin via PKC-mediated GRK2/Akt activation in aortas of ob/ob mice. Am J Physiol Heart Circ Physiol 301: H571–583.
22. Li X, Yang G, Zhao G, Wu B, Edin ML, et al. (2011) Rosuvastatin attenuates the elevation in blood pressure induced by overexpression of human C-reactive protein. Hypertens Res 34: 869–875.
23. Gual P, Le Marchand-Brustel Y, Tanti JF (2005) Positive and negative regulation of insulin signaling through IRS-1 phosphorylation. Biochimie 87: 99–109.
24. Huang A, Yang YM, Yan C, Kaley G, Hintze TH, et al. (2012) Altered MAPK signaling in progressive deterioration of endothelial function in diabetic mice. Diabetes 61: 3181–3188.
25. Boura-Halfon S, Zick Y (2009) Phosphorylation of IRS proteins, insulin action, and insulin resistance. Am J Physiol Endocrinol Metab 296: E581–591.
26. Guo AM, Arbab AS, Falck JR, Chen P, Edwards PA, et al. (2007) Activation of vascular endothelial growth factor through reactive oxygen species mediates 20-hydroxyeicosatetraenoic acid-induced endothelial cell proliferation. J Pharmacol Exp Ther 321: 18–27.
27. De Fea K, Roth RA (1997) Modulation of insulin receptor substrate-1 tyrosine phosphorylation and function by mitogen-activated protein kinase. J Biol Chem 272: 31400–31406.
28. Aguirre V, Werner ED, Giraud J, Lee YH, Shoelson SE, et al. (2002) Phosphorylation of Ser307 in insulin receptor substrate-1 blocks interactions with the insulin receptor and inhibits insulin action. J Biol Chem 277: 1531–1537.
29. Fleming I, Busse R (2003) Molecular mechanisms involved in the regulation of the endothelial nitric oxide synthase. Am J Physiol Regul Integr Comp Physiol 284: R1–12.
30. Andreozzi F, Laratta E, Procopio C, Hribal ML, Sciacqua A, et al. (2007) Interleukin-6 impairs the insulin signaling pathway, promoting production of nitric oxide in human umbilical vein endothelial cells. Mol Cell Biol 27: 2372–2383.
31. Shoelson SE, Lee J, Goldfine AB (2006) Inflammation and insulin resistance. J Clin Invest 116: 1793–1801.
32. Medhora M, Chen Y, Gruenloh S, Harland D, Bodiga S, et al. (2008) 20-HETE increases superoxide production and activates NAPDH oxidase in pulmonary artery endothelial cells. Am J Physiol Lung Cell Mol Physiol 294: L902–911.
33. Lukaszewicz KM, Lombard JH (2013) Role of the CYP4A/20-HETE pathway in vascular dysfunction of the Dahl salt-sensitive rat. Clin Sci (Lond) 124: 695–700.
34. Giacco F, Brownlee M (2010) Oxidative stress and diabetic complications. Circ Res 107: 1058–1070.
35. Elshenawy OH, Anwar-Mohamed A, El-Kadi AO (2013) 20-Hydroxyeicosatetraenoic acid is a potential therapeutic target in cardiovascular diseases. Curr Drug Metab 14: 706–719.
36. Ward NC, Rivera J, Hodgson J, Puddey IB, Beilin LJ, et al. (2004) Urinary 20-hydroxyeicosatetraenoic acid is associated with endothelial dysfunction in humans. Circulation 110: 438–443.
37. Hotamisligil GS, Shargill NS, Spiegelman BM (1993) Adipose expression of tumor necrosis factor-alpha: direct role in obesity-linked insulin resistance. Science 259: 87–91.

19

Association of Liver Enzymes and Computed Tomography Markers of Liver Steatosis with Familial Longevity

Michiel Sala[1]*, Lucia J. M. Kroft[1], Boudewijn Röell[1], Jeroen van der Grond[1,4], P. Eline Slagboom[3,4], Simon P. Mooijaart[2,4], Albert de Roos[1], Diana van Heemst[2,4]

1 Department of Radiology, Leiden University Medical Center, Leiden, the Netherlands, **2** Department of Gerontology and Geriatrics, Leiden University Medical Center, Leiden, the Netherlands, **3** Department of Molecular Epidemiology, Leiden University Medical Center, Leiden, the Netherlands, **4** Netherlands Consortium for Healthy Ageing, Leiden, the Netherlands

Abstract

Objective: Familial longevity is marked by enhanced peripheral but not hepatic insulin sensitivity. The liver has a critical role in the pathogenesis of hepatic insulin resistance. Therefore we hypothesized that the extent of liver steatosis would be similar between offspring of long-lived siblings and control subjects. To test our hypothesis, we investigated the extent of liver steatosis in non-diabetic offspring of long-lived siblings and age-matched controls by measuring liver enzymes in plasma and liver fat by computed tomography (CT).

Research Design and Methods:: We measured nonfasting alanine transaminase (ALT), aspartate aminotransferase (AST), and ϒ-glutamyl transferase (GGT) in 1625 subjects (736 men, mean age 59.1 years) from the Leiden Longevity Study, comprising offspring of long-lived siblings and partners thereof. In a random subgroup, fasting serum samples (n = 230) were evaluated and CT was performed (n = 268) for assessment of liver-spleen (L/S) ratio and the prevalence of moderate-to-severe non-alcoholic fatty liver disease (NAFLD). Linear mixed model analysis was performed adjusting for age, gender, body mass index, smoking, use of alcohol and hepatotoxic medication, and correlation of sibling relationship.

Results: Offspring of long-lived siblings had higher nonfasting ALT levels as compared to control subjects (24.3 mmol/L versus 23.2 mmol/L, $p = 0.03$), while AST and GGT levels were similar between the two groups. All fasting liver enzyme levels were similar between the two groups. CT L/S ratio and prevalence of moderate-to-severe NAFLD was similar between groups (1.12 vs 1.14, $p = 0.25$ and 8% versus 8%, $p = 0.91$, respectively).

Conclusions: Except for nonfasting levels of ALT, which were slightly higher in the offspring of long-lived siblings compared to controls, no differences were found between groups in the extent of liver steatosis, as assessed with liver biochemical tests and CT. Thus, our data indicate that the extent of liver steatosis is similar between offspring of long-lived siblings and control subjects.

Editor: Manlio Vinciguerra, University College London, United Kingdom

Funding: Funding was provided by Netherlands Genomics Initiative/Netherlands Organisation for Scientific Research (05040202 Netherlands Consortium for Healthy Aging) and by the European Community within the Seventh Framework Program under grant agreement no. Health-2013-INNOVATION-1-602757 (HUMAN). The funders had no role in study design, data collection and analysis, decision to publish, or preparation of the manuscript.

Competing Interests: The authors have declared that no competing interests exist.

* E-mail: M.L.Sala@lumc.nl

Introduction

Non-alcoholic fatty liver disease (NAFLD) is the most common chronic liver disease in Western countries and is associated with metabolic risk factors such as obesity, diabetes mellitus, and dyslipedimia [1]. NAFLD is prevalent in more than one-third of the elderly [2], while prevalence may increase up to 69% in type 2 diabetes patients [3].

Hepatocyte dysfunction due to liver fat accumulation may interfere with insulin action and cause hepatic insulin resistance [4]. Accordingly, the liver enzymes ϒ-glutamyl transferase (GGT) and alanine aminotransferase (ALT) correlate with liver fat content, and have been shown to predict impaired glucose metabolism and type 2 diabetes mellitus incidence [5]. On the other hand, secondary to insulin resistance, prolonged compensatory hyperinsulinemia may lead to the development of NAFLD [6]. From this point of view, NAFLD may be a consequence rather than a cause of age related insulin resistance.

Offspring of long-lived siblings exhibit an exceptional healthy glucose metabolism in middle age, including preservation of insulin sensitivity and increased glucose tolerance [7,8]. We have previously shown that these subjects had a higher insulin-mediated glucose disposal rate (peripheral insulin sensitivity), while the capacity of insulin to suppress endogenous glucose production (hepatic insulin sensitivity) was not different as compared to controls [8]. In line with enhanced peripheral glucose disposal, we have previously shown that lipid accumulation within muscle cells was lower in offspring of nonagenarian siblings as compared to controls [8,9]. Likewise, given the correlation between insulin resistance and liver steatosis [10], it can be questioned whether there is an association between the extent of liver steatosis and the healthy metabolic profile observed in familial longevity. One previous study found that nonfasting serum triglyceride levels were lower in offspring of long-lived siblings as compared to controls, albeit only in women [11]. Accordingly, while serum triglyceride levels correlate with liver fat content [12], this may suggest that the extent of liver steatosis is lower in offspring of long-lived siblings. However, triglyceride levels were determined in nonfasting samples, so results might have potentially been confounded by differences in food intake between groups. Moreover, it was previously shown that familial longevity is marked by enhanced peripheral but not hepatic insulin sensitivity [8]. Based on these considerations, we hypothesized that the extent of liver steatosis would be similar between offspring of long-lived siblings and control subjects. To test our hypothesis, we evaluated liver biochemical tests (aspartate aminotransferase [AST], ALT, and GGT) and computed tomography markers of liver steatosis in the non-diabetic offspring of long-lived siblings and age-matched controls.

Methods

Study Subjects

The Medical Ethical Committee of the Leiden University Medical Center approved the study, and written informed consent was obtained from all subjects according to the Declaration of Helsinki.

Subjects were included from the Leiden Longevity Study, which has been described in more detail elsewhere [13]. In short, 421 Dutch Caucasian families were enrolled in the study between 2002 and 2006 based on the following inclusion criteria: (1) there were at least two living siblings per family, who fulfilled the age criteria and were willing to participate, (2) men had to be aged ≥89 years and women had to be aged ≥91 years and (3) the sib pairs had to have the same parents. In 2002, only 0.5% of Dutch men were aged 89 and older, and only 0.5% of Dutch women aged 91 and older. Accordingly, siblings who meet these age criteria are even rarer and are estimated to represent far less than 0.1% of the population in the Netherlands [14]. Offspring of these long-lived siblings were included as they were shown to have a 35% lower mortality rate compared to the general population. Their partners, who share the same socio-economic and geographical background, were enrolled as age-matched control group [13]. Accordingly, there were no selection criteria on health or demographic characteristics.

In total, 2415 subjects comprising1671 offspring and 744 partners are included in the Leiden Longevity Study. For the current study, additional information was collected, including self-reported information on height, weight, alcohol intake and smoking habits. Information on past medical history was obtained from the participants' treating physicians. Subjects with diabetes (65 offspring and 53 partners) were excluded. Subjects were regarded as having diabetes if they had nonfasting glucose levels > 11.0 mmol/L, a previous medical history of diabetes and/or used glucose lowering agents. Of the remaining 2297 subjects, we excluded subjects with plasma levels more than threefold higher than the upper reference limit for GGT (18 offspring, 14 partners) or ALT (0 offspring, 1 partner). For the remaining subjects, all plasma AST levels were within the reference range. For the remaining 2264 subjects, plasma samples were not available for 35 subjects (25 offspring, 10 partners) and serum data on GGT or ALT were not available for 46 subjects (32 offspring, 14 partners). In total 8 subjects (8 offspring, 0 partners) were excluded based on presence of chronic hepatitis (n = 4), liver steatosis (n = 3, confirmed by ultrasound), or liver metastasis (n = 1) in past medical history. Accordingly, information on medication was lacking for 238 subjects (173 offspring, 65 partners), data on alcohol intake was missing for 293 subjects (214 offspring, 79 partners), information on smoking was lacking for 12 subjects (11 offspring, 1 partner), and information on BMI was lacking for 7 subjects (3 offspring, 4 partners). Hence, in total 1625 subjects (1122 offspring and 503 partners) were selected for the current analyses.

From the cohort of 2415 subjects, a subgroup of 234 was previously recruited, from which fasting serum samples were obtained and who participated in an oral glucose tolerance test (OGTT) [7]. From this group of 234 subjects, 4 subjects were excluded because GGT levels were more than threefold higher than the upper reference limit (2 offspring, 2 partners).

From the cohort of 2415 subjects, another random subgroup of 268 subjects was recruited for computed tomography (see below).

Biochemical Analysis and Plasma Parameters

Fasting blood samples were obtained between November 2006 and May 2008, as previously described [7]. Nonfasting blood samples were obtained between September 2002 and May 2006. All serum and plasma measurements were performed with fully automated equipment. For insulin, the Immulite 2500 from DPC (Los Angeles, CA, USA) was applied. All other measurements were implemented on an Abbott ci8200 (Roche, Almere, the Netherlands). ALT and AST were measured using the NADH (with P-5′-P) methodology and GGT by measuring the substrate L-Gamma-glutamyl-3-carboxy-4-nitroanilide methodology. Activated reagentia were based on the optimized formulation as recommended by the International Federation of Clinical Chemistry (IFCC). Reference values were 0–55 U/l for ALT, 5–34 U/l for ASAT, and sex specific reference values for GTT were 9–36 U/l women and 12–64 U/l for males. Coefficients of variation for these measurements were all below 9%.

Alcohol Consumption

Participants reported the number of alcoholic beverages they consumed on a weekly basis in each of the following 4 categories: beer, wine, liquor, and moderately strong alcoholic beverages such as port or sherry. Non-drinkers were considered abstainers. A drink was defined as 200 mL of beer that contained 8.0 g of alcohol, 100 mL of wine that contained 10.0 g of alcohol, 50 mL of liquor that contained 14.0 g of alcohol, or 75 mL of moderately strong alcohol types that contained 10.5 g of alcohol [15]. We added the amounts of alcohol in the four groups, and calculated the total alcohol consumption per participant in grams per day.

Medication Use

Detailed information on medication use according to the Anatomical Therapeutic Chemical (ATC) Classification System [16] was obtained from the participants' pharmacist. Hepatotoxic medication was defined as medication for which liver damage has been reported frequently at the National Center for Drug Safety [17].

Image Acquisition

Unenhanced Computed Tomography examinations were performed between September 2009 and December 2010 with an

Aquilion ONE (Toshiba Medical Systems, Otawara, Japan) 320 multi detector-row scanner, using the following parameters: tube voltage: 120 kV, tube current: 155 mAs, rotation time: 0.5 sec. A single cross-sectional 8-mm slice of the abdomen at the T12/L1 intervertebral disc was obtained. Imaging was performed during breath hold after expiration.

Image Analysis

Data were processed by a research fellow (M.S.) under direct supervision of an experienced radiologist (L.K., 13 years of experience).

To quantify hepatic steatosis, we measured the attenuation of the liver in Hounsfield Units (HU) by placing a region of interest (ROI) in the right peripheral liver lobe. The ROI was made as large as possible (at least 1 cm^2), avoiding the hepatic vessels or any focal lesions. Accordingly, as internal control, HU measures were performed in the spleen. Lower attenuation values correspond to lower tissue density, which indicates a greater fat content. One cross-sectional slice has been shown to adequately capture the majority of variance in hepatic fat content, and for a single versus three ROI measures in the liver, the intraclass coefficient has been shown 0.99 [18]. To measure liver fat content, liver-spleen ratio (L/S) was calculated, where L is the hepatic attenuation (HU) and S is the splenic attenuation (HU).

The definition of NAFLD requires that (a) there is evidence of hepatic steatosis, either by imaging or by histology and (b) there are no causes for secondary hepatic fat accumulation [1]. In previous imaging studies, hepatic steatosis has been defined as > 5.5% liver fat accumulation, as assessed by magnetic resonance proton spectroscopy (^{1}H-MRS) [19,20]. Although ^{1}H-MRS is the most accurate non-invasive method to quantify liver fat, CT imaging has been shown to be fairly accurate in identifying patients with moderate-to-severe liver steatosis (>30% liver fat), using histologic analysis as the reference standard [21]. Previous CT studies have defined NAFLD as L/S ratio <1 [22]. In addition, one recent study showed that L/S ratio <0.8 provides high performance in qualitative diagnosis of higher (>30%) degrees of liver steatosis with 100% specificity and 82% sensitivity using histologic analysis as the reference standard [23]. Therefore we also included this cut-off value in our analysis. In 21 subjects (7 offspring, 14 controls), ROI measurements in the spleen were not feasible (e.g. the spleen was not shown, or subjects had a splenectomy in the past medical history). These subjects were excluded from L/S ratio analyses. Accordingly, L/S ratio analysis was performed in 247 subjects.

Statistical Analyses

Continuous variables were tested for normality and, if appropriate, logarithmically transformed and used in all calculations (LnALT, LnAST, LnGGT, LnInsulin, and LnTriglyceride). For transformed variables, data are presented as geometric means with 95% confidence intervals.

Differences in subject demographics between offspring and control subjects were calculated using student's t-test and Pearson chi-square test. Differences in markers of lipid and glucose metabolism were assessed with the use of a linear mixed model, adjusting for age, gender, BMI, and correlation of sibling relationships. To assess the association between tertiles of liver enzymes and serum levels of glucose, linear regression analysis was performed, correcting for relation to descent (offspring of long-lived siblings or age-matched control subject), age, gender, smoking, alcohol use in g/day, and number of hepatotoxic medications. Differences in liver biochemical tests in offspring of long-lived siblings and control subjects were assessed with linear mixed model analysis, using different models. Model 1 was adjusted for age, gender, and correlation of sibling relationship. Model 2 included model 1 and was adjusted additionally for smoking, BMI, alcohol use in g/day, and number of hepatotoxic medications. Analyses were repeated after excluding all subjects with lipid-modifying agents.

Differences in CT markers of liver steatosis and NAFLD prevalence between offspring of long-lived siblings and control subjects were assessed with linear mixed models and logistic regression analysis, using the same models as in liver biochemical test analyses. For statistical analyses, Statistical Package for the Social Sciences (SPSS) software for windows (version 20.0) was used.

Results

Subject characteristics are shown in table 1. In total, 1122 offspring of long-lived siblings and 503 controls were included for the nonfasting analyses. The offspring of long-lived siblings were slightly older than their partners (mean age 59.3 years and 58.6 years, respectively, $p = 0.050$). Body mass index was similar between the two groups ($p = 0.25$).

Nonfasting glucose levels were lower in the offspring group as compared to control subjects ($p = 0.001$), while nonfasting insulin levels were not significantly different ($p = 0.25$). Sex specific analysis showed that compared to controls, both female offspring and male offspring had relatively lower mean nonfasting serum glucose (5.6 mmol/L vs 5.8 mmol/L, $p = 0.003$ for female offspring and partners respectively, and 5.8 mmol/L vs 5.9 mmol/L, $p = 0.05$ for male offspring and partners respectively). Subject characteristics for the fasted group are also shown in table 1. Differences between groups were comparable to those of the nonfasting group.

The association between liver biochemical tests parameters and serum TG levels with serum levels of glucose are shown in figure 1. After correcting for age, gender, smoking, use of alcohol and number of hepatotoxic medication, and correlation of sibling relationship, tertiles of nonfasting ALT ($p = 0.002$), GGT ($p < 0.001$), and TG ($p < 0.001$) were positively associated with serum levels of glucose. In the fasting group, tertiles of fasting GGT ($p = 0.004$) and TG ($p = 0.009$) were positively associated with serum levels of glucose.

Nonfasting liver biochemical tests in offspring of long-lived siblings and control subjects are shown in table 2. In both the minimally adjusted and the fully adjusted models, plasma AST and GGT were similar in offspring of long-lived siblings and control subjects. In both models, offspring of long-lived siblings had higher mean plasma ALT levels as compared to control subjects (24.3 vs 23.2 mmol/L, $p = 0.03$ after adjusting for age, gender, correlation of sibling relationship, smoking, BMI, and use of alcohol and hepatotoxic medications). Sex specific analysis showed that in both sexes a similar trend towards relatively higher levels of ALT in the offspring group was observed (19.9 vs 19.4 mmol/L, $p = 0.27$ for female offspring versus partners; 24.8 vs 21.1 mmol/L for male offspring versus partners, $p = 0.12$). In both the minimally adjusted and the fully adjusted models, nonfasting serumTG levels were lower in offspring of long-lived siblings and control subjects (table 2). Also after excluding all subjects with lipid-modifying agents, in both the minimally adjusted and the fully adjusted models, offspring of long-lived siblings had lower nonfasting serum triglyceride levels as compared to control subjects (offspring versus controls, 1.65 vs 1.78 mmol/L, $p = 0.01$ after adjusting for age, gender, correlation of sibling relationship, smoking, BMI, and use of alcohol and hepatotoxic

Table 1. Subject demographics.

	Nonfasting group (n = 1625)			Fasting group (n = 230)		
	Offspring	Controls	p-value	Offspring	Controls	p-value
Participants, n	1122	503		120	110	
Male gender, n (%)‡	521 (46%)	215 (43%)	0.17	58 (48%)	53 (44%)	0.98
Age in years (mean, SE)†	59.3 (0.2)	58.6 (0.3)	0.05	63.8 (0.6)	62.8 (0.7)	0.26
Alcohol consumption in g/day (mean, SE)†	11.7 (0.4)	11.8 (0.5)	0.83	13.8 (1.2)	13.6 (1.3)	0.91
Body mass index in kg/m^2, mean (SE)†	25.2 (0.1)	25.4 (0.2)	0.25	26.4 (0.4)	26.5 (0.4)	0.89
Hypertension yes/no, n (%)‡	214 (21%)	113 (25%)	0.11	26 (22%)	27 (25%)	0.47
Current smoking yes/no, n (%)‡	151 (13%)	74 (15%)	0.5	11 (9%)	11 (1%)	0.86
History of disease‡						
COPD n (%)	26 (3%)	12 (3%)	0.95	5 (4%)	6 (5%)	0.61
Stroke, n (%)	21 (2%)	13 (3%)	0.19	3 (3%)	0 (0%)	0.10
Myocard infarct, n (%)	20 (2%)	13 (3%)	0.24	1 (1%)	1 (1%)	0.94
Malignancy, n (%)	87 (6%)	34 (7%)	0.48	8 (7%)	9 (8%)	0.61
Number of hepatotoxic medications, n (%)‡			0.74			0.36
0	976 (87%)	444 (88%)		84 (82%)	76 (79%)	
1	129 (11%)	53 (11%)		17 (17%)	18 (19%)	
2	17 (2%)	6 (1%)		0 (0%)	2 (2%)	
3	0 (0%)	0 (0%)		1 (1%)	0 (0%)	
Use of lipid modifying agents, n (%)‡	76 (7%)	37 (7%)	0.67	7 (6%)	18 (16%)	0.01
Insulin in µIU/L (mean, 95% CI)^a	15.7 (15.0–16.5)	16.5 (15.4–17.7)	0.25	5.89 (5.31–6.54)	6.74 (6.04–7.52)	0.08
Glucose in mmol/L (mean, 95% CI)^a	5.68 (5.62–5.75)	5.87 (5.78–5.97)	0.001	5.00 (4.91–5.09)	5.13 (5.04–5.23)	0.04

Values are means (SE, standard error or 95% CI, confidence interval) or numbers (%). P values are from student's t-test (†), Pearson chi-square test (‡), and from linear mixed model analysis, correcting for age, gender, BMI, and correlation of sibling relationship (^{a}). Models were fitted for natural log-transformed values for insulin. For transformed variables, data are presented as geometric means with 95% confidence intervals.
Age: age at serum screening, Hypertension: systolic blood pressure ≥130 mmHg and/or diastolic pressure ≥85 mmHg, or administration of antihypertensive medication, COPD: chronic obstructive pulmonary disease, Insulin: nonfasting serum insulin levels, Glucose: nonfasting serum glucose levels.

medications). Sex specific analysis showed that after excluding all subjects with lipid-modifying agents, nonfasting triglyceride levels were lower in female offspring compared to controls (1.3 mmol/L vs 1.5 mmol/L, p = 0.001 respectively, but not in male offspring compared to controls (1.7 mmol/L vs 1.8 mmol/L, p = 0.42 respectively).

Liver biochemical test results from the fasting group are shown in table 3. In both the minimally adjusted and the fully adjusted models, fasting ALT, AST, GGT, and triglyceride levels were similar in offspring of long-lived siblings and control subjects. Also after excluding all subjects with lipid-modifying agents, triglyceride levels were similar between the two groups (offspring versus controls, 1.51 mmol/L vs 1.52 mmol/L, p = 0.90 after adjusting for age, gender, correlation of sibling relationship, smoking, BMI, and use of alcohol and hepatotoxic medications). Sex specific analysis showed that in both sexes triglyceride levels were similar between offspring of long-lived siblings and controls.

Computed tomography evaluation of liver steatosis in offspring of long-lived siblings and control subjects are shown for a random subgroup in table 4 and figure 2. In the subgroup for which computed tomography data were available, nonfasting glucose levels were lower in the offspring group as compared to the control subjects, although this difference was only borderline significant (5.7 and 6.0 mmol/L for offspring of long-lived siblings and partners respectively, p = 0.06). However, nonfasting triglyceride levels (1.6 and 1.6 mmol/L for offspring and partners, respectively, p = 0.62) were not different between the two groups in the computed tomography group. In both the minimally adjusted and the fully adjusted models, absolute liver HU values and L/S ratios were not different between the two groups (p = 0.23 and p = 0.25, respectively). Also, prevalence of moderate-to-severe NAFLD was similar between offspring of long-lived siblings and control subjects (18% and 21% for offspring of long-lived siblings versus controls respectively, L/S ratio <1; 8% and 8% for offspring of long-lived siblings versus controls respectively, L/S ratio <0.8).

Discussion

The main findings of this study are threefold. First, in a large nonfasting cohort we found that plasma ALT levels were relatively higher in the offspring of long-lived siblings as compared to controls, while nonfasting triglyceride levels were lower in offspring of long-lived siblings. In this group, plasma AST and GGT levels were similar between the two groups. Second, in our fasting subsample, all liver biochemical tests and serum triglyceride levels were similar between offspring of long-lived siblings as compared to controls. Third, computed tomography assessed liver-spleen ratios were not different between the two groups, indicating that the extent of liver fat is not different.

Consistent with the critical role for liver fat in the pathogenesis of hepatic insulin resistance and type 2 diabetes, recent studies showed that caloric restriction rapidly lowers hepatic fat content and improves hepatic insulin sensitivity in type 2 diabetes patients [10,24]. Insulin resistance is strongly correlated with liver steatosis, and interventions that ameliorate insulin resistance result in lower

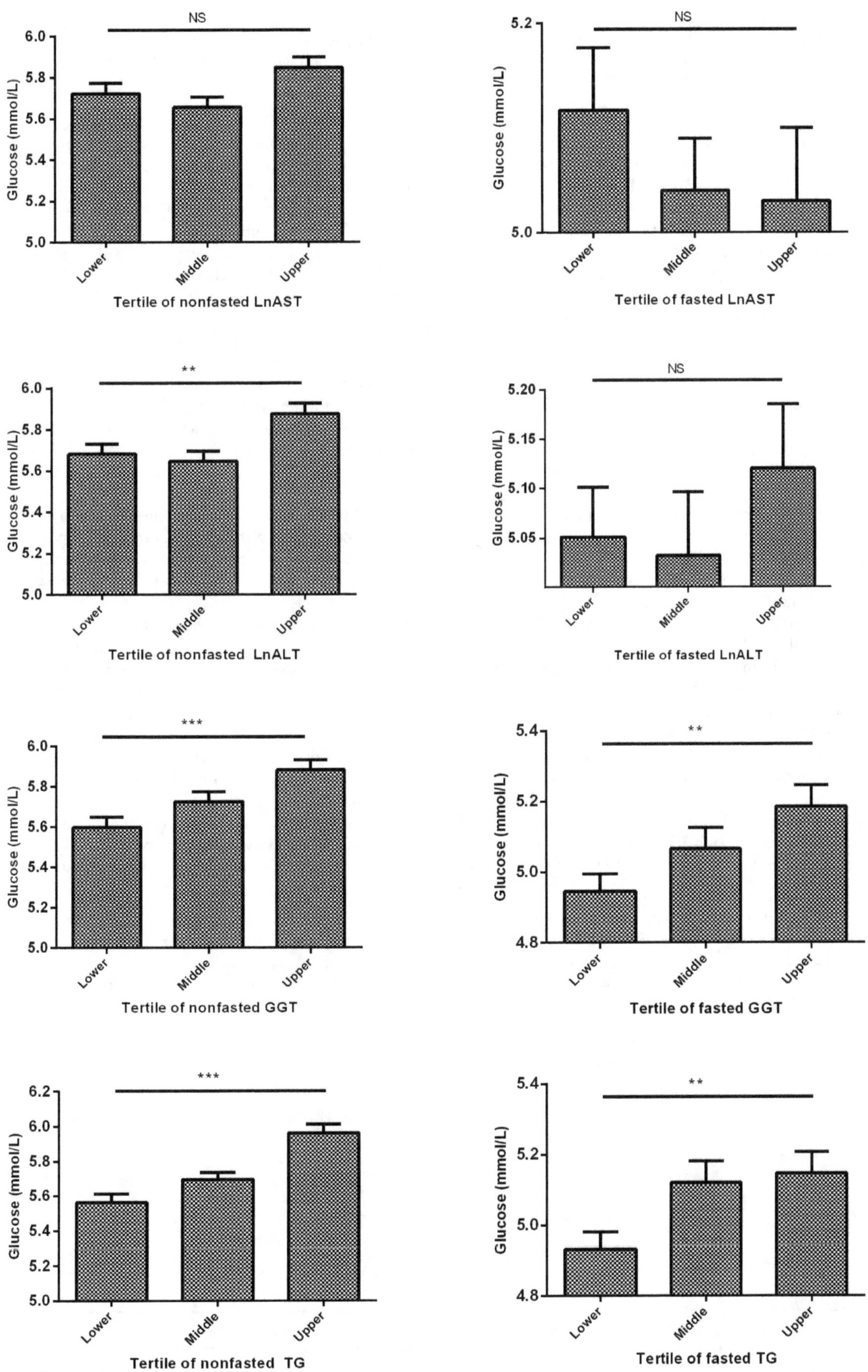
NS
Glucose (mmol/L)
Lower
Middle
Upper
Tertile of nonfasted LnAST
NS
Glucose (mmol/L)
Lower
Middle
Upper
Tertile of fasted LnAST
**
Glucose (mmol/L)
Lower
Middle
Upper
Tertile of nonfasted LnALT
NS
Glucose (mmol/L)
Lower
Middle
Upper
Tertile of fasted LnALT
***
Glucose (mmol/L)
Lower
Middle
Upper
Tertile of nonfasted GGT
**
Glucose (mmol/L)
Lower
Middle
Upper
Tertile of fasted GGT
***
Glucose (mmol/L)
Lower
Middle
Upper
Tertile of nonfasted TG
**
Glucose (mmol/L)
Lower
Middle
Upper
Tertile of fasted TG

Figure 1. Association between liver biochemical test parameters and serum glucose. Tertiles of plasma LnALT, LnAST, LnGGT and serum LnTriglyceride (TG) (mmol/L) in association with nonfasting serum levels (mmol/L) of glucose. Asterisks (*p<0.05, **p<0.01, ***p<0.001) represents significant difference between groups using linear regression analysis, correcting for relation to sibling relationship, age, gender, smoking, alcohol use in g/day, and number of hepatotoxic medication. NS: not significant.

insulin levels and decreased liver fat content [25]. While it has been demonstrated earlier that familial longevity is marked by better glucose tolerance and better peripheral insulin sensitivity [7,8], our data indicate that this healthy metabolic profile is not accompanied by differences in liver fat content. In line with this notion, it was previously shown that familial longevity is marked by enhanced peripheral but not hepatic insulin sensitivity [8]. Moreover, we previously found no differences in C-reactive protein levels, a marker of systemic inflammation, between offspring of long-lived siblings and control subjects [26]. While it has been suggested that NAFLD is characterized by a systemic low-grade inflammation [27], this may also support our finding that the extent of liver fat content is similar between the two groups.

We found that nonfasting plasma ALT levels were slightly higher in offspring of long-lived siblings as compared to age-matched control subjects. This is a surprising finding as it suggests a greater liver fat content in the offspring group. One potential explanation may be that we observed a statistically but not clinically significant difference in plasma ALT levels between the two groups. An alternative explanation is that the observed difference in ALT levels is clinically significant. In line with this explanation, another recent study found that lower serum ALT levels were associated with higher all-cause mortality in old age [28]. On the other hand, in our fasting subsample, we found that fasting ALT levels were similar between the two groups. Also, we found similar levels of both fasting and nonfasting serum GGT between groups. While GGT is more strongly associated with diabetes incidence than ALT [5], it may thus be a better marker of liver fat, although ALT is considered a more liver-specific marker than GGT [5].

In the postprandial condition, triglycerides in the plasma originate mainly from intestinal derived chylomicrons and to a smaller extent from very low density lipoproteins (VLDL) [29]. Plasma triglyceride levels can increase substantially postprandially, and elevated postprandial levels, via higher peak concentrations or delayed clearance, may represent an abnormal response to an oral fat load that reflects insulin resistance [30]. Although currently under debate [31], national guidelines recommend measuring lipid levels in a fasting state. In the fasting state plasma triglyceride levels are mainly determined by triglycerides within VLDL as secreted by the liver [32]. Accordingly, results from previous studies using fasting blood samples indicate that liver fat content correlates with fasting serum triglyceride levels [12,18,33]. Furthermore, excessive liver fat accumulation influences the VLDL production rate [34]. In our full cohort, nonfasting serum triglyceride levels were lower in offspring of long-lived siblings as compared to controls, while nonfasting serum triglyceride levels in the CT group were similar, which is in line with the similar extent of liver fat as assessed by L/S ratios in this group. However, the CT group may thus be not fully representative for the full nonfasting group. On the other hand, in the fasting group, fasting triglyceride levels were similar, although lack of statistical power to detect a difference due to the relatively small sample size may also have been a factor. Still, based on the considerations above, we believe that liver biochemical test results from the fasting samples are in fact most indicative in assessing liver fat content.

Our data support the notion that, although healthy longevity is marked by better glucose tolerance and better peripheral insulin sensitivity, this favourable metabolic condition is not accompanied by early differences in liver fat. This strongly suggests that differences in NAFLD will only be detectable later in the pathophysiology towards type 2 diabetes pathogenesis. This notion is in line with those of a study that addressed the time sequence of the various metabolic abnormalities associated with the development of type 2 diabetes by studying their reversal after bariatric surgery [35]. Within days after surgery, liver fat levels fell and normal hepatic insulin sensitivity was restored, arguing that

Table 2. Nonfasting liver enzymes and triglycerides in offspring of long-lived siblings and control subjects.

	Offspring (n = 1122)	Controls (n = 503)	p-value
ALT in mmol/L			
Model 1	22.2 (21.7–22.8)	21.2 (20.5–22.0)	0.04
Model 2	24.3 (22.8–25.9)	23.2 (21.6–24.8)	0.03
AST in mmol/L			
Model 1	26.2 (25.8–26.5)	25.9 (25.4–26.4)	0.36
Model 2	27.1 (26.1–28.1)	26.8 (25.7–27.9)	0.39
GGT in mmol/L			
Model 1	22.9 (22.2–23.6)	23.2 (22.1–24.3)	0.66
Model 2	27.9 (25.8–30.2)	27.9 (25.6–30.4)	0.96
Triglycerides in mmol/L			
Model 1	1.51 (1.47–1.56)	1.63 (1.55–1.70)	0.01
Model 2	1.55 (1.49–1.61)	1.65 (1.57–1.74)	0.02

Results are from linear mixed models, correcting for age, gender, and correlation of sibling relationship (model 1) and additionally for smoking, body mass index, alcohol use in g/day and number of hepatotoxic medications (model 2). Models were fitted for natural log-transformed values of alanine transaminase (ALT), aspartate transaminase (AST), gamma-glutamyltransferase (GGT), and LnTriglycerides. Geometric means (95% confidence interval) are reported for transformed variables.

Table 3. Fasting liver enzymes and triglycerides in offspring of long-lived siblings and control subjects.

	Offspring (n = 120)	Controls (n = 110)	p-value
ALT in mmol/L			
Model 1	16.3 (15.2–17.4)	15.9 (14.8–17.0)	0.64
Model 2	20.1 (15.6–25.8)	19.3 (15.0–24.9)	0.52
AST in mmol/L			
Model 1	21.2 (20.2–22.1)	20.7 (19.7–21.6)	0.45
Model 2	22.9 (19.5–27.0)	22.7 (19.2–26.8)	0.80
GGT in mmol/L			
Model 1	23.1 (21.0–25.4)	22.9 (20.7–25.3)	0.89
Model 2	35.5 (25.1–50.2)	34.8 (24.4–49.5)	0.80
Triglycerides in mmol/L			
Model 1	1.25 (1.16–1.35)	1.25 (1.16–1.36)	0.94
Model 2	1.47 (1.13–1.91)	1.47 (1.13–1.92)	0.99

Results are from linear mixed models, correcting for age, gender, and correlation of sibling relationship (model 1) and additionally for smoking, body mass index, alcohol use in g/day and number of hepatotoxic medications (model 2). Models were fitted for natural log-transformed values of alanine transaminase (ALT), aspartate transaminase (AST) and gamma-glutamyltransferase (GGT), and LnTriglycerides. Geometric means (95% confidence interval) are reported for transformed variables.

NAFLD is a late step in the pathophysiology towards type 2 diabetes. In contrast, muscle insulin sensitivity remained abnormal up to months after bariatric surgery, arguing that this is an earlier step and that muscle insulin resistance, caused by genetic and-or environmental factors, will facilitate the development of fatty liver at a later stage. Therefore, as previously proposed [8], it is plausible that longevity genes are involved in favourable muscle insulin sensitivity observed in familial longevity. The differences in peripheral insulin sensitivity are potentially related to the (epi)genetic differences previously observed in nutrient sensing pathways between groups [36,37].

A strength of the current study is the large sample size which enabled us to adjust for multiple factors affecting both liver biochemical test parameters and liver attenuation at computed tomography. Also, our control group comprises partners of offspring which did not differ on any major indicators of lifestyle, including level of education, current smoking, and BMI [14].

The liver function tests we used to evaluate the extent of liver steatosis (ALT, AST, and GGT) cannot confirm a diagnosis of NAFLD or distinguish between steatosis, steatohepatitis, and cirrhosis [38]. Also, although mildly elevated ALT levels are the primary abnormality seen in NAFLD patients, liver enzymes may be normal in up to 70% of patients with NAFLD [39]. Still, in epidemiological studies, liver fat content is commonly assessed by using these liver function tests, and ALT in particular is judged to be an acceptable marker of liver fat content [40]. Although magnetic resonance proton spectroscopy is the most accurate non-invasive method to quantitate liver fat, CT imaging provides visualization of the whole liver, by which liver steatosis can be detected with high reproducibility in clinically asymptomatic

Table 4. Computed tomography markers of liver steatosis in offspring of long-lived siblings and control subjects.

	Offspring (n = 138)	Controls (n = 130)	p-value
Liver attenuation (HU)			
Model 1, mean (95% CI)	60.8 (59.2–62.3)	62.0 (60.4–63.6)	0.28
Model 2, mean (95% CI)	60.8 (58.8–62.7)	62.1 (60.1–64.0)	0.23
Liver/spleen ratio			
Model 1, mean (95% CI)	1.12 (1.09–1.16)	1.15 (1.11–1.18)	0.34
Model 2, mean (95% CI)	1.12 (1.07–1.16)	1.14 (1.1–1.18)	0.25
NAFLD (L/S ratio <1), number (%)†	29 (18%)	32 (21%)	
Model 1, OR (95% CI)	1.10 (0.54–2.26)		0.79
Model 2, OR (95% CI)	1.01 (0.51–2.25)		0.85
NAFLD (L/S ratio <0.8), number (%)†	12 (8%)	12 (8%)	
Model 1, OR (95% CI)	1.06 (0.40 2.85)		0.90
Model 2, OR (95% CI)	0.94 (0.34–2.63)		0.91

Results are from linear mixed model and logistics regression analysis, correcting for age and gender (model 1) and additionally for smoking, body mass index, alcohol use in g/day, and number of hepatotoxic medications (model 2).

†LS ratio were available in 131 offspring and 116 controls.

NAFLD: moderate-to-severe non-alcoholic fatty liver disease, L/S ratio: liver/spleen ratio, 95% CI: 95% confidence interval, HU: hounsfield units.

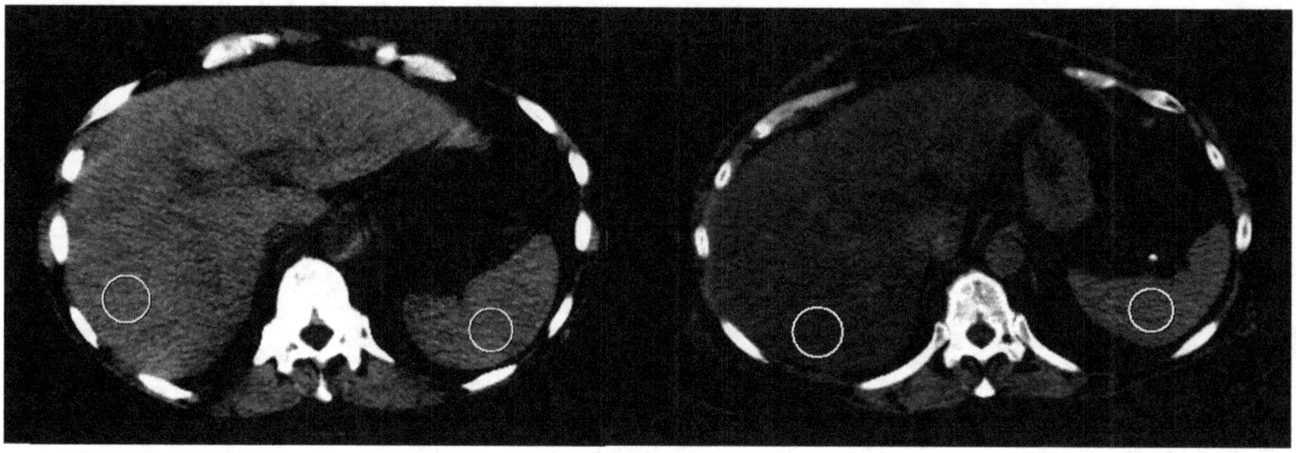

Figure 2. Unenhanced Computed Tomography (CT) scan of the upper abdomen, axial view. Normal liver in a 58-year-old female; liver attenuation is 62 HU, spleen is 55 HU, liver-spleen ratio is 1.1 (a). 64-year-old female with liver steatosis; the liver parenchyma (28 HU) is relatively hypodense compared to the spleen (55 HU), liver-spleen ratio is 0.5 (b). HU: hounsfield units.

individuals in the community [41]. For this purpose, CT is used to quantify liver steatosis in epidemiological studies [33,42,43] and clinical trials [22]. The time span between blood sampling and image acquisition is relatively large which is a potential limitation. On the other hand, we used liver biochemical test parameters and CT liver attenuation values as separate and independent (e.g. assessed at different times, with different group compositions) markers of liver steatosis in our analysis, which actually may be considered a strength of this study.

In our fasting sample we found no differences between groups in the extent of liver steatosis, as assessed with liver biochemical tests and serum triglyceride levels. These results are in line with our CT findings that liver-spleen ratios were similar between the two groups. We conclude that decreased liver steatosis is not an early metabolic phenotype that associates with the more favourable glucose metabolism in familial longevity.

Author Contributions

Conceived and designed the experiments: Conceived of the study and its initial design: LK SM DvH. Involved in data collection: LK JvdG DvH. Analyzed and interpreted the data: MS DvH JvdG. Provided support on data analysis and interpretation: AdR PES SM BR. Contributed to and edited the report: MS LK BR JvdG PES SM AdR DvH. Approved the report before submission: MS LK BR JvdG PES SM AdR DvH.

References

1. Chalasani N, Younossi Z, Lavine JE, Diehl AM, Brunt EM, et al. (2012) The diagnosis and management of non-alcoholic fatty liver disease: practice Guideline by the American Association for the Study of Liver Diseases, American College of Gastroenterology, and the American Gastroenterological Association. Hepatology 55: 2005–2023. 10.1002/hep.25762 [doi].
2. Koehler EM, Schouten JN, Hansen BE, van Rooij FJ, Hofman A, et al. (2012) Prevalence and risk factors of non-alcoholic fatty liver disease in the elderly: results from the Rotterdam study. J Hepatol 57: 1305–1311. S0168-8278(12)00604-6 [pii];10.1016/j.jhep.2012.07.028 [doi].
3. Leite NC, Salles GF, Araujo AL, Villela-Nogueira CA, Cardoso CR (2009) Prevalence and associated factors of non-alcoholic fatty liver disease in patients with type-2 diabetes mellitus. Liver Int 29: 113–119. LIV1718 [pii];10.1111/j.1478-3231.2008.01718.x [doi].
4. Farese RV, Jr., Zechner R, Newgard CB, Walther TC (2012) The problem of establishing relationships between hepatic steatosis and hepatic insulin resistance. Cell Metab 15: 570–573. S1550-4131(12)00099-X [pii];10.1016/j.cmet.2012.03.004 [doi].
5. Fraser A, Harris R, Sattar N, Ebrahim S, Davey SG, et al. (2009) Alanine aminotransferase, gamma-glutamyltransferase, and incident diabetes: the British Women's Heart and Health Study and meta-analysis. Diabetes Care 32: 741–750. dc08-1870 [pii];10.2337/dc08-1870 [doi].
6. Reaven GM (2005) Compensatory hyperinsulinemia and the development of an atherogenic lipoprotein profile: the price paid to maintain glucose homeostasis in insulin-resistant individuals. Endocrinol Metab Clin North Am 34: 49–62. S0889-8529(04)00106-9 [pii];10.1016/j.ecl.2004.12.001 [doi].
7. Rozing MP, Westendorp RG, de Craen AJ, Frolich M, de Goeij MC, et al. (2010) Favorable glucose tolerance and lower prevalence of metabolic syndrome in offspring without diabetes mellitus of nonagenarian siblings: the Leiden longevity study. J Am Geriatr Soc 58: 564–569. JGS2725 [pii];10.1111/j.1532-5415.2010.02725.x [doi].
8. Wijsman CA, Rozing MP, Streefland TC, le CS, Mooijaart SP, et al. (2011) Familial longevity is marked by enhanced insulin sensitivity. Aging Cell 10: 114–121. 10.1111/j.1474-9726.2010.00650.x [doi].
9. Wijsman CA, van Opstal AM, Kan HE, Maier AB, Westendorp RG, et al. (2012) Proton magnetic resonance spectroscopy shows lower intramyocellular lipid accumulation in middle-aged subjects predisposed to familial longevity. Am J Physiol Endocrinol Metab 302: E344–E348. ajpendo.00455.2011 [pii];10.1152/ajpendo.00455.2011 [doi].
10. Petersen KF, Dufour S, Befroy D, Lehrke M, Hendler RE, et al. (2005) Reversal of nonalcoholic hepatic steatosis, hepatic insulin resistance, and hyperglycemia by moderate weight reduction in patients with type 2 diabetes. Diabetes 54: 603–608. 54/3/603 [pii].
11. Vaarhorst AA, Beekman M, Suchiman EH, van Heemst D, Houwing-Duistermaat JJ, et al. (2011) Lipid metabolism in long-lived families: the Leiden Longevity Study. Age (Dordr) 33: 219–227. 10.1007/s11357-010-9172-6 [doi].
12. Marchesini G, Brizi M, Bianchi G, Tomassetti S, Bugianesi E, et al. (2001) Nonalcoholic fatty liver disease: a feature of the metabolic syndrome. Diabetes 50: 1844–1850.
13. Schoenmaker M, de Craen AJ, de Meijer PH, Beekman M, Blauw GJ, et al. (2006) Evidence of genetic enrichment for exceptional survival using a family approach: the Leiden Longevity Study. Eur J Hum Genet 14: 79–84. 5201508 [pii];10.1038/sj.ejhg.5201508 [doi].
14. Westendorp RG, van Heemst D, Rozing MP, Frolich M, Mooijaart SP, et al. (2009) Nonagenarian siblings and their offspring display lower risk of mortality and morbidity than sporadic nonagenarians: The Leiden Longevity Study. J Am Geriatr Soc 57: 1634–1637. JGS2381 [pii];10.1111/j.1532-5415.2009.02381.x [doi].
15. Vliegenthart R, Geleijnse JM, Hofman A, Meijer WT, van Rooij FJ, et al. (2002) Alcohol consumption and risk of peripheral arterial disease: the Rotterdam study. Am J Epidemiol 155: 332–338.
16. World Health Organization Collabarating Center for Drug Statistics Methodology. Guidelines for ATC classification and DDD assignment 2013. WHO: Oslo; 2013. Available at: http://www.whocc.no/atc_ddd_index/(accessed Feb 14, 2014).
17. Jessurun N, Hunsel van F (2013) Leverschade niet te onderschatten bijeffect. Pharmaceutisch Weekblad 148(5): 28–31.

18. Speliotes EK, Massaro JM, Hoffmann U, Foster MC, Sahani DV, et al. (2008) Liver fat is reproducibly measured using computed tomography in the Framingham Heart Study. J Gastroenterol Hepatol 23: 894–899. JGH5420 [pii];10.1111/j.1440-1746.2008.05420.x [doi].
19. Browning JD, Szczepaniak LS, Dobbins R, Nuremberg P, Horton JD, et al. (2004) Prevalence of hepatic steatosis in an urban population in the United States: impact of ethnicity. Hepatology 40: 1387–1395. 10.1002/hep.20466 [doi].
20. Szczepaniak LS, Nurenberg P, Leonard D, Browning JD, Reingold JS, et al. (2005) Magnetic resonance spectroscopy to measure hepatic triglyceride content: prevalence of hepatic steatosis in the general population. Am J Physiol Endocrinol Metab 288: E462–E468. 10.1152/ajpendo.00064.2004 [doi];00064.2004 [pii].
21. Saadeh S, Younossi ZM, Remer EM, Gramlich T, Ong JP, et al. (2002) The utility of radiological imaging in nonalcoholic fatty liver disease. Gastroenterology 123: 745–750. S001650850200166X [pii].
22. Foster T, Budoff MJ, Saab S, Ahmadi N, Gordon C, et al. (2011) Atorvastatin and antioxidants for the treatment of nonalcoholic fatty liver disease: the St Francis Heart Study randomized clinical trial. Am J Gastroenterol 106: 71–77. ajg2010299 [pii];10.1038/ajg.2010.299 [doi].
23. Park SH, Kim PN, Kim KW, Lee SW, Yoon SE, Pet al. (2006) Macrovesicular hepatic steatosis in living liver donors: use of CT for quantitative and qualitative assessment. Radiology 239: 105–112. 2391050361 [pii];10.1148/radiol.2391050361 [doi].
24. Lim EL, Hollingsworth KG, Aribisala BS, Chen MJ, Mathers JC, et al. (2011) Reversal of type 2 diabetes: normalisation of beta cell function in association with decreased pancreas and liver triacylglycerol. Diabetologia 54: 2506–2514. 10.1007/s00125-011-2204-7 [doi].
25. Hebbard L, George J (2011) Animal models of nonalcoholic fatty liver disease. Nat Rev Gastroenterol Hepatol 8: 35–44. nrgastro.2010.191 [pii];10.1038/nrgastro.2010.191 [doi].
26. Rozing MP, Mooijaart SP, Beekman M, Wijsman CA, Maier AB, et al. (2011) C-reactive protein and glucose regulation in familial longevity. Age (Dordr) 33: 623–630. 10.1007/s11357-011-9206-8 [doi].
27. Targher G (2006) Relationship between high-sensitivity C-reactive protein levels and liver histology in subjects with non-alcoholic fatty liver disease. J Hepatol 45: 879–881. S0168-8278(06)00502-2 [pii];10.1016/j.jhep.2006.09.005 [doi].
28. Ford I, Mooijaart SP, Lloyd S, Murray HM, Westendorp RG, et al. (2011) The inverse relationship between alanine aminotransferase in the normal range and adverse cardiovascular and non-cardiovascular outcomes. Int J Epidemiol 40: 1530–1538. dyr172 [pii];10.1093/ije/dyr172 [doi].
29. Redgrave TG (2004) Chylomicron metabolism. Biochem Soc Trans 32: 79–82. 10.1042/[doi].
30. Bansal S, Buring JE, Rifai N, Mora S, Sacks FM, et al. (2007) Fasting compared with nonfasting triglycerides and risk of cardiovascular events in women. JAMA 298: 309–316. 298/3/309 [pii];10.1001/jama.298.3.309 [doi].
31. Sidhu D, Naugler C (2012) Fasting time and lipid levels in a community-based population: a cross-sectional study. Arch Intern Med 172: 1707–1710. 1391022 [pii];10.1001/archinternmed.2012.3708 [doi].
32. Voshol PJ, Rensen PC, van Dijk KW, Romijn JA, Havekes LM (2009) Effect of plasma triglyceride metabolism on lipid storage in adipose tissue: studies using genetically engineered mouse models. Biochim Biophys Acta 1791: 479–485. S1388-1981(08)00239-4 [pii];10.1016/j.bbalip.2008.12.015 [doi].
33. Kim LJ, Nalls MA, Eiriksdottir G, Sigurdsson S, Launer LJ, et al. (2011) Associations of visceral and liver fat with the metabolic syndrome across the spectrum of obesity: the AGES-Reykjavik study. Obesity (Silver Spring) 19: 1265–1271. oby2010291 [pii];10.1038/oby.2010.291 [doi].
34. Adiels M, Taskinen MR, Packard C, Caslake MJ, Soro-Paavonen A, et al. (2006) Overproduction of large VLDL particles is driven by increased liver fat content in man. Diabetologia 49: 755–765. 10.1007/s00125-005-0125-z [doi].
35. Taylor R (2008) Pathogenesis of type 2 diabetes: tracing the reverse route from cure to cause. Diabetologia 51: 1781–1789. 10.1007/s00125-008-1116-7 [doi].
36. Deelen J, Uh HW, Monajemi R, van Heemst D, Thijssen PE, et al. (2013) Gene set analysis of GWAS data for human longevity highlights the relevance of the insulin/IGF-1 signaling and telomere maintenance pathways. Age (Dordr) 35: 235–249. 10.1007/s11357-011-9340-3 [doi].
37. Passtoors WM, Beekman M, Deelen J, van der Breggen R, Maier AB, et al. (2013) Gene expression analysis of mTOR pathway: association with human longevity. Aging Cell 12: 24–31. 10.1111/acel.12015 [doi].
38. Adams LA, Angulo P, Lindor KD (2005) Nonalcoholic fatty liver disease. CMAJ 172: 899–905. 172/7/899 [pii];10.1503/cmaj.045232 [doi].
39. Obika M, Noguchi H (2012) Diagnosis and evaluation of nonalcoholic fatty liver disease. Exp Diabetes Res 2012: 145754. 10.1155/2012/145754 [doi].
40. Schindhelm RK, Diamant M, Dekker JM, Tushuizen ME, Teerlink T, et al. (2006) Alanine aminotransferase as a marker of non-alcoholic fatty liver disease in relation to type 2 diabetes mellitus and cardiovascular disease. Diabetes Metab Res Rev 22: 437–443. 10.1002/dmrr.666 [doi].
41. Schwenzer NF, Springer F, Schraml C, Stefan N, Machann J, et al. (2009) Non-invasive assessment and quantification of liver steatosis by ultrasound, computed tomography and magnetic resonance. J Hepatol 51: 433–445. S0168-8278(09)00390-0 [pii];10.1016/j.jhep.2009.05.023 [doi].
42. Speliotes EK, Massaro JM, Hoffmann U, Vasan RS, Meigs JB, et al. (2010) Fatty liver is associated with dyslipidemia and dysglycemia independent of visceral fat: the Framingham Heart Study. Hepatology 51: 1979–1987. 10.1002/hep.23593 [doi].
43. Dick TJ, Lesser IA, Leipsic JA, Mancini GB, Lear SA (2013) The effect of obesity on the association between liver fat and carotid atherosclerosis in a multi-ethnic cohort. Atherosclerosis 226: 208–213. S0021-9150(12)00724-1 [pii];10.1016/j.atherosclerosis.2012.10.040 [doi].

20

Plasma Metabolomic Profiling Suggests Early Indications for Predisposition to Latent Insulin Resistance in Children Conceived by ICSI

Alexandra Gkourogianni[1], Ioanna Kosteria[1], Aristeidis G. Telonis[2,7], Alexandra Margeli[3], Emilia Mantzou[4], Maria Konsta[1], Dimitrios Loutradis[5], George Mastorakos[6], Ioannis Papassotiriou[3], Maria I. Klapa[2], Christina Kanaka-Gantenbein[1], George P. Chrousos[1]*

1 Division of Endocrinology, Diabetes and Metabolism, First Department of Pediatrics, University of Athens Medical School, Athens, Greece, **2** Metabolic Engineering and Systems Biology Laboratory, Institute of Chemical Engineering Sciences, Foundation for Research and Technology-Hellas (FORTH/ICE-HT), Patras, Greece, **3** Department of Clinical Biochemistry, "Aghia Sophia" Children's Hospital, Athens, Greece, **4** Endocrine Unit, Department of Endocrinology and Metabolism, Evgenidion Hospital, Athens, Greece, **5** Division of In Vitro Fertilization, First Department of Obstetrics and Gynecology, University of Athens Medical School, Athens, Greece, **6** Division of Endocrinology, Second Department of Obstetrics and Gynecology, University of Athens Medical School, Athens, Greece, **7** Graduate Program "Biological Technology", Department of Biology, University of Patras, Greece

Abstract

Background: There have been increasing indications about an epigenetically-based elevated predisposition of assisted reproductive technology (ART) offspring to insulin resistance, which can lead to an unfavorable cardio-metabolic profile in adult life. However, the relevant long-term systematic molecular studies are limited, especially for the IntraCytoplasmic Sperm Injection (ICSI) method, introduced in 1992. In this study, we carefully defined a group of 42 prepubertal ICSI and 42 naturally conceived (NC) children. We assessed differences in their metabolic profile based on biochemical measurements, while, for a subgroup, plasma metabolomic analysis was also performed, investigating any relevant insulin resistance indices.

Methods & Results: Auxological and biochemical parameters of 42 6.8±2.1 yrs old ICSI-conceived and 42 age-matched controls were measured. Significant differences between the groups were determined using univariate and multivariate statistics, indicating low urea and low-grade inflammation markers (YKL-40, hsCRP) and high triiodothyronine (T3) in ICSI-children compared to controls. Moreover, plasma metabolomic analysis carried out for a subgroup of 10 ICSI- and 10 NC girls using Gas Chromatography-Mass Spectrometry (GC-MS) indicated clear differences between the two groups, characterized by 36 metabolites linked to obesity, insulin resistance and metabolic syndrome. Notably, the distinction between the two girl subgroups was accentuated when both their biochemical and metabolomic measurements were employed.

Conclusions: The present study contributes a large auxological and biochemical dataset of a well-defined group of pre-pubertal ICSI-conceived subjects to the research of the ART effect to the offspring's health. Moreover, it is the first time that the relevant usefulness of metabolomics was investigated. The acquired results are consistent with early insulin resistance in ICSI-offspring, paving the way for further systematic investigations. These data support that metabolomics may unravel metabolic differences before they become clinically or biochemically evident, underlining its utility in the ART research.

Editor: Ioannis P. Androulakis, Rutgers University, United States of America

Funding: The study was funded by University of Athens, First Pediatric Clinic and FORTH/ICE-HT internal funds and a fellowship of Panhellenic Endocrinology Society to Dr. Alexandra Gkourogianni. The funders had no role in study design, data collection and analysis, decision to publish, or preparation of the manuscript.

Competing Interests: The authors have declared that no competing interests exist.

* E-mail: chrousog@mail.nih.gov

These authors contributed equally to this work.

Introduction

Assisted reproductive technology (ART) comprises the classic *in vitro* fertilization (IVF) and the intra-cytoplasmic sperm injection (ICSI), the latter primarily developed and indicated for the treatment of male infertility [1–3]. ICSI bypasses several natural selection barriers, as it involves the injection of a single spermatozoon or even spermatid directly into the oocyte through the *zona pellucida*. The spermatozoa and/or spermatids currently used in ICSI are usually obtained from oligozoospermic men [3]. The ovarian stimulation protocols and the *in vitro* manipulation of both gametes and the blastocyst raise serious concerns about the genetic, epigenetic and developmental risks of the ICSI method to the offspring [4–6]. Despite these concerns, the European Society of Human Reproduction and Embryology (ESHRE) reported a recent marked increase in the use of ICSI [1], even in cases of no apparent medical indication [7].

Presently, long-term detailed systematic prospective studies of the ART offspring regarding potential health risks are limited, especially for the ICSI method due to its recent (i.e. in 1992) introduction as ART method. The existing studies have mainly investigated auxological data, indicating a higher risk of preterm delivery and intrauterine growth restriction (IUGR) for the ART offspring, leading to children born prematurely and/or small for gestational age (SGA) [8]. Predisposition for adult disease is *per se* increased by being born SGA [9–11], further accentuated by the fact that ART pregnancies are characterized by older mothers, an increased anxiety level before and during pregnancy, and a higher rate of multiple gestations, all risk factors for numerous adverse effects [12]. However, our group as well as others have extended the investigation to cardiometabolic markers reporting that children born after classic IVF show early indices of cardiometabolic derangements, such as higher blood pressure (BP) or higher triglycerides, irrespectively of having been born SGA or not, indicating thus that ART *per se* is a predisposing factor for unfavorable cardiometabolic outcomes [13,14]. Glucocorticoids are considered the main mediators of the poor long-term outcome of an adverse intrauterine environment, by stimulating hepatic gluconeogenesis, inhibiting insulin actions on skeletal muscle and potentiating insulin's actions on visceral adipose tissue, ultimately promoting visceral adiposity and sarcopenia leading to metabolic syndrome [15]. Recent evidence suggests that ART may be associated with epigenetic modifications in several genes that could have long-term impact on the health of the offspring [16] and that both obesity and metabolic syndrome may have their basis in epigenetic modifications [17]. Thus, systematic studies of the ART offspring are required to validate and investigate the causes of the indicated increased predisposition to unfavorable cardiometabolic profiles later in life. Sensitive holistic methods of the metabolic profile that allow for the early detection of subtle metabolic differences are necessary.

In the systems biology era, high-throughput biomolecular omic analyses of biofluid compositions between two groups of subjects contribute to the identification of characteristically discriminatory multi-component molecular profiles. Compared to singling out specific biomarkers, in multivariate analyses, even subtle differences in a molecular quantity can carry significance if viewed in the context of the observed changes in the rest of the molecules. Thus, there is a higher probability for the identification of considerable variations in molecular profiles in complex medical cases, when conventional analyses fail to provide statistically significant results. Moreover, knowledge-based analysis of high-throughput biomolecular profiles in the context of biological networks lead to a broader perspective of the molecular cell physiology dynamics. In this context, omic analyses pave the way for in-depth systemic studies of human physiology [18]. Metabolomics refers to the analysis of the (relative) concentration profile of the free small metabolite pools of a biological system, providing a comprehensive metabolic signature and a direct link to the phenotype [19]. Untargeted blood metabolomics has been used in the context of disease diagnosis, as biological variation in human blood plasma mainly originates from the constant factors in a person's lifetime, i.e. heritable/familial effects and one's stable individual environment [20], metabolic profile being thus a significant component of the epigenetic fingerprint of an individual. In this context, the usefulness of metabolomics in ART research becomes apparent however there exists currently no published report for application of metabolomics in the analysis of ART offspring physiology.

The objective of this study is to explore in a cross-sectional design the presence of metabolic variation in pre-pubertal children born after ICSI compared to age- and demographically- matched naturally conceived (NC) controls, using medical history and biochemical data, along with untargeted metabolomic analysis of blood plasma in a subgroup of them, investigating any relevance of insulin resistance indices.

Materials and Methods

Subjects

The "ICSI group". Forty-two ICSI-conceived [19 boys (45.23%) and 23 girls (54.76%)] healthy prepubertal caucasian children with a mean age of 6.8±2.1 yrs were recruited randomly from the IVF Section of the First Department of Obstetrics-Gynaecology of the University of Athens (Table 1). Underlining the difficulty in recruiting such a large group of ART-conceived children and conducting this type of systematic studies, we report that only 20% of the families contacted were willing to participate in the study.

The "naturally conceived (NC) control group". Forty-two age- ($P = 0.93$) and gender- ($P = 0.99$) matched, naturally conceived healthy prepubertal caucasian children served as controls (Table 1). These children were selected among those referred to the Division of Endocrinology for growth assessment but found to be within the normal growth curves and willing to participate in the study.

From the initial cohort of the 84 children, a subgroup comprising 10 girls from each of the ICSI and NC groups (6.8 ± 2.1yrs) were studied using metabolomics. The girls were selected from the ICSI and NC groups in pairs matched for age, duration of gestation, birth weight and them being singletons or twins (Table 2). We opted for the first investigation of the usefulness of metabolomics in this type of research to be based on a single sex. Girls were selected over boys, since most cases of precocious adrenarche, an insulin resistance marker, occur in females [21,22]. Thus, we expected for any potential early metabolic variation between the ICSI and NC groups, in the form of differences in the plasma metabolite concentration profiles that were measured through metabolomics, could be more apparent in girls compared to boys, increasing the potential for them being detected even if subtle.

Ethical issues

The study was approved by the Ethics Committee of the "Aghia Sophia" Children's Hospital. Children were included in the study only after informed written consent had been obtained from their parents or guardians.

Medical History

A thorough medical history was obtained from all subjects and their parents. Specifically, the recorded data included: a) for the parents: maternal and paternal age at the time of conception, years and number of trials of IVF-ICSI in order to achieve a pregnancy, course of gestation, problems during the perinatal period, type of childbirth (vaginal delivery or cesarean section), chronic disease of the parents, b) for the children: gender, gestational age, twins or singletons, birth weight, birth length, head circumference at birth, duration of breastfeeding, as well as the child's personal and family medical history. Children were classified as SGA or AGA when birth weight was <10th or between the 10th and 90th centile,

Table 1. Demographic and anthropometric characteristics of ICSI and normal conception (NC) groups.

		ICSI (n = 42)	Control (n = 42)	P
Gender, n (%)	**Boys**	19 (45.2%)	19 (45.2%)	0.999[c]
	Girls	23 (54.8%)	23 (54.8%)	
Twins, n (%)	**Singletons**	13 (31%)	36 (85.7%)	<0.0001[c]
	Twins	29 (69%)	6 (14.3%)	
Pregnancy outcome	**Uneventful**	22 (52.4%)	27 (71%)	0.09[c]
	Complicated	20 (47.6%)	11 (29%)	
Type of delivery	**Normal**	5 (11.9%)	17 (40.5%)	0.003[c]
	Caesarean Section	37 (88.1%)	25 (59.5%)	
Perinatal outcome/complications	**Complicated**	19 (45.2%)	16 (38.1%)	0.5[c]
	Uneventful	23 (54.8%)	26 (61.9%)	
Breastfeeding	**YES**	30 (73.2%)	30 (71.4%)	0.86[c]
	NO	11 (26.8%)	12 (28.6%)	
Growth for Gestational age	**SGA**	18 (45%)	13 (34.2%)	0.33[c]
	AGA	22 (55%)	25 (65.8%)	
Gestational age (wk)		36 (35–37)	38 (37–40)	0.0001[a]
Birth weight-SDS		−0.39±0.95	0.42±0.9	0.0001[b]
Birth Length-SDS		−0.1 (−0.5–5)	0.5 (−0.3 0.7)	0.015[a]
Child's Age(yr)		7.2 (6.1–8.2)	7.2 (5.8–8.2)	0.93[a]
BMI-sds		−0.2 (−0.8–0.2)	−0.1 (−0.8–0.5)	0.4[a]
Height-sds		0.17±0.92	−0.11±0.99	0.17[b]
Weight-sds		−0.09±0.8	−0.03±0.96	0.7[b]
Waist/height (WHtR)		0.48 (0.45–0.5)	0.48 (0.44–0.52)	0.5[a]
Waist/hip (WHR)		0.96±0.06	0.94±0.06	0.4[b]
SBP-sds		0.006±0.9	0.83±1.02	0.0004[b]
DBP-sds		−0.5 (−0.7–0.009)	−0.26 (−0.6–0.14)	0.2[a]
Mother's Age (yr)		35.6±5.2	31.7±5.3	0.0013[b]
Father's Age (yr)		38 (33.5–40.5)	35.5 (31–40)	0.09[a]

Differences between ICSI-Control children using Pearson X^2 test, two sample Student t-test or Mann-Whitney U test, are depicted and expressed as mean±SD or median and IQR (interquartile range).
[a]: Mann-Whitney test,
[b]: Normal distribution, two-sample t-test,
[c]: Pearson X^2 test.
Abbreviations: AGA = Appropriate for Gestational Age; BMI = body mass index; SBP = systolic blood pressure DBP = diastolic blood pressure; ICSI = Intracytoplasmic Sperm Injection; SGA = Small for Gestational Age; W/H = waist-to hip ratio (WHR); WHtR = Waist-to-height ratio.

respectively, according to the individual centile calculator at www.gestation.net, which took into account birth weight, gestational age, parity, ethnic group, the child's gender, and the mother's height and weight. The children were examined by the same physicians. Demographic and physical examination data recorded are included in Table 1, including height, weight, head circumference, waist to hip ratio (W/H), BMI, pubertal status and systolic (SBP) and diastolic blood pressure (DBP). Girls with Breast Tanner stage (TS) I and boys with testicular size <4 ml were considered prepubertal, while girls with Breast TS≥II and boys with testicular size ≥4 ml pubertal.

Blood Sampling

Blood collection of all subjects was carried out at 8 AM after an overnight fast; both plasma and serum samples were collected and stored at −80°C until analysis. Biochemical data were obtained at the "Aghia Sophia" Children's Hospital. Metabolomic data acquisition and analysis of the 20 selected plasma samples was carried out at FORTH/ICE-HT.

Blood Chemistry

Standard blood biochemical, hematological and hormonal parameters as well as the non-conventional cardiometabolic markers High- sensitivity-Interleukin 6 (hsIL-6), YKL-40 and Hepsidin were assessed by standard methodology using standard equipment. Specifically, blood chemistry including serum glucose, total cholesterol, triglycerides, HDL-Cholesterol, LDL-Cholesterol, uric acid, urea, creatinine, SGOT, SGPT, γGT and iron were determined using the Siemens Advia 1800 Clinical Chemistry System (Siemens Healthcare Diagnostics, Tarrytown, NY, USA). The lipoproteins Apo A-I, Apo-B, Lp(a) and hs-CRP levels were quantified by means of latex-particle-enhanced immunonephelometric assays on the BN ProSpec nephelometer (Dade Behring, Siemens Healthcare Diagnostics, Liederbach, Germany). Serum insulin, cortisol and IGF1 levels were measured using the automated chemiluminescence Siemens ACS180 System Analyzer (Siemens Healthcare Diagnostics, Tarrytown, NY, USA). The intra-assay and interassay coefficients of variation (CV) for all measured variables was <5%, with the exception of the insulin

Table 2. Demographic and anthropometric characteristics of ICSI and normal conception (NC) girl subgroups used in metabolomics.

		ICSI (n = 10)	Control (n = 9)	P
Twins, n (%)	**Singletons**	7 (70%)	6 (66.7%)	0.87[c]
	Twins	3(30%)	3 (33.3%)	
Pregnancy outcome	**Uneventful**	7 (70%)	6 (75%)	0.8[c]
	Complicated	3 (30%)	2 (25%)	
Type of delivery	**Normal**	2 (20%)	3 (33.3%)	0.5[c]
	Caesarean Section	8 (80%)	6 (66.7%)	
Perinatal outcome/complications	**Uneventfull**	7 (70%)	6 (66.7%)	0.87[c]
	Complicated	3 (30%)	3 (33.3%)	
Breastfeeding	**YES**	3 (30%)	3 (33.3%)	0.87[c]
	NO	7 (70%)	6 (66.7%)	
Growth for Gestational age	**SGA**	5 (55.6%)	3 (33.3%)	0.34[c]
	AGA	4 (44.4%)	6 (66.7%)	
Gestational age (wk)		37 (36–39)	38 (36–38)	0.85[a]
Birth weight-sds		0.06±1.07	0.12±0.8	0.9[b]
Birth Length-sds		−0.14 (−0.26–0.5)	−0.26 (−0.4–0.5)	0.8[a]
Child's Age (yr)		6.25 (4.8–7.9)	5.5 (4.3–7.6)	0.6[a]
BMI-sds		0.01±0.9	−0.7±0.8	0.08[b]
Height-sds		−0.01±0.95	−0.5±0.7	0.2[b]
Weight-sds		0.04±0.9	0.095±0.6	0.9[b]
Waist/height (WHtR)		0.49±0.04	0.46±0.02	0.12[b]
Waist/hip (WHR)		0.96±0.06	0.94±0.04	0.4[b]
SBP-sds		−0.5 (−0.7–−0.25)	0.3 (−0.25 to 1.1)	0.1[a]
DBP-sds		−0.4±0.6	−0.2±0.3	0.4[b]
Mother's Age (yr)		34.1±3.3	33.6±6.1	0.8[b]
Father's Age (yr)		37.5 (36–40)	38 (30–39)	0.8[a]

Differences between ICSI-Control children using Pearson X^2 test, two sample Student *t*-test or Mann-Whitney *U* test, are depicted and expressed as mean±SD or median and IQR (interquartile range).
[a]:Mann-Whitney *U* test.
[b]: Normal distribution, two-sample Student *t*-test.
[c]: Pearson X^2 test.
Abbreviations: AGA = Appropriate for Gestational Age; BMI = body mass index; SBP = systolic blood pressure DBP = diastolic blood pressure; ICSI = Intracytoplasmic Sperm Injection; SGA = Small for Gestational Age; W/H = waist-to hip ratio (WHR); WHtR = Waist-to-height ratio.

assay, in which the CV was <10%. Complete blood counts were performed using the Siemens-ADVIA 120 whole blood auto-analyzer (Siemens Healthcare Diagnostics, Tarrytown, NY, USA). Ferritin levels were measured with the electrochemiluminescence immunoassay "ECLIA" using the Roche Elescys 2010 immuno-assay analyzer (Roche Diagnostics Mannheim, Germany). High-sensitivity-Interleukin (IL)-6 levels were measured by sandwich ELISA (R&D systems, Minneapolis, MN, USA) with a CV <6%. Serum concentrations of YKL-40 were determined by sandwich ELISA (Quidel, Santa Clara, CA, USA) with 3.6% and 5.3% intra- and inter-assay CVs, respectively. Hepcidin levels were measured by sandwich ELISA (DRG Instruments, Marburg, Germany), the intra- and inter-assay CVs, where 4.5% and 6.2%, respectively. Homeostasis model assessment (HOMA), as marker of insulin resistance, was calculated according to the original formula [23].

Metabolomic Data Acquisition and Normalization

The Gas Chromatography-Mass Spectrometry (GC-MS) metabolomic analysis of 300 μL blood plasma samples was carried out after appropriate adaptation of a previously described protocol [24]. After addition of 0.14 μg ribitol and 0.25 μg [U-^{13}C]-glucose as internal standards, each sample was derivatized with 100 μL of 20 mg/mL methoxyamine hydrochloride in pyridine and 200 μL of N-methyl-trimethylsylil-trifluoroacetamide (MSTFA), following the protocol. At least three measurements for each sample were acquired, while the experiment was carried out twice in consecutive weeks. After appropriate data normalization and filtering [24,25], the profiles of 70 (35 of known identity and 12 of known chemical class) metabolite relative peak areas (RPAs) were considered in the multivariate statistical analysis for the extraction of biologically relevant conclusions. Full description of the data normalization and filtering steps can be found in File S1 and the normalized metabolomic dataset is provided in Table S1.

Statistical Analyses

Differences of demographic and biochemical data between groups were evaluated by the two sample Student t-test or by the non-parametric Mann–Whitney U-test, according to the normality of the data. The Pearson chi-square (X^2) test was applied to examine the relations between categorical variables. A *p-value* of < 0.05 was considered significant. Analysis was conducted using the STATA-9 statistical software.

Multivariate statistical analysis of the metabolomic and biochemical data of the 20 subject subgroup was carried out using the significance analysis for microarrays (SAM) algorithm in the TM4 MeV (version 4.9.0) omic data analysis software [26], and the Partial Least Squares – Discriminant Analysis (PLS-DA) algorithm in the XLSTAT statistical software (version 2013.4.03). The biochemical profiles included the markers shown in Table 3 augmented by the children's age and BMI. The significant metabolic differences between the groups were visualized by positioning the metabolites, the concentration of which was identified as significantly different between the two groups based on SAM, on the inter-organ metabolic network that was reconstructed based on metabolic databases, human metabolism literature and our own metabolomic data, as described in File S2.

Results

Anthropometric & Biochemical Data

In the ICSI group, mothers'age [35.6±5.2 (ICSI) vs. 31.7±5.3 (NC), $p = 0.0013$], prevalence in twins [29 (ICSI) vs. 6 (NC), $p < 0.0001$] and cesarean sections [37 (ICSI) vs. 25 (NC), $p = 0.003$] were significantly higher than in NC. Moreover, gestational age [median: 36 wks (ICSI) vs. 38 (NC), $p = 0.0001$], birth weight Standard Deviation Score (SDS) [−0.39±0.95 (ICSI) vs. 0.42±0.9 (NC), $p < 0.0001$] and birth length SDS [median: −0.1 (ICSI) vs. 0.5 (NC), $p = 0.015$] were significantly lower in ICSI children than controls. No differences were identified regarding gender, pregnancy outcome, perinatal outcome/complications, breastfeeding, or fathers' age (Table 1).

Statistical analysis of the demographic data indicates a well selected and consistent group with no differences in the family and personal lifestyle or other demographic parameters that may

Table 3. Biochemical, hormonal and non-conventional cardiometabolic markers in ICSI and NC children groups.

		ICSI (n = 42)	Control (n = 42)	p-value**
Hematologic parameters	**Hct (%)**	39.5±2.9	38.4± 2.2	0.07*
	Hb (g/dL)	13.1± 1.1	12.8± 0.8	0.22*
	Fe (μg/dL)	71.9± 21.7	88.8±38.9	0.1*
	Ferritin (μg/L)	35 (20–48)	33 (26–45)	0.7
Biochemistry	**Glucose (mg/dL)**	81.5 (77–86)	83 (78–88)	0.36
	Urea (mg/dL)	31 (28–34)	34.5 (30–38)	0.04
	Creatinine (mg/dL)	0.62± 0.07	0.6±0.08	0.25*
	SGOT (U/L)	30 (27–32)	27 (24–32)	0.08
	SGPT (U/L)	20 (16–24)	14 (12–19)	<0.00001
	γ-GT (U/L)	12 (9–15)	11 (9–13)	0.6
	Uric Acid (mg/dL)	3.55±0.75	3.85±0.77	0.07*
	Total Cholesterol (mg/dL)	167.7±25.3	172.7±24.5	0.35*
	TG (mg/dL)	43 (36–50)	52 (36–66)	0.07
	HDL (mg/dL)	63.9±8.9	60.8±12	0.17*
	LDL (mg/dL)	94.6± 21.2	100.9±22	0.18*
	ApoA1 (mg/dL)	153±21.1	156.1±19.8	0.5*
	ApoB (mg/dL)	75.7±14.7	74.2± 14.9	0.65*
	Lp(a) (mg/dL)	6.2 (2.4–9.8)	7.2 (3.9–17.3)	0.16
	T3 (ng/dL)	182.6±25	156.7±30.1	0.0001*
Hormones	**T4 (μg/dL)**	8.7±1.2	8.9±1.3	0.3*
	TSH (μIU/mL)	2.99 (2.1–4)	2.4 (1.8–3.7)	0.22
	Insulin (μIU/mL)	5.2 (3.9–6.8)	4.75 (4.1–7.8)	0.9
	Cortisol (μg/dL)	11.2 (8.5–14.8)	11.5 (9.3–15.8)	0.4
	IGF-1 (ng/mL)	159 (112–226)	165 (133–221)	0.58
	HOMA	1.04 (0.8–1.4)	0.94 (0.8–1.6)	0.9
Inflammation markers	**YKL-40 (ng/mL)**	15.1 (7.3–22.8)	24.58 (16–33.7)	0.0002
	Hepcidin (ng/mL)	59.9 (44.2–84.8)	69.2 (52.5–101.7)	0.15
	hs-IL6 (pg/mL)	1.2 (0.7–1.9)	1.3 (0.5–1.9)	0.38
	hsCRP (mg/L)	0.44±0.04	0.78±0.14	0.022*

Differences are depicted as mean±SD or median and IQR (interquartile range), according to normality of the data.
*normal distribution, Student t-test for two independent samples;
**MannWhitney test.
Abbreviations:ALP = Alkaline Phosphatase; Apo-A1 = apolipoprotein-A1; Apo-B = apolipoprotein-B; hsCRP = high-sensitivity C-reactive protein; ICSI = Intracytoplasmic Sperm Injection; IGF1 = Insulin like Growth Factor 1; LDL = low-density lipoprotein; Lp(a) = lipoprotein(a); NC = naturally conceived; TG = triglycerides; YKL-40 = Human cartilage glycoprotein 39; hsIL-6 = high-sensitivity interleukin-6.

Table 4. Biochemical, hormonal and non-conventional cardiometabolic markers in ICSI and NC girl subgroups used in metabolomics.

		ICSI (n = 10)	Control (n = 9)	p-value**
Hematologic parameters	**Hct (%)**	39 (36.8–39.4)	37.4 (35.4–39.9)	0.9
	Hb (g/dL)	13.3 (12.2–13.3)	12.6 (11.8–13.3)	0.5
	Fe (μg/dL)	69.8±19.3	83±37.5	0.46*
	Ferritin (μg/L)	22.6±12.3	33±9.5	0.15*
Biochemistry	**Glucose (mg/dL)**	75.5 (71–82)	79 (78–86)	0.2
	Urea (mg/dL)	31.8±6	33.6±7.7	0.6*
	Creatinine (mg/dL)	0.57±0.05	0.59±0.06	0.5*
	SGOT (U/L)	32.3±7.2	28.1±7.7	0.2*
	SGPT (U/L)	18.8±5.6	16.2± 6.5	0.4*
	γ-GT (U/L)	8.7±2.3	10.4±1.8	0.09*
	Uric Acid (mg/dL)	3.7±1.1	4.1±0.95	0.4*
	Total Cholesterol (mg/dL)	170.2±22.7	168.7±22.3	0.88*
	TG (mg/dL)	47 (40–57)	45 (38–54)	0.46
	HDL (mg/dL)	58±7.6	61.3±12.5	0.48*
	LDL (mg/dL)	101.6±18.3	97.3±18.3	0.62*
	ApoA1 (mg/dL)	147.3± 20.3	156±26.1	0.4*
	ApoB (mg/dL)	78.3± 10.5	75±11.8	0.5*
	Lp(a) (mg/dL)	5.8 (3.1–7.6)	17.3 (3.6–33.5)	0.15
	T3 (ng/dL)	195.7±27.8	143.5± 25	0.0007*
Hormones	**T4 (μg/dL)**	8.9±0.8	9.15±1.2	0.7*
	TSH (μIU/mL)	2.86±0.99	2.9±1.4	0.9*
	Insulin (μIU/mL)	4.7 (2.4–6.1)	4.3 (4.1–8.2)	0.4
	Cortisol (μg/dL)	8.6 (5.9–11.9)	17.9 (11.2–22.3)	0.02
	IGF-1 (ng/mL)	130.5 (110–185)	129 (107–165)	0.87
	HOMA	0.9 (0.5–1.1)	0.91 (0.7–1.4)	0.5
Inflammation markers	**YKL-40 (ng/mL)**	20.4±10.8	21.8±8.2	0.75*
	Hepcidin (ng/mL)	68.3 (43.9–89.5)	71.6 (44–119.8)	0.77
	hs-IL6 (pg/mL)	1.6 (0.94–1.9)	0.95 (0.6–2.7)	0.44
	hsCRP (mg/L)	0.39 (0.18–0.66)	0.48(0.14–1.75)	0.7

Differences are depicted as mean±SD or median and IQR (interquartile range), according to the normality of the data.
*normal distribution, t-test for two independent samples;
**MannWhitney U test.
Abbreviations:ALP = Alkaline Phosphatase; Apo-A1 = apolipoprotein-A1; Apo-B = apolipoprotein-B; hsCRP = high-sensitivity C-reactive protein; ICSI = Intracytoplasmic Sperm Injection; IGF1 = Insulin like Growth Factor 1; LDL = low-density lipoprotein; Lp(a) = lipoprotein(a); TG = triglycerides; YKL-40 = Human cartilage glycoprotein 39; hsIL-6 = high-sensitivity interleukin-6.

influence the metabolic phenotype between ICSI-children and controls (Table 1). Moreover, from the physical examination, only the SBP-SDS was significantly lower in ICSI than controls ($p = 0.0004$). Similarly, significantly lower values in the non-conventional cardiometabolic markers YKL-40 [median: 15.1 (ICSI) vs. 24.6 (NC), $p = 0.0002$] and hs-CRP [0.44±0.3 (ICSI) vs. 0.78±0.87 (NC), $p = 0.022$] were observed in the ICSI group (Table 3). Among the biochemical and hormonal markers, SGPT and T3 were significantly higher in the ICSI than the NC group. Moreover, urea was lower in the ICSI than the NC group, even though less prominently in the girls' sub-set analyzed using metabolomics (Table 4) compared to the entire group of children (Table 3), due to the high standard deviation of the measurement combined with the smaller number of children in the girls' subset. In the subset of girls analyzed using metabolomics (Tables 2 and 4), only T3 was identified as significantly higher in the ICSI group. Finally, cortisol levels showed a notable decrease in the ICSI compared to the NC group in the subset of girls analyzed using metabolomics, while there was no difference between the two groups over the entire set of children.

Metabolomic analysis

The GC-MS metabolomics data of the 10 ICSI and 10 NC girls were analyzed using PLS-DA to investigate whether the two subgroups can be differentiated based on the 70 metabolite concentration profiles. The PLS-DA method projects the experimental space to a low-dimension perspective corresponding to maximal variance between the two investigated sets of measurements; in the PLS-DA graph, each point corresponds to the metabolic or biochemical profile of a subject. As shown in Figure 1A, the ICSI and NC groups were clearly differentiated based on their GC-MS metabolic profiles. The groups were

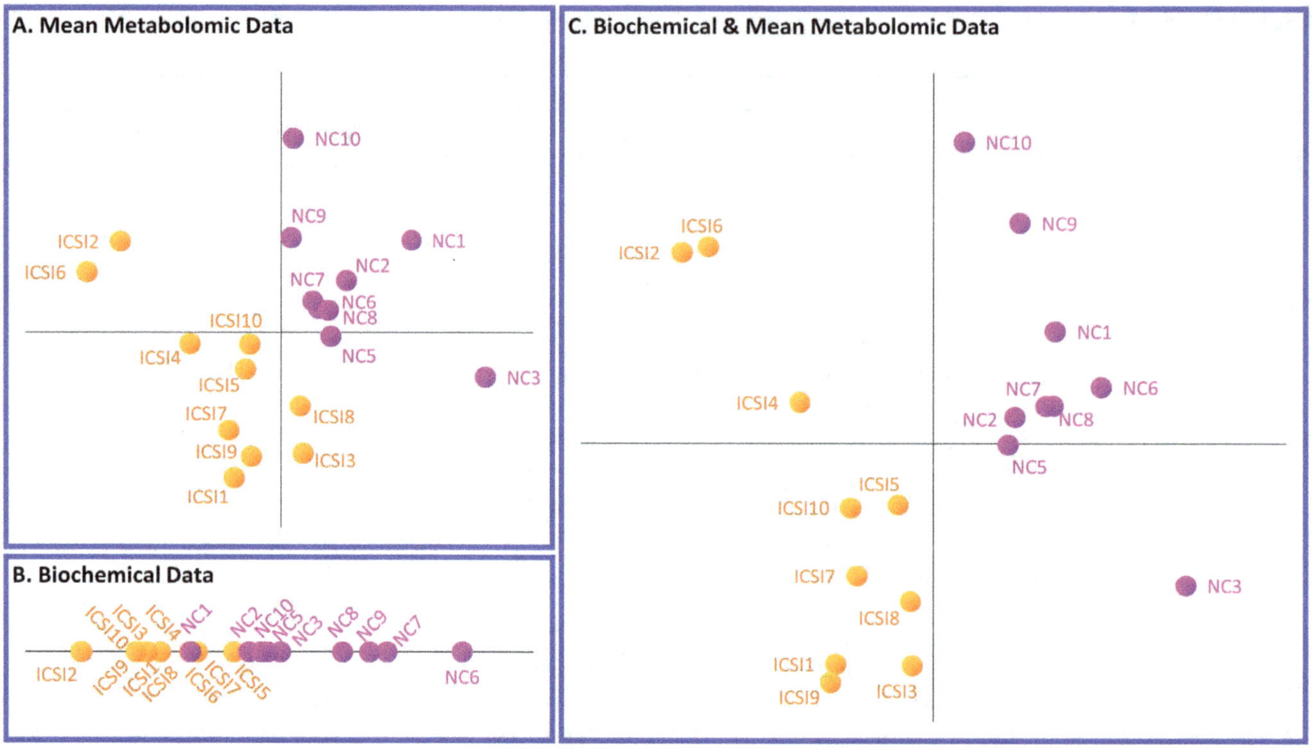

Figure 1. Multivariate statistical analysis of (A) metabolomic, (B) biochemical, (C) combined datasets for the girl subgroup. Partial Least Squares – Discriminant Analysis (PLS-DA) analysis indicates a fair discrimination between the ICSI and NC girl subgroups based on their (A) metabolic profiles, (B) biochemical profiles and (C) combined profiles. In these graphs, each point corresponds, respectively, to the metabolic, biochemical or combined profile of the subject, whose number is shown next to it. The axes of the graphs correspond to functions of multiple variables (i.e. metabolites and/or biochemical markers).

distinguished based on their biochemical profiles too, even though the discrimination was not as clear as in the metabolomic data analysis (Figure 1B). Notably, the observed difference between the two groups is markedly enhanced when both their metabolic and biochemical profiles were considered (Figure 1C).

Having established separation of the ICSI and NC groups based on their metabolic profiles, significance analysis (SAM) was applied to identify the metabolites with difference in the concentration characteristic of this separation. SAM is used for the significance analysis of omic data, as it has the advantage of not requiring them to follow a particular distribution. Full description of SAM analysis for the metabolomics and biochemical datasets is provided in File S3. It was found that among the 70 metabolites included in the analysis, 34 (18 of known identity and 9 of known chemical class) and 3 (urea, glycerol 3-phosphate and 1 unknown) metabolites were, respectively, of significantly higher (positively significant) or lower (negatively significant) concentration in the ICSI than the NC group (Table 5). Sugars, sugar alcohols, sugar acids and lipids dominate the list of the positively affected metabolites, with citrate and myo-inositol being the most discriminatory. Moreover, the total concentration of the 70 metabolites was higher in the ICSI group. The difference in the metabolic physiology of the ICSI compared to the NC subjects is visualized in the context of the appropriately color-coded inter-organ metabolic network, in which the names of the known positively and negatively affected metabolites are, respectively, shown in red and green (Figure 2). In accordance with the statistical analysis of biochemical markers discussed above, SAM analysis indicated T3 of significantly larger concentration in the ICSI 10-girl subgroup. The fact that SAM analysis of the metabolomic data indicated urea as the most negatively significant metabolite in the ICSI girls' subgroup compared to NC, while this decrease is not that prominent when only the biochemical measurements are considered, is an example of the significance of the multivariate statistical analysis on a profile of metabolite concentrations compared to the statistical analysis of a single measurement separately. In the biochemical analyses each of the indices is measured independently, with unique experimental handling from the other measurements, and is statistically evaluated in a univariate way. On the other hand, in the metabolomic analysis, the concentrations of the metabolites are measured simultaneously usually with a different protocol compared to the biochemical analysis, and the generated dataset is processed with algorithms of multivariate statistical analysis. Multivariate approaches consider the difference in the concentration of each given metabolite between the two (ICSI and NC) groups in the context of the respective variation of the rest of the metabolites, taking also into consideration the variance of all measurements among the multiple technical replicates considered in the metabolomic analysis. In this way, multivariate analysis can attribute statistical significance to differences in metabolite concentrations for which the standard deviation of the measurements in the two groups could hinder a statistically significant result if evaluated alone, independently of the other data. Therefore, the biochemical and metabolomic approaches differ both in the experimental procedures for metabolite quantification and in the statistical evaluation, which could justify any discrepancies between the two analyses for the common metabolites. As far as the biomedical conclusions are concerned, the two approaches are complementary, as it is shown in our study, as

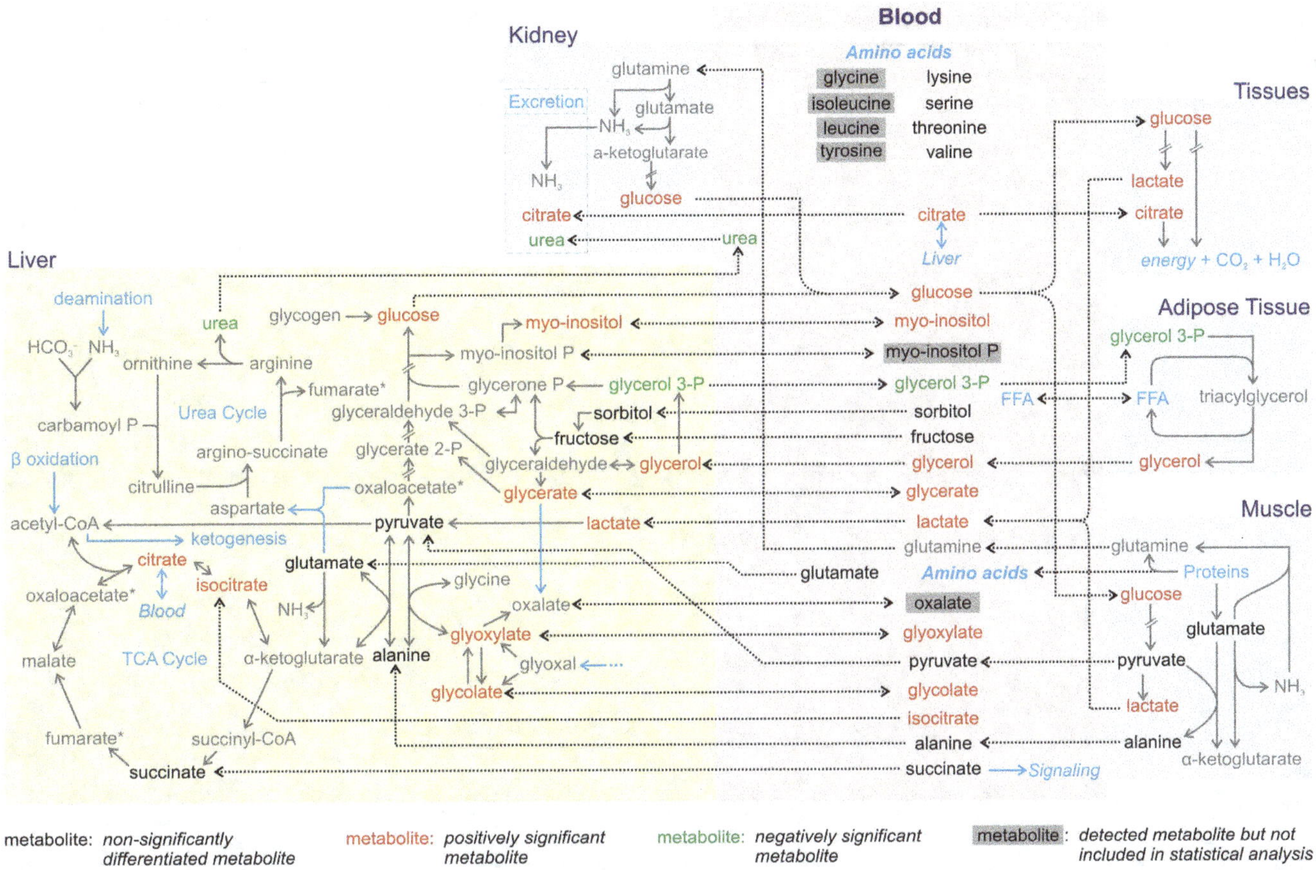

Figure 2. The significant metabolites between the ICSI and NC girl subgroups within the inter-organ metabolic network. Positioning the significant metabolites shown in Table 3 within the reconstructed network indicates metabolic physiology differences between the ICSI and NC girl subgroups. All known metabolites detected in the plasma GC-MS metabolic profiles are shown in the area of the figure named "blood"; among these, the metabolites which were not included in the analysis after the normalization and filtering steps are shown in gray boxes. The names of the positively and negatively significant metabolites (Table 3) are shown in red and green fonts, respectively, while the nonsignificant are shown in black. The plasma metabolites are connected with dashed lines with the same metabolite pool in any of the depicted tissues. The intra-tissue pools of the plasma positively and negatively significant metabolites are shown in red and green, respectively; it is noted that we cannot predict the intra-tissue metabolite concentration from its plasma concentration, but we have tried to include the most significant tissue "sources" and "sinks" that contribute to the observed plasma concentration.

combined the two provide a larger perspective of the physiological state, which cannot be provided from each dataset alone.

Discussion

We report the cardiometabolic profile of a well selected group of ICSI-conceived children with a mean age of 6.8±2.1 yrs in comparison to naturally-conceived age- and gender-matched controls, based on both the "conventional" biochemical and hormonal markers and metabolomic analysis for a subgroup of them. Notably, statistical analysis of the auxological and biochemical dataset for the entire group indicated low urea and low-grade inflammation markers (YKL-40, hsCRP) and high triiodothyronine (T3) in ICSI-children compared to controls. Low urea and high T3 was also validated by the combined analysis of the metabolomic and biochemical profiles of the girl subgroup. The identified significantly higher concentration of T3 in the ICSI group agrees with probable epigenetic changes in the hormonal profile in the ICSI children. Higher concentration of T3 may imply increased peripheral conversion of T4 to T3, already reported in obese subjects [27]. Hyperthyroidism increases the flux of gluconeogenesis, the Cori cycle and adipose tissue lipolysis [28], leading to glucose intolerance and insulin resistance [29]. Interestingly, no elevations of T3 were observed in children conceived by classic IVF; these children rather had elevated TSH with normal T3 and T4 values [30]. Urea was the most significant metabolite with reduced concentration in the ICSI-conceived children, validated very prominently in the metabolomic dataset of the girl subgroup. Urea is synthesized in the liver in order to detoxify the organism from $NH4^+$. The reduced urea concentration can be either explained by reduced amino acid breakdown or by nitrogen imbalance with increased disposal of N [31,32]. Further studies are needed to investigate this observation. The decreased levels of cortisol in the ICSI compared to the NC group within the subset of girls analyzed using metabolomics is consistent with a recent publication reporting lower salivary cortisol levels in the ICSI-conceived girls [33]. Moreover, there is growing evidence of hypothalamo-pituitary-adrenal axis dysfunction and blunted cortisol response in children born preterm or small for gestational age [34–35]. Interestingly, studying alone the non-conventional cardiometabolic markers, YKL-40 and hsCRP, would be characterized as improved in the ICSI- compared to the NC group.

Table 5. List of positively and negatively significant metabolites in the ICSI compared to the natural conception (NC) group.

Positively significant metabolites	Negatively significant metabolites	Order of Significance
citrate	urea	1 1[a]
myo-inositol	x_13	2 2[a]
U_083 (similar to U_088 & U_078)		3
U_041 (sugar acid)		4
U_046 (sugar – hexose)		5
U_010 (putatively α-hydroxyvalerate)		6
glycerate		7
α-tocopherol		8
phosphate		9
U_088 (similar to U_083 & U_078)		10
P2412 (sugar, marker ion 204)		11
(chiro- or) scyllo-inositol		12
U_078 (similar to U_083 & U_088)		13
lactate		14
unknown_no120/P2427 (sugar acid)		15
U_055 (sugar pyranose)		16
glycerol monostearate		17
glucose		18
P2400 (putatively alpha-ketoglutarate)		19
cholesterol		20
gluconate		21
9,12-(z,z)-octadecadienoate (linoleic acid)	*FDR (median) = 0 metabolites*	22
U_039 (sugar pyranose)		23
glyoxylate		24
glycerol		25
threonate		26
U_040 (sugar)		27
U_009 (putatively α-hydroxyisobutyrate)		28
U_014		29
U_048 (sugarpyranose)		30
glycolate		31
U_094 (putatively lipid; same marker ion as stearate)	*FDR (median) = 1.3 metabolites (3.8%)*	32
isocitrate		33
myristate	glycerol 3 –P	34 3[a]
erythritol	*FDR (median) = 2.2 metabolites (5.85%)*	35

[a]The first number in the column corresponds to the order of significance of the positively significant metabolites; the second number corresponds to the order of significance of the negatively significant metabolites.
The table shows the list of positively and negatively significant metabolites at three significance threshold cutoffs. Positively/Negatively Significant Metabolites: Metabolites the concentration of which is significantly larger in ICSI compared to the NC group; FDR (median): False Discovery Rate (median) at each significance threshold cutoff, shown in metabolite number and percentage of the total significant metabolite number (in parenthesis).

Specifically, for serum YKL-40, there is a growing body of evidence that its levels are increased in cases of low-grade inflammation. Moreover, it has been recently published that YKL-40 is also increased in obese prepubertal children suggesting that it represents a marker of insulin resistance not only in adulthood but in childhood as well. Therefore, YKL-40 was selected to be measured in our study as a potential marker of inflammation, endothelial dysfunction and diabetes and an independent predictor of overall cardiovascular mortality [36,37,38]. However, in the context of the other metabolic differences, the obtained values for YKL-40 and hsCRP could indicate a positive response of a part of the physiology to counteract the negative derangements in other processes, balancing a healthy state for these children. Obviously, negative predisposition to certain cardiometabolic diseases does not mean definite manifestation in adult life, but only in the case that certain environmental stimuli could trigger the particular physiological imbalance.

It should be noted, however, that combining the anthropometric and biochemical approach results with metabolomics analysis in the girl subgroup enabled a more prominent and informative differentiation between the ICSI and NC girls. More than half of the metabolites analyzed were identified with a statistically different concentration between the two groups based on the multivariate dataset significance analysis SAM. Such substantial metabolic difference cannot be viewed as coincidental due to the small number of considered subjects; it has of course to be validated in larger groups of children. The set of metabolites, which were identified with significantly higher concentration in the ICSI compared to the NC group, was dominated by sugars, sugar alcohols, sugar acids and fatty acids, with most of the known having been associated with obesity, insulin resistance and/or metabolic syndrome. The higher concentration of glucose (and other sugars) and lactate in the ICSI group is consistent with a higher activity of the Cori cycle [39], as shown in the reconstructed inter-organ metabolic network, this cycle having been associated with non-insulin-dependent diabetes in obese subjects [40]. The higher concentration of glycerol and four fatty acids (myristate, linoleic acid, glycerol monostearate and unknown U_094) followed by the lower concentration of the glycerol-3-phosphate, imply a higher lipolysis flux in the ICSI than the control group [41]. Higher glycerol and free fatty acid levels in the blood have been implicated in metabolic disorders [42] and obesity [43]. This state is consistent with the observed higher concentration of alpha-tocopherol, the biologically active form of the lipophilic vitamin E [44], which is positively correlated with blood lipid levels [45] and adiposity [46]. Glyoxylate and its precursor glycolate are directly implicated in lipid β-oxidation. These measurements are consistent with the higher concentration of citrate in the ICSI group, the accumulation of which in the post-absorptive state, along with that of isocitrate, represents higher rates of lipid β-oxidation [47]. The presented metabolomic analysis results are the first reported in the context of the ART effect on the cardiometabolic profile of the offspring. It strongly indicates the usefulness of this approach in detecting early indices of metabolic derangements which could contribute to predisposition to metabolic diseases in adult life.

This study has clearly produced indications that ICSI children, like classic IVF-children, have a metabolic profile compatible with insulin resistance. This similarity ends with this though. In contrast to classic IVF children who have increased nonconventional indices of inflammation, ICSI offspring appear to have an improved inflammatory profile [48]. Why and how this will translate in the future is not known. Certainly though it appears that the actual ART procedure employed may have distinct biochemical effects in the offspring.

Conclusions

The present study contributes a large auxological and biochemical dataset of a consistent group of pre-pubertal ICSI-conceived subjects to the research of the ART effect to the health of the offspring. The importance of this contribution becomes more apparent considering that such systematically collected data are even more sporadic for the ICSI compared to the IVF method. Moreover, it provides the first GC-MS metabolomics dataset for a subgroup of subjects in the context of this type of research. The acquired results support the concerns for increased predisposition of ICSI offspring for cardiometabolic disorders in later life. Moreover, the data demonstrate the value of metabolomic analysis in providing a high resolution perspective of the metabolic state, enabling the determination of characteristic metabolic profiles in complex cases even before impairment can be clearly demonstrated at the biochemical level. Thus, the metabolomics approach could significantly contribute to the research of the ART cardiometabolic effects. The obtained metabolomic findings should be further confirmed in a larger group of children with comparative analysis of both sexes.

Supporting Information

Table S1 Normalized Metabolomic Dataset. This excel file contains the normalized metabolomic dataset of the girl subgroup, which was used in the multivariate statistical analysis.

File S1 Metabolomic data normalization and filtering process. This textfile describes the methods and criteria based on which the normalization and filtering of the metabolomics data was carried out.

File S2 Inter-organ metabolic network reconstruction. This textfile describes which prior biological knowledge reported in the literature and metabolic databases was used to reconstruct an inter-organ metabolic network connecting the metabolites measured in the blood plasma with the metabolic networks of various organs, including liver, muscle, kidney, adipose and other tissues, shown in Figure 2.

File S3 Multivariate statistical analysis of metabolomic and biochemical datasets of the girl subgroup. This file describes the application of the Significance Analysis of Microarrays (SAM) method for the analysis of the metabolomic and biochemical datasets. Figures A and B in File S3 depict, respectively, the SAM graph for the metabolomics and the biochemical datasets.

Acknowledgments

The authors are indebted to all the children and their families that participated in this study.

Author Contributions

Conceived and designed the experiments: GPC CK-G MIK DL GM. Performed the experiments: AG IK AGT EM AM. Analyzed the data: AG IK AGT MK. Contributed reagents/materials/analysis tools: IP MIK GPC. Wrote the paper: AG IK AGT GPC CK-G MIK. Coordinated the biochemical analyses: IP. Coordinated the metabolomics analyses: MIK.

References

1. Ferraretti AP, Goossens V, de Mouzon J, Bhattacharya S, Castilla JA, et al. (2012) Assisted reproductive technology in Europe, 2008: results generated from European registers by ESHRE. Hum Reprod 27: 2571–2584.
2. Palermo G, Joris H, Devroey P, Van Steirteghem AC (1992) Pregnancies after intracytoplasmic injection of single spermatozoon into an oocyte. Lancet 340: 17–18.
3. Van Steirteghem A, Devroey P, Liebaers I (2002) Intracytoplasmic sperm injection. Mol Cell Endocrinol 186: 199–203.
4. Maher ER (2005) Imprinting and assisted reproductive technology. Hum Mol Genet 14 Spec No 1: R133–138.
5. Kanaka-Gantenbein C, Sakka S, Chrousos GP (2010) Assisted reproduction and its neuroendocrine impact on the offspring. Prog Brain Res 182: 161–174.
6. Wen J, Jiang J, Ding C, Dai J, Liu Y, et al. (2012) Birth defects in children conceived by in vitro fertilization and intracytoplasmic sperm injection: a meta-analysis. Fertil Steril 97: 1331–1337 e1331–1334.
7. Nyboe Andersen A, Carlsen E, Loft A (2008) Trends in the use of intracytoplasmatic sperm injection marked variability between countries. Hum Reprod Update 14: 593–604.
8. Grace KS, Sinclair KD (2009) Assisted reproductive technology, epigenetics, and long-term health: a developmental time bomb still ticking. Semin Reprod Med 27: 409–416.

9. Kanaka-Gantenbein C, Mastorakos G, Chrousos GP (2003) Endocrine-related causes and consequences of intrauterine growth retardation. Ann N Y Acad Sci 997: 150–157.
10. Saenger P, Czernichow P, Hughes I, Reiter EO (2007) Small for gestational age: short stature and beyond. Endocr Rev 28: 219–251.
11. Gluckman PD, Hanson MA, Cooper C, Thornburg KL (2008) Effect of in utero and early-life conditions on adult health and disease. N Engl J Med 359: 61–73.
12. McDonald SD, Han Z, Mulla S, Murphy KE, Beyene J, et al. (2009) Preterm birth and low birth weight among in vitro fertilization singletons: a systematic review and meta-analyses. Eur J Obstet Gynecol Reprod Biol 146: 138–148.
13. Sakka SD, Loutradis D, Kanaka-Gantenbein C, Margeli A, Papastamataki M, et al. (2010) Absence of insulin resistance and low-grade inflammation despite early metabolic syndrome manifestations in children born after in vitro fertilization. Fertil Steril 94: 1693–1699.
14. Ceelen M, van Weissenbruch MM, Vermeiden JP, van Leeuwen FE, Delemarre-van de Waal HA (2008) Cardiometabolic differences in children born after in vitro fertilization: follow-up study. J Clin Endocrinol Metab 93: 1682–1688.
15. Chrousos GP (2000) The role of stress and the hypothalamic-pituitary-adrenal axis in the pathogenesis of the metabolic syndrome: neuro-endocrine and target tissue-related causes. Int J Obes Relat Metab Disord 24 Suppl 2: S50–55.
16. Laprise SL (2009) Implications of epigenetics and genomic imprinting in assisted reproductive technologies. Mol Reprod Dev 76: 1006–1018.
17. Youngson NA, Morris MJ (2013) What obesity research tells us about epigenetic mechanisms. Philos Trans R Soc Lond B Biol Sci 368: 20110337.
18. Vidal M (2009) A unifying view of 21st century systems biology. FEBS Lett 583: 3891–3894.
19. Patti GJ, Yanes O, Siuzdak G (2012) Innovation: Metabolomics: the apogee of the omics trilogy. Nat Rev Mol Cell Biol 13: 263–269.
20. Nicholson G, Rantalainen M, Maher AD, Li JV, Malmodin D, et al. (2011) Human metabolic profiles are stably controlled by genetic and environmental variation. Mol Syst Biol 7: 525.
21. Mittelstrass K, Ried JS, Yu Z, Krumsiek J, Gieger C, et al. (2011) Discovery of sexual dimorphisms in metabolic and genetic biomarkers. PLoS Genet 7: e1002215.
22. Ucar A, Saka N, Bas F, Bundak R, Gunoz H, et al. (2012) Precocious adrenarche in children born appropriate for gestational age: is there a difference between genders? Eur J Pediatr 171: 1661–1666.
23. Matthews DR, Hosker JP, Rudenski AS, Naylor BA, Treacher DF, et al. (1985) Homeostasis model assessment: insulin resistance and beta-cell function from fasting plasma glucose and insulin concentrations in man. Diabetologia 28: 412–419.
24. Kanani HH, Klapa MI (2007) Data correction strategy for metabolomics analysis using gas chromatography-mass spectrometry. Metab Eng 9: 39–51.
25. Spagou K, Theodoridis G, Wilson I, Raikos N, Greaves P, et al. (2011) A GC-MS metabolic profiling study of plasma samples from mice on low- and high-fat diets. J Chromatogr B Analyt Technol Biomed Life Sci 879: 1467–1475.
26. Saeed AI, Bhagabati NK, Braisted JC, Liang W, Sharov V, et al. (2006) TM4 microarray software suite. Methods Enzymol 411: 134–193.
27. Ortega FJ, Jilkova ZM, Moreno-Navarrete JM, Pavelka S, Rodriguez-Hermosa JI, et al. (2012) Type I iodothyronine 5′-deiodinase mRNA and activity is increased in adipose tissue of obese subjects. Int J Obes (Lond) 36: 320–324.
28. Mitrou P, Raptis SA, Dimitriadis G (2010) Insulin action in hyperthyroidism: a focus on muscle and adipose tissue. Endocr Rev 31: 663–679.
29. Brenta G (2011) Why can insulin resistance be a natural consequence of thyroid dysfunction? J Thyroid Res 2011: 152850.
30. Sakka SD, Malamitsi-Puchner A, Loutradis D, Chrousos GP, Kanaka-Gantenbein C (2009) Euthyroid hyperthyrotropinemia in children born after in vitro fertilization. J Clin Endocrinol Metab 94: 1338–1341.
31. Barber T, Vina JR, Vina J, Cabo J (1985) Decreased urea synthesis in cafeteria-diet-induced obesity in the rat. Biochem J 230: 675–681.
32. Herrero MC, Remesar X, Arola L, Blade C (1999) Ammonium uptake and urea production in hepatocytes from lean and obese Zucker rats. Mol Cell Biochem 200: 163–167.
33. Belva F, Painter RC, Schiettecatte J, Bonduelle M, Roelants M, et al. (2013) Gender-specific alterations in salivary cortisol levels in pubertal intracytoplasmic sperm injection offspring. Horm Res Paediatr 80:350–355.
34. Kaseva N, Wehkalampi K, Pyhälä R, Moltchanova E, Feldt K, et al. (2014) Blunted hypothalamic-pituitary-adrenal axis and insulin response to psychosocial stress in young adults born preterm at very low birth weight. Clin Endocrinol (Oxf) 80:101–106.
35. Kajantie E, Feldt K, Räikkönen K, Phillips DI, Osmond C, et al. (2007) Body size at birth predicts hypothalamic-pituitary-adrenal axis response to psychosocial stress at age 60 to 70 years. J Clin Endocrinol Metab 92:4094–4100.
36. Kyrgios I, Galli-Tsinopoulou A, Stylianou C, Papakonstantinou E, Arvanitidou M, et al. (2012) Elevated circulating levels of the serum acute-phase protein YKL-40 (chitinase 3-like protein 1) are a marker of obesity and insulin resistance in prepubertal children. Metabolism 61:562–568.
37. Rathcke CN, Thomsen SB, Linneberg A, Vestergaard H (2012) Variations of CHI3L1, levels of the encoded glycoprotein YKL-40 and prediction of fatal and non-fatal ischemic stroke. PLoS One 7(8):e43498.
38. Lin CH, Li HY, Jiang YD, Chang TJ, Chuang LM (2013) Plasma YKL-40 predicts 10-year cardiovascular and all-cause mortality in individuals with type 2 diabetes.Clin Endocrinol (Oxf). 79(2):185–191.
39. Cori CF (1981) The glucose-lactic acid cycle and gluconeogenesis. Curr Top Cell Regul 18: 377–387.
40. Zawadzki JK, Wolfe RR, Mott DM, Lillioja S, Howard BV, et al. (1988) Increased rate of Cori cycle in obese subjects with NIDDM and effect of weight reduction. Diabetes 37: 154–159.
41. Sabin MA, De Hora M, Holly JM, Hunt LP, Ford AL, et al. (2007) Fasting nonesterified fatty acid profiles in childhood and their relationship with adiposity, insulin sensitivity, and lipid levels. Pediatrics 120: e1426–1433.
42. Schaffer JE (2003) Lipotoxicity: when tissues overeat. Curr Opin Lipidol 14: 281–287.
43. Le Stunff C, Bougneres PF (1992) Glycerol production and utilization during the early phase of human obesity. Diabetes 41: 444–450.
44. Traber MG (2007) Vitamin E regulatory mechanisms. Annu Rev Nutr 27: 347–362.
45. Bieri JG, Evarts RP (1975) Effect of plasma lipid levels and obesity on tissue stores of alpha-tocopherol. Proc Soc Exp Biol Med 149: 500–502.
46. Manolescu B, Atanasiu V, Cercasov C, Stoian I, Oprea E, et al. (2008) So many options but one choice: the human body prefers alpha-tocopherol. A matter of stereochemistry. J Med Life 1: 376–382.
47. Muoio DM, Newgard CB (2006) Obesity-related derangements in metabolic regulation. Annu Rev Biochem 75: 367–401.
48. Sakka SD, Margeli A, Loutradis D, Chrousos GP, Papassotiriou I, et al. (2013) Gender dimorphic increase in RBP-4 and NGAL in children born after IVF: an epigenetic phenomenon? Eur J Clin Invest 43: 439–448.

21

Effects of Prolonged Exposure to Hypobaric Hypoxia on Oxidative Stress, Inflammation and Gluco-Insular Regulation: The Not-So-Sweet Price for Good Regulation

Mario Siervo[1], Heather L. Riley[2], Bernadette O. Fernandez[3,4], Carl A. Leckstrom[3], Daniel S. Martin[5,6], Kay Mitchell[5,7], Denny Z. H. Levett[5,7,8], Hugh E. Montgomery[5], Monty G. Mythen[5], Michael P. W. Grocott[4,5,7,8☯], Martin Feelisch[2,3,4,8*☯], for the Caudwell Xtreme Everest Research Group[¶]

1 Human Nutrition Research Centre, Institute for Ageing and Health, Newcastle University, Newcastle on Tyne, United Kingdom, **2** Warwick Systems Biology Centre, University of Warwick, Coventry, United Kingdom, **3** Warwick Medical School, University of Warwick, Coventry, United Kingdom, **4** University of Southampton, Clinical & Experimental Sciences, Faculty of Medicine, Southampton General Hospital, Southampton, United Kingdom, **5** Centre for Altitude Space and Extreme Environment Medicine, Portex Unit, UCL Institute of Child Health, London, United Kingdom, **6** Division of Surgery and Interventional Science, University College London, Royal Free Hospital, London, United Kingdom, **7** University Hospital Southampton NHS Foundation Trust, Southampton General Hospital, Southampton, United Kingdom, **8** Southampton NIHR Respiratory Biomedical Research Unit, Southampton, United Kingdom

Abstract

Objectives: The mechanisms by which low oxygen availability are associated with the development of insulin resistance remain obscure. We thus investigated the relationship between such gluco-insular derangements in response to sustained (hypobaric) hypoxemia, and changes in biomarkers of oxidative stress, inflammation and counter-regulatory hormone responses.

Methods: After baseline testing in London (75 m), 24 subjects ascended from Kathmandu (1,300 m) to Everest Base Camp (EBC;5,300 m) over 13 days. Of these, 14 ascended higher, with 8 reaching the summit (8,848 m). Assessments were conducted at baseline, during ascent to EBC, and 1, 6 and 8 week(s) thereafter. Changes in body weight and indices of gluco-insular control were measured (glucose, insulin, C-Peptide, homeostasis model assessment of insulin resistance [HOMA-IR]) along with biomarkers of oxidative stress (4-hydroxy-2-nonenal-HNE), inflammation (Interleukin-6 [IL-6]) and counter-regulatory hormones (glucagon, adrenalin, noradrenalin). In addition, peripheral oxygen saturation (SpO_2) and venous blood lactate concentrations were determined.

Results: SpO_2 fell significantly from 98.0% at sea level to 82.0% on arrival at 5,300 m. Whilst glucose levels remained stable, insulin and C-Peptide concentrations increased by >200% during the last 2 weeks. Increases in fasting insulin, HOMA-IR and glucagon correlated with increases in markers of oxidative stress (4-HNE) and inflammation (IL-6). Lactate levels progressively increased during ascent and remained significantly elevated until week 8. Subjects lost on average 7.3 kg in body weight.

Conclusions: Sustained hypoxemia is associated with insulin resistance, whose magnitude correlates with the degree of oxidative stress and inflammation. The role of 4-HNE and IL-6 as key players in modifying the association between sustained hypoxia and insulin resistance merits further investigation.

Editor: Darcy Johannsen, Pennington Biomed Research Center, United States of America

Funding: The research was funded from a variety of sources, including Mr. John Caudwell, BOC Medical (now part of Linde Gas therapeutics), Eli Lilly Critical Care, The London Clinic, Smiths Medical, Deltex Medical, and The Rolex Foundation (unrestricted grants). Peer reviewed research grants were awarded by the Association of Anaesthetists of Great Britain and Ireland (AAGBI), the UK Intensive Care Foundation, and the Sir Halley Stewart Trust. The CXE volunteers who trekked to Everest base camp also kindly donated to support the research. Some of this work was undertaken at University College Hospitals–University College London Comprehensive Biomedical Research Centre, which received a portion of funding from the UK Department of Health Research Biomedical Research Centres funding scheme. All funding was unrestricted. Part of the biomarker work was supported by the Medical Research Council (Strategic Appointment Scheme, to MF) and funds from the Faculty of Medicine, University of Southampton (to MF). The funders had no role in study design, data collection and analysis, decision to publish, or preparation of the manuscript.

Competing Interests: This project was partly funded by grants from BOC Medical (now Linde Gas Therapeutics), Lilly Critical Care, The London Clinic, Smiths Medical, Deltex Medical, and The Rolex Foundation. All monies were given as unrestricted grants: the funders had no role in study design, data collection and analysis, decision to publish, or preparation of the manuscript.

* E-mail: m.feelisch@soton.ac.uk

☯ These authors contributed equally to this work.

¶ Membership of the Caudwell Xtreme Everest Research Group is provided in the Acknowledgments.

Introduction

Ascent to high altitude is associated with a fall in barometric pressure, and with it a reduction in oxygen availability ('hypobaric hypoxia'). Such exposure, whether in the short- or long-term) leads to diverse endocrine responses (e.g. in insulin signalling, thyroid function and sympatho-adrenal activity [1–12]).

Hypobaric hypoxia may also affect the gluco-insular axis. However, data have been inconsistent or contradictory [3–6,12–14]: beneficial effects of hypoxia on peripheral insulin action and body weight regulation have, for instance, been suggested [5,6,15] whereas a deterioration of insulin signalling has been reported in other studies [3,7]. The source of such conflicting data may relate to inter-study differences in 1) sample size, 2) intensity of exposure to hypoxia (rate of ascent and maximum height gained: ascent profile) 3) duration of exposure to hypoxia, 4) subjects' phenotypic characteristics, 5) exposure to other environmental stressors (e.g. physical exertion and altered energy balance), and 6) testing conditions (chamber, high-altitude) [16]. Operation Everest II (simulated ascent of Mount Everest over 40 days in a hypobaric chamber) tried to obviate the effect of some of these confounders, with homogenous ascent profile, diet and exercise regime. A key finding was that some endocrine responses were more marked during the last week of the intervention when subject were exposed to the lowest oxygen concentrations [14,17]. Of note, insulin concentrations at the end of the study were typically 2-fold greater than those at the start, while glucose levels remained unaltered, suggesting the development of insulin resistance [14].

Such findings are of possible importance to the pathogenesis of disease at sea level: there is renewed interest in the role of chronic hypoxia as a potential causative factor in the pathogenesis of insulin resistance. Indeed, chronic intermittent hypoxia (CIH) due to obstructive sleep apnea (OSA) may contribute to the development and progression of insulin resistance and diabetes [18–21]. OSA appears to be a predictor of abnormal glucose metabolism in chronically sleep deprived obese adults [19].

Such effects on insulin resistance may be specifically mediated through the genesis of associated adipose tissue hypoxia (ATH) [22], This, in turn, may related to the occurrence of enhanced adipocyte growth, which may not be accompanied by a parallel, functional expansion of stromal and vascular tissue to adequately satisfy the nutritive requirements of the newly formed tissue [23–25]. A consequent decrease in convective and diffusive oxygen flux may result in reduced cellular oxygen availability leading to a progressive impairment of oxidative energetic reactions [26]. Prolonged cell/tissue hypoxia induces adaptive mechanisms including production of reactive oxygen species (ROS), inflammatory adipokines and adipose tissue macrophage infiltration. In addition, hypoxic exposure may also affect gluco-insular homeostasis by increasing systemic inflammation [27] and modification of pancreatic β-cell function [28].

Progressive exposure of human volunteers to hypobaric hypoxia at high altitude provides an opportunity to explore associations between hypoxia, oxidative stress, inflammation and gluco-insular deregulation as well as to identify novel mechanistic targets. The 2007 Caudwell Xtreme Everest (CXE) expedition [16] provided such an opportunity. We evaluated whether sustained hypoxemia was associated with alterations in glucose and insulin homeostasis. Specifically, patterns of change in indices of insulin resistance (homeostasis model assessment of insulin resistance, HOMA-IR) [29], insulin secretion (C-Peptide) and hepatic insulin extraction (C-Peptide/Insulin Ratio) [30] were evaluated. In addition, we investigated the role of oxidative stress (Isoprostanes (8-iso-prostaglandin F-2α) and 4-hydroxy-2-nonenal (4-HNE), Total Glutathione, Reduced Glutathione (GSH), Oxidized Glutathione (GSSG)) and inflammatory biomarkers (Interleukin 6 (IL-6), C Reactive Protein (CRP), Macrophage Migration Inhibitory Factor (MIF), Tumour Necrosis Factor Alpha (TNF-Alpha) and counter-regulatory hormones (Glucagon, Adrenalin, Noradrenalin) as putative causal factors linking hypobaric hypoxia to changes in gluco-insular action.

Methods

The study was approved by the University College of London (UCL) Research Ethics committee, in accordance with the Declaration of Helsinki. Verbal and written informed consent was obtained from all subjects. The study took place between January and June 2007.

Subjects

Twenty-four healthy subjects (18 male; mean age 35.2 y; range 19–59 y) who were investigators on the CXE 2007 research expedition to Mount Everest participated in this study [16]. All subjects were sea level natives free of cardiovascular or respiratory disease and took no medication. Criteria for participation have been described elsewhere [16].

Study Protocol

The design and conduct of this study is described elsewhere [16]. Briefly, subjects underwent baseline testing in London (altitude 75 m) before travelling by plane to Kathmandu, Nepal (1,300 m). From there they flew to Lukla (2,800 m) on expedition day 1 and then trekked to Everest Base Camp (EBC; 5,300 m), arriving on expedition day 13. The ascent profile is detailed in **Table S1 in File S1**. Testing was repeated during the ascent in field laboratories in Kathmandu (1,300 m; day −3 to 0), Namche (3,500 m; day 4 to 6), Pheriche (4,250 m; day 9 to 10), and at EBC (5,300 m; day 15 to 17, EBC week 1). The subjects were then divided into two subgroups: Group 1 (laboratory staff) subsequently remained at EBC for the duration of the expedition (n = 10), whilst Group 2 (climbers; n = 14) subsequently ascended above 5,300 m, to a maximum of 8,848 m on Mount Everest. Measurements were repeated in both groups at EBC (5,300 m) at week 6 and week 8. Ambient temperatures were well controlled during testing [16].

Plasma Biomarker Analyses

Blood sampling. All blood samples were taken prior to exercise testing and drawn from the antecubital vein. Plasma was separated from blood cells by centrifugation of whole blood at 800×g for 15 min and immediately frozen in 1 ml aliquots in liquid nitrogen. Samples were stored in liquid nitrogen for the duration of the expedition (including carriage back to Kathmandu), transported back to the UK on dry ice, then stored at −80°C in a commercial cryostorage facility until analysis. A summary of the number of samples available for each biomarker is reported in **Table S2 in File S1**.

Peripheral oxygen saturation. SpO_2 was measured in the morning of the same day that blood was analyzed, after 10 minutes of rest, using a pulse oximeter (Onyx 9500, Nonin, USA). Measurements were taken by independent individuals, with the subject blind to oximeter data (thus preventing feedback to alter respiratory rate, and hence SpO_2).

Oxidative Stress Markers. Isoprostanes (8-iso-prostaglandin F-2α) and 4-hydroxy-2-nonenal (4-HNE) were quantified using direct competitive enzyme immunoassay (Assay Designs, Ann Arbor, MI) and ELISA (OxiSelect HNE-His Adduct ELISA kit, Cell Biolabs, San Diego, CA), respectively. Reduced and oxidized glutathione were determined spectrofluorimetrically (DetectX, Arbor Assays, Ann Arbor, MI). For methodological reasons, this assay overestimates oxidized glutathione; thus reported values should not be misinterpreted to reflect true circulating concentrations.

Inflammatory Markers. Interleukin-6, TNF-α and MIF were quantified using xMAP technology (Human-Cytokines-12-plex-panel, BioRad) on a Luminex/Bio-Plex-200 System with high-throughput fluidics (BioRad).

Glucose, Insulin and C-Peptide. Plasma glucose levels were measured with the glucose oxidase method. Insulin and C-Peptide levels were determined using the Bio-Plex-Pro-Human-Diabetes 12-plex panel (BioRad).

Counter-regulatory hormones. Glucagon was measured with the Bio-Plex-Pro-Human-Diabetes 12-plex panel (BioRad). Adrenalin and Noradrenalin were quantified using a direct competitive enzyme immunoassay (Bi-CAT ELISA, Alpco Diagnostics, Salem, NH).

Lactate, Creatinine and Osmolality. Lactate and creatinine concentrations were determined colorimetrically by coupled enzymatic reactions using commercial assay kits (Sigma). Plasma osmolality was measured using freezing point depression (Model 3320 Micro-Osmometer, Advanced Instruments, Inc).

Assessment of insulin resistance. The degree of insulin resistance was estimated by the homeostasis model assessment of insulin resistance (HOMA-IR) and the fasting glucose/insulin ratio (FGIR). HOMA-IR was computed as follows: fasting insulin (μIU/ml) × fasting glucose (mmol/ml)/22.5 [29]. C-Peptide is a fragment cleaved from pro-insulin and secreted in amounts equimolar to those of insulin [31]. The longer half-life and the minimal hepatic first-pass extraction compared to insulin support the utilisation of C-Peptide as a measure of β-cell secretion [32]. The fasting C-peptide–to–insulin ratio was calculated as a measure of hepatic insulin extraction (C-peptide–to–insulin ratios decrease as hepatic insulin extraction decreases) [30].The C-Peptide/Insulin ratio can be used as a surrogate measure of hepatic insulin clearance which is correlated with hepatic insulin effects [33]. The glucagon-insulin ratio was calculated as an index of the pancreatic endocrine response [34].

Statistical Analysis

Variables were inspected for normality of distribution using the Q-Q and the Shapiro-Wilk tests, and appropriate transformations were utilised (where necessary) to normalise the data before statistical analysis. However, we also reported untransformed values so as to provide more interpretable information on the changes of the various biomarkers; median and inter-quartile range (25th and 75th percentile) were used as descriptive statistics. A general linear model for repeated measures was used to analyse changes in biomarker concentrations during the expedition. The Bonferroni post-hoc test was used to evaluate significant changes relative to baseline (London). The method proposed by Bland and Altman was utilised to calculate within-subject coefficients of correlation to evaluate significant associations between variables [35]. Multiple-testing was taken into account and the criterion for statistical significance was therefore set at a p value <0.001. Analyses were conducted using SPSS-19 for Windows and Sigmaplot-11 for Windows.

Results

Baseline Characteristics and Weight Changes

Twenty-four subjects participated in the expedition; 2 subjects were excluded because biomarkers data were missing, leaving data from 22 subjects (17 males) included in the final analysis. Subjects were stratified according to their main task during the expedition: Group 1 (EBC laboratory staff; n = 10) and Group 2 (climbers; n = 12). The two groups were well matched for BMI and circulating levels of biomarkers involved in glycaemic control, indices of insulin resistance, inflammation (IL-6, CRP, TNF-α, MIF), oxidative stress and SpO_2. While glucose levels were within the normal range, levels of fasting insulin, C-Peptide and HOMA-IR exceeded expected physiological levels (**Table 1**). Subjects lost body weight during the expedition (-7.3±5.0 kg, $p<0.001$), with climbers losing more weight than EBC residents (−9.0 kg vs −4.3 kg respectively, p = 0.03) (**Figure S1 in File S1**). The average rate of weight loss during the expedition was 173 g/day.

Evidence of Hypoxemia, and Lactate, Osmolality and Creatinine Changes

During ascent, median peripheral oxygen saturation (SpO_2) fell from 98.0% at sea level to 82.0% on arrival at 5,300 m ($p<0.001$) and improved marginally with time spent at that altitude (87.0% on EBC day 71; **Table S1 in File S1**). SpO_2 measured at EBC was not different between climbers and EBC team during the entire expedition.

Baseline lactate levels were within the normal range (1.39±0.42 mmol/L). They progressively increased during the ascent, peaked at EBC week 1 (2.12±0.89 mmol/L; $p<0.001$) and remained elevated at EBC week 6 (1.78±0.53 mmol/L; $p<0.05$) and week 8 (1.89±0.48 mmol/L; $p<0.05$). Osmolality did not change during the expedition (Baseline: 292.9±5.8 mOsm/kg; EBC week 8: 291.1±12.5 mOsm/kg; $p>0.05$). Creatinine levels were unmodified until EBC week 6 but showed a significant increase in both groups at the end of the study (baseline: 0.82±0.11 mg/dl; EBC week 8: 1.03±0.16 mg/dl, $p<0.001$).

Hypoxemia and Gluco-Insular Homeostasis

Glucose levels were maintained within the normal range throughout the expedition and no differences were observed between the two groups (**Figure 1a**). Low glucose levels (< 3 mmol/L) were mostly observed during the ascent phase (6 measurements) whereas only one low value was observed at high altitude (EBC week 6, climbers). A different pattern was observed for insulin axis responses. Insulin levels increased slightly during the ascent and returned to baseline values at the end of the first week at EBC. However, fasting insulin levels increased by 250% after 6 weeks at EBC ($p<0.001$) and this was maintained until the end of the expedition ($p<0.001$, EBC 8 weeks) (**Figure 1b**). Changes of comparable magnitude were observed for C-Peptide (**Figure 1c**), HOMA-IR (**Figure 1d**) and FIGR (reversed changes, **Figure 1e**). The C-Peptide/Insulin ratio appeared to be minimally affected by the prolonged exposure to hypoxia (**Figure 1f**).

Counter-Regulatory Hormones

Glucagon levels had risen significantly by week 6 ($p<0.001$) and week 8 ($p<0.001$), albeit to a lesser proportional extent than those of insulin and C-peptide. No differences in the responses were found between climbers and EBC residents (**Figure 2a**). One week after arrival at EBC, Adrenalin and Noradrenalin concentrations changed in opposite directions, and the response to sustained hypoxia was greater for Adrenalin (**Figure 2b**) com-

Table 1. Baseline characteristics of the CXE 2007 Expedition Team and comparison between team members reaching the summit and members residing at Everest Base Camp during the 8-week expedition.

	All	Climbers	Everest Base Camp	p
N	22	12	10	-
Gender (M/F)	17/5	11/1	6/4	-
Age, years	34.05 (24.02, 40.62)	36.15 (31.35, 40.67)	30.85 (25.37, 42.25)	NS
Weight, kg	76.0 (66.8, 83.8)	79.5 (70.0, 89.0)	71.0 (63.8, 80.3)	<0.05
Height, cm	178.8 (171.5, 181.0)	180.0 (176.4, 182.1)	174.0 (165.5, 180.3	<0.05
BMI, kg/m^2	24.40 (22.82, 26.07)	24.90 (22.82, 26.37)	23.65 (22.65, 24.92)	NS
Glucose, mM/L	4.50 (3.80, 4.90)	4.34 (3.55, 4.84)	4.64 3.85 4.97	NS
Insulin, mU/mL	29.38 (26.55, 34.26)	30.52 (27.51 37.10)	27.91 24.09 32.48	NS
C-peptide, pg/mL	1590.53 (1353.74, 1819.91)	1726.26 (1483.78 1945.38)	1403.26 1302.69 1617.22	NS
HOMA-IR	5.46 (4.56, 6.38)	5.36 (4.61, 6.87)	5.53 (3.92, 6.34)	NS
FIGR	2.65 (2.03, 3.39)	2.23 (1.90, 3.10)	3.20 (2.15, 3.41)	NS
C-Peptide/Insulin Ratio	1.28 (1.20, 1.43)	1.33 (1.21, 1.58)	1.24 (1.12, 1.32)	NS
Glucagon (pg/mL)	339.06 (307.81, 392.21)	351.89 (314.00, 406.17)	334.69 (294.22, 368.83)	NS
Adrenalin (ng/mL)	0.02 (0.008, 0.05)	0.01 (0.003, 0.04)	0.02 (0.01, 0.05)	NS
Noradrenalin (ng/mL)	0.13 (0.07, 0.16)	0.14 (0.10, 0.17)	0.09 (0.06, 0.16)	NS
8-isoPGF, ng/mL	36.20 (28.64, 47.38)	33.94 (29.34, 40.79)	43.45 (27.64, 47.92)	NS
4-HNE, mg/mL	108.22 (91.54, 141.28)	105.72 (91.08, 154.09)	110.72 (97.24, 134.77)	NS
GSH, μM$^¥$	0.53 (0.47, 0.57)	0.53 (0.44, 0.56)	0.53 (0.47, 0.60)	NS
GSSG, μM$^¥$	0.20 (0.07, 0.29)	0.17 (0.03, 0.25)	0.27 (0.14, 0.45)	NS
GSH/GSSG$^¥$	2.07 (1.15, 3.98)	2.29 (1.14, 5.84)	1.87 (1.14, 2.77)	NS
Total Glutathione, μM$^¥$	0.91 (0.68, 1.13)	0.88 (0.52, 1.03)	1.07 (0.89, 1.50)	NS
IL-6, pg/mL	11.75 (10.11, 14.90)	11.31 (10.04, 15.52)	12.07 (10.13, 14.15)	NS
CRP, ng/mL	626.6 (306.2, 2085.4)	480.8 (305.0, 1614.9)	670.08 (452.0, 3043.1)	NS
TNF-α, pg/mL	31.31 (27.53, 38.92)	32.89 (27.65, 38.92)	28.85 (26.14, 36.21)	NS
MIF (pg/mL)	6714.3 (5503.8, 7047.8)	6806.9 (5816.2, 7260.7)	6316.3 (5306.1, 7004.8)	NS
Lactate (mmol/L)	1.30 (1.22, 1.64)	1.35 (1.11, 1.60)	1.27 (1.12, 1.79)	NS
SpO_2 (%)	97.0 (98.0, 99.0)	97.0 (98.0, 99.0)	97.0 (98.0, 99.0)	NS

Data are presented as median (25th and 75th percentile). N = number of subjects; M = Male; F = Female; BMI = body mass index; HOMA-IR = homeostasis model of assessment-insulin resistance; 8-isoPGF = 8-iso-Prostaglandin F_2alpha; 4-HNE = 4-Hydroxynonenal; GSH = reduced glutathione; GSSG = oxidized glutathione; IL-6 = interleukin 6; CRP = C-reactive protein; TNF-α = tumour necrosis factor alpha; MIF = macrophage migration inhibitory factor; SpO_2 = peripheral oxygen saturation. Data were transformed before analysis. T test was used to determine differences between the two groups. NS = not statistically significant. ¥Data for these biomarkers were not available from the samples collected in London; therefore we have used the data derived from the samples collected in Kathmandu as baseline levels.

pared to Noradrenalin (**Figure 2c**). The glucagon-insulin ratio decreased significantly during the last two weeks of the expedition ($p<0.001$) (**Figure 2d**).

Biomarkers of Oxidative Stress

We have previously reported some of these data [36]. Levels of total glutathione and related biomarkers (GSH, GSSG, GSH/GSSG) were compared to the values taken at the start of the ascent (Kathmandu, 1,300 m), due to unavailability of baseline measures for London. responses varied substantially between individuals, with a non-significant trend for total glutathione and GSH to increase at high altitude (**Figure 3a–d**). Marked inter-individual variation in Isoprostane levels (8-isoPGF) was also identified, with a complex pattern of response to ascent (**Figure 3e**). By contrast, 4-HNE showed much smaller inter-individual variability and a direct association with the duration of hypoxia. Changes in circulating levels were significantly elevated during the ascent and had increased almost 3-fold by EBC week 6 and week 8 ($p<0.001$) (**Figure 3f**).

Biomarkers of Inflammation

CRP levels did not change significantly (**Figure 4a**) whilst TNF-α levels showed a tendency to decline (**Figure 4b**). MIF increased only at EBC week 8 ($p<0.001$) (**Figure 4c**) whereas the profile of IL-6 mirrored changes in insulin levels. Specifically, IL-6 levels showed no changes until after EBC week 1 but had increased by ~250% by EBC week 6 and week 8 ($p<0.001$) (**Figure 4d**).

Correlation Analysis

The main aim of this analysis was to evaluate the associations between hypoxemia, oxidative stress and inflammatory biomarkers with glucose, insulin and indices of insulin resistance. A correlation matrix has been provided in **Table S3 in File S1**. In addition, a mechanistic-model of insulin resistance based on the correlation of HOMA-IR with biomarkers of inflammation and oxidative stress has been proposed (**Figure 5**). The model suggests a non-significant role of CRP whereas a strong and significant association with HOMA-IR was observed for IL-6 ($r = 0.74$, $p<0.001$). The

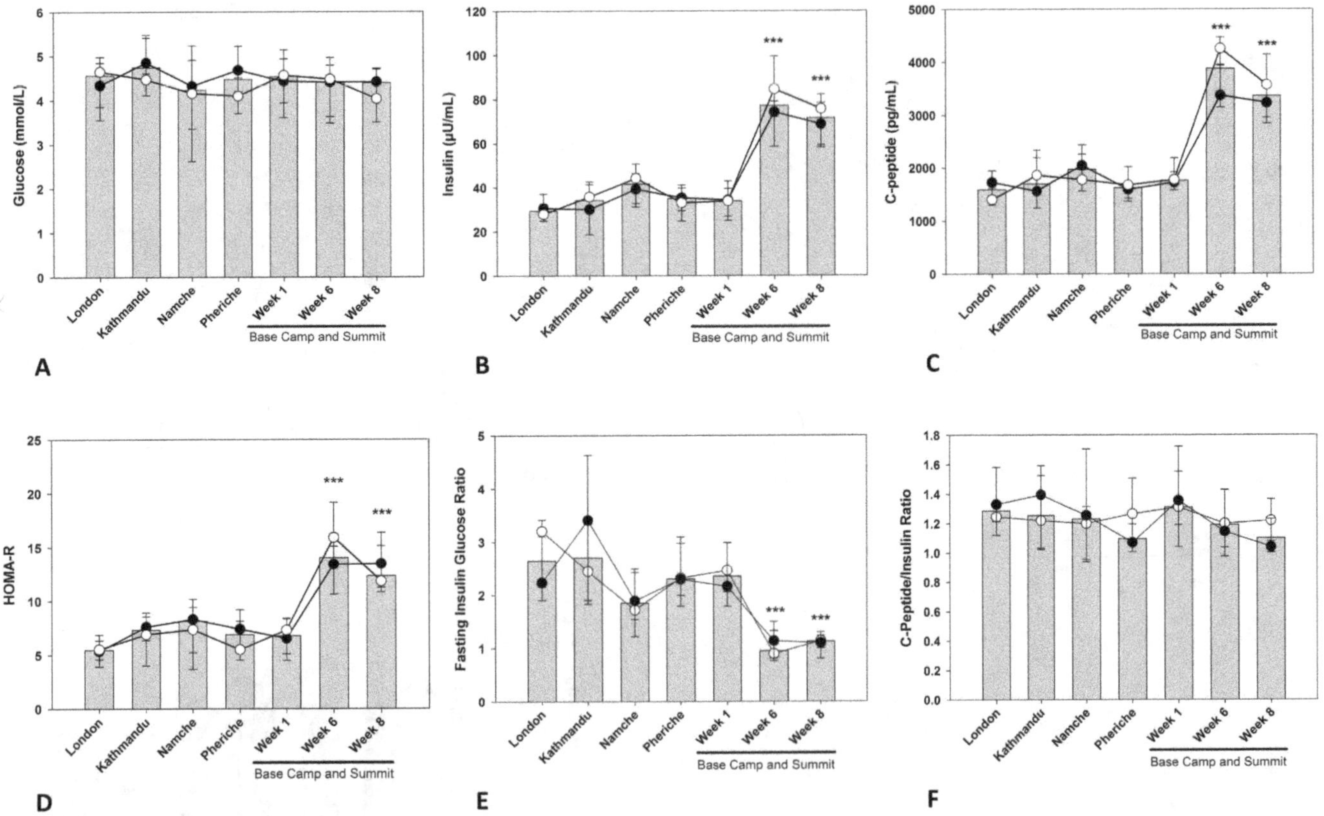

Figure 1. Gluco-insulin axis regulation in members of the research team reaching the summit (●) or remaining at base camp (○) during the expedition. Homeostatic model of assessment was calculated as a proxy indicator of systemic insulin resistance (HOMA-IR). C-Peptide/Insulin Ratio was calculated as a measure of hepatic insulin extraction. Median data are presented for the two groups (lines) and all subjects (bars). Error bars are 25th and 75th percentiles. Significant differences were flagged in each graph: ***$p<0.001$. No significant differences were observed between climbers and base camp at either time point.

correlation of oxidative stress with inflammation revealed an important relationship between IL-6 with 4-HNE ($r = 0.48$, $p < 0.001$). 4-HNE was the only oxidative stress biomarkers strongly correlated with HOMA-IR ($r = 0.42$, $p<0.001$) (**Figure 5**). The strongest association with insulin and indices of gluco-insular regulation were observed for glucagon, IL-6 and 4-HNE. SpO_2 was weakly associated with biomarkers of insulin resistance (**Table S3 in File S1**).

Discussion

The key finding of the present study is that sustained hypoxia induced a significant increase in IL-6 and 4-HNE concentrations which were correlated with insulin concentrations and HOMA-IR levels.

Gluco-Insular Response

Our results are in accord with those from the (hypobaric chamber-based) simulated ascent of Everest in Operation Everest II, whose study duration (40 days) and intensity of exposure to hypoxia was similar for the 6 healthy male participants to that which our subjects faced [12]: in both studies, glucose- insulin response was dependent on the duration and intensity of exposure to hypoxia, with a paradoxical increase in insulin levels during weight loss [14]. These data are consistent with an increase in insulin resistance at altitude, resulting in a compensatory increase in insulin secretion. Such an increase in insulin levels may also help compensate for the increase in hepatic glucose output induced by counter-regulatory hormones (glucagon, adrenalin), whose levels rose by ~70% and ~300%, respectively during the last two weeks at altitude.

Results from other studies testing the association between hypoxia and insulin function are conflicting. Short-term exposure to hypoxia for two days at high altitude was characterised by increased glucose and insulin levels which progressively returned to baseline levels within one week [3]. Simulated short-term (16 hours) exposure to hypoxia (4,300 m) induced a decline in insulin sensitivity in both women and men [37]. Endocrine responses to hypoxia have also been investigated in longer studies. Plasma glucose and insulin levels increased in fifteen healthy subjects after seven days at 5,080 m but returned to baseline values at the end of the 41-day expedition. Decreased glycaemia and stable insulin levels were observed in nine male elite climbers during their ascent of Mt. Everest [1].

The Operation Everest II study resembles the Caudwell Xtreme Everest Expedition for study duration and intensity of exposure to hypoxia. Weight loss in the 6 healthy men making a simulated (hypobaric chamber) ascent of Mt. Everest over 40days [12] was similar to that seen in our study (-7.4 kg). This study reported a two-fold rise of insulin levels with ascent to 335Torr (25days; altitude equivalent = ~5700 m) and 282Torr (32days, altitude equivalent = ~7000 m) that remained elevated until the end of the study (40days, 282Torr). Plasma glucose concentrations were unchanged throughout the study [12]. Operation Everest II did

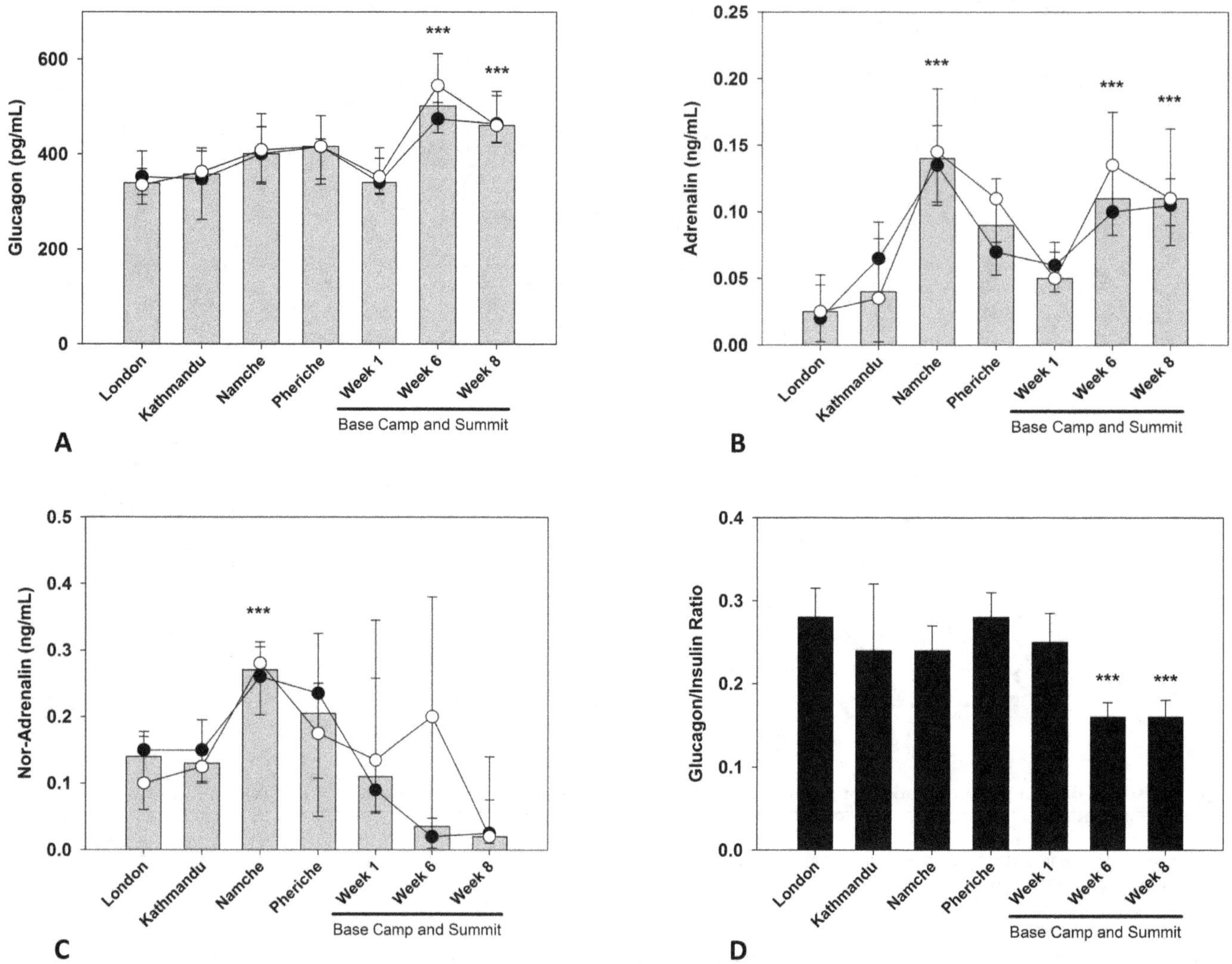

Figure 2. Changes in concentration of counter-regulatory hormones (glucagon, adrenalin, Noradrenalin) and glucagon-insulin ratio in members of the research team reaching the summit (●) or remaining at base camp (○) during the expedition. Median data are presented for the two groups (lines) and all subjects (bars). Error bars are 25th and 75th percentiles. Significant differences were flagged in each graph: ***$p<0.001$ No significant differences were observed between climbers and EBC lab team members at either time point.

not, however, report significant changes in either glucagon or adrenalin concentrations [12]. Larsen et al measured glucagon and adrenalin levels in healthy subjects after seven days at high altitude and found no change in the blood concentrations of either hormone [3]. In our study, Noradrenalin concentrations peaked as soon as subjects had to face the first substantial environmental stressor represented by the ascent to Namche Bazaar at the start of the trekking expedition [16]. Subsequently, Noradrenalin levels progressively declined, returning to baseline levels during the last two weeks of the expedition. A similar pattern for Noradrenalin concentrations was observed in the Operation Everest II study [14]. The physiological meaning of the reciprocal changes in adrenalin and Noradrenalin concentrations at the end of the study is not clear. Perhaps the elevated metabolic stress occurring during the last part of the expedition may have posed a greater demand on systemic functions (metabolic, respiratory) regulated by adrenalin and, therefore, a reduction of the adrenalin/Noradrenalin ratio may have enhanced these responses.

The role of hepatic insulin resistance and neo-glucogenesis had been previously investigated in healthy men exposed to 7-day high altitude hypoxia (4,559 m) utilising hyperglycaemic euglycaemic clamps to determine peripheral and hepatic insulin resistance [3]. Insulin action decreased after two days of hypobaric hypoxia but improved with more prolonged exposure. No effects of hypoxia were observed on hepatic gluconeogenesis [3]. Glucose and insulin levels were unchanged during the ascent and the first week at EBC, suggesting that a longer exposure to hypoxia is needed to induce changes in insulin signalling.

The effects of prolonged hypoxia exposure on gluco-insular regulation may be contextualised within a pathogenetic allostatic metabolic model [38]. Chronic hypoxia represents the allostatic metabolic load, which initiates a series of adaptive responses leading to maintenance of physiological function (allostasis). Over time, the allostatic hypoxic load can accumulate and activate neural, endocrine, and immune stress responses which in turn modify glucose and insulin regulation. This concept has been previously proposed to explain the pathogenesis of hyperglycemia and insulin resistance [39].

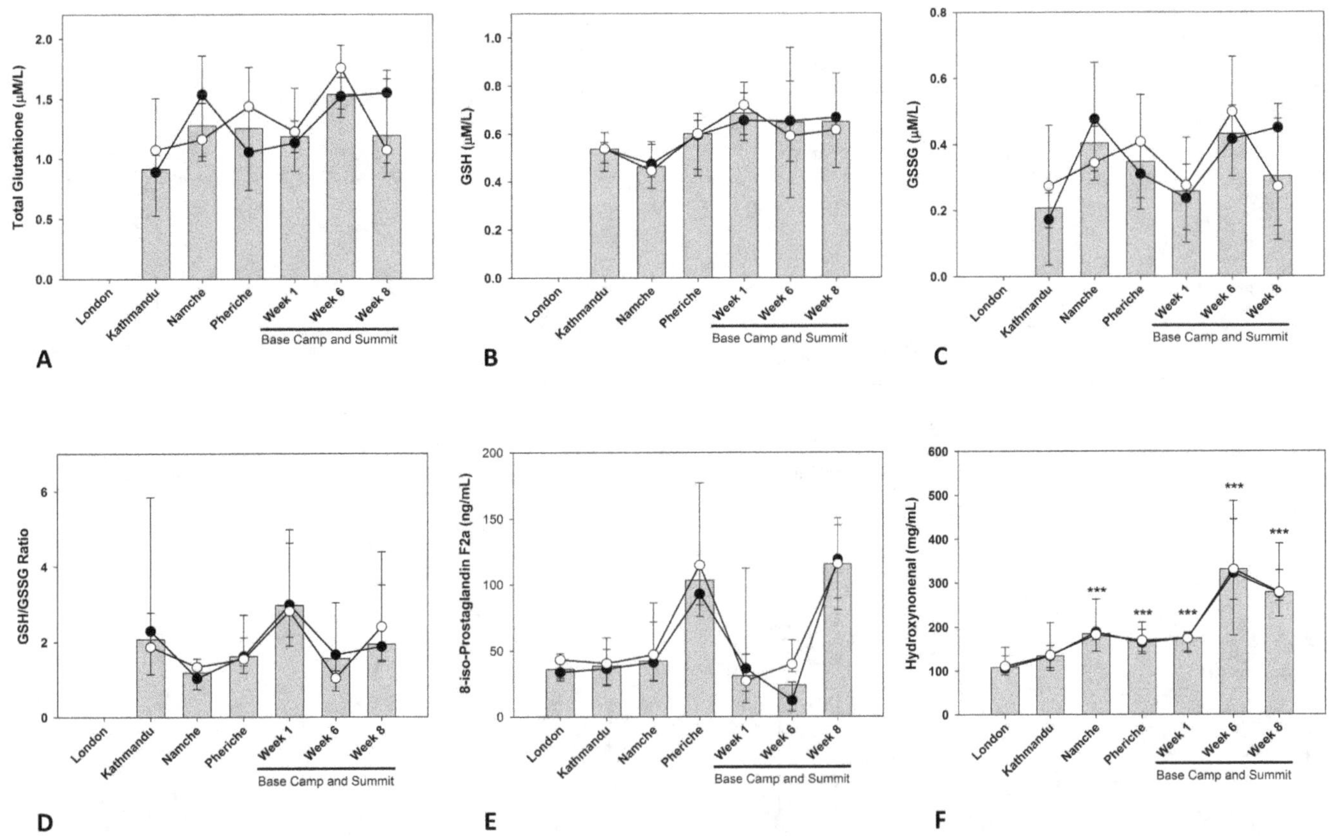

Figure 3. Changes in biomarkers of oxidative stress in members of the research team reaching the summit (●) or remaining at base camp (○) during the expedition. Median data are presented for the two groups (lines) and all subjects (bars). Error bars are 25th and 75th percentiles. Data for Total Glutathione, GSH, GSSG and GSH/GSSG were not available from the samples collected in London. Therefore we have used the data derived from the samples collected in Kathmandu as baseline levels. Significant differences were flagged in each graph: ***$p<0.001$ No significant differences were observed between climbers and EBC lab team members at either time point.

Changes in 4-HNE and IL-6

The uniqueness of our results is in the identification of a consistent association between 4-HNE, IL-6 and insulin resistance (i.e., HOMA-IR), which suggests the existence of a mechanistic link between these molecules and the development of insulin resistance during exposure to hypoxia. The two oxi-inflammatory biomarkers (4-HNE and IL-6) may represent the stress mediators of chronic exposure to hypoxia. In addition, the associations appeared to be minimally affected by changes in energy balance as the oxidative-inflammatory and glucose-insular responses to hypoxia were similar in both groups, despite the significant differences in weight changes and physical activity between groups during the last two weeks of the expedition. These changes coincided temporally with the increases in insulin concentrations and HOMA-IR. IL-6 also showed a strong correlation with glucagon, which suggests that the mechanistic link between the prolonged exposure to hypoxia and pancreatic endocrine function may be modified by IL-6.

This study is the first to report the association between sustained hypoxia, IL-6 and gluco-insular hormones. Hartmann et al reported increased IL-6 levels in healthy volunteers who spent 3 nights at an elevation above 3,400 m [40]. However, this acute response was not observed in our study. IL-6 is secreted by enlarged, activated adipocytes which may result in a systemic elevation of IL-6 plasma levels leading to insulin resistance [41]. In muscular tissue, IL-6 may be secreted during physical activity to act as an energy sensor by activating AMP-kinase and enhancing glucose disposal. The evidence suggests an association between chronic elevations of IL-6 and hepatic insulin resistance. IL-6 also appears to impede maturation of pre-adipocytes and deregulate the insulin pathway [42]. Therefore, the association of IL-6 with insulin function is still controversial; our results suggest that, under chronic hypoxic conditions, IL-6 may be influencing the physiology of pancreatic endocrine hormones. However, the causality of the associations and the physiological mechanisms underpinning these associations remain to be established. Pedersen et al have summarised the role of IL-6 as a metabolic modulator of muscular function during exercise [43]. IL-6 concentrations scaled with exercise duration and intensity but concentrations returned to basal levels shortly after cessation of exercise [43]. The investigators concluded that IL-6 plays a physiological role during muscle contraction as it seems to have anti-inflammatory effects and a role in fat oxidation, and improved insulin-stimulated glucose uptake [43]. The metabolic role of IL-6 cannot be ignored in the interpretation of our results. However, the effects of muscle contraction on circulating IL-6 concentrations are likely to have been limited because 1) samples were collected in the morning after subjects had rested overnight, and 2) plasma IL-6 levels of base camp residents and climbers were overlapping in spite of very different physical activity levels during the last part of the expedition.

Hypoxia is associated with mitochondrial dysfunction and production of ROS [44]. This is also caused by a reduced capacity

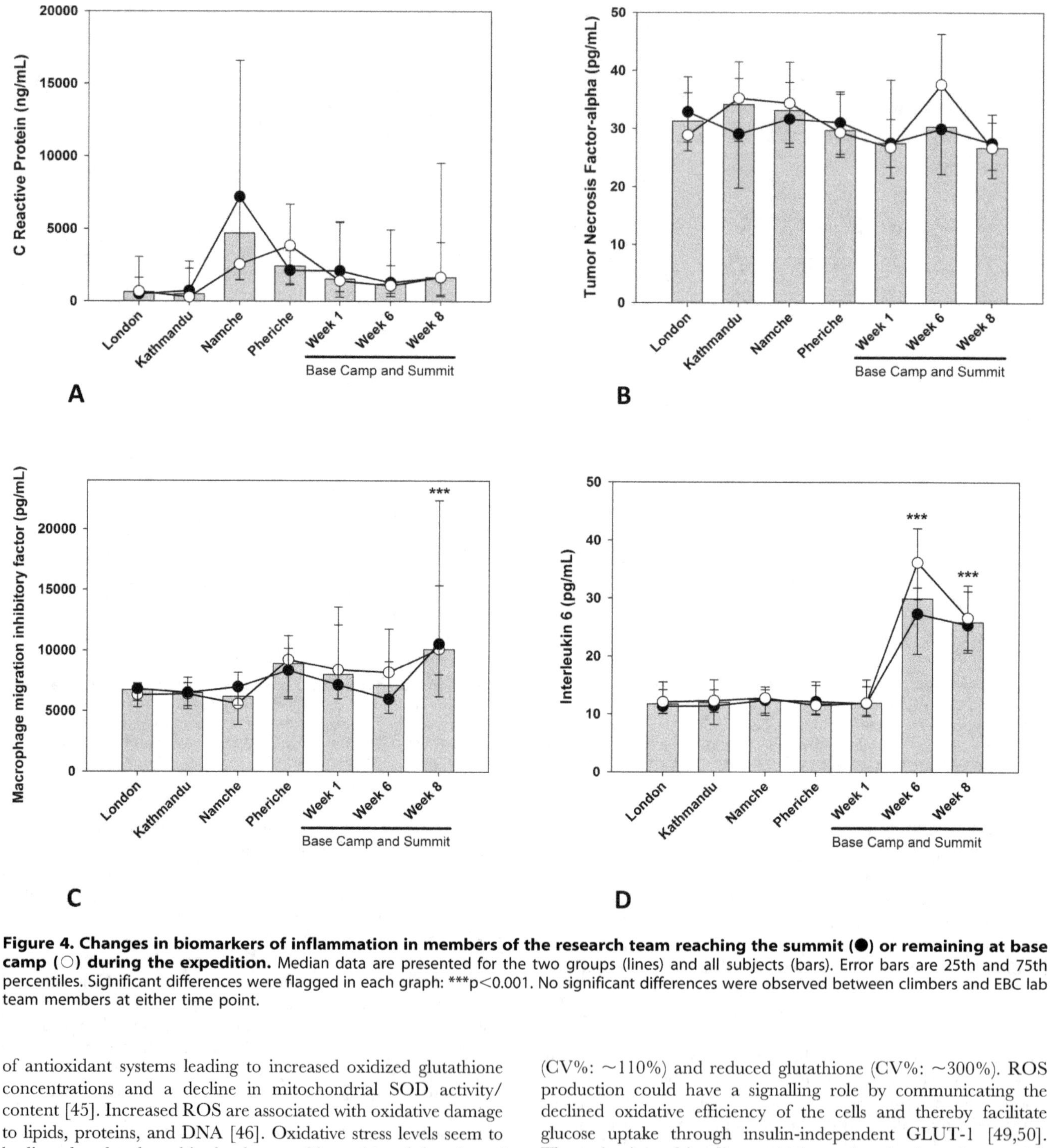

Figure 4. Changes in biomarkers of inflammation in members of the research team reaching the summit (●) or remaining at base camp (○) during the expedition. Median data are presented for the two groups (lines) and all subjects (bars). Error bars are 25th and 75th percentiles. Significant differences were flagged in each graph: ***p<0.001. No significant differences were observed between climbers and EBC lab team members at either time point.

of antioxidant systems leading to increased oxidized glutathione concentrations and a decline in mitochondrial SOD activity/content [45]. Increased ROS are associated with oxidative damage to lipids, proteins, and DNA [46]. Oxidative stress levels seem to be linearly related to altitude, degree of hypoxia and duration of exposure. The Operation Everest III study suggested a direct association as lipid peroxidation increased by 23% at 6,000 m and 79% at 8,848 m [47]. Vij *et al* studied acclimatization to high-altitude hypoxia over a period of 13 months, and it appeared that a period of 3 months was sufficient to increase lipid peroxidation and decrease enzymatic and non-enzymatic antioxidant defences [48]. In our study, hypoxia induced progressive changes in biomarkers of oxidative stress. In particular, 4-HNE levels increased significantly during the last phase of the expedition and, interestingly, the inter-subject variability of these responses was relatively low (CV%: ~45%) compared to isoprostanes (CV%: ~110%) and reduced glutathione (CV%: ~300%). ROS production could have a signalling role by communicating the declined oxidative efficiency of the cells and thereby facilitate glucose uptake through insulin-independent GLUT-1 [49,50]. The reduction of insulin sensitivity and activation of anaerobic oxidative pathways could therefore represent an energy-buffer mechanism to reroute glucose and oxygen towards vital organs such as brain and heart. Increased insulin secretion during hypoxia may therefore be a reflection of the increased reliance of cellular metabolism on glycolysis [26].

Limitations

Subjects were exposed to other extreme environmental conditions (low temperature, physical exertion) in addition to hypoxia which may confound the associations with metabolic outcomes. However, although climbers experienced much harsher conditions

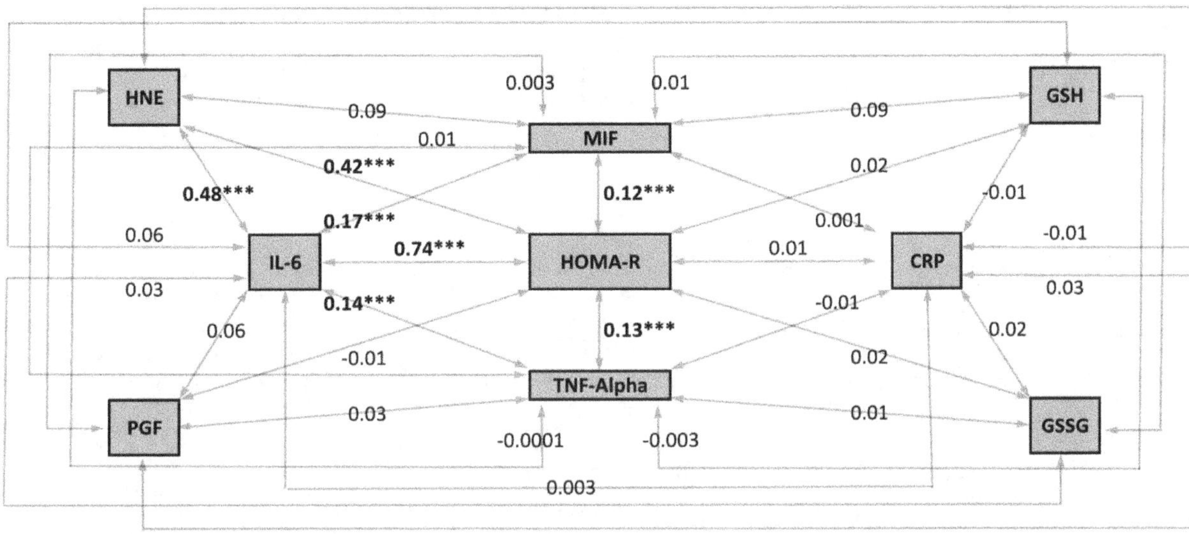

Figure 5. Correlation between Homeostatic Model of Assessment of insulin resistance (HOMA-IR) with biomarkers of inflammation and oxidative stress during the 2007 Caudwell Xtreme Everest Expedition. The pathogenic model is centripetal (direction of causality is towards the centre of the diagram) implying that the position of the biomarkers reflects the hypothesised order of activation of the responses to hypoxia (Oxidative Stress → Inflammation → Insulin Resistance (HOMA-IR)). Within-subject correlation analysis was performed and correlation coefficients are reported. Significant results have been highlighted: ***$p<0.001$. Acronyms: 4-HNE = 4-Hydroxynonenal; PGF = 8-iso-Prostaglandin F_2alpha; IL-6 = interleukin 6; MIF = macrophage migration inhibitory factor; GSH = reduced glutathione; TNF-α = tumour necrosis factor alpha; CRP = C-reactive protein; GSSG = oxidized glutathione.

than EBC residents, they did not show higher levels of oxidative stress, inflammation or insulin levels. This suggests that metabolic derangements were essentially driven by the prolonged exposure to hypoxia. We were unable to determine the exact time of onset of the metabolic derangements as no measurements were taken between week 1 and week 6 at EBC. Cortisol levels were not measured during the expedition and any possible association with changes in insulin and glucagon concentrations cannot therefore be assessed. Finally, subjects were initially of normal weight and thence in negative energy balance, which may limit the transferability of the results to obese subjects in positive energy balance as a mechanistic model of insulin resistance. However, in consideration of the established insulin sensitising effects of weight loss we argue that this study supports the role of systemic hypoxia in the impairment of gluco-insular action as well as defines a potential pathogenetic trajectory that may link tissue hypoxia to insulin resistance in obese subjects.

Conclusions

Healthy humans exposed to sustained hypobaric hypoxia at high-altitude appear to become insulin-resistant while they are in negative energy balance. Normo-glycemia was maintained by a compensatory increase in β-cell secretion and reduced hepatic extraction leading to sustained hyperinsulinemia during the last two weeks of the expedition. Previous cellular and animal models of hypoxia-induced insulin resistance have identified two core causal mechanisms: over-production of ROS and inflammation [22]. Our results are aligned with this mechanistic paradigm and provide evidence to support a causal relationship between hypoxia and insulin resistance in humans. The role of 4-HNE and IL-6 as mediators of these effects should be corroborated in future studies. Ideally, these studies should be conducted in simulated-hypoxic environments where other factors can be constrained to control for the confounding effects of weight loss while utilising dedicated experimental protocols for the assessment of peripheral and hepatic insulin resistance.

Supporting Information

File S1 Supporting information figure and tables. Figure S1, Cumulative mean changes in body weight occurred at the end of the Caudwell Everest Expedition in climbers and in members residing at base camp (EBC). Mann-Whitney test was used to determine between-group differences in weight loss after EBC 8 weeks. **Table S1, Ascent profile and residence at high altitude of the team remaining at Everest Base Camp (EBC, N = 10) and those climbing higher (Climbers, N = 14)*.** Information on altitude (m), barometric pressure (mmHg) and inspired partial pressure of oxygen (PiO_2, mmHg) is reported for each phase. Hemoglobin concentrations (g/dl) and arterial oxygen saturation (SaO_2, %) are reported in each group during the different phases of the expedition. **Table S2, Summary of the number of samples included in the analyses for each biomarker. Table S3, Correlation matrix to look at association between biomarkers of inflammation, oxidative stress and counter-regulatory hormones with glucose, insulin, C-peptide and HOMA-R.**

Acknowledgments

The Caudwell Xtreme Everest Research Group contributed to designing and conducting the experiments. The members of the Caudwell Xtreme Everest Research Group are as follows: Investigators—V. Ahuja, G. Aref-Adib, R. Burnham, A. Chisholm, K. Clarke, D. Coates, M. Coates, D. Cook, M. Cox, S. Dhillon, C. Dougall, P. Doyle, P. Duncan, M. Edsell, L. Edwards, L. Evans, P. Gardiner, M. Grocott, P. Gunning, N. Hart, J. Harrington, J. Harvey, C. Holloway, D. Howard, D. Hurlbut, C. Imray, C. Ince, M. Jonas, J. van der Kaaij, M. Khosravi, N. Kolfschoten, D. Levett, H. Luery, A. Luks, D. Martin, R. McMorrow, P. Meale, K.

Mitchell, H. Montgomery, G. Morgan, J. Morgan, A. Murray, M. Mythen, S. Newman, M. O'Dwyer, J. Pate, T. Plant, M. Pun, P. Richards, A. Richardson, G. Rodway, J. Simpson, C. Stroud, M. Stroud, J. Stygal, B. Symons, P. Szawarski, A. Van Tulleken, C. Van Tulleken, A. Vercueil, L. Wandrag, M. Wilson, J. Windsor; Scientific Advisory Group—B. Basnyat, C. Clarke, T. Hornbein, J. Milledge, J. West.

Author Contributions

Conceived and designed the experiments: MS HLR BOF CAL HEM MGM DSM DZHL KM MPWG MF. Performed the experiments: HLR BOF CAL HEM DSM DZHL KM MPWG MF. Analyzed the data: MS MPWG MF. Wrote the paper: MS HLR BOF CAL HEM MGM DSM DZHL KM MPWG MF.

References

1. Benso A, Broglio F, Aimaretti G, Lucatello B, Lanfranco F, et al. (2007) Endocrine and metabolic responses to extreme altitude and physical exercise in climbers. Eur J Endocrinol 157: 733–740.
2. Kelly KR, Williamson DL, Fealy CE, Kriz DA, Krishnan RK, et al. (2010) Acute altitude-induced hypoxia suppresses plasma glucose and leptin in healthy humans. Metabolism 59: 200–205.
3. Larsen JJ, Hansen JM, Olsen NV, Galbo H, Dela F (1997) The effect of altitude hypoxia on glucose homeostasis in men. J Physiol 504 (Pt 1): 241–249.
4. Louis M, Punjabi NM (2009) Effects of acute intermittent hypoxia on glucose metabolism in awake healthy volunteers. J Appl Physiol 106: 1538–1544.
5. Mackenzie R, Maxwell N, Castle P, Brickley G, Watt P (2011) Acute hypoxia and exercise improve insulin sensitivity (S(I) (2*)) in individuals with type 2 diabetes. Diabetes Metab Res Rev 27: 94–101.
6. Mackenzie R, Maxwell N, Castle P, Elliott B, Brickley G, et al. (2012) Intermittent Exercise with and without Hypoxia Improves Insulin Sensitivity in Individuals with Type 2 Diabetes. J Clin Endocrinol Metab 97: E546–555.
7. Oltmanns KM, Gehring H, Rudolf S, Schultes B, Rook S, et al. (2004) Hypoxia causes glucose intolerance in humans. Am J Respir Crit Care Med 169: 1231–1237.
8. Polotsky VY, Li J, Punjabi NM, Rubin AE, Smith PL, et al. (2003) Intermittent hypoxia increases insulin resistance in genetically obese mice. J Physiol 552: 253–264.
9. Rafacho A, Gonçalves-Neto LM, Ferreira FBD, Protzek AOP, Boschero AC, et al. (2013) Glucose homeostasis in rats exposed to acute intermittent hypoxia. Acta Physiologica: n/a-n/a.
10. Sawhney RC, Malhotra AS, Singh T (1991) Glucoregulatory hormones in man at high altitude. Eur J Appl Physiol Occup Physiol 62: 286–291.
11. Sawhney RC, Malhotra AS, Singh T, Rai RM, Sinha KC (1986) Insulin secretion at high altitude in man. Int J Biometeorol 30: 231–238.
12. Young PM, Rose MS, Sutton JR, Green HJ, Cymerman A, et al. (1989) Operation Everest II: plasma lipid and hormonal responses during a simulated ascent of Mt. Everest. J Appl Physiol 66: 1430–1435.
13. Chen M, Lee W, Chen S, Chen C, Chen C, et al. (2010) Effect of a Prolonged Altitude Expedition on Glucose Tolerance and Abdominal Fatness. Research Quarterly for Exercise and Sport 81: 472–477.
14. Young PM, Rose MS, Sutton JR, Green HJ, Cymerman A, et al. (1989) Operation Everest II: plasma lipid and hormonal responses during a simulated ascent of Mt. Everest. J Appl Physiol (1985) 66: 1430–1435.
15. Lippl FJ, Neubauer S, Schipfer S, Lichter N, Tufman A, et al. (2010) Hypobaric hypoxia causes body weight reduction in obese subjects. Obesity (Silver Spring) 18: 675–681.
16. Levett DZ, Martin DS, Wilson MH, Mitchell K, Dhillon S, et al. (2010) Design and conduct of Caudwell Xtreme Everest: an observational cohort study of variation in human adaptation to progressive environmental hypoxia. BMC Med Res Methodol 10: 98.
17. Rose MS, Houston CS, Fulco CS, Coates G, Sutton JR, et al. (1988) Operation Everest. II: Nutrition and body composition. J Appl Physiol (1985) 65: 2545–2551.
18. Wang XIA, Bi Y, Zhang Q, Pan F (2013) Obstructive sleep apnoea and the risk of type 2 diabetes: A meta-analysis of prospective cohort studies. Respirology 18: 140–146.
19. Cizza G, Piaggi P, Lucassen EA, de Jonge L, Walter M, et al. (2013) Obstructive Sleep Apnea Is a Predictor of Abnormal Glucose Metabolism in Chronically Sleep Deprived Obese Adults. PLoS One 8: e65400.
20. Odegaard JI, Chawla A (2008) Mechanisms of macrophage activation in obesity-induced insulin resistance. Nat Clin Pract End Met 4: 619–626.
21. Drager LF, Jun JC, Polotsky VY (2010) Metabolic consequences of intermittent hypoxia: Relevance to obstructive sleep apnea. Best Practice & Research Clinical Endocrinology & Metabolism 24: 843–851.
22. Trayhurn P (2013) Hypoxia and adipose tissue function and dysfunction in obesity. Physiol Rev 93: 1–21.
23. Cao Y (2010) Adipose tissue angiogenesis as a therapeutic target for obesity and metabolic diseases. Nat Rev Drug Discov 9: 107–115.
24. Halberg N, Khan T, Trujillo ME, Wernstedt-Asterholm I, Attie AD, et al. (2009) Hypoxia-inducible factor 1alpha induces fibrosis and insulin resistance in white adipose tissue. Mol Cell Biol 29: 4467–4483.
25. Khan T, Muise ES, Iyengar P, Wang ZV, Chandalia M, et al. (2009) Metabolic dysregulation and adipose tissue fibrosis: role of collagen VI. Mol Cell Biol 29: 1575–1591.
26. Wheaton WW, Chandel NS (2011) Hypoxia. 2. Hypoxia regulates cellular metabolism. American Journal of Physiology - Cell Physiology 300: C385–C393.
27. Greenberg H, Ye X, Wilson D, Htoo AK, Hendersen T, et al. (2006) Chronic intermittent hypoxia activates nuclear factor-κB in cardiovascular tissues in vivo. Biochemical and Biophysical Research Communications 343: 591–596.
28. Wang N, Khan SA, Prabhakar NR, Nanduri J (2013) Impaired Pancreatic Beta Cell Function by Chronic Intermittent Hypoxia. Exp Physiol.
29. Matthews DR, Hosker JP, Rudenski AS, Naylor BA, Treacher DF, et al. (1985) Homeostasis model assessment: insulin resistance and beta-cell function from fasting plasma glucose and insulin concentrations in man. Diabetologia 28: 412–419.
30. Polonsky KS, Rubenstein AH (1984) C-peptide as a measure of the secretion and hepatic extraction of insulin. Pitfalls and limitations. Diabetes 33: 486–494.
31. Wahren J, Ekberg K, Johansson J, Henriksson M, Pramanik A, et al. (2000) Role of C-peptide in human physiology. American Journal of Physiology - Endocrinology And Metabolism 278: E759–E768.
32. Faber OK, Binder C (1986) C-peptide: An index of insulin secretion. Diabetes/Metabolism Reviews 2: 331–345.
33. Duckworth WC, Bennett RG, Hamel FG (1998) Insulin Degradation: Progress and Potential. Endocrine Reviews 19: 608–624.
34. Unger RH (1971) Glucagon and the Insulin:Glucagon Ratio in Diabetes and Other Catabolic Illnesses. Diabetes 20: 834–838.
35. Bland JM, Douglas GA (1995) Statistics notes: Calculating correlation coefficients with repeated observations: Part 1—correlation within subjects. BMJ 310: 446.
36. Levett DZ, Fernandez BO, Riley HL, Martin DS, Mitchell K, et al. (2011) The role of nitrogen oxides in human adaptation to hypoxia. Sci Rep 1: 109.
37. Braun B, Rock PB, Zamudio S, Wolfel GE, Mazzeo RS, et al. (2001) Women at altitude: short-term exposure to hypoxia and/or alpha(1)-adrenergic blockade reduces insulin sensitivity. J Appl Physiol 91: 623–631.
38. McEwen BS, Wingfield JC (2003) The concept of allostasis in biology and biomedicine. Horm Behav 43: 2–15.
39. Virtue S, Vidal-Puig A (2010) Adipose tissue expandability, lipotoxicity and the Metabolic Syndrome — An allostatic perspective. Biochimica et Biophysica Acta (BBA) - Molecular and Cell Biology of Lipids 1801: 338–349.
40. Hartmann G, Tschöp M, Fischer R, Bidlingmaier C, Riepl R, et al. (2000) High Altitude Increases Circulating Interleukin-6, Interleukin-1 Receptor Antagonist And C-Reactive Protein. Cytokine 12: 246–252.
41. Kim JH, Bachmann RA, Chen J (2009) Chapter 21 Interleukin-6 and Insulin Resistance. In: Gerald L, editor. Vitamins & Hormones: Academic Press. pp. 613–633.
42. Glund S, Krook A (2008) Role of interleukin-6 signalling in glucose and lipid metabolism. Acta Physiologica 192: 37–48.
43. Pedersen BK, Febbraio MA (2008) Muscle as an Endocrine Organ: Focus on Muscle-Derived Interleukin-6. Physiological Reviews 88: 1379–1406.
44. Peng Y, Yuan G, Overholt J, Kumar G, Prabhakar N (2003) Systemic and Cellular Responses to Intermittent Hypoxia: Evidence for Oxidative Stress and Mitochondrial Dysfunction. In: Pequignot J-M, Gonzalez C, Nurse C, Prabhakar N, Dalmaz Y, editors. Chemoreception: Springer US. pp. 559–564.
45. Dosek A, Ohno H, Acs Z, Taylor AW, Radak Z (2007) High altitude and oxidative stress. Respir Physiol Neurobiol 158: 128–131.
46. Bergamini CM, Gambetti S, Dondi A, Cervellati C (2004) Oxygen, reactive oxygen species and tissue damage. Curr Pharm Des 10: 1611–1626.
47. Joanny P, Steinberg J, Robach P, Richalet JP, Gortan C, et al. (2001) Operation Everest III (Comex'97): the effect of simulated severe hypobaric hypoxia on lipid peroxidation and antioxidant defence systems in human blood at rest and after maximal exercise. Resuscitation 49: 307–314.
48. Vij AG, Dutta R, Satija NK (2005) Acclimatization to oxidative stress at high altitude. High Alt Med Biol 6: 301–310.
49. Ouiddir A, Planès C, Fernandes I, VanHesse A, Clerici C (1999) Hypoxia Upregulates Activity and Expression of the Glucose Transporter GLUT1 in Alveolar Epithelial Cells. American Journal of Respiratory Cell and Molecular Biology 21: 710–718.
50. Semenza GL (1999) Regulation Of Mammalian O2 Homeostasis By Hypoxia-Inducible Factor 1. Annual Review of Cell and Developmental Biology 15: 551–578.

Monocytes Expand with Immune Dysregulation and is Associated with Insulin Resistance in Older Individuals with Chronic HIV

Cecilia M. Shikuma[1]*, Dominic C. Chow[1], Louie Mar A. Gangcuangco[1], Guangxiang Zhang[1], Sheila M. Keating[2], Philip J. Norris[2,3], Todd B. Seto[1,4], Nisha Parikh[1,4], Kalpana J. Kallianpur[1], Beau K. Nakamoto[1,5], Lorna S. Nagamine[1], Lishomwa C. Ndhlovu[1], Jason D. Barbour[1]

1 Hawaii Center for AIDS, University of Hawaii, Honolulu, Hawaii, United States of America, **2** Blood Systems Research Institute, San Francisco, California, United States of America, **3** University of California San Francisco, San Francisco, California, United States of America, **4** Queen's Medical Center, Honolulu, Hawaii, United States of America, **5** Straub Clinic and Hospital, Honolulu, Hawaii, United States of America

Abstract

Background: Rates of insulin resistance are increased in HIV-infected patients on stable antiretroviral therapy (ART). Such increase may partially be due to HIV-induced immune dysregulation involving monocytes (MO) and its subsets.

Materials and Methods: Cross-sectional analysis of 141 HIV-infected subjects age $\geq$ 40 years on stable ART. Homeostatic model assessment–insulin resistance (HOMA-IR) and rates of metabolic syndrome were calculated. Subjects were classified by fasting glucose and oral glucose tolerance test (OGTT) into clinical diabetes categories. Multi-parametric flow cytometry was used to determine MO subset percentages: [classical ($CD14^{++}CD16^{-}$), intermediate ($CD14^{++}CD16^{+}$), non-classical ($CD14^{low/+}CD16^{++}$), and a recently identified fourth ($CD14^{low/+}CD16^{-}$) 'transitional' MO subset] and percentage of activated ($CD38^{+}HLA\text{-}DR^{+}$) CD8 T cells. Absolute levels of cells were calculated using clinical CBC and T cell subset data. Multiple plasma soluble biomarkers were assessed by Luminex technology.

Results: Median age 50 years, CD4 count (percent) 505 cells/μL (29%), and 89% male. Total MO ($r = -0.23$, $p = 0.006$) and classical and non-classical MO subsets correlated negatively with CD4 percent. No correlations were seen with CD4 count as absolute values. Log-total MO and log-classical MO predicted HOMA-IR independently of HIV immuno-virologic and diabetes risk factors ($\beta = 0.42$, $p = 0.02$ and $\beta = 0.35$, $p = 0.02$, respectively) and were increased in subjects with metabolic syndrome ($p = 0.03$ and $p = 0.05$ respectively). Total and/or subset MO levels correlated with multiple soluble plasma biomarkers including CRP, IL-6, MMP-9, MPO, SAA, SAP and tPAI-1, with tPAI-1 independently predicting HOMA-IR ($\beta = 0.74$, $p < 0.001$).

Conclusions: MO levels increase with worsening HIV immune dysregulation as assessed by CD4 percent. CD4 percent may provide additional information about MO and metabolic risk in this population beyond absolute values. MO, and specifically classical MO, may contribute to insulin resistance and metabolic syndrome during chronic HIV infection. Multiple soluble plasma biomarkers including tPAI-1 increase with increase in MO. Levels of tPAI-1 independently predict the development of insulin resistance.

Editor: Derya Unutmaz, New York University, United States of America

Funding: This study was supported by grants R01HL095135, U54RR026136, U54MD007584,and G12MD007601. The content is solely the responsibility of the authors and does not necessarily represent the official views of the National Institutes of Health. The funders had no role in study design, data collection and analysis, decision to publish, or preparation of the manuscript.

Competing Interests: The authors have declared that no competing interests exist.

* E-mail: shikuma@hawaii.edu

Introduction

Abnormalities of glucose metabolism occur commonly among HIV infected patients on stable antiretroviral therapy (ART) [1] and may contribute to increased rates of cardio-metabolic complications. The etiologies for the higher prevalence of insulin resistance and diabetes among ART-treated individuals with chronic HIV are likely multifactorial including the possible effects of various antiretroviral medications, presence of lipodystrophy, co-infection with hepatitis C virus (HCV), higher rates of hypogonadism, and higher rates of traditional risk factors in some HIV populations such as obesity and physical inactivity [1]. HIV-induced immune dysregulation and inflammation may also play a role in the increased prevalence of insulin resistance and diabetes. Low CD4 count is an independent risk factor for altered insulin sensitivity [2]. Higher systemic levels of C-reactive protein (CRP), and soluble receptors of tumor necrosis factor-alpha (TNF-α), sTNF1 and sTNF2, accompany incident diabetes after initiation of HIV antiretroviral therapy [3].

While studies of HIV-induced immune activation have traditionally focused on the role of CD8 T cells, there is increasing interest in the role that MO may play in non-infectious complications seen among individuals with chronic HIV. MO originate in the bone marrow and circulate in the peripheral blood for 1−3 days before differentiating into macrophages within various tissues. MO are a heterogeneous population of cells, and are classified by international consensus into several subsets on the basis of their CD14 and CD16 surface expression: classical MO lacking CD16 expression ($CD14^{++}CD16^{-}$) and those expressing CD16 comprised of intermediate ($CD14^{++}CD16^{+}$) and non-classical ($CD14^{low/+}CD16^{++}$) MO [4]. We have recently published data reporting the identification of a fourth MO subset which we have termed 'transitional' MO. This transitional MO subset is characterized by reduced but still detectable levels of CD14 ($CD14^{+}CD16^{-}$) and is associated within our cohort of HIV-infected individuals on stable ART with increases in carotid intima-media thickness, a well-established marker of arterial injury [5,6]. Classical MO account for roughly 80−90% of circulating MO in normal healthy individuals. This population has been reported to increase in acute inflammation and to be rapidly recruited to sites of infection [7,8,9]. The CD16-containing population increases with aging and chronic inflammatory disorders, and compared to classical MO, shows higher expression of pro-inflammatory cytokines, higher potency in antigen presentation, and is more permissive for productive HIV infection [10,11,12]. The CD16-containing MO subset expands with HIV infection and is increased in subjects with HIV-associated neurocognitive disorders [13,14]. An increase in non-classical MO has been reported to correlate with HIV disease progression in ART-naïve subjects [15]. Increases in both non-classical and intermediate MO subsets similar in pattern to those in HIV-uninfected subjects with acute coronary syndrome have been reported in HIV-infected individuals with uncontrolled HIV disease [14]. In the general population, increases in circulating MO have been observed in diabetic subjects compared to nondiabetic controls [16,17,18]. CD16-bearing MO subsets have been reported to be increased in patients with type 2 diabetes and in particular in those with diabetic complications such as renal disease [16,19]. Taken together these data indicate a potentially important role for MO populations in the pathogenesis of HIV-associated cardio-metabolic disorders.

This study sought to understand how HIV-induced immune dysregulation influences MO and its subsets, and to then assess the relationship of these MO to insulin resistance and glucose dysregulation among HIV infected individuals on stable ART. We also assessed CD8 T cell activation levels and levels of various soluble plasma biomarkers as these parameters are known to play a substantial role in HIV immune dysregulation. We found that HIV immune dysregulation, as assessed specifically by CD4 percent but not as absolute CD4 count, is associated with an increase in MO with a very modest increase in the percentage represented by non-classical MO. In turn, we found that an increase in MO, primarily accounted for by an increase in classical MO, is associated with insulin resistance independent of HIV immuno-virologic and traditional diabetes risk factors and with metabolic syndrome. We further found that multiple positive correlations exist between numbers of total MO and/or its subsets and levels of various soluble plasma biomarkers including CRP, interleukin-6 (IL-6), matrix metallopeptidase-9 (MMP-9), myeloperoxidase (MPO), serum amyloid A (SAA), serum amyloid P component (SAP) and tissue plasminogen activator inhibitor-1 (tPAI-1). Levels of tPAI-1 increase as CD4 percent decreases and predict insulin resistance in an adjusted model.

Materials and Methods

Subjects and Study Design

We analyzed entry data of participants enrolled into the Hawaii Aging with HIV-Cardiovascular (HAHC-CVD) cohort, a 5-year longitudinal study investigating the role of immune activation and mitochondrial-specific oxidative stress on the pathogenesis of cardiovascular disease among HIV-infected patients on ART. The study was approved by the Committee on Human Subjects of the University of Hawaii and written informed consents were obtained from all participants.

Entry criteria required subjects to have documented HIV infection, be at least 40 years old, and be on stable ART for ≥ 6 months. Blood pressure and waist and hip measurements were obtained in triplicate and averaged. Body mass index (kg/m^2) was calculated. CBC, T cell subsets, plasma HIV RNA assessments, chemistries and metabolic labs (glucose, insulin, total, directly measured LDL and HDL cholesterol, and triglycerides) were obtained at entry in a fasted state (nothing by mouth except water for 12 hours). Subjects were assessed for past and current tobacco use. All subjects without known history of diabetes underwent an oral glucose tolerance test (OGTT). Homeostatic Model Assessment of Insulin Resistance (HOMA-IR) was calculated using the formula: [pre-OGTT glucose (mg/dL) X pre-OGTT insulin (uIU)]/405.

Subjects were grouped by glucose dysregulation according to the American Diabetic Association Guidelines utilizing fasting glucose and results of the OGTT [20]. Impaired fasting glucose (IFG) was defined as fasting glucose between 100 and 125 mg/dL and impaired glucose tolerance (IGT) as a 2-hour OGTT glucose level between 140−199 mg/dL. Diabetes was defined as self-reported history of diabetes, use of diabetic medications, fasting blood glucose ≥ 126 mg/dL or a 2-hour OGTT glucose level >200 mg/dL. Subjects were categorized as having metabolic syndrome utilizing the parameters as proposed by the National Cholesterol Education Program's Adult Treatment Panel III report (ATP III) [21].

Cell Flow Cytometry

Blood was separated within 30 minutes of the blood draw and peripheral blood mononuclear cells (PBMC) were isolated using Ficoll-Hypaque density gradient centrifugation (Pfizer, Inc., New York, NY). Separated PBMC and plasma were cryopreserved for future phenotypic analyses of cells and plasma cytokines. Banked PBMC were phenotyped based on CD14 and CD16 cell surface expression into 4 MO subsets [classical ($CD14^{++}CD16^{-}$), intermediate ($CD14^{++}CD16^{+}$), non-classical ($CD14^{+/low}CD16^{++}$), and transitional ($CD14^{+}CD16^{-}$)] and CD14-CD16- cells using a multiparametric panel of conjugated monoclonal antibodies that identified the $HLA\text{-}DR^{+}$ PBMC live cell population and excluded T lymphocytes, B cells, NK cells ($CD3^{-}CD19^{-}CD14^{-}CD20^{-}CD56^{-}$) and dead cells (aqua amine reactive dye [$AARD^{+}$]) as shown in Figure 1. Cells are washed twice and fixed with 1% paraformaldehyde solution (PFA) before acquiring on a custom 4 laser BD Fortessa flow cytometer (BD Biosciences, San Jose, CA). Data were analyzed using Flowjo software (Treestar Inc Ashland, OR).

The total MO count was calculated using white blood cell count (WBC) and percent MO values on the CBC conducted as part of entry evaluations on the same blood specimen as that utilized for flow cytometry. The CBC was performed by Diagnostic Laboratory Services (DLS), Inc., a local commercial Clinical Laboratory Improvement Amendments ACT (CLIA)-certified laboratory. Total numbers in each MO subset were then derived by

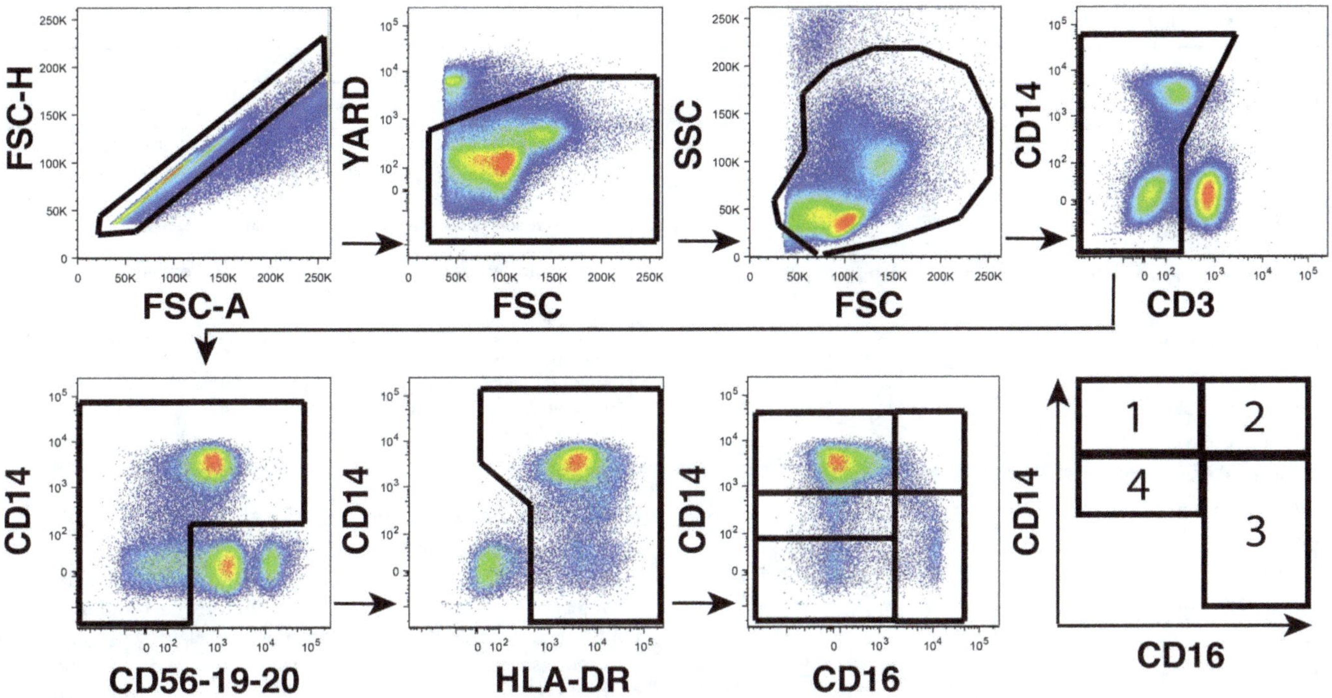

Figure 1. Multiparametric flow cytometry protocol utilized for identification of classical, intermediate, non-classical, and transitional monocyte subsets from peripheral blood mononuclear cells. Banked PBMC were phenotyped based on CD14 and CD16 cell surface expression into four MO subsets: [classical ($CD14^{++}CD16^{-}$); intermediate ($CD14^{++}CD16^{+}$), non-classical ($CD14^{+/low}CD16^{++}$), and transitional ($CD14^{+}CD16^{-}$)] and CD14-CD16- cells using a multiparametric panel of conjugated monoclonal antibodies that identified the HLA-DR^{+} PBMC live cell population.

multiplying the number of total MO by the percent of total MO representing each MO subset as derived from cell flow cytometry.

Similarly, the number of total CD8 T lymphocytes was obtained from T cell subset analyses performed by DLS as part of entry evaluations. The number of activated $CD38^{+}$HLA-DR^{+} CD8 T cells was derived by multiplying the total number of CD8 T cells by the percentage of CD8 T cells co-expressing CD38 and HLA-DR as assessed by flow cytometry.

Plasma Soluble Biomarkers

Testing was conducted using Milliplex Human Cardiovascular Disease panels (EMD Millipore, USA) as outlined in the manufacturer's protocols. Soluble biomarkers assessed included MMP-9, MPO, tPAI-1, CRP, SAA, SAP, IL-1β, IL-6, IL-8, IL-10, TNF-α, soluble E-selectin (sE-selectin), soluble vascular cell adhesion molecule-1 (sVCAM-1), soluble intercellular cell adhesion molecule-1 (sICAM-1), monocyte chemoattractant protein-1 (MCP-1), vascular endothelial growth factor (VEGF), interferon-gamma (IFN-γ), and N-terminal pro-brain natriuretic peptide (NT-proBNP).

Statistical Analyses

Demographic, clinical and immunologic information was summarized by median (quartile1, quartile3) values for continuous variables and frequency (percentage) for categorical variables. Continuous variables were first $\log_{10}$-transformed to improve normality before further analyses if their distributions were skewed. Correlations between variables were performed by Pearson correlation. The relationships between HOMA-IR and various immune variables were assessed by univariate and multivariate linear regression analyses, adjusting for immuno-virologic and HIV specific factors as well as for risk factors for insulin resistance and diabetes. For soluble plasma biomarkers, biomarkers were examined by multivariate analysis if the univariate analysis produced a $p<0.10$. MO differences by diabetes categories and by presence or absence of metabolic syndrome were assessed by ANOVA and ANCOVA. All statistical analyses were conducted in SPSS (IBM, Version 21). A two-sided p-value < 0.05 was regarded as statistically significant.

Results

Patient Characteristics

A total of 141 subjects enrolled into the HAHC-CVD cohort who had available MO phenotype data were included in this analysis. The demographic, clinical, and immunologic characteristics of the subjects are summarized in Table 1. The majority of the subjects were male and of Caucasian ethnicity. Entry criteria for the cohort required subjects to be on ART and 86.5% of these subjects were virologically suppressed at a plasma HIV RNA level of $<$ 50 copies/mL. The study recruited subjects age 40 or older, and the median age of the selected subjects in this dataset was 50 years. The median current CD4 count (percent) was relatively high at 505 cells/μL (29%) but the median self-reported nadir CD4 was relatively low at 150 cells/μL. A total of 22.3% of the population had evidence of glucose dysregulation. The median MO percent was 8%, and the median total MO count was 400 cells/μL. By subsets, the classical MO comprised the majority (76%) of the MO population with intermediate, non-classical and transitional MO comprising the rest in our gating strategy.

Table 1. Baseline characteristics of the subjects.

Clinical and Demographic Information	
Age	50 [45, 57]
Males, n (%)	125 (88.6%)
Race/ethnicity	
White	85 (60.3%)
Full or part Hawaiian/Pacific Islander (NH/PI)	18 (12.8%)
Asian	8 (5.7%)
African-American	5 (3.6%)
Native American/Alaskan	3 (2.1%)
Mixed (other than NH/PI)	22 (15.6%)
Hepatitis C, n (%)[a]	16 (11.3%)
Body mass index (kg/m^2)	25.8 [23.7, 27.9]
Waist to hip ratio	
Male	0.94 [0.91, 0.98]
Female	0.94 [0.79, 0.95]
Systolic BP/diastolic BP	120 [113, 129]/75 [69, 82]
History of smoking, n (%)	93 (66.4%)
Glucose metabolism[b]	
Normal	109 (77.8%)
Impaired fasting glucose(IFG)/glucose tolerance(IGT)	16 (11.4%)
Diabetes	15 (10.7%)
Fasting glucose (mg/dL)	87 [81, 94]
HOMA-IR	1.49 [0.81, 2.50]
Total cholesterol (mg/dL)	177 [155, 202]
LDL cholesterol (mg/dL)	107 [89, 130]
HDL cholesterol (mg/dL)	42 [33, 53]
Triglyceride (mg/dL)	113 [82, 166]
Metabolic Syndrome n(%)[c]	25 (17.7%)
Immunologic Parameters	
WBC count ($\times 10^9$ cells/L)	5.3 [4.3, 6.3]
Monocyte (%)	8 [7,9]
% undetectable HIV RNA (< 50 copies/mL)	122 (86.5%)
Nadir CD4 count (cells/μL)[d]	150 [50, 245]
Current CD4 count (cells/μL)	505 [341, 640]
Current CD4%	29 [21,36]
Current CD8%	44 [36, 52]
CD38+HLA-DR CD8 T-lymphocytes (%)	10.5 [7.7, 16.8]
CD38+HLA-DR CD8 T-lymphocytes (cells/μL)	76.6 [47.8, 124.1]
Monocyte Subsets (%)[e]	
Classical ($CD14^{++}CD16^{-}$)	76 [71.7, 81.9]
Intermediate ($CD14^{++}CD16^{+}$)	1.6 [0.60, 4.1]
Transitional $CD14^{+}CD16^{-}$)	14.1 [9.3, 18.9]
Non-classical ($CD14^{+/low}CD16^{++}$)	5.9 [4.0, 8.7]
Absolute monocyte count (cells/μL)	400 [329, 530]
Classical ($CD14^{++}CD16^{-}$)	310 [231, 410]
Intermediate ($CD14^{++}CD16^{+}$)	6.3 [2.5, 15.8]
Transitional $CD14^{+}CD16^{-}$)	55.8 [38.6, 81.3]
Non-classical ($CD14^{+/low}CD16^{++}$)	24.6 [13.7, 35.3]

All values reported are median [quartile1, quartile 3], except for frequency counts [n (%)].
HOMA-IR: Homeostatic Model Assessment of Insulin Resistance.
[a]By self-report, one patient with unknown HCV status.
[b]One patient with missing data.
[c]Based on the United States Cholesterol Education Program Adult Treatment Panel Guidelines (2001).
[d]Nadir CD4 count based on self-report (data available from 132 subjects).
[e]The sum may not necessarily add to 100% as the median percentage rather than the mean is reported.

Relationship of CD4 and CD8 T cell Parameters to MO and Plasma Soluble Biomarkers

Self-reported nadir CD4 T cell count did not correlate with numbers of total MO or MO subsets. Similarly current CD4 T cell count as an absolute value did not correlate with any MO parameters. However, multiple correlations were seen between current CD4 T cells examined as a percentage of lymphocytes and various MO parameters. Current CD4 percent correlated negatively with log-total MO ($r = -0.23$, $p = 0.006$) and MO subsets log-classical MO ($r = -0.19$, $p = 0.023$) and log-non-classical MO ($r = -0.23$, $p = 0.005$) with a trend for log-transitional MO ($r = -0.15$, $p = 0.080$). No correlation was found between current CD4 percent and log-intermediate MO ($r = 0.05$, $p = 0.561$).

The association between CD4 percent and MO can be seen visually in Figure 2 which shows the median total and subset MO numbers categorized by CD4 percent quartiles. Total MO increased in stepwise fashion with lower CD4 percent quartiles. All MO subsets contributed to this increase, although with a slightly higher contribution from non-classical MO. This could be demonstrated by the negative correlation between CD4 percent and percent (rather than the absolute value) of MO comprising non-classical MO ($r = -0.19$, $p = 0.024$).

Because decreases in CD4 percent can result not only from a decrease in the number of CD4 T cells but by an increase in other lymphocyte cell types including CD8 T cells, we assessed the relationship between CD4 percent and CD8 T cell parameters. CD4 percent correlated negatively with log-total CD8 T cells ($r = -0.45$, $p < 0.001$) and with log-total CD38+HLA-DR+CD8 T cells ($r = -0.49$, $p < 0.001$). In turn, log-total CD8 T cell count correlated positively with log-total MO ($r = 0.35$, $p < 0.001$), log-classical MO ($r = 0.27$, $p = 0.001$), and log-transitional MO ($r = 0.29$, $p = 0.001$), with marginal significance with log-non-classical MO ($r = 0.16$, $p = 0.061$). Similar relationships were seen for activated CD8 T cells. Log-$CD38^{+}HLA\text{-}DR^{+}CD8$ T cells correlated with log-total MO ($r = 0.36$, $p < 0.001$), log-classical MO ($r = 0.29$, $p < 0.001$), log-transitional MO ($r = 0.29$, $p = 0.001$), and log-non-classical MO ($r = 0.20$, $p = 0.018$). No correlation was seen between log-CD38+HLA-DR+CD8 T cells and log-intermediate MO ($r = -0.02$, $p = 0.81$).

The database was examined for any correlations between CD4 percent and various soluble plasma biomarkers. Total CD4 count

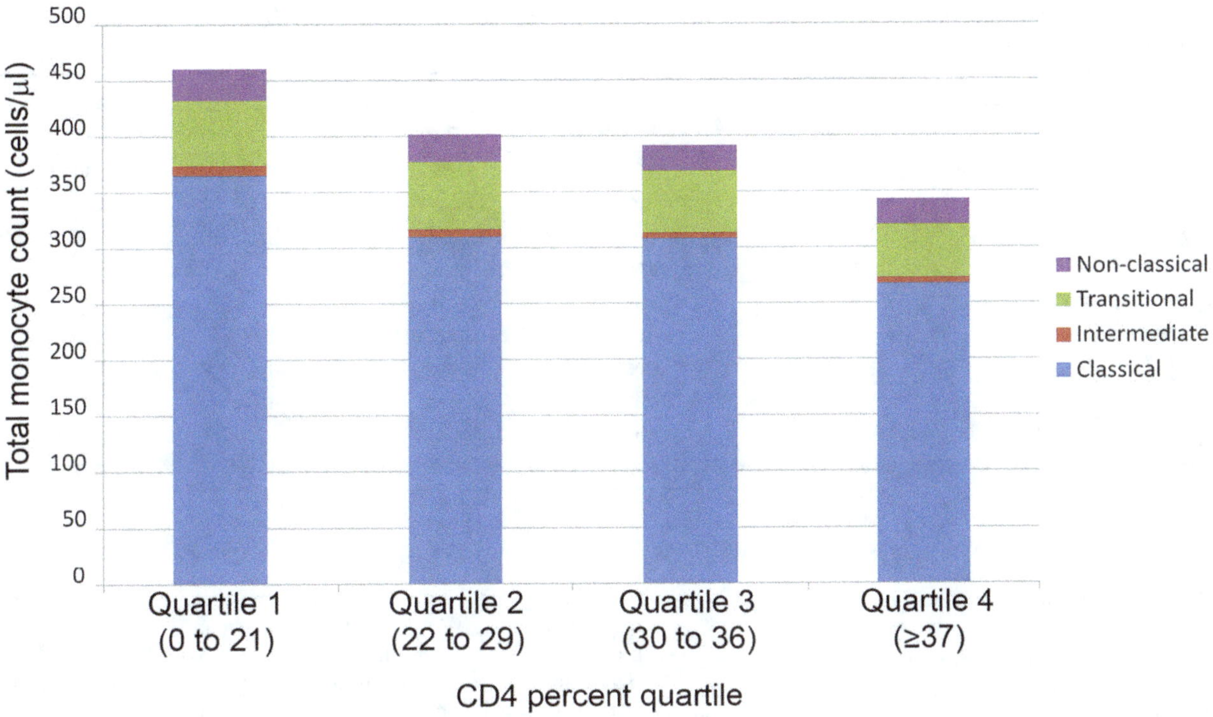

Figure 2. Absolute counts (cells/µL) of total monocytes by classical, intermediate, transitional and non-classical monocyte subset components by CD4 T cell percent quartiles.

did not correlate with any soluble plasma biomarkers assessed. CD4 percent correlated negatively with log-transformed values of tPAI-1 ($r = -0.19$, $p = 0.032$) and TNF-α ($r = -0.20$, $p = 0.028$). Total CD8 T cell count correlated with log-sVCAM ($r = 0.20$, $p = 0.026$). CD8 T cell percent correlated with log-TNF-α ($r = 0.19$, $p = 0.040$).

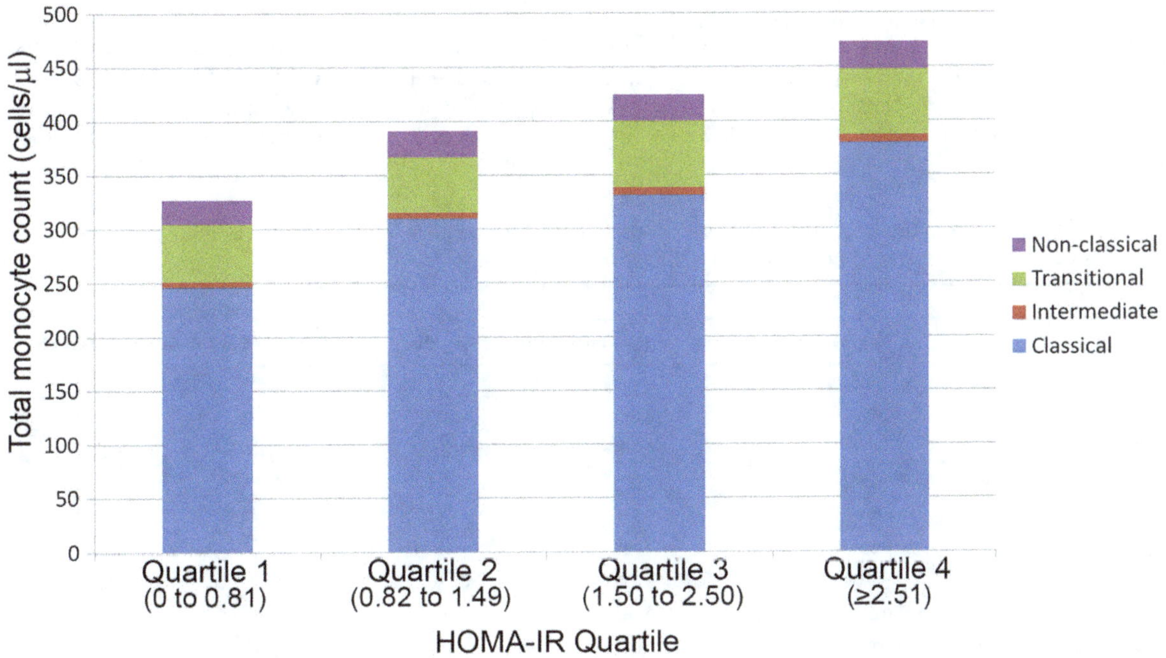

Figure 3. Absolute counts (cells/µL) of total monocytes by classical, intermediate, transitional and non-classical monocyte subset components by HOMA-IR quartiles.

Table 2. Multivariate linear regression analysis of the relative contribution of total monocyte count to HOMA-IR adjusting for various HIV-associated and diabetes risk factors.

	Regression coefficient	Standard Error	p-value	95% Confidence	Interval
Age, years	0.004	0.003	0.239	−0.003	0.011
Male (yes or no)	−0.028	0.086	0.743	−0.198	0.141
Caucasian (yes or no)	−0.021	0.055	0.710	−0.129	0.088
Hepatitis C (yes or no)	0.132	0.080	0.103	−0.027	0.290
Past or current smoking (yes or no)	−0.032	0.055	0.565	−0.140	0.077
Body Mass Index (kg/m^2)	0.035	0.006	<0.001*	0.023	0.047
Current protease inhibitor use (yes or no)	−0.012	0.057	0.834	−0.124	0.100
Current CD4%	−0.001	0.003	0.788	−0.006	0.004
Plasma HIV RNA <50 copies/mL (yes or no)	0.036	0.080	0.652	−0.123	0.195
Log-total monocyte count	0.424	0.177	0.018*	0.073	0.775

*statistically significant.

Relationship of Cellular and Soluble Plasma Biomarkers to HOMA-IR

No associations were seen between CD4 percent or log-total CD4 count and HOMA-IR ($r = -0.08$, $p = 0.359$ and $r = 0.05$, $p = 0.581$ respectively). Similarly, there was no association between CD8 T cell parameters (CD8 percent, log-total CD8 T cells, log-total CD38+HLA-DR+CD8 T cells) or log-CD4/CD8 ratio and HOMA-IR. However, log-total MO ($r = 0.26$, $p = 0.002$) and log-total classical MO ($r = 0.26$, $p = 0.002$) correlated positively with HOMA-IR. These associations are shown graphically in Figure 3 which depicts the quantity of total MO and its subsets by increasing HOMA-IR quartiles. The increase in total MO with higher HOMA-IR quartiles was contributed primarily by an increase in classical MO.

The relationship of MO to HOMA-IR was examined further in multivariate linear regression models with HOMA-IR as the dependent variable, adjusting for immuno-virologic and HIV specific factors (CD4 percent, presence/absence of plasma HIV RNA, and current protease inhibitor use) as well as for traditional risk factors for diabetes (age, gender, race, hepatitis C, smoking, body mass index [BMI]). Of these parameters, BMI ($\beta = 0.03$, $p < 0.001$) and self-reported hepatitis C co-infection ($\beta = 0.21$, $p = 0.021$) were significantly associated in univariate linear regression with log-HOMA-IR. As shown in Table 2 using our multivariate model, log-total MO ($\beta = 0.42$, $p = 0.018$) remained a significant predictor of log-HOMA-IR. When this relationship was examined individually by specific MO subsets, log-classical MO was also a significant predictor ($\beta = 0.35$, $p = 0.023$), but not the other subsets.

Univariate linear regression was used to identify soluble plasma biomarkers associated with log-HOMA-IR to select biomarkers for testing in multivariate models. The following biomarkers were associated with log-HOMA-IR in a univariate model at $p < 0.10$ level: sE-selectin, tPAI-1, CRP, SAP, IL-6, and IL-8. When examined by multivariate linear regression adjusting for immuno-virologic and cardio-metabolic parameters as performed for MO, log-tPAI-1 ($\beta = 0.74$, $p < 0.001$) alone remained associated with log-HOMA-IR (Table 3).

Relationship of Cellular and Soluble Plasma Biomarkers to Fasting Glucose and Clinical Diabetes Classification

The only associations found between cellular biomarkers and fasting glucose values was that between log-total CD4 count and log-fasting glucose ($r = 0.17$, $p = 0.043$). This association was no

Table 3. Multivariate linear regression analysis of the relative contribution of tissue plasminogen activator inhibitor-1 (tPAI-1) to HOMA-IR adjusting for various HIV-associated and diabetes risk factors

	Regression coefficient	Standard Error	p-value	95% Confidence	Interval
Age, years	0.008	0.003	0.019*	0.001	0.015
Male (yes or no)	−0.051	0.081	0.530	−0.211	0.109
Caucasian (yes or no)	−0.029	0.054	0.598	−0.136	0.079
Hepatitis C (yes or no)	0.164	0.085	0.055	−0.004	0.332
Past or current smoking (yes or no)	−0.035	0.054	0.514	−0.142	0.072
Body Mass Index, (kg/m^2)	0.030	0.006	<0.001*	0.018	0.042
Current protease inhibitor use (yes or no)	−0.031	0.057	0.589	−0.143	0.082
Current CD4%	0.0003	0.002	0.895	−0.005	0.005
Plasma HIV RNA < 50 copies/mL (yes or no)	−0.019	0.082	0.812	−0.182	0.143
Log-tPAI-1	0.745	0.133	<0.001*	0.480	1.010

*statistically significant.

Table 4. Correlation table of absolute counts of total monocytes, monocyte subsets and $CD38^{+}HLA\text{-}DR^{+}CD8$ T cells with various plasma cytokines.

	Total monocyte count	Classical $CD14^{++}CD16^{-}$	Intermediate $CD14^{++}CD16^{+}$	Transitional $CD14^{+}CD16^{-}$	Non-classical $CD14^{+/low}CD16^{++}$	$CD38^{+}HLA\text{-}DR^{+}$ CD8 T cells
CRP	0.23**	0.27**	0.47**	−0.10	0.15	−0.09
IFN-γ	0.02	−0.06	0.10	0.12	0.01	0.13
IL-1β	0.22*	0.18	−0.06	0.20*	0.15	0.02
IL-6	0.29**	0.35**	0.20*	0.03	0.04	0.03
IL-8	0.16	0.16	0.05	0.04	−0.05	−0.10
IL-10	0.21*	0.24**	0.05	0.10	0.09	0.20*
MCP-1	0.14	0.12	0.21*	−0.05	0.29**	0.10
MMP-9	0.30**	0.30**	0.31**	0.08	0.05	−0.02
MPO	0.29**	0.30**	0.42**	−0.01	0.14	0.18*
NT-proBNP	0.16	0.12	−0.02	0.14	0.04	0.12
SAA	0.29**	0.31**	0.43**	−0.05	0.23*	0.07
SAP	0.17	0.18*	0.45**	−0.17	0.26**	−.04
sE-selectin	0.11	0.11	0.22*	−0.07	0.09	−.08
sICAM-1	0.08	0.11	0.10	−0.07	−0.06	0.25**
sVCAM-1	0.08	0.10	0.27**	−0.12	0.19*	0.18*
TNF-α	0.19*	0.17	−0.06	0.16	0.03	0.29**
tPAI-1	0.32**	0.28**	0.18*	0.20*	0.12	0.003
VEGF	0.13	0.13	−0.02	0.23*	−0.08	0.02

Values were log-transformed prior to analysis.
Pearson Correlation was utilized.
*Correlation significant at the 0.05 level (2-tailed).
** Correlation significant at the 0.01 level (2-tailed).

longer present when adjusted for immuno-virologic and diabetes risk factors.

Log-transformed sE-selectin ($\beta = 0.08$, $p = 0.007$), MPO ($\beta = 0.04$, $p = 0.089$), tPAI-1 ($\beta = 0.08$, $p = 0.050$), IL-8 ($\beta = 0.08$, $p = 0.053$), and IL-10 ($\beta = 0.02$, $p = 0.064$) values were associated with log-fasting blood glucose at $p<0.10$ level using simple linear regression. Analyses by multivariate linear regression adjusting for immuno-virologic and diabetes risk parameters showed weak associations of uncertain significance [log-sE-selectin ($\beta = 0.07$, $p = 0.044$), log-tPAI-1 ($\beta = 0.09$, $p = 0.035$), and log-IL-10 ($\beta = 0.02$, $p = 0.037$)].

No differences by diabetes clinical classification (normal, IFG/IGT, or diabetes) were found for any cellular parameter except for total CD8 T cell count (cells/μL) [means(SD): normal 796.1 (361.8), IFG/IGT 1017.6 (590.2), diabetes: 661 (304.6), $p = 0.034$]. In terms of soluble biomarkers, differences by diabetes clinical classification were found for various biomarkers (pg/mL): sICAM [means(SD): normal 151.2 (61.0), IFG/IGT 242.5 (298.6), diabetes: 144.9 (117.0); $p = 0.026$], MPO [normal 19.0 (14.7), IFG/IGT: 16.3 (6.0), diabetes 44.1 (SD 81.6); $p = 0.014$], MCP-1 [normal 144.4 (51.6), IFG/IGT 146.7 (52.3), diabetes 186.8 (64.5); $p = 0.045$], and VEGF [normal 37.4 (34.6), IFG/IGT 36.8 (42.9), diabetes 79.7 (110.2); $p = 0.019$]. Comparisons by t-test showed that MPO ($p = 0.004$), MCP-1 ($p = 0.013$), and VEGF ($p = 0.009$) were significantly higher among diabetic subjects compared to subjects with normal glucose levels.

Relationship of Immune Parameters to Metabolic Syndrome

No differences were found for individuals with or without metabolic syndrome by CD4 or CD8 parameters. Higher total MO levels were found in subjects with metabolic syndrome: [mean (SD): 504 (143) cells/μL in subjects with vs 427 (161) cells/μL in subjects without metabolic syndrome, $p = 0.029$]. This result remained significant when adjusted for age, gender and ethnicity ($p = 0.013$). By subsets, a trend towards significance was seen for difference in classical MO ($p = 0.051$) and for intermediate MO ($p = 0.059$). Soluble biomarkers sE-selectin ($p = 0.007$) and sICAM ($p = 0.041$) were higher in subjects with metabolic syndrome.

Correlations between Monocytes and Activated CD8 T Cells and Soluble Plasma Biomarkers

The correlations between MO and activated CD8 T cells and soluble plasma biomarkers are shown in Table 4. Correlations at $p<0.01$ were seen between $CD38^{+}HLA\text{-}DR^{+}CD8$ T cells and sICAM and TNF-α. A larger number of positive correlations were found between MO and/or MO subsets and various plasma biomarkers. Specifically, correlations at $p<0.01$ were found between total MO and CRP, IL-6, MMP-9, MPO, SAA and tPAI-1. Associations between classical MO and intermediate MO and various biomarkers overall mirrored the correlations seen with total MO. Non-classical MO showed correlations at $p<0.01$ with MCP-1 and SAP.

DISCUSSION

Our study found that HIV-associated immune dysregulation, as assessed by a decrease in CD4 percent is characterized by an increase in the total MO population with a small rise in the percentage accounted for by non-classical MO. This association was seen specifically with CD4 T cells assessed as a percentage of CD4 T cells and not as an absolute value of total CD4 T cells. In turn, we found that an increase in total MO, comprised largely of classical MO, accompanies insulin resistance. This association remained after adjustment for HIV immuno-virologic and traditional diabetes risk factors. Higher levels of MO were seen in subjects with metabolic syndrome. Positive correlations were detected between MO and many plasma biomarkers. Included among these biomarkers was tPAI-1 which also correlated inversely with CD4 percent, positively with MO levels, and predicted insulin resistance.

Insulin resistance is increasingly recognized as a state of chronic, low-level inflammation [22,23,24]. Immune activation and inflammation also occur in the context of HIV and are predictors of HIV disease progression and mortality, and of multiple non-infectious chronic complications [25,26,27]. Such activation may be secondary to HIV itself, to co-pathogens such as CMV or hepatitis C, or be secondary to microbial translocation across a damaged gut mucosa [28]. There is also increasing recognition that in addition to CD8 T cells, MO may play a role in the immune activation and inflammation that drive many of these disease processes [29].

Our study found an association between low CD4 percent and MO increase and, in turn MO increase and increase in insulin resistance. One potential interpretation of the data is that an increase in MO is part of HIV-induced immune activation, and that such increase in turn may drive the increased risk of insulin resistance seen in chronic HIV. While our study did not show a direct association between CD4 count, either as a percent or as total numbers, and insulin resistance or diabetes as shown in larger epidemiologic studies [2,33,34,35], it is consistent with a study that demonstrated a higher prevalence of elevated sCD14, a marker of MO activation, among HIV-infected veterans with a CD4 cell count <200 cells/μL [33]. Our inability to find a direct link between CD4 percent and insulin resistance may be related to the small sample size of our cohort.

By subsets, classical, non-classical and transitional MO, but not intermediate MO, contributed to the increase in MO with falling CD4 percent. Non-classical MO represented a slightly larger percentage of this MO increase. The association between CD4 T cells and MO was specifically related to CD4 percent and not to total numbers of CD4 T cells. Decrease in CD4 percent may represent a decrease in total CD4 count or, may also be secondary to increase(s) in other lymphocyte subsets including CD8 T cells. Our study did find a negative correlation between CD4 percent and total numbers of CD8 T cells. However, neither total CD8 T cells nor total activated CD8 T cells explained insulin resistance, while a clear association was seen between total MO or classical MO and insulin resistance in adjusted models. It is worthy of note that a number of studies in the literature have found independent predictive values for percentage of CD4 T cells and CD4 absolute count in respect to HIV disease progression or death [30,31,32]. One study explored the role of CD8 T cells as a potential explanation for the association between CD4 percent and disease progression and found that it did not explain this relationship [31]. We speculate that CD4 percent may provide additional information on increased risk for cardio-metabolic complications mediated in part through MO immune activation. Analysis of large cohort datasets to determine whether CD4 percent and MO levels are related to such complications might be considered.

The association between MO and glucose metabolism identified in our study was primarily with insulin resistance with little or no relationship to fasting glucose levels or to diabetes classification. When examined by subsets, we found that classical MO, the largest subset represented, played the most prominent role in the MO increase associated with insulin resistance.

Metabolic syndrome is a constellation of inter-related metabolic risk factors associated with increased risk for the development of diabetes and cardiovascular disease. While its limitations and significance in the context of HIV is uncertain, the metabolic syndrome is closely related to the presence of insulin resistance, and, given the association between MO and insulin resistance found in our study, the finding of increased MO with metabolic syndrome is not surprising, and adds to the likelihood that MO do indeed play a pathologic role in increasing both diabetes and cardiovascular disease risk in the HIV-infected population.

Our study found multiple positive correlations between MO and/or its subsets and plasma biomarkers CRP, IL-6, MMP-9, MPO, SAA, SAP and tPAI-1. Significant correlations were also found between $CD38^{+}HLA\text{-}DR^{+}CD8$ T cells and biomarkers sICAM and TNF-α. Interestingly we also found correlations between low CD4 percent and TNF-α and tPAI-1, and correlations between HOMA-IR and CRP, IL-6, SAP, and tPAI-1. This suggests that cellular immune parameters and soluble plasma biomarkers are likely inter-related in the roles they play in HIV immune dysregulation and insulin resistance. These results are furthermore consistent with studies that have found higher levels of hs-CRP and sTNF1 and sTNF2 in association with insulin resistance and diabetes in the context of HIV [3], [36].

The associations found for tPAI-1 are worthy of particular attention. TPAI-1 is an inhibitor of fibrinolysis and believed to play a crucial role in the development of atherothrombotic disease. In our study, higher levels of tPAI-1 were associated with lower CD4 percent and predicted insulin resistance in an adjusted model. Our findings are consistent with studies in the general population that have demonstrated associations between high levels of circulating PAI-1 and insulin resistance, diabetes and cardiovascular disease [37,38]. Levels of PAI-1 have been reported to be higher in HIV infected individuals than in seronegative controls [39], and to be associated with insulin resistance [40]. It has been linked to protease inhibitor-containing ART [41], and, in contrast to some other plasma markers of inflammation, have been reported to not improve after the initiation of ART [42]. Our finding of a negative correlation between tPAI-1 and CD4 percent suggests that in addition to the potential role of antiretroviral medications, HIV-associated immune dysregulation may play a role in high tPAI-1 levels seen in the treated population. Furthermore our study links tPAI-1 with total and classical MO but not with T cell activation.

This study is limited by its cross sectional nature and the relatively modest size of the cohort. However the strengths of the study are the careful clinical and metabolic characterization performed in the cohort in association with detailed phenotypic characterization of MO and CD8 T cells, and biomarker assays performed in plasma. We conclude that chronic HIV in subjects on stable ART is characterized not only by dysregulation and immune activation of CD8 T cells but also of MO, and that higher levels of MO may contribute to the increased rates of insulin resistance and metabolic syndrome seen in this population. MO may therefore play a substantial role in the increased risk of cardio-metabolic disease during chronic HIV. CD4 percent may provide additional information beyond absolute values about MO and metabolic risk in the HIV-infected population. Increase in MO is associated with increase in multiple plasma soluble biomarkers, including tPAI-1 which also predicts insulin resistance in adjusted models.

Acknowledgments

The authors thank the clinical and laboratory staff of the Hawaii Center for AIDS, University of Hawaii and the many patients of the Hawaii Aging with HIV cohort study who made this study possible.

Author Contributions

Conceived and designed the experiments: CMS DCC SMK PJN LCN JDB. Performed the experiments: SMK PJN LCN JDB. Analyzed the data: CMS LMG GXZ DCC KJK. Contributed reagents/materials/analysis tools: SMK PJN LCN JDB KJK BKN LSN TBS NP. Wrote the paper: CMS. Created the tables and figures: LMG. Contributed to the drafting and approval of the final manuscript submitted: All.

References

1. Gutierrez AD, Balasubramanyam A (2012) Dysregulation of glucose metabolism in HIV patients: epidemiology, mechanisms, and management. Endocrine 41: 1–10.
2. Boufassa F, Goujard C, Viard JP, Carlier R, Lefebvre B, et al. (2012) Immune deficiency could be an early risk factor for altered insulin sensitivity in antiretroviral-naive HIV-1-infected patients: the ANRS COPANA cohort. Antivir Ther 17: 91–100.
3. Brown TT, Tassiopoulos K, Bosch RJ, Shikuma C, McComsey GA (2010) Association between systemic inflammation and incident diabetes in HIV-infected patients after initiation of antiretroviral therapy. Diabetes Care 33: 2244–2249.
4. Ziegler-Heitbrock L, Ancuta P, Crowe S, Dalod M, Grau V, et al. (2010) Nomenclature of monocytes and dendritic cells in blood. Blood 116: e74–80.
5. Jalbert E, Crawford TQ, D'Antoni ML, Keating SM, Norris PJ, et al. (2013) IL-1Beta Enriched Monocytes Mount Massive IL-6 Responses to Common Inflammatory Triggers among Chronically HIV-1 Infected Adults on Stable Anti-Retroviral Therapy at Risk for Cardiovascular Disease. PLoS One 8: e75500.
6. Barbour JD, Jalbert EC, Chow DC, Gangcuangco LM, Norris PJ, et al. (2014) Reduced CD14 expression on classical monocytes and vascular endothelial adhesion markers independently associate with carotid artery intima media thickness in chronically HIV-1 infected adults on virologically suppressive anti-retroviral therapy. Atherosclerosis 232: 52–58.
7. Gordon S, Taylor PR (2005) Monocyte and macrophage heterogeneity. Nat Rev Immunol 5: 953–964.
8. Strauss-Ayali D, Conrad SM, Mosser DM (2007) Monocyte subpopulations and their differentiation patterns during infection. J Leukoc Biol 82: 244–252.
9. Geissmann F, Jung S, Littman DR (2003) Blood monocytes consist of two principal subsets with distinct migratory properties. Immunity 19: 71–82.
10. Ziegler-Heitbrock L (2007) The CD14+ CD16+ blood monocytes: their role in infection and inflammation. J Leukoc Biol 81: 584–592.
11. Seidler S, Zimmermann HW, Bartneck M, Trautwein C, Tacke F (2010) Age-dependent alterations of monocyte subsets and monocyte-related chemokine pathways in healthy adults. BMC Immunol 11: 30.
12. Ellery PJ, Tippett E, Chiu YL, Paukovics G, Cameron PU, et al. (2007) The CD16+ monocyte subset is more permissive to infection and preferentially harbors HIV-1 in vivo. J Immunol 178: 6581–6589.
13. Kusao I, Shiramizu B, Liang CY, Grove J, Agsalda M, et al. (2012) Cognitive performance related to HIV-1-infected monocytes. J Neuropsychiatry Clin Neurosci 24: 71–80.
14. Funderburg NT, Zidar DA, Shive C, Lioi A, Mudd J, et al. (2012) Shared monocyte subset phenotypes in HIV-1 infection and in uninfected subjects with acute coronary syndrome. Blood 120: 4599–4608.
15. Han J, Wang B, Han N, Zhao Y, Song C, et al. (2009) CD14(high)CD16(+) rather than CD14(low)CD16(+) monocytes correlate with disease progression in chronic HIV-infected patients. J Acquir Immune Defic Syndr 52: 553–559.
16. Min D, Brooks B, Wong J, Salomon R, Bao W, et al. (2012) Alterations in monocyte CD16 in association with diabetes complications. Mediators Inflamm 2012: 649083.
17. Corrales JJ, Almeida M, Burgo RM, Hernandez P, Miralles JM, et al. (2007) Decreased production of inflammatory cytokines by circulating monocytes and dendritic cells in type 2 diabetic men with atherosclerotic complications. J Diabetes Complications 21: 41–49.
18. Pandzic Jaksic V, Gizdic B, Miletic Z, Trutin-Ostovic K, Jaksic O (2013) Association of monocyte CCR2 expression with obesity and insulin resistance in postmenopausal women. Clin Invest Med 36: E24–31.
19. Yang M, Gan H, Shen Q, Tang W, Du X, et al. (2012) Proinflammatory CD14+CD16+ monocytes are associated with microinflammation in patients with type 2 diabetes mellitus and diabetic nephropathy uremia. Inflammation 35: 388–396.
20. (2013) Executive summary: standards of medical care in diabetes—2013. Diabetes Care 36 Suppl 1: S4–S10.
21. Grundy SM, Brewer HB Jr, Cleeman JI, Smith SC Jr, Lenfant C (2004) Definition of metabolic syndrome: Report of the National Heart, Lung, and Blood Institute/American Heart Association conference on scientific issues related to definition. Circulation 109: 433–438.
22. Scarpellini E, Tack J (2012) Obesity and metabolic syndrome: an inflammatory condition. Dig Dis 30: 148–153.
23. Skalicky J, Muzakova V, Kandar R, Meloun M, Rousar T, et al. (2008) Evaluation of oxidative stress and inflammation in obese adults with metabolic syndrome. Clin Chem Lab Med 46: 499–505.
24. Fernandez-Real JM, Ricart W (2003) Insulin resistance and chronic cardiovascular inflammatory syndrome. Endocr Rev 24: 278–301.
25. Kuller LH, Tracy R, Belloso W, De Wit S, Drummond F, et al. (2008) Inflammatory and coagulation biomarkers and mortality in patients with HIV infection. PLoS Med 5: e203.
26. Sandler NG, Wand H, Roque A, Law M, Nason MC, et al. (2011) Plasma levels of soluble CD14 independently predict mortality in HIV infection. J Infect Dis 203: 780–790.
27. Deeks SG, Phillips AN (2009) HIV infection, antiretroviral treatment, ageing, and non-AIDS related morbidity. BMJ 338: a3172.
28. Deeks SG (2011) HIV infection, inflammation, immunosenescence, and aging. Annu Rev Med 62: 141–155.
29. Jalbert E CT, D'Antoni ML, Keating SM, Norris PJ, Nakamoto BK, et al. (2013) IL-1b Enriched Monocytes Mount Massive IL-6 Responses to Common Inflammatory Triggers among Chronically HIV-1 Infected Adults on Stable Anti-Retroviral Therapy at Risk for Cardiovascular Disease. PLoS ONE in press.
30. Hulgan T, Raffanti S, Kheshti A, Blackwell RB, Rebeiro PF, et al. (2005) CD4 lymphocyte percentage predicts disease progression in HIV-infected patients initiating highly active antiretroviral therapy with CD4 lymphocyte counts >350 lymphocytes/mm3. J Infect Dis 192: 950–957.
31. Hulgan T, Shepherd BE, Raffanti SP, Fusco JS, Beckerman R, et al. (2007) Absolute count and percentage of CD4+ lymphocytes are independent predictors of disease progression in HIV-infected persons initiating highly active antiretroviral therapy. J Infect Dis 195: 425–431.
32. Moore DM, Hogg RS, Yip B, Craib K, Wood E, et al. (2006) CD4 percentage is an independent predictor of survival in patients starting antiretroviral therapy with absolute CD4 cell counts between 200 and 350 cells/microL. HIV Med 7: 383–388.
33. Armah KA, McGinnis K, Baker J, Gibert C, Butt AA, et al. (2012) HIV status, burden of comorbid disease, and biomarkers of inflammation, altered coagulation, and monocyte activation. Clin Infect Dis 55: 126–136.
34. El-Sadr WM, Mullin CM, Carr A, Gibert C, Rappoport C, et al. (2005) Effects of HIV disease on lipid, glucose and insulin levels: results from a large antiretroviral-naive cohort. HIV Med 6: 114–121.
35. Petoumenos K, Worm SW, Fontas E, Weber R, De Wit S, et al. (2012) Predicting the short-term risk of diabetes in HIV-positive patients: the Data Collection on Adverse Events of Anti-HIV Drugs (D:A:D) study. J Int AIDS Soc 15: 17426.
36. Limone P, Biglino A, Valle M, Degioanni M, Paola Servato M, et al. (2003) Insulin resistance in HIV-infected patients: relationship with pro-inflammatory cytokines released by peripheral leukocytes. J Infect 47: 52–58.
37. Hamsten A, Wiman B, de Faire U, Blomback M (1985) Increased plasma levels of a rapid inhibitor of tissue plasminogen activator in young survivors of myocardial infarction. N Engl J Med 313: 1557–1563.
38. Erzen B, Sabovic M (2013) In young post-myocardial infarction male patients elevated plasminogen activator inhibitor-1 correlates with insulin resistance and endothelial dysfunction. Heart Vessels 28: 570–577.
39. Guzman-Fulgencio M, Medrano J, Rallon N, Echeverria-Urabayen A, Miguel Benito J, et al. (2011) Soluble markers of inflammation are associated with Framingham scores in HIV-infected patients on suppressive antiretroviral therapy. J Infect 63: 382–390.
40. De Larranaga G, Galich A, Puga L, Alonso B, Benetucci J (2004) Insulin resistance status is an important determinant of PAI-1 levels in HIV-infected patients, independently of the lipid profile. J Thromb Haemost 2: 532–534.
41. Koppel K, Bratt G, Schulman S, Bylund H, Sandstrom E (2002) Hypofibrinolytic state in HIV-1-infected patients treated with protease inhibitor-containing highly active antiretroviral therapy. J Acquir Immune Defic Syndr 29: 441–449.
42. van Vonderen MG, Hassink EA, van Agtmael MA, Stehouwer CD, Danner SA, et al. (2009) Increase in carotid artery intima-media thickness and arterial stiffness but improvement in several markers of endothelial function after initiation of antiretroviral therapy. J Infect Dis 199: 1186–1194.

Adiponectin Alleviates Genioglossal Mitochondrial Dysfunction in Rats Exposed to Intermittent Hypoxia

Hanpeng Huang[1]⁹, Xiufeng Jiang[2]⁹, Yanbin Dong[3], Xiaofeng Zhang[3], Ning Ding[3], Jiannan Liu[4], Sean Z. Hutchinson[5], Gan Lu[4]*, Xilong Zhang[3]*

1 Department of Respirology, Affiliated Hospital of Jiangsu University, Zhenjiang, China, **2** Department of Respirology, Nanjing Medical University affiliated Wuxi People's Hospital, Wuxi, China, **3** Department of Respirology, The First Affiliated Hospital with Nanjing Medical University, Nanjing, China, **4** Department of Respiratory Diseases, Jangsu Geriatric Hospital, Nanjing, China, **5** Morsani College of Medicine, Tampa, FL, United States of America

Abstract

Background: Genioglossal dysfunction is involved in the pathophysiology of obstructive sleep apnea hypoxia syndrome (OSAHS) characterized by nocturnal chronic intermittent hypoxia (CIH). The pathophysiology of genioglossal dysfunction and possible targeted pharmacotherapy for alleviation of genioglossal injury in CIH require further investigation.

Methodology/Principal Findings: Rats in the control group were exposed to normal air, while rats in the CIH group and CIH+adiponectin (AD) group were exposed to the same CIH condition (CIH 8 hr/day for 5 successive weeks). Furthermore, rats in CIH+AD group were administrated intravenous AD supplementation at the dosage of 10 µg, twice a week for 5 consecutive weeks. We found that CIH-induced genioglossus (GG) injury was correlated with mitochondrial dysfunction, reduction in the numbers of mitochondrias, impaired mitochondrial ultrastructure, and a reduction in type I fibers. Compared with the CIH group, impaired mitochondrial structure and function was significantly improved and a percentage of type I fiber was elevated in the CIH+AD group. Moreover, compared with the control group, the rats' GG in the CIH group showed a significant decrease in phosphorylation of LKB1, AMPK, and PGC1-α, whereas there was significant rescue of such reduction in phosphorylation within the CIH+AD group.

Conclusions: CIH exposure reduces mitochondrial biogenesis and impairs mitochondrial function in GG, while AD supplementation increases mitochondrial contents and alleviates CIH-induced mitochondrial dysfunction possibly through the AMPK pathway.

Editor: Victor Sanchez-Margalet, Virgen Macarena University Hospital, School of Medicine, University of Seville, Spain

Funding: This work is supported by National Natural Science Foundation of China 81370184, 81400066 and Chinese Jiangsu Provincial Program of Medical Science (BL2012012), 81400066. The funders had no role in study design, data collection and analysis, decision to publish, or preparation of the manuscript.

Competing Interests: The authors have declared that no competing interests exist.

* Email: zhangxilong1952@163.com (XLZ); lugan0121@163.com (GL)

⁹ These authors contributed equally to this work.

Introduction

Recent studies have suggested that chronic intermittent hypoxia (CIH), a key pathological hallmark of obstructive sleep apnea hypoxia syndrome (OSAHS), is responsible for hypoadiponectinemia revealed in OSAHS patients [1,2]. Further research also indicates that hypoadiponectinemia induced by CIH is associated with genioglossal dysfunction, which has been recognized as a crucial cause of OSAHS and could be improved by adiponectin (AD) supplementation [3]. However, the molecular mechanism of this process has not been fully elucidated.

AD, as an adipocyte-specific protein, plays an important role in the regulation of glucose and lipid metabolism, specifically inflammatory and oxidative stress [4–6]. Plasma AD levels are found to be decreased in OSAHS, obesity, type 2 diabetes, and insulin resistance [7,8]. Supplementation of AD in contrast has been shown to increase mitochondria numbers and oxidative metabolism [9,10]. Conversely, AD-deficient mice exhibited decreased mitochondrial number and increased mitochondrial dysfunction [11]. The mechanism behind these effects is related to AMP-activated protein kinase (AMPK) [9,11]. Our previous study showed that CIH could cause ultrastructural degenerative changes and mitochondrial dysfunction in gengioglossus [3]. However, the exact mechanisms of mitochondrial injury have yet to be ascertained.

The aim of this study is to further investigate the mechanisms by which CIH induces mitochondrial injury of genioglossus, and whether AD supplementation can protect CIH-induced genioglossal mitochondrial injury and involved pathways.

Materials and Methods

This study was approved by the Animal Ethic Committee of Nanjing Medical University.

Animals

45 healthy male Wistar rats (aged 8 weeks) were bought from Shanghai Silake Ltd. Inc. of Animal Experiment. Rats were

randomly distributed into three groups of 15. Rats in the control group were kept in a normoxic environment, rats in the CIH group were maintained under CIH condition for 35 days, and rats in the CIH+AD group were exposed to the same milieu as the CIH group with the addition of regularly administrated AD (R&D Inc., USA) via tail vein. Rats in the control group and CIH group were given saline through tail vein instantaneously. On day 35 of the experiment, the rats were anesthetized by using 1–2% isoflurane. After successful anesthesia, the rats had their abdominal cavitites quickly incised, blood drawn from the abdominal aorta followed by removal of the abdominal aorta. Subsequent acute hemorrhage resulted in rapid and non-violent exsanguination of the rats.

CIH exposure

The exposure of CIH was performed as previously described [3]. During the different exposures, the rats were placed in 2.5-liter separately sealed spaces. Rats were allowed to move and obtain water and food freely in the sealed spaces. During the CIH exposure, each cycle of intermittent hypoxia lasted for 2 minutes-with an initial minute of hypoxic exposure followed by a minute of reoxygenation. During the hypoxic period, the O_2 concentration in the CIH chambers was rapidly decreased to 5~6% by prompt flushing with 99% N_2. The nadir O_2 lasted for 15~20 s per the cycle. During the reoxygenation period, the O_2 concentration was increased to 21% at maximum by rapidly filling the room with room airoxygen. Rats in the three groups were exposed to each condition daily for 8 daylight hours for 5 consecutive weeks. Rats in the control group and CIH group were given saline at the dose of 500 μl per time via tail vein, and rats in the CIH+AD group were administered AD through tail vein at the dosage of 10 μg per time, twice a week for 5 successive weeks.

Observation of genioglossal ultrastructure

As soon as the rats were euthanized, their genioglossi were rapidly detached and sliced into small approximate 1.0 mm^3 pieces at and fixed in 5% glutaraldehyde phosphate buffer at 4°C for 2 hours. The samples were hereafter postfixed in 1% Osmium tetroxide at 4°C for 1 hour, dehydrated in graded alcohol, and embedded in Epon at either a transverse or longitudinal direction. The samples were cut by the RMC/MTX ultramicrotome (Elexience), the sections (between 60 and 80 nm each) were transferred to copper grids, and observed using transmission electron microscope (JEOL, JEM-101, Japan). The analysis was carried out by Soft Imaging System.

Western blot analysis

Cytoplasmic proteins were extracted from the GG, and immunoblots were implemented as previously described [12]. Protein homogenates were subjected to Western blot analysis with antibodies against phosphor-LKB1 (Cell Signaling Technology, USA), phosphor-AMPK (Cell Signaling Technology, USA), PGC1-α (Santa Cruz Biotechnology, USA), Troponin I (Santa Cruz Biotechnology, USA), Myosin chain 1 (Vectorlabs, USA) and GAPDH (Santa Cruz Biotechnology, USA),followed by incubation with a peroxidase-conjugated secondary antibody. The signals were detected with the electrochemiluminescence ECL system (Bio-Rad Laboratories Inc., USA) and quantification was carried out by measuring the densitometry of the signals with the Image J software.

Quantitative real-time PCR

The mRNAs of genes involved in this study are listed in Table 1. Rats were anesthetized and the genioglossi was sectioned and frozen in liquid nitrogen. Isolation of total RNA was extracted from the GG with Trizol reagent (Takara Bio Inc., Japan). Quantitative detection of gene expression was carried out on a ABI 7900 Real Time PCR System (Applied Biosystems Inc., USA). Primer sequences (Table 1) were designed by Invitrogen (Shanghai, China). Quantities of all genes were normalized to the rat GAPDH. Values were relative to each expression in control group respectively.

Table 1. Primer sequences.

Gene(Rat)	forward	reverse
Hmox1	GTCAAGCACAGGGTGACAGA	CTGCAGCTCCTCAAACAGC
Cycs	GATGCCAACAAGAACAAAGGT	TGGGATTTTCCAAATACTCCAT
NQO1	AGCGCTTGACACTACGATCC	CAATCAGGGCTCTTCTCACC
Cox4i1	CACTGCGCTTGTGCTGAT	CGATCAAAGGTATGAGGGATG
OGG1	ATGGCTTCCCAAACCTTCAT	CAACTTCCTGAGGTGGGTCT
Ant1	GTAGGATGATGATGCAGTCTGG	CGTCCTTCATCTTTTGCAATC
Cs	GCACGCCAGTGCTTCTTC	CATGCTGCTGTCTGAAGGTC
Esrrα	CTTCCCTGCTGGTCCTCTG	CACCAGGGCGTTAACTGG
Nrf1	CCAAACCCACAGAGAACAGAA	TCCATGCATGAACTCCATCT
PGC1-a	GATGCCAACAAGAACAAAGGT	TCTGGGGTCAGAGGAAGAGA
MHC1	CACCAACAACCCCTACGATT	AGCACATCAAAGGCGCTATC
MHC2a	TCAAATCATCAGTGCCAACC	TGCCAAAGTGAATCCTGATG
MHC2x	AGAGGCCAAAAGGAAAGAGC	TCAGCATCAGCCAAGCTGT
MHC2b	CCAGTTGAACCATGCCAAC	TCTGAGAGCATCGTCCAGGT
GAPDH	GCAAGTTCAATGGCACAG	CATTTGATGTTAGCGGGAT

Hmox1, heme oxygenase; Cycs, cytochrome C; NQO1, NAD(P)H dehydro-genase-quinone-1; Cox4i1, cytochrome oxidase subunit IV isoform 1; OGG1, 8-oxoguanine DNA glycosylase; Ant1, Adenine nucleotide translocator 1; Cs, citrate synthase; Esrrα, estrogen-related receptorα; Nrf1, nuclear respiratory factor 1; PGC1-α, peroxisome proliferative activated receptor gamma coactivator 1-α; MHC, myosin heavy chain; GAPDH, glyceraldehyde-3-phosphate dehydrogenase.

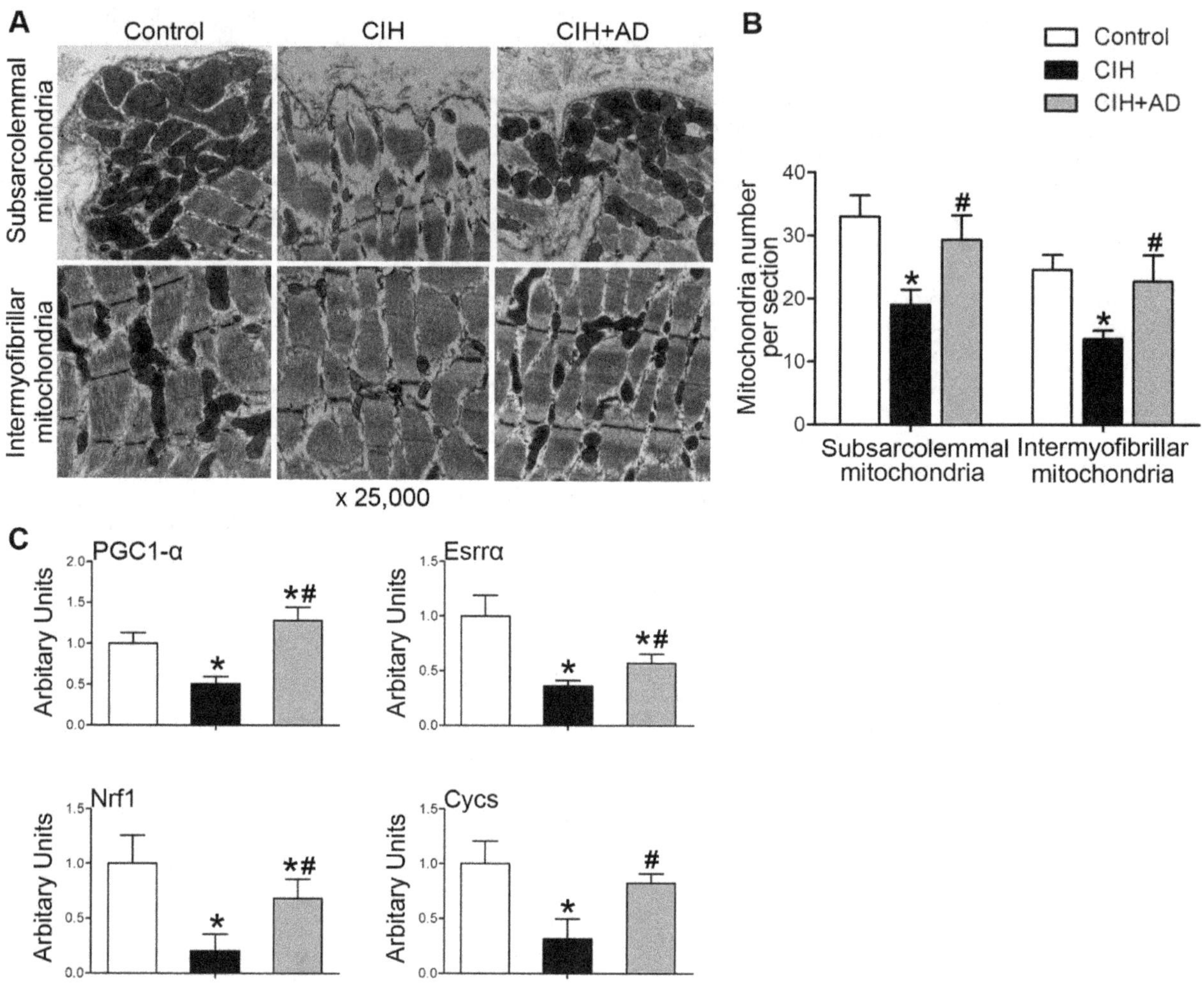

Figure 1. Changes of mitochondrial biogenesis in the three groups. (A) Mitochondrial density assessed by electron microscopy in the genioglossus muscle of rats from three groups. Original magnification, ×25,000. (B) Quantification of subsarcolemmal and intermyofibrillar mitochondria number per image area in the genioglossus muscle of rats from three groups (analysis of 5 images in 3 rats per group). *: P<0.05, CIH or CIH+AD compared with control, #: P<0.05, CIH+AD compared with CIH. (C) Levels of mRNAs implicated in mitochondrial biogenesis based on quantitative real-time RT-PCR performed on RNA isolated from genioglossus muscle from three groups (n = 6–8 per group). Results were normalized by the mean value for the control rats set to 1 unit.

Histological analyses

Samples of the GG were frozen down in liquid nitrogen-cooled isopentane. Enzyme histochemical staining for cytochrome oxidase activity (COX) [13] and succinate dehydrogenase (SDH) activity [14] were performed as described. We assessed COX and SDH activities by enzyme histochemistry.

Statistic analysis

Normal distributed data are expressed as mean ± SEM while non-normal distributed date are expressed as median ± inter-quartile. For normal distributed continuous variables, One-Way ANOVA was used, with a Newman-Keuls test to determine post hoc differences. For non-normal distributed variables, Kruskal-Wallis test was used with a post-hoc Dunn's multiple comparison.

Results

Changes of mitochondrial biogenesis

As shown in Figure 1A and 1B, the amounts of both subsarcolemmal and intermyofibrillar mitochondria were lower in CIH group than those in both control group and CIH+AD group ($p<0.05$), with no significant differences between control group and CIH+AD group ($p>0.05$).

To ascertain the mechanisms associated with the reduction of mitochondrial density in the GG of the CIH group, we measured the mRNA levels of genes such as PGC1-α, estrogen-related α receptor (Esrrα), nuclear respiratory factor 1(Nrf1), and cytochrome C (Cycs) since they usually reflect the degree of mitochondrial biogenesis (Figure 1C). The mRNA levels of PGC1-α, Esrrα, Nrf1 and Cycs in GGi were all significantly lower in CIH group than both control group and CIH+AD group ($p<0.05$). Comparison between control and CIH+AD groups showed that a) no significant difference in Cycs levels; b) a statistically higher PGC1-α level in CIH+AD group; c) a significantly lower Esrrα and Nrf1 levels in CIH+AD group.

Comparison of genioglossal mitochondrial ultrastructure

In addition to the reduction in mitochondrial density, marked alterations in mitochondrial morphology was also seen under transmission electron microscopy in the CIH group. Areas of both

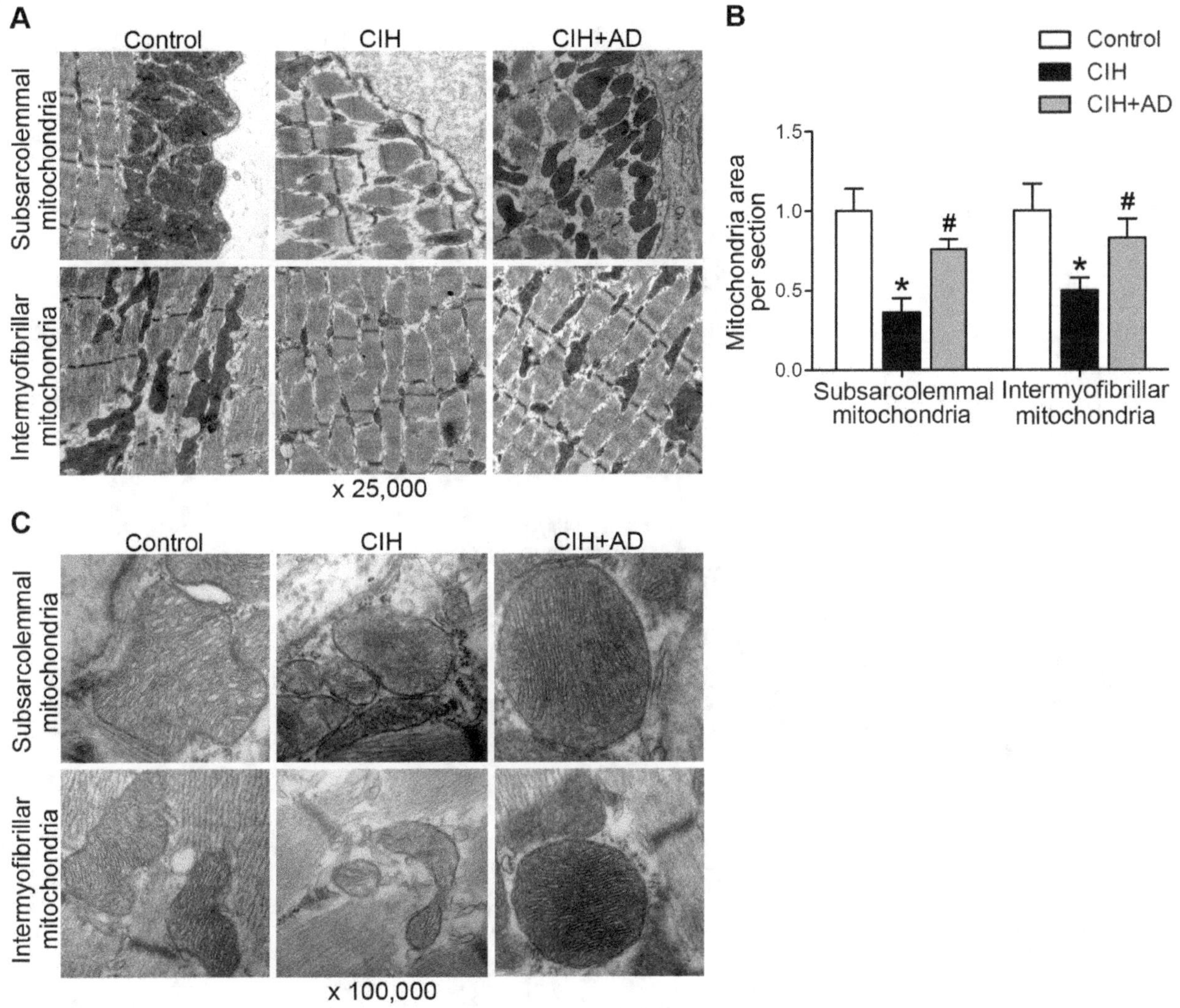

Figure 2. Alteration of mitochondrial ultrastructure in the genioglossus of the three groups. (A and C) Transmission electron microscopy images at original magnifications of ×25,000 (A) and ×100,000 (C) in subsarcolemmal and intermyofibrillar mitochondria from the genioglossus muscle of rats from three groups. (B) Quantification of subsarcolemmal and intermyofibrillar mitochondria area in the genioglossus muscle of rats from three groups (analysis of 5 images in 3 rats per group). *: P<0.05, CIH or CIH+AD compared with control, #: P<0.05, CIH+AD compared with CIH.

subsarcolemmal and intramyofibrillar mitochondria were notably lower in the CIH group than those in both control and CIH+AD group (Figures 2A and 2B). Swelling of mitochondria, a reduced electron density of the matrix, and an increased number of disarrayed cristae were shown only in the CIH group upon higher magnification (X100, 000) (Figure 2C).

Comparison of mitochondrial function

To detect whether changes in ultrastructure and mitochondrial density resulted in genioglossal mitochondrial dysfunction in the CIH group, we measured the expression of genes associated with mitochondrial function including the TCA cycle, OXPHOS, electron transport chain, and mitochondrial membrane organization with quantitative RT-PCR. The mRNA levels of genes related to mitochondrial function, such as heme oxygenase (Hmox1), citrate synthase (Cs), cytochrome oxidase subunit IV isoform 1 (Cox4i1), Adenine nucleotide translocator 1 (Ant1), 8-oxoguanine DNA glycosylase (OGG1), and NAD(P)H dehydrogenase-quinone-1 (NQO1) were all markedly lower in the genioglossus of CIH group than both control and CIH+AD groups (Figure 3A). Mitochondrial function was evaluated by estimating the enzymatic activities of succinate dehydrogenase (SDH) and Cox to further verify the changes in mitochondrial functions. Stained genioglossi sections demonstrated a lower number of Cox- and SDH-positive muscle fibres and a reduced intensity of SDH and Cox staining in CIH group (Figures 3B and 3C). In addition, the mRNA levels of Hmox1, Cs, Cox4i1, Ant1, OGG1, and NQO1 were remarkably higher in the GG of the CIH+AD group than those in the CIH group (Figure 3A). Stained genioglossi sections also showed a higher number of SDH- and Cox-positive muscle fibres and an increased intensity of SDH and Cox staining in the CIH+AD group than those in CIH group (Figures 3B and 3C).

Comparison of genioglossal fiber-types

As shown in Figure 4A, the mRNA levels of MHC1 was remarkably lower in the CIH group than those in control and CIH+AD groups ($p<0.05$). However, the levels of 2a, 2x, and 2b mRNA were not different among the three groups ($p>0.05$). The expression of markers of type I fibers such as myosin chain 1 and

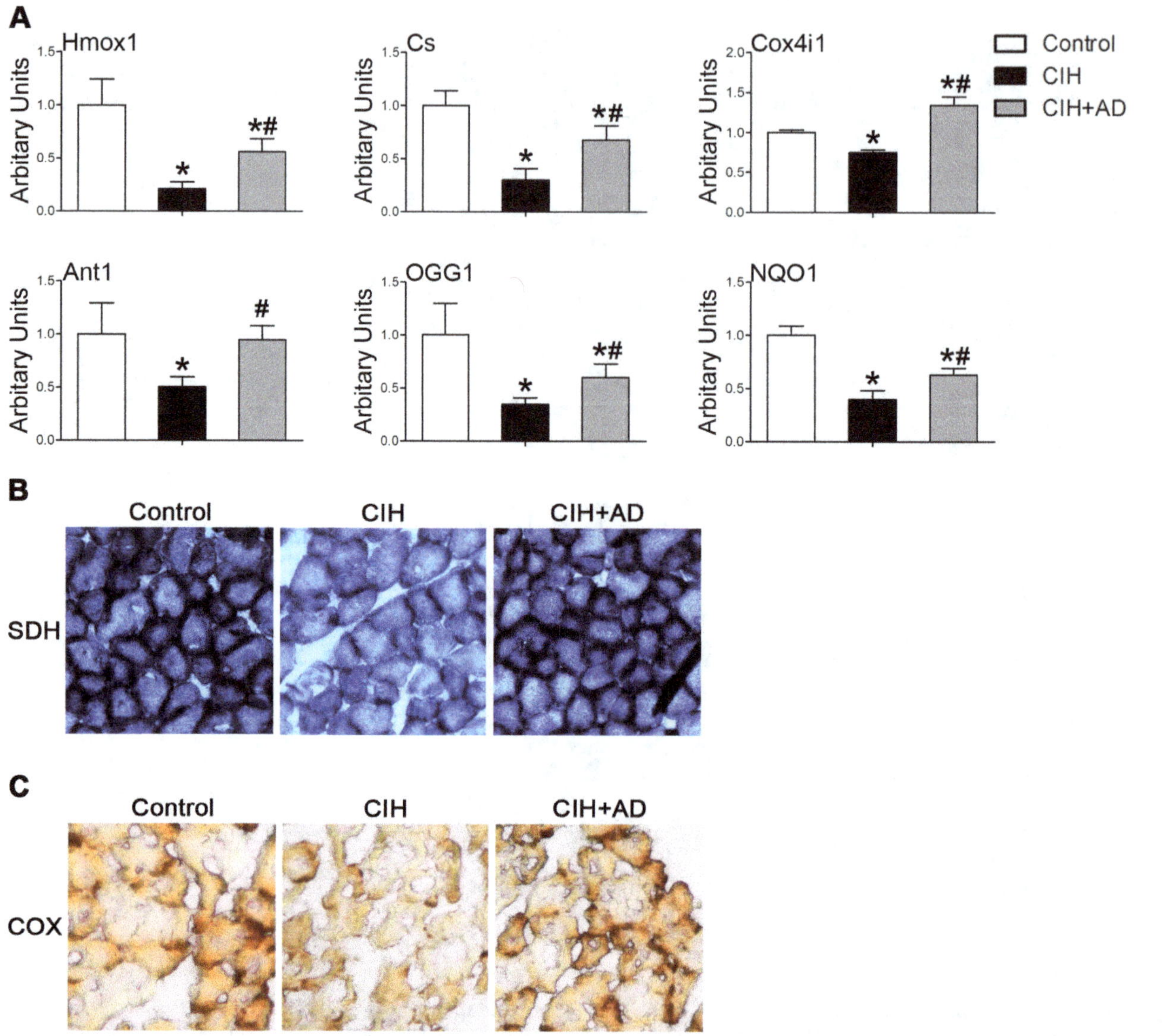

Figure 3. Changes of mitochondrial function in the three groups. (A) Levels of mRNAs implicated in mitochondrial function based on quantitative real-time RT-PCR performed on RNA isolated from the genioglossus muscle of three groups (n = 6–8 per group). Results were normalized by the mean value for the control rats set to 1 unit. (B) Succinate dehydrogenase (SDH) activity staining was performed on sections of the genioglossus muscle of three groups (n = 6–8 per group). (C) Cox activity staining was performed on sections of the genioglossus muscle of three groups (n = 6–8 per group). *: $P<0.05$, CIH or CIH+AD compared with control, #: $P<0.05$, CIH+AD compared with CIH.

troponin I was reduced in CIH groups, compared with the control and CIH+AD groups (Figures 4B, 4C, and 4D).

Adiponectin-mediated signaling

AMPK, as a pathway, is allosterically activated by alterations in the ratio of AMP/ATP and covalently phosphorylated at Thr172 by upstream kinase AMPK kinase. Adiponectin can activate the LKB1/AMPK/PGC1-α signaling pathway, which has impact on mitochondrial contents and function [9]. Therefore, we examined the effect of CIH and CIH+AD on AMPK activation. As shown in Figure 5A, 5B, and 5C, phosphorylation of LKB1, AMPK, and PGC1-α was significantly decreased in the CIH group, compared with the control group ($p<0.05$). Such weakened phosphorylation of LKB1, AMPK, and PGC1-α in the CIH group was so significantly increased in CIH+AD group that there was no statistical difference in degree of phosphorylation between control and CIH+AD groups.

Discussion

Upper airway dilator muscles (UADM) play a crucial role in the regulation of airway patency [15,16]. Dysfunction of UADM renders the organism susceptible to upper airway collapse. Impairment of UADM's structure and function occur in patients with OSAHS, and functional injury of UADM results in collapsibility of upper airway causing CIH in patients with OSAHS [15,17]. In our current study, we focused on the mitochondrion of the genioglossus (GG) because GG is one of the most important UADM [18,19] and the mechanisms driving genioglossal dysfunction might be related to impaired energy metabolism. Abnormal function of the GG can cause increased upper airway resistance and even induce its collapse [19]. Recent studies shown that the impairment of the GG's structure and function may be in association with abnormal energy metabolism in GG of OSAHS patients [15,17,20]. However, the specific

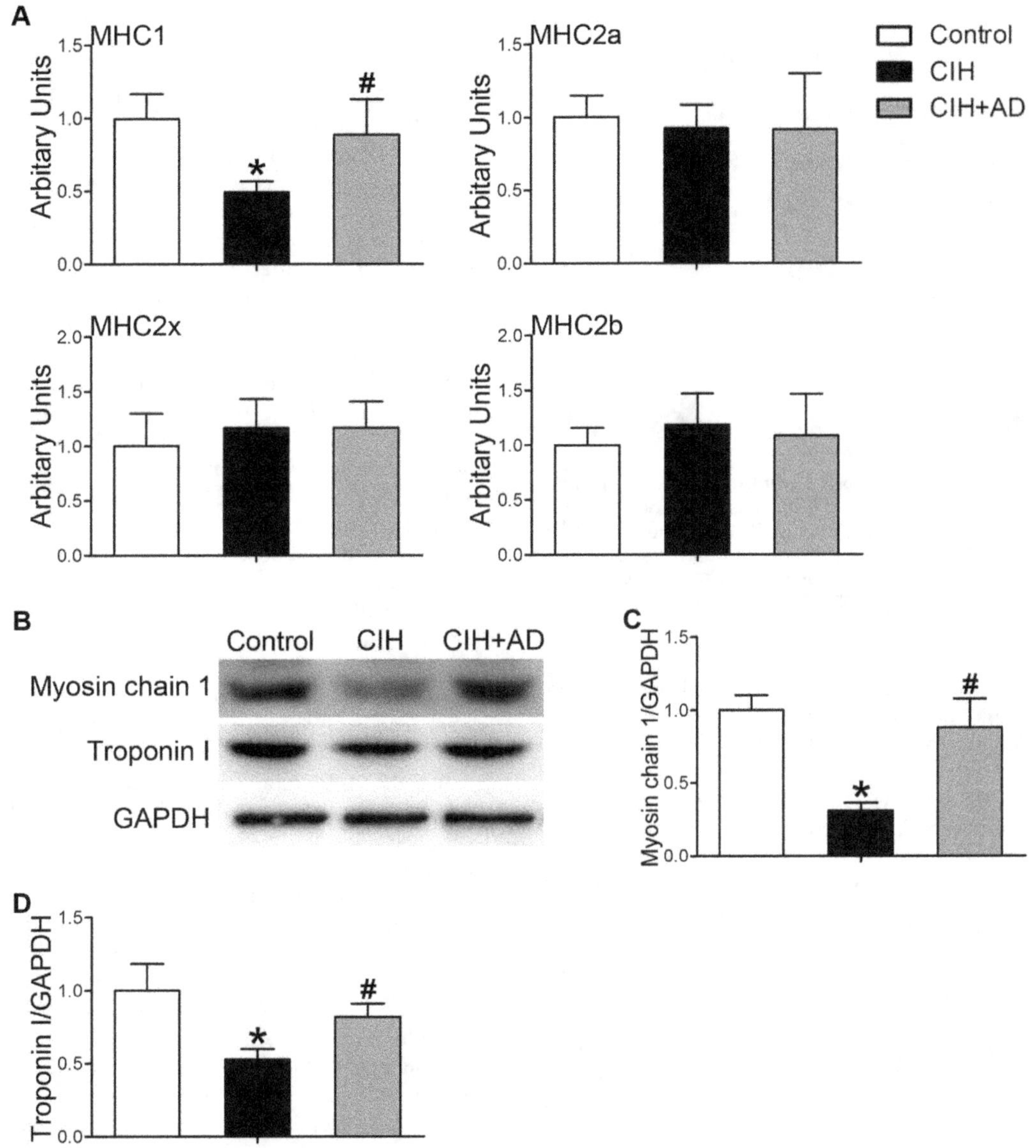

Figure 4. Genioglossus fiber-type changes in three groups. (A) Levels of MHC1, 2a, 2x and 2b mRNA based on quantitative real-time RT-PCR performed on RNA isolated from the genioglossus muscle homogenates in three groups. (n = 6–8 per group). (B) Western blot analysis of myosin chain 1, troponin I and GAPDH using the genioglossus muscle homogenates in three groups. (C and D) Densitometric analysis of Western blots (n = 5 per group). Results were normalized by the mean value for the control rats set to 1 unit. *: $P<0.05$, CIH or CIH+AD compared with control, #: $P<0.05$, CIH+AD compared with CIH.

mechanism is not yet clarified. Mitochondrium, as the central base for cellular energy metabolism, can better reflect the conditions of energy production and transmission within cells [21]. Here, we explore the structure, quantity, and function of genioglossal mitochondria in rats exposed to CIH.

PGC1-α is a key regulator of mitochondrial biogenesis [22–24]. Our study found that under CIH conditions, PGC1-α mRNA and PGC1-α protein levels were significantly reduced. Likewise, the mRNA levels of other genes associated with mitochondrial biogenesis, such as Esrrα, Nrf1 and Cycs, were all significantly lower in the CIH group. Furthermore, we observed the structure of the GG mitochondria under electron microscopy and found that the mitochondria appeared swollen, with fewer cristae and lower matrix density, severely destroyed inner and outer membrane integrity, and significantly reduced mitochondrial area in the rats of the CIH group. These mitochondrial abnormalities implicate CIH as a driving force in the impairment of GG mitochondrial content and structure. It has been reported that intermittent hypoxia could also cause brain mitochondrial dysfunction [25]. Shin-Da Lee et al found that CIH additionally weakened the mitochondrial oxidative capacity of cardiomyocytes [26]. In our study, we found that the expression levels of several genes involved in mitochondrial function were significantly reduced in the CIH group. In addition, the stained genioglossal sections revealed the decrease in the enzymatic activities of Cox and SDH. Moreover, CIH resulted in a remarkable decrease of genioglossal type I fibers [27,28], which might explain why the proportion of upper airway dilator muscle type I fibers was significantly reduced in OSAHS patients. Collectively, the data suggest that CIH induces mitochondrial dysfunction of the GG.

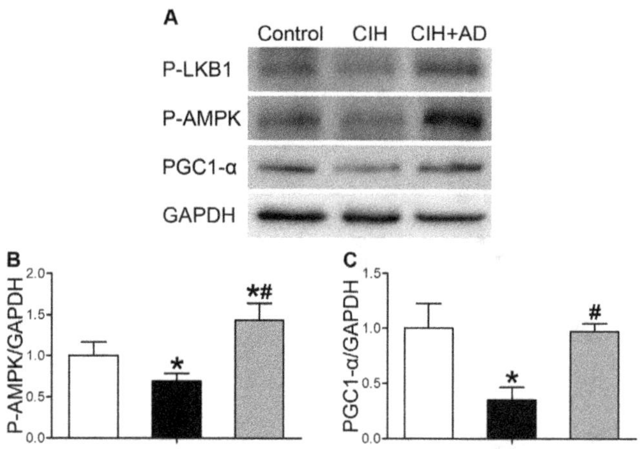

Figure 5. Adiponectin-mediated signaling. (A)Western blot analysis of P-LKB1, P-AMPK, PGC1-α and GAPDH using the genioglossus muscle homogenates in three groups. (B and C) Densitometric analysis of Western blots (n = 5 per group). Results were normalized by the mean value for the control rats set to 1 unit. *: $P<0.05$, CIH or CIH+AD compared with control, #: $P<0.05$, CIH+AD compared with CIH.

The mitochondrial dysfunction and reduced type I muscle fibers are likely to contribute to pathogenesis of contractile dysfunction of GG, as affirmed by other studies [15,29].

Previous studies have demonstrated that blood AD levels are decreased in OSAHS patients [1,3,15]. However, the relation between AD and mitochondrial function of the GG has not been fully elucidated. The current study revealed that AD supplementation could reverse hypoadiponectinemia and mitochondrial dysfunction associated with CIH [3]. Anthony E. and other studies have shown that AD could increase PGC1-α expression to promote mitochondrial content in skeletal muscle cells [9,11]. Consistent with our results, AD supplementation could promote GG mitochondrial synthesis even under CIH conditions. Moreover, after AD intervention, CIH-induced mitochondrial ultrastructural damage was significantly alleviated. Mitochondrial ultrastructural damage can substantially interrupt mitochondrial oxidative phosphorylation, and thereby decrease mitochondrial ATP generation. In mice with AD gene knockdown, reduced mitochondrial content and mitochondrial enzyme activity in skeletal muscle was reported, while AD treatment could improve mitochondrial biogenesis and mitochondrial enzyme activity [9]. In our study, we clearly demonstrated that exogenous AD supplementation could enhance the activity of cytochrome oxidase and succinate dehydrogenase, and improve the mRNA levels of Hmox1, Cs, Cox4i1, Ant1, OGG1 and of NQO1. Anthony E. et al found that AD could additionally switch type II fibers into type I fibers [9]. Our finding also showed that AD could significantly increase the expression level of PGC1-α. Overexpression of PGC1-α in muscle can result in a remarkable increase in the expression of troponin-1 protein and type I fiber [30]. In accordance with previous studies, we found that AD treatment increased the troponin-1 protein expression and type I muscle fiber content. These findings indicate that AD could improve the CIH-induced mitochondrial dysfunction and increase the type I muscle fiber content.

The AMP-activated protein kinase (AMPK) is a conserved sensor of cellular energy state, and it is reported that the AMPK pathway plays a pivotal role in regulating energy balance [31,32]. Chronic activation of AMP kinase can result in enhanced mitochondrial biogenesis and oxidative capacity [33]. AD can stimulate glucose utilization and fatty acid oxidation by activating AMP-activated protein kinase [11,34]. Our study demonstrated that CIH partially inhibited the expression of AMPK pathway, whereas AD supplementation could imminently elevate the expression of LKB1 (AMPKK)/AMPK/PGC1-α. Therefore, it is implied that AD rescues CIH-induced reductions in mitochondrial synthesis and oxidative capability through the AMPK pathway.

In spite of the fact that CIH is a consequence of apneas and hypopneas and cannot be the primum movens of genioglossal dysfunction, our results seemed to be able to explain that the OSAHS frequently becomes more severe during aging and when metabolic and cardiovascular comorbidities are associated with OSAHS.

It is also possible that CIH induced hypoadiponectinemia can further lead to reduced mitochondrial biogenesis and impaired mitochondrial function in genioglossus through insulin resistance, because the association between AD and insulin resistance is evident in clinical studies by showing that hypoadiponectinemia is a risk factor for insulin resistance represented by HOMA index [35,36]. It is unfortunate that the HOMA index was not tested in the current study. Since insulin resistance is a metabolic condition characterized by an impaired ability of plasma insulin to regulate glucose homeostasis in target tissue, such as skeleton muscle or adipose tissue [37], further studies are needed to investigate the relationship between AD and insulin resistance at a mitochondrial level within genioglossal tissue.

In conclusion, the present study demonstrated a) CIH could reduce mitochondrial biogenesis and impair mitochondrial function; b) AD supplementation could increase mitochondrial contents and alleviate mitochondrial dysfunction induced by CIH; c) AD might mediate the mitochondrial contents and function through the AMPK pathway. Our data strongly suggest that AD supplementation is a feasible novel therapeutic approach to prevent CIH-induced self-aggravation of genioglossal dysfunction in human OSAHS. Further clinical studies are therefore needed.

Author Contributions

Conceived and designed the experiments: XLZ GL. Performed the experiments: HPH XFJ YBD XFZ JNL. Analyzed the data: ND. Contributed reagents/materials/analysis tools: HPH YBD XFZ JNL. Wrote the paper: HPH XLZ SZH.

References

1. Zhang XL, Yin KS, Mao H, Wang H, Yang Y (2004) Serum adiponectin level in patients with obstructive sleep apnea hypopnea syndrome. Chin Med J (Engl) 117: 1603–1606.
2. Kanbay A, Kokturk O, Ciftci TU, Tavil Y, Bukan N (2008) Comparison of serum adiponectin and tumor necrosis factor-alpha levels between patients with and without obstructive sleep apnea syndrome. Respiration 76: 324–330.
3. Huang H, Zhang X, Ding N, Li Q, Min Y, et al. (2012) Effects of chronic intermittent hypoxia on genioglossus in rats. Sleep Breath 16: 505–510.
4. Shehzad A, Iqbal W, Shehzad O, Lee YS (2012) Adiponectin: regulation of its production and its role in human diseases. Hormones (Athens) 11: 8–20.
5. Yamauchi T, Nio Y, Maki T, Kobayashi M, Takazawa T, et al. (2007) Targeted disruption of AdipoR1 and AdipoR2 causes abrogation of adiponectin binding and metabolic actions. Nat Med 13: 332–339.
6. Ohashi K, Ouchi N, Matsuzawa Y (2012) Anti-inflammatory and anti-atherogenic properties of adiponectin. Biochimie 94: 2137–2142.

7. Arita Y, Kihara S, Ouchi N, Takahashi M, Maeda K, et al. (1999) Paradoxical decrease of an adipose-specific protein, adiponectin, in obesity. Biochem Biophys Res Commun 257: 79–83.
8. Illan-Gomez F, Gonzalvez-Ortega M, Orea-Soler I, Alcaraz-Tafalla MS, Aragon-Alonso A, et al. (2012) Obesity and inflammation: change in adiponectin, C-reactive protein, tumour necrosis factor-alpha and interleukin-6 after bariatric surgery. Obes Surg 22: 950–955.
9. Civitarese AE, Ukropcova B, Carling S, Hulver M, DeFronzo RA, et al. (2006) Role of adiponectin in human skeletal muscle bioenergetics. Cell Metab 4: 75–87.
10. Qiao L, Kinney B, Yoo HS, Lee B, Schaack J, et al. (2012) Adiponectin increases skeletal muscle mitochondrial biogenesis by suppressing mitogen-activated protein kinase phosphatase-1. Diabetes 61: 1463–1470.
11. Iwabu M, Yamauchi T, Okada-Iwabu M, Sato K, Nakagawa T, et al. (2010) Adiponectin and AdipoR1 regulate PGC-1alpha and mitochondria by Ca(2+) and AMPK/SIRT1. Nature 464: 1313–1319.
12. Zhu XD, Zhuang Y, Ben JJ, Qian LL, Huang HP, et al. (2011) Caveolae-dependent endocytosis is required for class A macrophage scavenger receptor-mediated apoptosis in macrophages. J Biol Chem 286: 8231–8239.
13. Seligman AM, Karnovsky MJ, Wasserkrug HL, Hanker JS (1968) Nondroplet ultrastructural demonstration of cytochrome oxidase activity with a polymerizing osmiophilic reagent, diaminobenzidine (DAB). J Cell Biol 38: 1–14.
14. Nachlas MM, Tsou KC, De Souza E, Cheng CS, Seligman AM (1957) Cytochemical demonstration of succinic dehydrogenase by the use of a new p-nitrophenyl substituted ditetrazole. J Histochem Cytochem 5: 420–436.
15. Carrera M, Barbe F, Sauleda J, Tomas M, Gomez C, et al. (1999) Patients with obstructive sleep apnea exhibit genioglossus dysfunction that is normalized after treatment with continuous positive airway pressure. Am J Respir Crit Care Med 159: 1960–1966.
16. Trinder J, Jordan AS (2011) Activation of the upper airway dilator muscle genioglossus during sleep is largely dependent on an interaction between chemical drive and mechanoreceptor feedback. Sleep 34: 983–984.
17. Young T, Palta M, Dempsey J, Skatrud J, Weber S, et al. (1993) The occurrence of sleep-disordered breathing among middle-aged adults. N Engl J Med 328: 1230–1235.
18. Jordan AS, White DP, Owens RL, Eckert DJ, Rahangdale S, et al. (2010) The effect of increased genioglossus activity and end-expiratory lung volume on pharyngeal collapse. J Appl Physiol 109: 469–475.
19. Bailey EF (2011) Activities of human genioglossus motor units. Respir Physiol Neurobiol 179: 14–22.
20. Oliven A, Tov N, Geitini L, Steinfeld U, Oliven R, et al. (2007) Effect of genioglossus contraction on pharyngeal lumen and airflow in sleep apnoea patients. Eur Respir J 30: 748–758.
21. Bonnard C, Durand A, Peyrol S, Chanseaume E, Chauvin MA, et al. (2008) Mitochondrial dysfunction results from oxidative stress in the skeletal muscle of diet-induced insulin-resistant mice. J Clin Invest 118: 789–800.
22. Li L, Muhlfeld C, Niemann B, Pan R, Li R, et al. (2011) Mitochondrial biogenesis and PGC-1alpha deacetylation by chronic treadmill exercise: differential response in cardiac and skeletal muscle. Basic Res Cardiol 106: 1221–1234.
23. Kong X, Wang R, Xue Y, Liu X, Zhang H, et al. (2010) Sirtuin 3, a new target of PGC-1alpha, plays an important role in the suppression of ROS and mitochondrial biogenesis. PLoS One 5: e11707.
24. Scarpulla RC (2011) Metabolic control of mitochondrial biogenesis through the PGC-1 family regulatory network. Biochim Biophys Acta 1813: 1269–1278.
25. Douglas RM, Ryu J, Kanaan A, Del Carmen Rivero M, Dugan LL, et al. (2010) Neuronal death during combined intermittent hypoxia/hypercapnia is due to mitochondrial dysfunction. Am J Physiol Cell Physiol 298: C1594–1602.
26. Lee SD, Kuo WW, Lin JA, Chu YF, Wang CK, et al. (2007) Effects of long-term intermittent hypoxia on mitochondrial and Fas death receptor dependent apoptotic pathways in rat hearts. Int J Cardiol 116: 348–356.
27. Sutlive TG, Shall MS, McClung JR, Goldberg SJ (2000) Contractile properties of the tongue's genioglossus muscle and motor units in the rat. Muscle Nerve 23: 416–425.
28. Kadi F, Karlsson C, Larsson B, Eriksson J, Larval M, et al. (2002) The effects of physical activity and estrogen treatment on rat fast and slow skeletal muscles following ovariectomy. J Muscle Res Cell Motil 23: 335–339.
29. Boyd JH, Petrof BJ, Hamid Q, Fraser R, Kimoff RJ (2004) Upper airway muscle inflammation and denervation changes in obstructive sleep apnea. Am J Respir Crit Care Med 170: 541–546.
30. Lin J, Wu H, Tarr PT, Zhang CY, Wu Z, et al. (2002) Transcriptional co-activator PGC-1 alpha drives the formation of slow-twitch muscle fibres. Nature 418: 797–801.
31. Hardie DG, Ross FA, Hawley SA (2012) AMPK: a nutrient and energy sensor that maintains energy homeostasis. Nat Rev Mol Cell Biol 13: 251–262.
32. Fritah A, Steel JH, Parker N, Nikolopoulou E, Christian M, et al. (2012) Absence of RIP140 reveals a pathway regulating glut4-dependent glucose uptake in oxidative skeletal muscle through UCP1-mediated activation of AMPK. PLoS One 7: e32520.
33. Bergeron R, Ren JM, Cadman KS, Moore IK, Perret P, et al. (2001) Chronic activation of AMP kinase results in NRF-1 activation and mitochondrial biogenesis. Am J Physiol Endocrinol Metab 281: E1340–1346.
34. Ix JH, Sharma K (2010) Mechanisms linking obesity, chronic kidney disease, and fatty liver disease: the roles of fetuin-A, adiponectin, and AMPK. J Am Soc Nephrol 21: 406–412.
35. Bonneau GA, Pedrozo WR, Berg G.(2013) Adiponectin and waist circumference as predictors of insulin-resistance in women. Diabetes Metab Syndr. 8(1): 3–7.
36. de Almeida AR, Monte-Alegre S, Zanini MB, Souza AL, Etchebehere M, et al.(2014) Association between prehypertension, metabolic and inflammatory markers,decreased adiponectin and enhanced insulinemia in obese subjects. Nutr Metab (Lond). 11: 25.
37. Miniello VL, Faienza MF, Scicchitano P, Cortese F, Gesualdo M, et al. (2014) Insulin resistance and endothelial function in children and adolescents. Int J Cardiol.174: 343–347.

Permissions

All chapters in this book were first published in PLOS ONE, by The Public Library of Science; hereby published with permission under the Creative Commons Attribution License or equivalent. Every chapter published in this book has been scrutinized by our experts. Their significance has been extensively debated. The topics covered herein carry significant findings which will fuel the growth of the discipline. They may even be implemented as practical applications or may be referred to as a beginning point for another development.

The contributors of this book come from diverse backgrounds, making this book a truly international effort. This book will bring forth new frontiers with its revolutionizing research information and detailed analysis of the nascent developments around the world.

We would like to thank all the contributing authors for lending their expertise to make the book truly unique. They have played a crucial role in the development of this book. Without their invaluable contributions this book wouldn't have been possible. They have made vital efforts to compile up to date information on the varied aspects of this subject to make this book a valuable addition to the collection of many professionals and students.

This book was conceptualized with the vision of imparting up-to-date information and advanced data in this field. To ensure the same, a matchless editorial board was set up. Every individual on the board went through rigorous rounds of assessment to prove their worth. After which they invested a large part of their time researching and compiling the most relevant data for our readers.

The editorial board has been involved in producing this book since its inception. They have spent rigorous hours researching and exploring the diverse topics which have resulted in the successful publishing of this book. They have passed on their knowledge of decades through this book. To expedite this challenging task, the publisher supported the team at every step. A small team of assistant editors was also appointed to further simplify the editing procedure and attain best results for the readers.

Apart from the editorial board, the designing team has also invested a significant amount of their time in understanding the subject and creating the most relevant covers. They scrutinized every image to scout for the most suitable representation of the subject and create an appropriate cover for the book.

The publishing team has been an ardent support to the editorial, designing and production team. Their endless efforts to recruit the best for this project, has resulted in the accomplishment of this book. They are a veteran in the field of academics and their pool of knowledge is as vast as their experience in printing. Their expertise and guidance has proved useful at every step. Their uncompromising quality standards have made this book an exceptional effort. Their encouragement from time to time has been an inspiration for everyone.

The publisher and the editorial board hope that this book will prove to be a valuable piece of knowledge for researchers, students, practitioners and scholars across the globe.

List of Contributors

Samuele De Minicis, Laura Agostinelli, Chiara Rychlicki, Stefania Saccomanno, Cinzia Candelaresi, Luciano Trozzi, Irene Pierantonelli, Eleonora Mingarelli, Marco Marzioni and Antonio Benedetti
Università Politecnica delle Marche, Department of Gastroenterology, Ancona, Italy

Gianluca Svegliati-Baroni
Università Politecnica delle Marche, Department of Gastroenterology, Ancona, Italy
Università Politecnica delle Marche, Obesity Center, Ancona, Italy

Giovanna Muscogiuri
Università Cattolica del Sacro Cuore, Policlinico Gemelli, Division of Endocrinology and Metabolic Disease, Rome, Italy

Gian Pio Sorice
Università Cattolica del Sacro Cuore, Policlinico Gemelli, Division of Endocrinology and Metabolic Disease, Rome, Italy
Diabetic Care Clinics, ACISMOM, Rome, Italy

Andrea Giaccari
Università Cattolica del Sacro Cuore, Policlinico Gemelli, Division of Endocrinology and Metabolic Disease, Rome, Italy
Don Gnocchi Foundation Onlus, Milan, Italy

Melania Gaggini and Amalia Gastaldelli
Institute of Clinical Physiology, Head of Cardiometabolic Risk Unit, Pisa, Italy

Maria Guido
Università di Padova, Department of Medicine Anatomic Pathology Unit, Padova, Italy

Kai-Chun Cheng, Akihiro Asakawa, Ying-Xiao Li, Haruka Amitani and Akio Inui
Department of Psychosomatic Internal Medicine, Kagoshima University Graduate School of Medical and Dental Sciences, Kagoshima, Japan

Hsien-Hui Chung
Institute of Basic Medical Sciences, College of Medicine, National Cheng Kung University, Tainan City, Taiwan

Takatoshi Ueki
Department of Neuroanatomy, Hamamatsu University School of Medicine. Hamamatsu, Japan

Juei-Tang Cheng
Department of Medical Research, Chi-Mei Medical Center, Yong Kang, Tainan City, Taiwan

Angela Sciacqua, Marta Letizia Hribal, Francesco Perticone and Giorgio Sesti
Department of Medical and Surgical Sciences, University "Magna Graecia" of Catanzaro, Catanzaro, Italy

Maria Adelaide Marini
Department of Internal Medicine, University of Rome-Tor Vergata, Rome, Italy

Maki Goto and Atsushi Goto
Department of Diabetes Research, Diabetes Research Center, National Center for Global Health and Medicine, Tokyo, Japan
Department of Endocrinology and Metabolism, Yokohama City University Graduate School of Medicine, Yokohama, Japan
National Institute of Health and Nutrition, Tokyo, Japan

Mitsuhiko Noda
Department of Diabetes Research, Diabetes Research Center, National Center for Global Health and Medicine, Tokyo, Japan
Department of Diabetes and Metabolic Medicine, Center Hospital, National Center for Global Health and Medicine, Tokyo, Japan

Yasuo Terauchi
Department of Endocrinology and Metabolism, Yokohama City University Graduate School of Medicine, Yokohama, Japan

Motohiko Miyachi and Shaw Watanabe
National Institute of Health and Nutrition, Tokyo, Japan

Akemi Morita
National Institute of Health and Nutrition, Tokyo, Japan
Department of Nutrition, College of Nutrition, Koshien University, Hyogo, Japan

Kijo Deura
Saku Central Hospital, Nagano, Japan

Satoshi Sasaki
Department of Social and Preventive Epidemiology, School of Public Health, University of Tokyo, Tokyo, Japan

Naomi Aiba
Department of Nutrition and Life Science, Kanagawa Institute of Technology, Kanagawa, Japan

Takuro Shimbo
Department of Clinical Research and Informatics, National Center for Global Health and Medicine, Tokyo, Japan

Miguel Debono, Richard J. Ross and John Newell-Price
Academic Unit of Diabetes, Endocrinology and Reproduction, Department of Human Metabolism, University of Sheffield, Sheffield, United Kingdom

Richard Eastell
Academic Unit of Bone Metabolism, Department of Human Metabolism, University of Sheffield, Sheffield, United Kingdom

Rita Chadarevian
HRA Pharma, Paris, France

Chao-Qun Cen and Kai-Yun Chen
Department of Pediatrics, the Third Affiliated Hospital of Sun Yat-sen University, Guangzhou, China

Hong-Zhu Deng
Department of Pediatrics, the Third Affiliated Hospital of Sun Yat-sen University, Guangzhou, China
Department of Pediatrics, the First Affiliated Hospital of Sun Yat-sen University, Guangzhou, China

Hong Deng
Department of Infectious diseases, the Third Affiliated Hospital of Sun Yat-sen University, Guangzhou, China

Min-Lian Du
Department of Pediatrics, the First Affiliated Hospital of Sun Yat-sen University, Guangzhou, China

Danielle M. Guizoni, Dijon H. S. Campos, Marina P. Okoshi, Katashi Okoshi and Antonio C. Cicogna
Botucatu Medical School, São Paulo State University, Botucatu, Brazil

Silvio A. Oliveira-Junior and Paula F. Martinez
Botucatu Medical School, São Paulo State University, Botucatu, Brazil
School of Physiotherapy, Federal University of Mato Grosso do Sul, Campo Grande, Brazil

Tiago Fernandes and Edilamar M. Oliveira
School of Physical Education and Sport, University of São Paulo, São Paulo, Brazil

Carlos R. Padovani
Botucatu Biosciences Institute, São Paulo State University, Botucatu, Brazil

Fei Jing, Masaki Mogi, Li-Juan Min, Kousei Ohshima, Hirotomo Nakaoka, Kana Tsukuda, Xiaoli Wang, Jun Iwanami and Masatsugu Horiuchi
Department of Molecular Cardiovascular Biology and Pharmacology, Ehime University Graduate School of Medicine, Ehime, Japan

Silvia Savastio, Giulia Genoni and Roberta Ricotti
Division of Pediatrics, Department of Health Sciences, University of "Piemonte Orientale Amedeo Avogadro", Novara, Italy

Flavia Prodam and Simonetta Bellone
Division of Pediatrics, Department of Health Sciences, University of "Piemonte Orientale Amedeo Avogadro", Novara, Italy
Endocrinology, Department of Clinical and Experimental Medicine, University of Piemonte Orientale, Novara, Italy
I.C.O.S. (Interdisciplinary Center for Obesity Study), Novara, Italy

Gianni Bona
Division of Pediatrics, Department of Health Sciences, University of "Piemonte Orientale Amedeo Avogadro", Novara, Italy
I. C. O. S. (Interdisciplinary Center for Obesity Study), Novara, Italy

Gianluca Aimaretti
Endocrinology, Department of Clinical and Experimental Medicine, University of Piemonte Orientale, Novara, Italy

Mara Giordano
I. C. O. S. (Interdisciplinary Center for Obesity Study), Novara, Italy
Laboratory of Human Genetics, Department of Health Sciences, University of Piemonte Orientale, Novara, Italy

Deepak Babu
Laboratory of Human Genetics, Department of Health Sciences, University of Piemonte Orientale, Novara, Italy

Thine Hvid and Thomas Grøndahl
Centre of Inflammation and Metabolism, Department of Infectious Diseases, Rigshospitalet, Copenhagen, Denmark
Copenhagen Muscle Research Centre, Rigshospitalet, Copenhagen, Denmark

Birgitte Lindegaard, Pernille Hojman and Bente Klarlund Pedersen
Centre of Inflammation and Metabolism, Department of Infectious Diseases, Rigshospitalet, Copenhagen, Denmark
Copenhagen Muscle Research Centre, Rigshospitalet, Copenhagen, Denmark
Department of Infectious Diseases, Rigshospitalet, Copenhagen, Denmark

Christian Frosig
Copenhagen Muscle Research Centre, Rigshospitalet, Copenhagen, Denmark
Institute of Exercise and Sport Sciences, Department of Human Physiology, Copenhagen, Denmark

Jan Gerstoft
Department of Infectious Diseases, Rigshospitalet, Copenhagen, Denmark

Sung Hee Choi, Kyoung Min Kim, Hak Chul Jang and Soo Lim
Department of Internal Medicine, Seoul National University College of Medicine and Seoul National University Bundang Hospital, Seongnam, Korea

Cheng Ji Jin
Department of Internal Medicine, Seoul National University College of Medicine and Seoul National University Bundang Hospital, Seongnam, Korea
Department of Endocrinology, The ZhongShan Hospital, aLian University, Dalian, China

Sung Hoon Yu
Department of Internal Medicine, Seoul National University College of Medicine and Seoul National University Bundang Hospital, Seongnam, Korea
Department of Internal Medicine, Hallym University Hangang Sacred Hospital, Seoul, Korea

Se Joon Woo
Department of Ophthalmology, Seoul National University College of Medicine and Seoul National University Bundang Hospital, Seongnam, Korea

Hyo Jin Park
Department of Pathology, Seoul National University College of Medicine and Seoul National University Bundang Hospital, Seongnam, Korea

Xiao-Mei Wang
Department of Endocrinology, The ZhongShan Hospital, aLian University, Dalian, China

Hyun Chul Lee
Department of Internal Medicine, Yonsei niversity College of Medicine, Seoul, Korea

Jung Hee Kim and Kyong Soo Park
Department of Internal Medicine, Seoul National University College of Medicine, Seoul, Korea

Veera R. Konda, Anuradha Desai, Gary Darland, Neile Grayson and Jeffrey S. Bland
KinDex Therapeutics, LLC, Seattle, Washington, United States of America

Xiuqing Huang, Yajun Lin, Tao Shen, Beidong Chen, Yong Man, Shu Wang and Jian Li
Key Laboratory of Geriatrics, Beijing Institute of Geriatrics & Beijing Hospital, Ministry of Health, Beijing, China

Hangxiang Zhang
Key Laboratory of Geriatrics, Beijing Institute of Geriatrics & Beijing Hospital, Ministry of Health, Beijing, China
Department of Gerontology, Xi-Jing Hospital, Fourth Military Medical University, Xian, China

Jiaojiao Chu
Key Laboratory of Geriatrics, Beijing Institute of Geriatrics & Beijing Hospital, Ministry of Health, Beijing, China
Zhejiang Hospital, Hangzhou, Zhejiang Province, China

Mohamed M. Elmazar
British Universityin Cairo (BUE), Cairo, Egypt

Hanan S. El-Abhar
Department of Pharmacology & Toxicology, Faculty of Pharmacy, Cairo University, Cairo, Egypt

Mona F. Schaalan
Department of Biochemistry, Faculty of Pharmacy, Misr International University (MIU), Cairo, Egypt

Nahla A. Farag
Department of Pharmaceutical Medicinal Chemistry, Faculty of Pharmacy, Misr International University (MIU), Cairo, Egypt

Khanrin P. Vashum, Mark McEvoy, Abul Hasnat Milton, Stephen Hancock and John Attia
Centre for Clinical Epidemiology and Biostatistics (CCEB), School of Medicine and Public Health, The University of Newcastle, and Hunter Medical Research Institute, Newcastle, New South Wales, Australia

Md. Rafiqul Islam
Centre for Clinical Epidemiology and Biostatistics (CCEB), School of Medicine and Public Health, The University of Newcastle, and Hunter Medical Research Institute, Newcastle, New South Wales, Australia
Ministry of Health and Family Welfare, Government of Bangladesh, Dhaka, Bangladesh

Heidi N. Boyda, Catherine C. Y. Pang, Erin Hawkes, Daniel Wong and Chen Helen Jin
Department of Anesthesiology, Pharmacology and Therapeutics, University of British Columbia, Vancouver, British Columbia, Canada

Alasdair M. Barr
Department of Anesthesiology, Pharmacology and Therapeutics, University of British Columbia, Vancouver, British Columbia, Canada
British Columbia Mental Health and Addictions Services, British Columbia Mental Health and Addictions Research Institute, Vancouver, British Columbia, Canada

Ric M. Procyshyn and William G. Honer
Department of Psychiatry, University of British Columbia, Vancouver, British Columbia, Canada
British Columbia Mental Health and Addictions Services, British Columbia Mental Health and Addictions Research Institute, Vancouver, British Columbia, Canada

Akinobu Ochi, Katsuhito Mori, Masanori Emoto, Shinya Nakatani, Tomoaki Morioka, Koka Motoyama, Shinya Fukumoto, Yasuo Imanishi, Eiji Ishimura and Masaaki Inaba
Department of Metabolism, Endocrinology and Molecular Medicine, Osaka City University Graduate School of Medicine, Osaka, Japan

Hidenori Koyama
Department of Internal Medicine, Division of Endocrinology and Metabolism, Hyogo College of Medicine, Nishinomiya, Japan

Xuguang Li, Jiang Hong and Shaowen Liu
Department of Cardiology, Shanghai First People's Hospital, School of Medicine, Shanghai Jiao Tong University, Shanghai, People's Republic of China

Gang Zhao, Ben Ma, Rui Li and Dao Wen Wang
Department of Internal Medicine, Tongji Hospital, Tongji Medical College, Huazhong University of Science and Technology, Wuhan, People's Republic of China

Michiel Sala, Lucia J. M. Kroft, Boudewijn Röell and Albert de Roos
Department of Radiology, Leiden University Medical Center, Leiden, the Netherlands

Jeroen van der Grond
Department of Radiology, Leiden University Medical Center, Leiden, the Netherlands
Netherlands Consortium for Healthy Ageing, Leiden, the Netherlands

Simon P. Mooijaart and Diana van Heemst
Department of Gerontology and Geriatrics, Leiden University Medical Center, Leiden, the Netherlands
Netherlands Consortium for Healthy Ageing, Leiden, the Netherlands

P. Eline Slagboom
Department of Molecular Epidemiology, Leiden University Medical Center, Leiden, the Netherlands
Netherlands Consortium for Healthy Ageing, Leiden, the Netherlands

Alexandra Gkourogianni, Ioanna Kosteria, Maria Konsta, Christina Kanaka-Gantenbein and George P. Chrousos
Division of Endocrinology, Diabetes and Metabolism, First Department of Pediatrics, University of Athens Medical School, Athens, Greece

Maria I. Klapa
Metabolic Engineering andSystems Biology Laboratory, Institute of Chemical Engineering Sciences, Foundation for Research and Technology-Hellas (FORTH/ICE-HT), Patras, Greece

Aristeidis G. Telonis
Metabolic Engineering andSystems Biology Laboratory, Institute of Chemical Engineering Sciences, Foundation for Research and Technology-Hellas (FORTH/ICE-HT), Patras, Greece
Graduate Program "Biological Technology", Department of Biology, University of Patras, Greece

Alexandra Margeli and Ioannis Papassotiriou
Department ofClinical Biochemistry, "Aghia Sophia" Children's Hospital, Athens, Greece

Emilia Mantzou
Endocrine Unit, Department of Endocrinology and Metabolism, Evgenidion Hospital, Athens, Greece

Dimitrios Loutradis
Division of In Vitro Fertilization, First Department of Obstetrics and Gynecology, University of Athens Medical School, Athens, Greece

George Mastorakos
Division ofEndocrinology, Second Department of Obstetrics and Gynecology, University of Athens Medical School, Athens, Greece

Mario Siervo
Human Nutrition Research Centre, Institute for Ageing and Health, Newcastle University, Newcastle on Tyne, United Kingdom

Heather L. Riley
Warwick Systems Biology Centre,University of Warwick, Coventry, United Kingdom

Martin Feelisch
Warwick Systems Biology Centre,University of Warwick, Coventry, United Kingdom
Warwick Medical School, University of Warwick, Coventry, United Kingdom
University of Southampton, Clinical &Experimental Sciences, Faculty of Medicine, Southampton General Hospital, Southampton, United Kingdom
Southampton NIHR Respiratory Biomedical Research Unit, Southampton, United Kingdom

Carl A. Leckstrom
Warwick Medical School, University of Warwick, Coventry, United Kingdom

Bernadette O. Fernandez
Warwick Medical School, University of Warwick, Coventry, United Kingdom
University of Southampton, Clinical &Experimental Sciences, Faculty of Medicine, Southampton General Hospital, Southampton, United Kingdom

Michael P. W. Grocott
University of Southampton, Clinical &Experimental Sciences, Faculty of Medicine, Southampton General Hospital, Southampton, United Kingdom
Centre for Altitude Space and Extreme Environment Medicine, Portex Unit, UCL Institute of Child Health, London, United Kingdom
University Hospital Southampton NHS Foundation Trust, Southampton General Hospital, Southampton, United Kingdom
Southampton NIHR Respiratory Biomedical Research Unit, Southampton, United Kingdom

Hugh E. Montgomery and Monty G. Mythen
Centre for Altitude Space and Extreme Environment Medicine, Portex Unit, UCL Institute of Child Health, London, United Kingdom

Daniel S. Martin
Centre for Altitude Space and Extreme Environment Medicine, Portex Unit, UCL Institute of Child Health, London, United Kingdom
Division of Surgery and Interventional Science, University College London, Royal Free Hospital, London, United Kingdom

Kay Mitchell
Centre for Altitude Space and Extreme Environment Medicine, Portex Unit, UCL Institute of Child Health, London, United Kingdom
University Hospital Southampton NHS Foundation Trust, Southampton General Hospital, Southampton, United Kingdom

Denny Z. H. Levett
Centre for Altitude Space and Extreme Environment Medicine, Portex Unit, UCL Institute of Child Health, London, United Kingdom
University Hospital Southampton NHS Foundation Trust, Southampton General Hospital, Southampton, United Kingdom
Southampton NIHR Respiratory Biomedical Research Unit, Southampton, United Kingdom

Cecilia M. Shikuma, Dominic C. Chow, Louie Mar A. Gangcuangco, Guangxiang Zhang, Kalpana J. Kallianpur, Lorna S. Nagamine, Lishomwa C. Ndhlovu and Jason D. Barbour
Hawaii Center for AIDS, University of Hawaii, Honolulu, Hawaii, United States of America

Todd B. Seto and Nisha Parikh
Hawaii Center for AIDS, University of Hawaii, Honolulu, Hawaii, United States of America,
Queen's Medical Center, Honolulu, Hawaii, United States of America

Beau K. Nakamoto
Hawaii Center for AIDS, University of Hawaii, Honolulu, Hawaii, United States of America,
Straub Clinic and Hospital, Honolulu, Hawaii, United States of America

Sheila M. Keating
Blood Systems Research Institute, San Francisco, California, United States of America

Philip J. Norris
Blood Systems Research Institute, San Francisco, California, United States of America
University of California San Francisco, San Francisco, California, United States of America

Hanpeng Huang
Department of Respirology, Affiliated Hospital of Jiangsu University, Zhenjiang, China

Xiufeng Jiang
Department of Respirology, Nanjing Medical University affiliated Wuxi People's Hospital, Wuxi, China

Yanbin Dong, Xiaofeng Zhang, Ning Ding and Xilong Zhang
Department of Respirology, The First Affiliated Hospital with Nanjing Medical University, Nanjing, China

Jiannan Liu and Gan Lu
Department of Respiratory Diseases, Jangsu Geriatric Hospital, Nanjing, China

Sean Z. Hutchinson
Morsani College of Medicine, Tampa, FL, United States of America

Index

N

O

P

R

S

T

V

Z

www.ingramcontent.com/pod-product-compliance
Lightning Source LLC
LaVergne TN
LVHW060942220926
848485LV00015B/1374
9781632419088